RESPIRATORY DISEASE

A Case Study Approach to Patient Care

THIRD EDITION

RESPIRATORY DISEASE

A Case Study Approach to Patient Care

Robert L. Wilkins, PhD, RRT, FAARC
Professor and Chair
Department of Respiratory Care
School of Allied Health Sciences
The University of Texas Health Science Center at San Antonio
San Antonio, Texas

James R. Dexter, MD, FACP, FCCP
Associate Clinical Professor
School of Medicine
Loma Linda University
Loma Linda, California
and
Chair, Division of Pulmonary, Critical Care, Sleep Medicine
Beaver Medical Group
Redlands, California

Philip M. Gold, MD, MACP, FCCP
Executive Vice Chair and Professor
Department of Medicine
Chief, Division of Pulmonary and Critical Care Medicine
School of Medicine
Loma Linda University
Loma Linda, California

THIRD EDITION

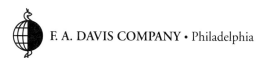
F. A. DAVIS COMPANY • Philadelphia

F. A. Davis Company
1915 Arch Street
Philadelphia, PA 19103
www.fadavis.com

Printed in the United States of America

Last digit indicates print number: 10 9 8 7 6 5 4 3 2 1

Acquisitions Editor: Andy McPhee
Manager of Content Development: Deborah Thorp
Developmental Editor: Karol-Lee Trakalo
Design Manager: Carolyn O'Brien

As new scientific information becomes available through basic and clinical research, recommended treatments and drug therapies undergo changes. The author(s) and publisher have done everything possible to make this book accurate, up to date, and in accord with accepted standards at the time of publication. The author(s), editors, and publisher are not responsible for errors or omissions or for consequences from application of the book, and make no warranty, expressed or implied, in regard to the contents of the book. Any practice described in this book should be applied by the reader in accordance with professional standards of care used in regard to the unique circumstances that may apply in each situation. The reader is advised always to check product information (package inserts) for changes and new information regarding dose and contraindications before administering any drug. Caution is especially urged when using new or infrequently ordered drugs.

Library of Congress Cataloging-in-Publication Data

Respiratory disease : a case study approach to patient care / [edited by] Robert L. Wilkins, James R. Dexter, Philip M. Gold—3rd ed.
    p. ; cm.
Includes bibliographical references and index.
ISBN 13: 978-0-8036-1374-4
ISBN 10: 0-8036-1374-1
1. Respiratory organs—Diseases—Case studies.   I. Wilkins, Robert L.   II. Dexter, James R., 1948—   III. Gold, Philip M.
    [DNLM: 1. Respiratory Tract Diseases—Case Reports. WF 140 R4341022 2006]
    RC731.R466 2007
    616.2—dc22

                                                              2006015190

To Joyce W. Hopp, PhD: You have been a wonderful mentor, colleague, and friend over the past 20 years. Your energy and leadership have moved me forward in ways I didn't think possible.

R.L.W.

In memory of Geoffrey Chaucer, good friend and pioneer in sleep research.

J.R.D.

To Roberta, my strongest supporter.

P.M.G.

Preface

The role of the respiratory therapist in health care has changed dramatically over the past several decades. Originally, "inhalation therapists" were primarily employed by hospitals to provide expertise in the equipment needed to care for patients with lung disease. If a patient needed oxygen, the IT would roll an oxygen cylinder into the room, attach a reducing valve, and apply oxygen per the physician's order. Inhalation therapists were not expected to understand the pathophysiology associated with the variety of lung diseases seen in the hospital. They were not expected to assist the physician in making the diagnosis or apply therapy with a critical eye to identify the effectiveness of the treatment plan. If complications occurred, they were not expected to recognize them or implement corrective measures. Today, however, the respiratory therapist has become an important member of the medical team. Physicians now depend on RTs to provide a second opinion, monitor the patient, suggest new therapy as needed, think critically, and give notification when the patient has taken a turn for the worse. The goal of this book is to help RTs become knowledgeable about the diseases they see in the hospital and other health care facilities and to better understand how these diseases affect lung function. This knowledge will improve patient care and provide better job satisfaction for the RT.

This third edition has changed in numerous ways when compared to the second edition. We have eliminated the neonatal and pediatric diseases because reviewers of the second edition indicated that such topics are well covered in pediatric textbooks. This allows us to focus primarily on adult disorders in this edition. Each chapter has been updated to reflect the latest research related to incidence and treatment. The number of case studies has been increased to help the reader better apply important concepts to patient care. Learning tools have been added to help the student engage with the information. For insurance, chapter objectives are listed at the start of each chapter to provide the learner with expected learning outcomes. "Side Bars" have been placed strategically throughout the chapters to emphasize key points. The side bars represent important issues associated with the surrounding content. Bulleted chapter summaries have been added at the end of each chapter to provide a concise overview for those who want a quick review of each topic.

The intended audience of this book continues to be students enrolled in a respiratory care program. Practitioners in respiratory care, nursing, physician assistants, and junior and senior medical students will find the content applicable to their discipline when caring for patients with pulmonary disease. Respiratory care students and practitioners preparing for the National Board for Respiratory Care exams, especially the clinical simulation examination, will find this text helpful. As with the clinical simulation examination, the case studies in this text emphasize patient assessment (information gathering) and treatment (decision making).

Readers of this text should study the background material presented before the case studies. This material will provide information that is useful for answering the questions presented in the cases. Next, the reader should read the case study and ponder the questions presented periodically throughout the case presentation. Readers should attempt to answer the questions in writing before looking at the provided answers. This exercise will develop critical thinking skills and will better prepare the reader for clinical practice.

As with any major project, this book would not have been possible without the assistance of many individuals. Our contributors did a wonderful job of updating the chapters and writing interesting case studies that highlight relevant points associated with each disease. Their research and writing are the backbone of this text and we are most appreciative. Our developmental editor, Kelly Trakalo, did an excellent job of making the manuscript consistent from one chapter to the next and helping us prepare a book that students can read and understand. Our editor, Andy McPhee, engineered the entire project and kept us on task and focused on our audience. We are grateful to these two key individuals for their professional work with this educational endeavor.

Finally, we hope readers find this book useful in developing their understanding of cardiopulmonary diseases and in improving the care of patients with these disorders. Quality patient care is the ultimate goal of this project, and if this book helps that cause in any way, we have been successful.

Robert L. Wilkins
James R. Dexter
Philip M. Gold

Contributors

Gregory A.B. Cheek, MD, FCCP, MSPH
Clinical Instructor
Department of Internal Medicine
Pulmonary/Critical Care Fellow
Loma Linda University
Loma Linda, California

James R. Dexter, MD, FACP, FCCP
Associate Clinical Professor
School of Medicine
Loma Linda University
Loma Linda, California
and
Chair, Division of Pulmonary, Critical
    Care, Sleep Medicine
Beaver Medical Group
Redlands, California

Carl A. Eckrode, MPH, RRT
Instructor
Respiratory Care Program
Mt. Hood Community College
Gresham, Oregon

William F. Galvin, MSEd, RRT, CPFT,
FAARC
Program Director/Assistant Professor
Respiratory Care Program
Gwynedd Mercy College
Gwynedd Valley, Pennsylvania

Enrique Gil, MD, FCCP
Pulmonary, Critical Care, and Sleep
    Medicine
Beaver Medical Group
Redlands, California

Philip M. Gold, MD, MACP, FCCP
Executive Vice Chair and Professor
Department of Medicine
Chief, Division of Pulmonary and Critical
    Care Medicine
Loma Linda University School of
    Medicine
Loma Linda, California

George H. Hicks, MS, RRT
Instructor/Clinical Coordinator
Respiratory Care Program
Mt. Hood Community College
Gresham, Oregon

Thomas P. Malinowski, BS, RRT,
FAARC
Director, Respiratory Care Services
Inova Fairfax Hospital
Falls Church, Virginia

Arthur B. Marshak, MS, RRT, RPFT
Instructor/Clinical Coordinator
Department of Cardiopulmonary Sciences
School of Allied Health Professions
Loma Linda University
Loma Linda, California

N. Lennard Specht, MD, FACP
Medical Director
Department of Cardiopulmonary Sciences
School of Allied Health Professions
Loma Linda University
Loma Linda, California

Rebekah Bartos Specht, MSN, FNP
Instructor
School of Medicine
Loma Linda University
Loma Linda, California

Robert L. Wilkins, PhD, RRT, FAARC
Professor and Chair
Department of Respiratory Care
School of Allied Health Sciences
The University of Texas Health
    Science Center at San Antonio
San Antonio, Texas

Reviewers

Randall W. Anderson, AS, RRT, CRTT
Department Head
Respiratory Care
Spartanburg Technical College
Spartanburg, South Carolina

Helen S. Corning, RRT
Registered Respiratory Therapist
Respiratory Care
St. Luke's Hospital
Jacksonville, Florida

Juanita Davis, RRT
Instructor
Health and Public Safety
Southern Alberta Institute of Technology
Calgary, Alberta, Canada

Robert W. Hooper, RRT, MALS
Program Director
Respiratory Care
University of Southern Indiana
Evansville, Indiana

Thomas J. Johnson, MS, RRT
Director and Assistant Professor
Respiratory Care
Long Island University
Brooklyn, New York

Brian Keller, MS, RRT, RPFT
Director
Respiratory Care
West Chester University
West Chester, Pennsylvania
Bryn Mawr Hospital
Bryn Mawr, Pennsylvania

Richard A. Patze, MEd, RRT
Division Dean
Health Related Professions
Pima Community College
Tucson, Arizona

Georgette Rosenfeld, MEd, RRT, RN
Department Chair
Respiratory Care
Indian River Community College
Fort Pierce, Florida

Robert Walsh, BS, RRT, P-EMT
Director
Respiratory Therapy
Indian River Community College
Fort Pierce, Florida

William Wojciechowski, MS, RRT
Chairman and Associate Professor
Cardiorespiratory Care
University of South Alabama
Mobile, Alabama

Contents

Introduction to Patient Assessment

Robert L. Wilkins, PhD, RRT, FAARC

Philip M. Gold, MD, MACP, FCCP

CHAPTER OBJECTIVES:

After reading this chapter you will be able to state or identify the following:

- The role of the respiratory therapist in patient assessment.
- The most common symptoms associated with cardiopulmonary disease and the common causes of each.
- The common physical examination procedures performed to evaluate patients with cardiopulmonary disease and the implications of abnormalities.
- The laboratory tests done to evaluate patients with diseases of the chest and common causes of abnormalities.

INTRODUCTION

Patient assessment is a vital part of patient care. Whether in the emergency department, intensive care unit (ICU), or home-care setting, patient assessment skills make the difference between inadequate and effective patient care. The purpose of this chapter is to provide the reader with an overview of how patient assessment is done, with an emphasis on assessment skills for the respiratory therapist (RT). The therapist does not evaluate patients to make a diagnosis, but assists the physician to determine the appropriate therapy and to monitor the effects of that therapy. In many cases, modifications in the treatment plan are based on observations by the RT.

The clinicians who are best at patient assessment are those who are rigorous in their daily patient care. This entails asking all relevant questions, examining all sides of the patient's chest, and reviewing other data such as the chest x-ray. Clinicians who take a superficial approach to patient assessment are likely to miss important clues to changes in the patient's condition and render inappropriate care.

This chapter is divided into three parts. First, the patient interview and the medical history are reviewed and a brief case study is presented to show how the interview is applied in practice. Second, use of the physical examination is presented; this is followed by continuation of the case study to illustrate use of the examination. Finally, use of laboratory data is described, followed by continuation of the illustrative case study.

THE MEDICAL HISTORY AND THE INTERVIEW

Most patient evaluations begin with the interview. The interview is done to gather important information about what is currently wrong with the patient. It is also useful because it allows you to establish a rapport with the patient before other procedures such as a physical examination are done. As an interviewer, you must be knowledgeable about diseases and typical patterns of diseases in order to ask the most appropriate questions. For this reason, the study of cardiopulmonary diseases, as presented in this text, will make you a better interviewer. Examples of basic questions to ask your patient, regardless of the symptoms, include the following:

- When did the problem start?
- Have you ever had this problem before?
- How severe is the problem? How has the severity changed since onset?
- What seemed to provoke the problem, and does anything seem to aggravate it or make it better?
- What region of the body is affected by the problem? If pain is the symptom, exactly where is the pain, and does it radiate to any other part of the body?

> RTs are not called on to perform complete health histories but must be able to interview the patient to assess their symptoms and the changes that occur with treatment.

Answers to these questions will help determine a differential diagnosis, what further tests may be needed, and what initial therapy may be appropriate. The length of the interview is often determined by the severity of the patient's illness. Patients who are acutely ill may need immediate care (e.g., oxygen therapy or metered-dose inhaler treatment) before you can conduct a lengthy interview or examination.

Symptoms

The following are among the most common symptoms that patients with cardiopulmonary disease experience:

- Shortness of breath (dyspnea)
- Cough
- Sputum production
- Chest pain
- Coughing up bloody sputum (hemoptysis)
- Fever
- Wheeze

Each of these symptoms will be described in detail to give you a better background and allow you to ask the right questions when your patient mentions these problems during your interview.

Shortness of Breath

Shortness of breath, as perceived by the patient, is known as **dyspnea.** It is a common problem in patients with cardiopulmonary disease. Patients who experience dyspnea are often anxious because of the fear associated with feeling short of breath. Dyspnea usually worsens with exertion (termed exertional dyspnea) and improves with rest. Patients with minimal cardiopulmonary reserve will be dyspneic even at rest. If the dyspnea occurs only during exertion, you should identify the level of exertion at which the patient must stop to catch his breath. Is it after climbing one flight of stairs or after walking a certain distance on a flat surface? You also can ask the patient to rate his dyspnea on a scale from 1 to 10, 10 being the worst. This type of questioning helps identify the severity of the dyspnea and the urgency of therapy.

Dyspnea may be more severe in certain positions. Patients experiencing shortness of breath only in the reclining (supine) position are said to have **orthopnea.** Orthopnea is most commonly associated with heart failure and occurs when increased venous return adds to the pulmonary vascular congestion associated with congestive heart failure. **Platypnea** refers to dyspnea in the upright position. This may occur after lung surgery to remove a diseased segment or lobe and is the result of severe ventilation perfusion mismatching. Dyspnea occurring with any change in position is abnormal and should be reported to the patient's attending physician.

> **p**atients will complain of dyspnea when they sense that their work of breathing is excessive for the level of activity. Factors that increase the drive to breathe or reduce the patient's ventilatory capacity (i.e., neuromuscular disease) add to the sensation of dyspnea.

The physiologic mechanisms causing dyspnea are not well understood. Most experts believe it occurs when the patient senses that his work of breathing is excessive for the level of activity in which he is engaged. Any pathologic lung change (e.g., bronchospasm or lung consolidation) that increases the work of breathing usually will lead to dyspnea, especially during exertion. Patients with severe disease, or with an acute problem superimposed on a chronic problem (e.g., pneumonia in a patient with chronic obstructive lung disease), tend to have dyspnea with very little activity or even at rest. Abnormalities that stimulate the drive to breathe (e.g., metabolic acidosis) also lead to dyspnea (Box 1.1).

Box 1.1 Causes of Dyspnea

INCREASES IN THE DRIVE TO BREATHE
- Significant hypoxemia
- Acidosis
- Fever
- Exercise

INCREASES IN AIRWAY RESISTANCE
- Asthma
- Acute bronchitis
- Croup and epiglottitis
- Chronic obstructive pulmonary disease

DECREASES IN LUNG OR CHEST WALL COMPLIANCE
- Severe pneumonia
- Severe pulmonary edema
- Adult respiratory distress syndrome
- Atelectasis
- Kyphoscoliosis
- Pneumothorax
- Pulmonary fibrosis

Cough

Cough is one of the most frequent symptoms observed in patients with cardiopulmonary disease. It typically occurs when the cough receptors of the larger airways are stimulated. These receptors respond to stimulation from mechanical, chemical, inflammatory, and thermal sources. Mechanical stimulation occurs when foreign bodies touch the airway wall. Food, liquid, and suction catheters are examples of mechanical stimulators of the cough receptors. Chemical stimulation of the cough receptors occurs when the patient inhales an irritating gas, such as cigarette smoke. Infection and inflammation of the larger airways can irritate the cough receptors and are common causes of coughing. Breathing extremely cold air can also stimulate the cough receptors. Cough receptors are also located in the pleural lining of the lung and may be stimulated when pleural inflammation is present as in congestive heart failure.

Cough is often associated with airway disease. Common causes of cough include acute upper respiratory infections, asthma, gastroesophageal reflux, and bronchitis. Other causes include sinusitis or postnasal drip and reactive airway disease not severe enough to be classified as asthma.

> Coughing in chronic obstructive pulmonary disease (COPD) patients is often weak and ineffective because of high airway resistance, reduced lung recoil, and weakness in the muscles of breathing.

You should identify the severity of the cough, when and how often it occurs, and whether it is productive. A productive cough can occur with infection of the airways or pneumonia. A weak cough may indicate thoracic or abdominal pain or neuromuscular disease. Emphysema patients often have a weak cough because of poor respiratory muscle mechanics, increased airway resistance, and reduced lung recoil. Patients with chronic bronchitis often cough and produce sputum for the first hour or two after getting out of bed in the morning. Heart failure may be associated with a dry cough.

Sputum Production

Sputum refers to excessive production of secretions from the lung. Sputum is often contaminated with oral secretions and may not accurately reflect the microbiology occurring in the lung. Mucus is normally produced in small amounts in the airways as part of the lungs' defense against invasion by germs. It is moved to the larynx by cilia (tiny waving fingers on the cells lining the airways). It is not normally noticed by healthy people.

Noticeable sputum production is a sign of disease of the airways or lungs. The most common cause of excessive mucus production is cigarette smoking. Cigarette smoke is irritating to the airways and causes them to produce excessive mucus as a reflex response. This in turn causes the smoker to cough and produce mucus every day, especially in the morning. Other causes of increased sputum production include inflammation associated with asthma and infection associated with pneumonia.

Sputum is described as **mucoid** when it is clear and thick, **fetid** when it is foul smelling, **purulent** when it contains pus, and **copious** when it is present in large amounts. Mucoid sputum is a common finding in airway disease without infection. Bacterial infections cause the sputum to become purulent and colored, often green or yellow. Some bacteria, especially anaerobes, cause fetid sputum. Copious mucus production most often is seen in patients with bronchiectasis (see Chapter 5).

> Patients with COPD who have an infection often note a change in sputum color, consistency, or volume with the onset of the infection.

Ask questions to clarify any recent changes in the amount and color of the patient's sputum. Increases in the amount and changes in the color from clear to yellow or green often indicate acute infection. Stagnation of the mucus in the airways also will lead to discoloration of the sputum. Patients who have trouble coughing up excessive mucus tend to retain it longer than normal and produce discolored sputum, even when infection is not present. Patients with asthma and extensive inflammation in the airways have so many eosinophils in their sputum that it appears purulent when no infection is present.

Chest Pain

Chest pain often is divided into two types: pleuritic and nonpleuritic. Pleuritic chest pain is made worse by breathing, coughing, sneezing, or moving the chest wall. It is usually sharp in nature. Diseases that affect the lining of the lung (e.g., pleurisy, pneumothorax, pulmonary embolism, pneumonia) may cause pleuritic chest pain.

Nonpleuritic chest pain is often located centrally in the chest and is usually not affected by respiratory efforts. It may radiate to the shoulder, arm, jaw, or back and is more often a dull pressure type of sensation. It is often associated with diseases such as ischemic heart disease and tends to increase with exertion. Patients with chest pain should be evaluated by a physician especially if heart disease is the likely cause (e.g., patient over the age of 40 years).

Hemoptysis

Hemoptysis refers to the spitting up of blood from the tracheobronchial tree or lungs. When hemoptysis is caused by an infectious disease, the blood is often mixed with sputum. The presence of blood-tinged sputum is strong evidence that the blood is coming from the respiratory tract, rather than the gastrointestinal tract. Pneumonia, trauma, bronchitis/bronchiectasis, bronchogenic carcinoma, tuberculosis, and pulmonary

> The patient with hemoptysis and a significant smoking history must be evaluated for lung cancer.

embolism are common causes of hemoptysis. Even after extensive evaluation, the cause of massive hemoptysis (more than 200 to 600 mL of blood in 24 hours) is undetermined 20% to 30% of the time. Chronic hemoptysis that has been occurring over many years is usually associated with a relatively benign condition, such as bronchiectasis. Acute hemoptysis also may be harmless when associated with acute bronchitis, but the potentially life-threatening causes of hemoptysis (e.g., carcinoma) must be ruled out before it is assumed that the problem is self-limited.

Fever

Fever is an abnormal increase in body temperature caused by disease. It is a nonspecific response to many problems, but most often occurs in response to an infection. Pulmonary infections are a common cause of infection-related fever and should always be considered in the evaluation of fever. Fevers tend to increase in the afternoon and evening and decrease in the early morning.

Fever causes an increase in oxygen consumption and carbon dioxide production. Patients with high fever need to take deeper breaths at a faster rate in order to accommodate the fever-related increase in metabolism. Some patients report having a fever when they feel warm even though they have not measured their temperature. This subjective sensation of feeling warm may simply reflect the temperature of their environment. It is important to know whether the report of fever is based on actual temperature measurements.

Common respiratory problems associated with fever include viral infections, bacterial bronchitis, bacterial pneumonia, fungal infections, and tuberculosis. The degree of fever in any illness depends on the severity of the infection and the patient's ability to respond to the infection. A patient with a compromised immune system may not generate a significant fever despite having a severe infection.

Box 1.2 Outline of the Medical History

I. PATIENT IDENTIFICATION
   A. Name of patient
   B. Address of patient
   C. Age of patient
   D. Date and place of birth
   E. Marital status
   F. Current occupation
   G. Religious preference

II. CHIEF COMPLAINT(S)
   A. List of patient complaints in the order of severity

III. HISTORY OF PRESENT ILLNESS
   Chronological description of each symptom including:
   A. When it started and what seemed to provoke it
   B. Severity
   C. Location on the body
   D. Aggravating/alleviating factors
   E. Frequency (how often it occurs)

IV. PAST MEDICAL HISTORY
   A. Childhood illnesses and development
   B. Hospitalizations, surgeries, injuries, and major illnesses
   C. Allergies/immunizations
   D. Drugs and medications
   E. Smoking history and attempts at quitting

V. FAMILY HISTORY
   A. List of living close relatives and their health conditions
   B. List of close relatives who are deceased and the causes of death
   C. Marital history

VI. SOCIAL AND ENVIRONMENTAL HISTORY
   A. Education level
   B. Military experience
   C. Occupational history
   D. Hobbies and recreation activities
   E. Current life situation, including stresses from employment and relationship problems
   F. Recent travel that might have an impact on the patient's health

VII. REVIEW OF SYSTEMS

Wheeze

Wheeze is a common complaint in patients with asthma, congestive heart failure, and bronchitis. It is often associated with shortness of breath and is caused by rapid airflow through one or more narrowed airways. Airway walls vibrate between a partially open and closed position as air passes through at high speed. Wheezing may be associated with cough, sputum, and dyspnea when airway disease is present. More information about wheezing is presented in the Physical Examination section of this chapter.

Outline for the Medical History

In addition to interviewing the patient to evaluate the onset and relief of symptoms, you will need to examine the patient's chart to identify the previously documented medical history. This requires familiarity with the outline used to document the patient's medical history. The typical outline and the common information listed in each category are presented in Box 1.2.

The most important category is the history of present illness. This section describes the crucial information that the physician obtains for each of the patient's complaints. All clinicians should be familiar with this section before caring for any patient. Each symptom is described as to when it started, what may have provoked it, how severe it is, and what seems to relieve it. The symptoms are usually arranged in chronological perspective, and the effect of the illness on the patient's life is often also described. Your responsibility is to read this section before seeing the patient so that you can be apprised of the initial symptoms and their severity. Changes in these symptoms may occur with the therapy you provide, and you will recognize such changes more easily if you are familiar with the history of the present illness.

In addition to learning the details surrounding each of the patient's pertinent complaints, the interviewer should ask about the possible presence of other symptoms. This helps define the problem better, as well as clarify a possible diagnosis. For example, if the patient comes to the doctor complaining of cough, the interviewer should ask about fever, sputum production, shortness of breath, hemoptysis, or recent exposure to tuberculosis. If the patient denies the existence of any of these other symptoms, they become a list of pertinent negatives. The list is presented in the history of present illness as "the patient denies fever, sputum production," and so on.

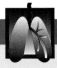

Mr. B

HISTORY

Mr. B is a 49-year-old white man who came to the emergency department at 2 a.m. complaining of chest pain and shortness of breath. The chest pain started about 12 hours previously when Mr. B was mowing the grass. The shortness of breath started while Mr. B was reclining, which was about 2 hours before he came to the emergency department.

QUESTIONS	ANSWERS
1. What details about the chest pain need to be identified?	Mr. B should be asked where his chest pain is located and to point to the spot. Constant chest pain under the sternum is consistent with cardiac ischemia. Chest pain located laterally or posteriorly is more consistent with pleuritic involvement. Questions should be asked about the effect of breathing on the chest pain: Does the chest pain increase with a deep breath? Does the pain radiate to other parts of the body? How severe is the pain? Is it associated with nausea, indigestion, diaphoresis, weakness, or faintness?
2. What details about the shortness of breath need to be identified?	The severity of the shortness of breath needs to be clarified. Does it occur at rest or only with exertion? Has Mr. B ever had this shortness of breath before? Did the dyspnea occur only when he was supine and, if so, did it improve when he sat upright?
3. What term is used to describe dyspnea in a reclining position?	Dyspnea in the reclining position is known as orthopnea.

4. What other possible symptoms need to be asked about in order to define the problem better?	The interviewer should ask Mr. B if he has any other symptoms, such as fever, cough, sputum production, hemoptysis, recent exposure to tuberculosis, or swollen or sore calf muscles. His cholesterol level, family history of heart disease, stress levels, and personal history of heart disease should be evaluated.
5. What social habits need to be identified?	Mr. B's cigarette smoking history must be identified. His symptoms could be consistent with a myocardial infarction, which occurs more often among patients with a significant smoking history.

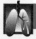

More on Mr. B

Mr. B explains that the chest pain is centrally located and radiates to his left shoulder and jaw. The chest pain started when he was pushing a lawn mower. The pain decreased with rest but did not subside totally. It is not affected by breathing. He has not taken any medication for the chest pain. On a scale from 1 to 10, Mr. B says that at its worst the pain was a 7. Currently he rates the chest pain as a 3.

The shortness of breath is described as severe; it awakened Mr. B from sleep about 2 hours after going to bed. It improved when he sat upright. He has never experienced shortness of breath before. He describes it as a feeling of suffocation.

Mr. B denies cough, sputum production, hemoptysis, fever, or exposure to tuberculosis. He does admit to having some diaphoresis, weakness, and nausea but denies having vomited. He states that he smokes about two packs of cigarettes per day and has been smoking since the age of 16. He has tried to quit on several occasions but was never successful for more than 6 weeks.

QUESTIONS	ANSWERS
6. What pathology probably is responsible for the chest pain?	Centrally located chest pain that worsens with exertion and radiates to the shoulder is the classic description of cardiac pain. Mr. B's coronary vessels are probably narrowed, preventing adequate blood flow to the heart muscle, resulting in an ischemic myocardium. Exertion increases the difference between the amount of oxygen needed by the heart and the amount that can be supplied by the narrowed coronary arteries. As a result, exertion causes the chest pain to worsen.
7. What pathology probably is responsible for the shortness of breath?	The shortness of breath is probably related to buildup of fluid in the lung. Left ventricular failure causes an increased hydrostatic pressure in the pulmonary capillaries, which leads to pulmonary edema. This makes it more difficult for the lung to expand and increases the work of breathing. In such

cases, the patient often complains of labored breathing. Oxygenation of the arterial blood also will be reduced as a result of the pulmonary edema, which causes an increase in the drive to breathe via the carotid bodies and adds to the sensation of dyspnea. The entire process is worsened when the patient lies flat in bed. Reclining causes the venous return to the heart to increase, which in turn increases the hydrostatic pressure in the pulmonary capillaries.

8. What problems are decreased in likelihood by the list of pertinent negatives?

The lack of fever, cough, and sputum helps rule out pneumonia. The lack of leg tenderness, swelling, hemoptysis, or pleuritic chest pain helps rule out pulmonary embolism. The acute onset and lack of exposure help rule out tuberculosis.

9. If Mr. B had a dry, nonproductive cough, what pathology would probably explain it?

A dry, nonproductive cough is common in heart failure patients with pleural effusion.

10. Should Mr. B be admitted to the hospital?

Yes, Mr. B should be admitted to the telemetry ward or ICU for close monitoring and treatment.

PHYSICAL EXAMINATION

Once you have established a rapport with the patient during the interview, you and the patient will usually find the physical examination a more comfortable experience. The physical examination is done to confirm or rule out certain illnesses suspected based on the results of the interview. For example, in the case above, it is suspected that Mr. B has ischemic heart disease and pulmonary edema. The clinician should perform the physical examination with this tentative diagnosis in mind and seek evidence of heart failure and pulmonary edema. The physical examination is also done to identify all abnormalities, some of which may be very important but unrelated to the current problem. RTs most often use the physical examination to evaluate the patient's response to therapy. This calls for a brief and well-focused examination, primarily centered around the cardiopulmonary system. For this reason, this section will emphasize examination of the cardiopulmonary system.

The physical examination is simple, quick, and inexpensive. In many cases, it also is sensitive, resulting in the identification of the initial evidence of disease. The examination may need to be brief when the patient is in serious distress and initial treatment is needed. A more thorough examination can be done when the patient is stable. A typical outline for documentation of a complete physical examination is listed in Box 1.3.

Vital Signs and Sensorium

In general, the vital signs provide an index of the patient's acute condition. Most acute medical problems will be reflected by abnormal vital signs that become more abnormal as the problem

Box 1.3 Format for Documenting the Physical Examination

INITIAL IMPRESSION

    Age, height, weight, and general appearance

VITAL SIGNS

    Heart rate, respiratory rate, temperature, and blood pressure

HEAD, EARS, EYES, NOSE, AND THROAT (HEENT)

NECK

    Evidence of jugular venous distention; position of the trachea; any lymphadenopathy

THORAX

    Heart: Evidence of heaves or lifts, heart sounds, and murmurs

    Lungs: Lung sounds, breathing pattern, chest configuration, percussion findings, etc.

ABDOMEN

    Evidence of distention and hepatomegaly

    Degree of obesity

EXTREMITIES

    Evidence of cyanosis, clubbing, and pedal edema

Acute onset of tachycardia and tachypnea at rest suggest the onset of a significant cardiopulmonary problem. The patient should be evaluated by a physician.

Box 1.4 Common Causes of Abnormal Heart Rate

TACHYCARDIA

- Anxiety
- Stress
- Response to medications, such as bronchodilators
- Hypoxemia
- Heart failure
- Fever

BRADYCARDIA

- Hypothermia
- Myocardial infarction with damaged SA node
- Stimulation of the vagus nerve

---

increases in severity. Chronic conditions may not result in abnormal vital signs as compensatory mechanisms take effect.

The four basic vital signs are heart rate, respiratory rate, blood pressure, and body temperature. A heart rate greater than 100/minute is known as **tachycardia**. A heart rate less than 60/minute is known as **bradycardia**. Common causes of tachycardia and bradycardia are listed in Box 1.4. The heart rate is determined by counting the rate of the peripheral pulse or by using a cardiac monitor.

A respiratory rate higher than 20/minute in the adult is known as **tachypnea** and is a common finding in patients with cardiopulmonary disease. Common causes of tachypnea are disorders of the lung that cause a reduction in lung volume and increased stiffness of the lung (e.g., restrictive defect). This forces the patient to breathe with smaller tidal volumes and more rapidly in order to compensate for the shallow breaths. Disorders such as atelectasis, pulmonary edema, pneumonia, pneumothorax, and pulmonary fibrosis cause loss of lung volume and result in an increase in respiratory rate. Other causes of tachypnea include hypoxemia, pain, anxiety, fever, and exertion.

Bradypnea, a respiratory rate in the adult of less than 10/minute, is not common but may be seen with hypothermia and central nervous system (CNS) disorders. Hypothermia causes a decrease in the amount of oxygen consumed and carbon dioxide produced by the body and results in a reduced need for breathing. CNS disorders may interfere with the brain activity responsible for breathing and cause bradypnea or even a complete lack of breathing, known as **apnea**.

Normal blood pressure is approximately 120/80 mm Hg in the adult patient. A blood pressure less than 90/60 mm Hg is known as **hypotension**. Mild levels of hypotension may be seen in normal persons or healthy athletes. Severe hypotension occurs when the heart fails as a pump, when peripheral vasculature dilates excessively, or when the circulating blood volume is severely reduced. Severe hypotension is to be avoided at all costs because it indicates that blood flow to important vascular beds is inadequate.

Hypertension is present when the blood pressure exceeds 140/90 mm Hg. Hypertension is a common problem in adults. The exact cause is often unknown, but it leads to numerous health problems including heart failure and stroke. It is treated most often with medications that reduce the contractility of the heart (negative inotropics) or medications that dilate peripheral blood vessels.

Normal body temperature is approximately 37°C $\pm$ 0.5°C (98.6°F $\pm$ 1°F). Elevation of body temperature caused by disease is known as **fever**. Fever is common in patients with infections, such as respiratory infections from viral, fungal, or bacterial organisms. Fever causes the metabolic rate of the patient to increase slightly, and this results in an increase in the oxygen consumption and carbon dioxide production each minute. As a result, a febrile patient needs to breathe at a slightly faster rate to accommodate the increased metabolic rate.

A low body temperature is referred to as **hypothermia**. It is not common but does occur in patients with head injuries that damage the hypothalamus and in those who have been exposed to cold temperatures for long periods of time. Near-drowning victims are frequently admitted to the hospital in a hypothermic condition. Some medications make patients more likely to become hypothermic. Although hypothermic patients need less oxygen to survive, the heart and some other body systems do not function well when body temperature is severely reduced. Blood flow is shunted to vital organs in hypothermic patients, which is why resuscitation of the hypothermic patient often requires special procedures and slow warming of the patient.

Sensorium assessment is done by evaluating the patient's level of consciousness. It is an important parameter in monitoring the patient with cardiopulmonary disease because it reflects the adequacy of blood flow and oxygenation of the brain as well as the net effect of acid-base imbalance, electrolyte imbalance, nutritional deficiency, and failure of other organ systems. The patient who is alert and oriented as to time, place, and person is said to be "oriented times 3"; that is, the patient knows the correct date and time, where he is physically located, and who he is. Confusion with regard to any of these items indicates that the patient is disoriented. As cerebral function continues to deteriorate, the patient will become semiconscious and eventually comatose.

> An acute decline in sensorioum requires immediate investigation.

Pulse oximetry has become a very popular noninvasive technique for monitoring the patient with acute cardiopulmonary disease. The popularity of pulse oximetry has caused some clinicians to refer to it as the "fifth vital sign." It can be used intermittently or continuously to monitor the oxygenation status of the patient. The probe is attached to the patient's finger or ear lobe and shines an infrared light through the tissues. Red, oxygenated blood absorbs infrared light differently in comparison to bluish, deoxygenated blood. The oximeter reads the amount of light absorption and determines the degree of oxygenation.

Although pulse oximetry has proved useful in a variety of settings, it does not evaluate the patient's ability to ventilate, fails when peripheral circulation is poor, and can

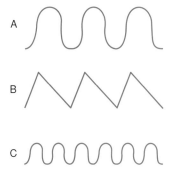

FIGURE 1.1 Patterns of breathing. (A) Normal. (B) Prolonged expiratory time. (C) Rapid and shallow.

read falsely high when the hemoglobin is saturated with carbon monoxide. For these reasons, pulse oximetry should not be the only parameter used to evaluate the respiratory status of the patient suspected of having circulatory problems, ventilatory problems, or carbon monoxide poisoning. Clinical examination and arterial blood gases (see later discussion) are needed in such cases.

Chest Inspection

An important parameter to evaluate during chest inspection is breathing pattern, because it can provide important clues regarding the underlying lung pathology. Patients who breathe with a prolonged expiratory phase usually have narrowed intrathoracic airways. Patients with acute asthma, bronchitis, or emphysema tend to breathe with a prolonged expiratory phase when airway obstruction is severe (Fig. 1.1). Patients with a narrowed upper airway (e.g., epiglottitis) breathe with a prolonged inspiratory phase. The upper airway tends to narrow more during inspiratory efforts, making gas flow into the lung more difficult. Patients with restrictive lung disease (i.e., loss of lung volume) breathe with a rapid and shallow breathing pattern. The greater the loss of lung volume, the faster the respiratory rate.

> Patients with atelectasis assume a rapid and shallow breathing pattern with a rate that is proportional to the degree of atelectasis.

Abdominal paradox is an abnormal breathing pattern seen in patients who have diaphragm fatigue. It is recognized by observing the abdomen sink inward with each inspiratory effort. Fatigue of the diaphragm, which is the major muscle for breathing, occurs when it has been overworked and underfed. These circumstances are common in patients with acute exacerbations of COPD. The abdomen sinks inward with each breath because the negative intrathoracic pressure created by the accessory respiratory muscles causes the diaphragm and abdomen contents to be pulled upward into the chest during inspiration. This, in turn, causes the flaccid abdomen to sink inward during each respiratory inspiration.

Inspection of the chest includes notation of the degree of symmetrical chest expansion. Normally, both sides of the chest expand evenly with each inspiratory effort. Unilateral chest diseases, such as pneumonia or pneumothorax, may result in better expansion of the healthy side of the chest compared to the diseased side. The diseased side is said to "lag behind" the normal side.

Inspection of the chest wall for possible deformities is important. Abnormal curvature of the spine can cause poor lung expansion and significant restrictive lung disease. Lateral curvature of the spine is termed scoliosis, and anteroposterior curvature of the spine is termed kyphosis. The term kyphoscoliosis is used when both are present. Older patients with emphysema and osteoporosis develop kyphosis. A premature anteroposterior increase in the diameter of the chest (referred to as barrel chest)

> A barrel chest indicates that the patient has emphysema and a significant air trapping.

often develops in the adult COPD patient (Fig. 1.2). Barrel chest occurs when the lung loses its elastic recoil and can no longer appropriately oppose the outward spring of the ribs. Other chest deformities to inspect for include pectus excavatum (abnormal

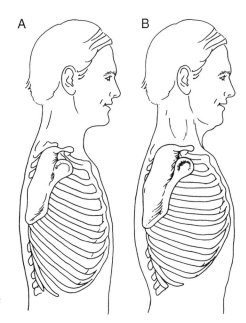

FIGURE 1.2 (A) Normal chest configuration vs. (B) increased AP diameter consistent with a barrel chest. Note the hypertrophy of the accessory muscles in B.

permanent depression of the sternum) and **pectus carinatum** (abnormal prominence of the sternum).

Palpation and Percussion of the Chest

Palpation of the chest wall is done in certain circumstances to evaluate lung disorders. Palpation of the chest wall for tactile fremitus can be helpful in detecting significant changes in the pathology of the lung. The patient is asked to repeat the phrase "1-2-3" or "99" while the examiner palpates the chest wall comparing side to side. Diseases of the lung that cause it to become more dense (e.g., pneumonia) cause an increase in tactile fremitus over the affected area. The vibrations created by the patient's larynx travel more rapidly through consolidated lung tissue and result in a noticeable increase in fremitus. Diseases that cause the lung to become less dense (e.g., emphysema, pneumothorax) cause a decrease in tactile fremitus, as will interposition of fluid (pleural effusion) or air (pneumothorax) between the lung and chest wall.

The chest wall is also palpated to detect evidence of air leakage into the skin around the chest in certain circumstances. Air may leak into the surrounding tissues when chest trauma has occurred or when the patient has been mechanically ventilated with high pressure. Air leakage into the chest wall results in subcutaneous emphysema; this is detected by palpating the chest wall for areas that produce a distinctive crackling sound and sensation known as **crepitations**.

Tapping on the chest wall for the purpose of evaluating underlying lung pathology is known as chest percussion. Chest percussion is done when major changes in the density of the lung are suspected based on the history and previous physical examination findings. Normal lung tissue is air filled and produces a resonant sound in response to percussion. Diseases that produce increased lung density, such as pneumonia, result in decreased resonance upon percussion. This also is present with pleural effusion. Air trapped in the pleural space and emphysema cause increased resonance upon percussion. Chest percussion for evaluation of changes in lung pathology is not done routinely by health-care providers but can be very useful in some circumstances.

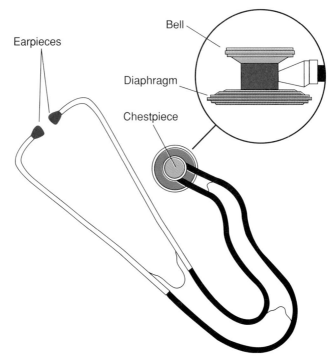

Bell

Earpieces

Diaphragm

Chestpiece

FIGURE 1.3 Diagram of a stethoscope used to auscultate the heart and lungs.

Chest Auscultation

The majority of health-care providers routinely listen to the chest to evaluate the sounds of breathing. Chest auscultation provides immediate information about the patency of the airways and condition of the lung parenchyma. It is inexpensive and reliable and is done with a stethoscope (Fig. 1.3). To detect unilateral changes in lung pathology, the clinician compares the sounds of breathing on one side to those at the same location on the opposite side (Fig. 1.4).

Breath sounds are the normal sounds of breathing. There are three different types of breath sounds: **tracheal** (or **bronchial**), **bronchovesicular**, and **vesicular**. Tracheal, or bronchial, breath sounds are heard directly over the trachea and are loud and high pitched. They have a relatively equal inspiratory and expiratory phase and are produced by the turbulent flow in the trachea and main bronchi (Fig. 1.5).

Bronchovesicular breath sounds are heard around the sternum on the anterior chest wall and between the scapulae on the posterior chest wall. They are softer in intensity and their pitch is reduced when compared to tracheal or bronchial breath sounds. The expiratory phase is not quite equal to the inspiratory phase. These sounds are also produced by turbulent flow in the larger airways, but they are not as loud or high pitched as tracheal or bronchial breath sounds because they are filtered by healthy lung tissue, which lies between the area of sound production and the surface of the chest wall.

Vesicular breath sounds are heard over the areas of the chest wall overlying lung parenchyma. These sounds are very soft and primarily heard on inspiration. Their expiratory component is normally minimal and heard only during the initial one-fourth of the expiratory phase. Vesicular breath sounds are lower pitched than tracheal breath sounds and are also produced by turbulent flow in the larger airways. Vesicular breath sounds are

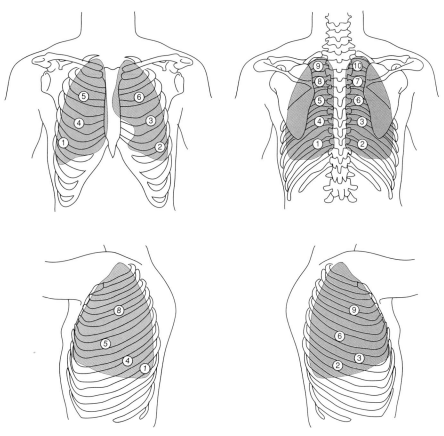

FIGURE 1.4 Sequence for chest auscultation. Note that examiner begins in the bases and compares side to side.

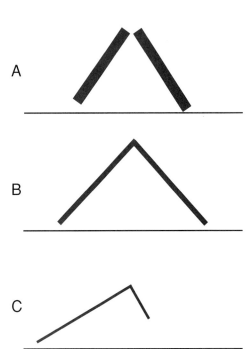

FIGURE 1.5 Diagram of (A) tracheobronchial, (B) bronchovesicular, and (C) vesicular breath sounds. The upstroke represents inspiration and the downstroke expiration. The thickness of the line represents the intensity of the sound.

significantly softer and lower pitched because they represent the turbulent flow sounds heard after they have passed through normal lung tissue. Normal lung tissue attenuates sound traveling through it and changes normal bronchial breath sounds to normal vesicular breath sounds. Changes in lung-tissue density resulting from disease (e.g., pneumonia) cause the normal attenuation characteristics of the lung to be altered.

Lung diseases that cause the parenchyma to become denser result in less attenuation of the turbulent flow sounds of the larger airways as they pass through the lung. This causes the normal vesicular breath sounds to be replaced with a harsher version that is louder and more bronchial in character. Peripheral atelectasis, pulmonary fibrosis, and pneumonia are examples of lung disorders that can cause harsh breath sounds called **bronchial breath sounds** over the affected region.

> The normal lung attenuates sounds as it passes through. This causes the sound waves to be lower in pitch and intensity.

Disorders of the lung that result in a loss of lung tissue density, such as emphysema, result in excessive attenuation of the turbulent flow sounds of the larger airways. This causes the normal breath sounds to be replaced by **diminished** breath sounds that are much harder to hear. Diseases of the chest wall can also cause diminished or absent breath sounds when excessive fluid or air build up in the pleural space, resulting in an acoustical sound barrier that prevents the transmission of normal breath sounds through the chest wall. Finally, diminished breath sounds can be present when the patient's breathing is excessively shallow. This is common in cases of drug overdose, which suppress the patient's drive to breathe.

Chest auscultation may reveal adventitious lung sounds, which are abnormal noises superimposed on the breath sounds. There are two basic types of adventitious lung sounds: *continuous* and *discontinuous* (Fig. 1.6). This categorization is based on acoustical recordings of the sounds. Study of these recordings reveals that the continuous type has a consistent sound pattern for at least one tenth of a second, whereas the discontinuous type has no such pattern.

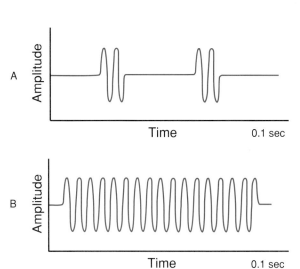

FIGURE 1.6 Time-expanded wave-form anaylsis of (A) discontinuous adventitious lung sound (wheeze) (B) continuous adventitious lung sound (crackles).

The continuous type of adventitious lung sounds often have a musical quality and are associated with narrowed intrathoracic airways. Rapid airflow through a site of obstruction is believed to cause the airway wall to flutter rapidly between a partially open and closed position. This rapid fluttering causes a continuous type of whistling sound, known as a **wheeze**. Wheezes are most often heard during exhalation because this is when the intrathoracic airways naturally narrow.

Wheezing produced by multiple airways fluttering, which produces numerous musical notes that begin and end simultaneously, is known as *polyphonic* wheezing. Wheezing resulting from one airway's becoming partially obstructed produces a single note and is known as a *monophonic* wheeze. Some clinicians refer to low-pitched wheezes as rhonchi.

Partial upper airway obstruction can cause a wheezing type of sound to come from the neck. This sound is most often heard during inspiration and is referred to as **stridor**. Stridor is a serious abnormality, since it signifies that the major airway into the lung is compromised; patients with stridor must be carefully monitored and treated. Not all patients with upper airway compromise present with stridor. In patients with partial upper airway obstruction, fatigue or the use of sedatives, or both, reduce the degree of air movement past the site of obstruction and cause the absence of stridor. Clinicians should never assume the upper airway is patent simply because the patient lacks noisy breathing.

Discontinuous adventitious lung sounds are termed **crackles**. Crackles are believed to be produced by two mechanisms: (1) sudden opening of small airways and (2) movement of excessive airway secretions with breathing. Sudden opening of small airways occurs when a patient with collapsed small airways inhales deeply enough to overcome the surface tension of fluid, causing the airways to stay collapsed. Such crackles are typically heard late in inspiration and occur most often in patients with congestive heart failure and in the lower lung fields of bedridden patients. Crackles from the movement of excessive airway secretions are lower pitched (coarse) and occur during inhalation and exhalation. They may clear with a strong cough or if the airway is aspirated with a suction catheter (Table 1.1).

> The majority of adventitious lung sounds are crackles or wheezes. Late-inspiratory crackles indicate restrictive lung disease, while expiratory wheezes suggest obstructive lung disease.

Examination of Other Parts of the Body

Inspect the patient's neck for evidence of jugular venous distention (JVD) when you suspect right heart failure. Failure of the right ventricle can occur with chronic lung disease or when chronic left heart failure is severe enough to affect the right heart. Failure of the right ventricle leads to backup of blood into the jugular vein, causing it to distend. Before examining the patient for JVD, you should ensure that the head of the patient's bed is elevated to a 45 degree angle each time the JVD is assessed. This assures a consistent

Table 1.1 Interpreting Abnormal Lung Sounds

Name of Sound	Mechanism	Characteristics
Bronchial BS	Increased sound transmission	Equal inspiratory and expiratory components
Diminished BS	Decreased sound transmission	Soft and low pitched
Wheezes	Airflow through narrowed airway	Musical, with a continuous pattern
Crackles	Sudden opening of closed airways or movement of airway secretions	Fine, late-inspiratory Coarse, inspiratory and expiratory
Stridor	Upper airway narrowing	Often high pitched

BS = breath sounds.

gravitational effect on the blood returning to the heart. The level of elevation should be recorded if it is different than the standard 45 degree angle.

The area of the chest overlying the heart is known as the **precordium**. You should inspect and palpate this area for abnormal pulsations when cardiac abnormalities are suspected. Enlargement of the right ventricle usually results in an abnormal pulsation around the sternum, known as a right ventricular **heave**, which occurs with each systolic heart beat. Left ventricular enlargement causes an abnormal heave in the left anterior axillary region.

> A gallop rhythm is associated with congestive heart failure in patients over age 45 years.

To identify the heart sounds, you auscultate over the precordium. Normally the heart sounds are soft and maintain a consistent "lub-dub" rhythm. The first heart sound (S1) is produced by closure of the mitral and tricuspid valves during systole, whereas the second heart sound (S2) is produced by closure of the aortic and pulmonary valves during diastole. The heart sounds may take on a "galloping" rhythm when added sounds are produced by abnormal cardiac pathology. For example, when the left ventricle becomes stiff after a myocardial infarction, an additional sound may be produced by the sudden filling of the ventricle with blood from the atrium during diastole. This added sound causes an additional heart sound, known as an S_3 gallop.

Murmurs are adventitious heart sounds that may also be heard during auscultation over the heart. They are caused by turbulent blood flow through a narrow opening. For example, when one of the heart valves becomes stenotic, rapid blood flow through the constriction causes an abnormal sound similar to a low-pitched blowing sound. Murmurs are typically described by their location and position in the cardiac cycle and rated on a scale from 1 to 6, according to their loudness.

Examine the extremities for possible digital clubbing and for their color and temperature. **Digital clubbing** is a nonspecific sign that occurs in a variety of chronic cardiopulmonary diseases such as COPD and lung cancer. You will recognize it by inspecting the fingers and toes for enlargement of soft tissue at the base of the nails and by examining the nails for abnormal lateral and longitudinal curvature (Fig. 1.7). A bluish discoloration of the skin caused by poorly oxygenated blood is known as

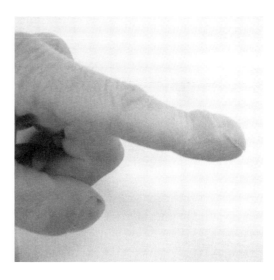

FIGURE 1.7 Example of digital clubbing.

cyanosis. Peripheral cyanosis indicates suboptimal circulation or oxygenation or both. Extremities that are cyanotic as a result of poor circulation are usually also cool to the touch.

Inspect and palpate the abdomen for evidence of distention. Abdominal distention can limit function of the diaphragm and further increase the severity of respiratory failure in the patient with a compromised respiratory condition. An enlarged liver, known as **hepatomegaly**, is often present in the patient with right ventricular failure. Right heart failure occurs as a result of chronic left heart failure or when cor pulmonale is present as a result of chronic lung disease.

Inspect the mouth for evidence of cyanosis. A cyanotic oral mucosa indicates the presence of central cyanosis. This is a sign of severe hypoxemia and indicates that the respiratory system is not fulfilling its obligations to the body. The presence of central cyanosis strongly suggests that the patient needs oxygen therapy and that you should investigate the respiratory system further.

Examination of the mouth may also reveal pursed-lip breathing. This breathing technique is naturally adopted by COPD patients as they attempt to maintain patency of distal airways during exhalation. COPD patients often have difficulty exhaling fully because of premature collapse of distal airways. Pursed-lip breathing helps these patients exhale more fully and maintain better gas exchange.

 More on Mr. B

PHYSICAL EXAMINATION

- **Vital Signs** (in the emergency department). Heart rate 112/minute, respiratory rate 28/minute, blood pressure 90/66 mm Hg, and temperature 36.7°C (98.0°F); alert but disoriented

- **HEENT.** Normal

- **Neck.** JVD noted at mid neck with the head of the bed at 45 degree angle

- **Chest.** A heave is noted at the left anterior axillary line; S_3 gallop rhythm noted on auscultation; no murmurs heard

- **Lungs.** Fine, late-inspiratory crackles are noted in the bases bilaterally; respiratory rate rapid and shallow

- **Extremities.** Digits mildly cyanotic and cool to the touch

QUESTIONS	ANSWERS
11. How would you interpret the vital signs and sensorium? What could be the cause of the blood pressure finding?	The heart rate and respiratory rate are increased. Blood pressure is reduced, while body temperature is essentially normal. The reduced sensorium suggests that the brain may not be getting adequate blood flow and may not be well oxygenated. The low blood pressure is probably the result of poor pumping ability of the heart because of acute ischemia.

12. What pathophysiology explains the JVD?	The JVD is probably related to left heart failure. As the left ventricle fails to pump blood forward into the aorta, the blood backs up into the lungs. This puts a heavy load on the right heart, which also fails and causes the blood to back up and distend the jugular veins.
13. What pathophysiology explains the heave at the left anterior axillary line and the gallop rhythm?	The heave at the left anterior axillary line is caused by left ventricular distention. The gallop rhythm is the result of a stiffened left ventricular wall following the myocardial injury. This stiff left ventricle causes turbulence and an added heart sound as blood from the left atrium fills the ventricle. The sudden deceleration of blood entering the left ventricle produces a third sound in a rhythm similar to a horse's gallop.
14. Why does this patient have fine, late-inspiratory crackles in the bases?	The fine, late-inspiratory crackles in the lung bases are due to the accumulation of pulmonary edema fluid in the small airways. Left heart failure increases the blood pressure in the capillaries, causing fluid to leak into the interstitial space and from there into the small airways. The airways collapse on exhalation and are stuck shut by the surface tension of the fluid within them. Subsequent inspiration will cause these collapsed units to pop open, making characteristic crackling sounds.
15. What probably explains Mr. B's cool and cyanotic extremities?	Mr. B's cool and cyanotic extremities are probably related to poor cardiac output. Poor perfusion of the extremities causes them to become cool to the touch, and the cyanosis is related to the presence of deoxygenated hemoglobin.

INTERPRETATION OF CLINICAL LAB DATA

Laboratory data are used for general evaluation of the patient, to diagnose specific problems, and to determine the effectiveness of therapy. This section focuses on those tests that are most frequently ordered for patients with cardiopulmonary disease.

Common Blood and Fluid Tests

The most common laboratory test is the complete blood count (CBC). The CBC measures the number and type of circulating white blood cells (WBCs) and the number and size of red blood cells (RBCs). The WBCs primarily fight invading organisms, such as bacteria, in

Table 1.2 Interpretation of the White Blood Cell Count Differential

Cell Type	Normal Values	Cause of Increase	Description
Neutrophil	40%–60%	Acute illness/stress	Neutrophilia
Lymphocyte	20%–40%	Viral infections	Lymphocytosis
Eosinophil	0%–6%	Allergic reaction	Eosinophilia
Monocyte	2%–10%	Chronic infection, malignancies	Monocytosis
Basophil	0%–1%	Bone marrow disease	Basophilia

a process known as phagocytosis. Elevation of the WBC count is known as **leukocytosis** and is a common finding in patients with pneumonia and other infections. Leukocytosis occurs when the bone marrow releases larger numbers of stored white cells in response to infection or acute stress (e.g., trauma).

A decrease in the WBC count is termed **leukopenia** and is less common than leukocytosis. It is seen in cases of bone marrow disease and overwhelming infection, especially in elderly patients or those with a compromised immune system. Leukopenia is an ominous sign in the patient with severe pneumonia and indicates that the body cannot respond adequately to the infection and the patient is at high risk for death.

The WBC count represents the total number of circulating WBCs per cubic millimeter. Five different cells make up the WBCs (Table 1.2). Neutrophils are the most common type of WBC and are primarily responsible for fighting bacterial organisms. Two types of neutrophils are counted: the segmented neutrophils (segs) and the immature segs (bands). Segs are the first line of defense against infection, but when they cannot be produced rapidly enough, bands are

> **S**ignificant elevation of the WBC count is usually the result of neutrophilia or lymphocytosis, as these two cells account for about 90% of the circulating WBCs.

called into action. Bands are stored in the bone marrow and are released in larger numbers when acute bacterial infection is present. Thus, the presence of a high number of bands usually means an acute bacterial infection is present. Lymphocytes, another common type of WBC, are mostly responsible for fighting viral infections. Eosinophils help the body deal with allergic reactions; thus, an elevation in eosinophils often indicates the presence of an allergic stimulus. Most mature eosinophils (99%) are located in the tissues of the lung, G.I. tract, or skin. See Appendix A for tables on normal values for laboratory tests.

The RBC count helps determine the ability of the blood to carry oxygen. A low RBC count is termed **anemia**, whereas a high RBC count is called **polycythemia**. Anemia is common after surgery or hemorrhage and it decreases the oxygen-carrying capacity of the blood. Secondary polycythemia is seen most often in cases of chronically low blood oxygen levels owing either to lung disease, cyanotic congenital heart disease, or living at high altitudes. Chronically low oxygen levels stimulate the bone marrow to produce more RBCs to compensate for low oxygen availability. This allows an increased quantity of oxygen to be carried in the blood despite a reduced partial pressure of oxygen.

In addition to the total RBC count, the amount of hemoglobin per 100 mL of blood is reported. In cases of microcytic, hypochromic anemia, the total number of circulating RBCs is normal, but their size is small and the amount of hemoglobin is reduced. This disorder is common among patients with iron-deficient diets or chronic blood loss.

Serum electrolytes are also frequently measured as a routine test for patients with cardiopulmonary disease. Most often, the serum sodium (Na^+), potassium (K^+), chloride (Cl^-), and total (HCO_3^-) are evaluated. Normal values are listed for these tests in Appendix A. Electrolyte abnormalities are associated with a large number of diseases; they can also occur as a complication of certain medications. In most cases, electrolytes are measured not to confirm suspicion of a specific disease, but to evaluate the general health condition of the patient and potential side effects of therapy. For example, the patient with heart failure may have a reduced serum sodium (hyponatremia) as a result of retaining too much water and a reduced serum potassium (hypokalemia) as a side effect of diuretic therapy. If either abnormality is present, the heart may pump suboptimally until the problem is corrected.

The clinical laboratory department has a microbiology section that evaluates the type of organisms present in body fluids. An example would be the patient with pneumonia who produces a sputum sample for laboratory evaluation. The laboratory technician attempts to identify the type of organisms present in the lung sputum. This can be very helpful for selecting an appropriate course of antibiotics. The Gram stain is used to initially evaluate sputum, and it is usually followed by a bacterial culture.

> Sputum samples that contain numerous epithelial cells have been contaminated with saliva from the mouth and should be discarded.

The Gram stain helps identify whether the sample consists of sputum from the lung or just secretions from the mouth. True sputum from the infected airways has few epithelial cells and numerous pus cells. Once the sample has been found to represent lower airway secretions, a portion of the sample is placed in an appropriate nutrient container and warmed to promote growth. In about 48 to 72 hours, the sample will reveal the identity of the organisms present in the specimen and the antibiotics to which they are most sensitive.

Cardiac enzymes are measured in patients suspected of having a myocardial infarction. Acute injury to the myocardium causes the heart muscle cells to release excessive amounts of enzymes into the circulating blood. For example, creatine phosphokinase (CPK) and troponin enzymes are usually elevated within hours of a heart attack. If the chest pain is not due to ischemia of the heart muscle, the enzymes will not be released into the blood. Other laboratory tests performed periodically in the patient with cardiopulmonary disease are listed in Table 1.3.

Arterial Blood Gases

Another common test done to evaluate patients with cardiopulmonary disease is the arterial blood gas (ABG). This test measures the ability of the lungs to oxygenate the blood and remove carbon dioxide from it. When the lungs are working well, the arterial oxygen tension (Pao_2) will be 90 to 100 mm Hg. **Hypoxemia** is present when the blood oxygen level is below normal. Mild hypoxemia is present when the Pao_2 is below normal for the age of the patient but above 59 mm Hg. Moderate hypoxemia is present when the Pao_2 is 40 to 59 mm Hg, and severe hypoxemia is defined as a Pao_2 of less than 40 mm Hg.

The normal carbon dioxide level is about 35 to 45 mm Hg. Elevation of the $Paco_2$ above 45 mm Hg is termed **hypercapnia** (or **hypercarbia**). It indicates that the degree of ventilation is inadequate to keep up with the rate of carbon dioxide production. Hypercarbia is common with hypoventilation caused by drug overdose, severe airways obstruction, and neuromuscular disease.

Hypocapnia (or **hypocarbia**) is present when the arterial tension of carbon dioxide ($Paco_2$) is less than 35 mm Hg. This indicates that the rate of ventilation is excessive for

Table 1.3 Other Laboratory Tests

Test Name	Purpose	Implications of Results
Platelet count	Assess blood clotting ability	Reduced with bone marrow dysfunction and chemotherapy
Sweat chloride	Assess excretory function of sweat glands	60–80 mEq/liter consistent with cystic fibrosis
Blood glucose	Measure blood sugar	Increased with diabetes; decreased with inadequate food intake or excessive use of insulin
BUN	Measure BUN level	Increased with renal disease and heart failure severe enough to cause renal dysfunction
Creatinine	Assess renal function	Increased with renal failure; more specific test
Serum protein/ albumin	Assess protein synthesis	Decreased with liver disease and malnutrition; decreased serum albumin may contribute to pulmonary edema
PTT	Test blood clotting ability	Lengthened with heparin therapy, coagulation disorders
PT	Test blood clotting ability	Lengthened with warfarin, but not heparin therapy, severe liver disease
INR	Test blood clotting ability	More accurate calculation of the PT
Urinalysis	Assess urine for:	
	WBCs	Many WBCs indicate infection
	RBCs	Many RBCs indicate kidney inflammation or infection
	Protein	Protein indicates renal disease
	Glucose	Presence of sugar may indicate diabetes

BUN = blood urea nitrogen; INR = international normalized ratio; PT = prothrombin time; PTT = partial thromboplastin time; RBCs = red blood cells; WBCs = white blood cells

the rate of carbon dioxide production. It is common with acute pain, anxiety, pregnancy, metabolic acidosis, sepsis, severe liver disease, and CNS disorders.

ABG measurements also evaluate the acid-base status of the patient. Normal arterial blood pH is 7.35 to 7.45. A pH of less than 7.35 is termed **acidosis** (or **acidemia**) and is caused by elevation of the arterial blood CO_2 (**respiratory acidosis**) or by reduction in blood bicarbonate (**metabolic acidosis**). Respiratory acidosis, also called ventilatory failure, is caused by failure of the lungs to provide adequate gas exchange between the blood and the environment. Disorders that result in neuromuscular weakness or obstruct the airways commonly cause ventilatory failure (Table 1.4). Reduction in blood bicarbonate occurs in conditions such as diarrhea, toxicity by some poisons, diabetes, renal failure, and anaerobic metabolism.

An arterial blood pH of greater than 7.45 is termed **alkalosis** (or **alkalemia**) and occurs with hyperventilation, which causes a reduction of $Paco_2$ (**respiratory alkalosis**), and with elevation of arterial blood bicarbonate (**metabolic alkalosis**). Respiratory alkalosis is frequently caused by anxiety, pain, acidosis,

> Metabolic acidosis is a potent stimulus to the respiratory center and causes hyperventilation that is proportional to the degree of acidosis.

Table 1.4 Common Causes of Respiratory Acidosis

Category of Problem	Clinical Examples
Decreased drive to breathe	Drug overdose; head trauma
Neuromuscular defect	Guillain-Barré syndrome, myasthenia gravis, muscular dystrophy, cervical neck injury
Thoracic cage defect	Kyphoscoliosis, chest trauma/flail chest
Airway obstruction	Asthma, chronic obstructive pulmonary disease, epiglottitis

or hypoxemia. Metabolic alkalosis can occur with a loss of acid (e.g., nasogastric suctioning, vomiting).

Pulmonary Function Tests

Pulmonary function tests are done to evaluate lung volumes and airway patency. The vital capacity is a measure of all usable lung volume. The patient inhales maximally and then exhales maximally into the spirometer; the amount of gas fully exhaled after a maximum inhalation is the **vital capacity**. Reductions in the vital capacity can be due to low lung volumes (**restrictive disease**) or narrowed airways with air trapping (**obstructive disease**).

The most common measures of airway patency are the forced expiratory volume in 1 second (FEV_1) and the forced expiratory flow during the middle half of the forced vital capacity ($FEF_{25\%-75\%}$). These measures of flow help determine whether obstructive lung disease is present. An FEV_1 of less than 80% of predicted is abnormally low, and an $FEF_{25\%-75\%}$ of less than 60% of predicted is abnormally low. Low FEV_1 and $FEF_{25\%-75\%}$ in the presence of a normal forced vital capacity document airway obstruction. Low FEV_1 and $FEF_{25\%-75\%}$ with a reduced vital capacity could be caused by either restrictive lung disease or by obstructive lung disease with air trapping. Further testing with a body box or helium dilution would be necessary to determine the exact cause. A bronchodilator is usually given to the patient with reduced flow measurements to see if it has a therapeutic effect. If the flow measurements increase significantly (i.e., by greater than 12%) after bronchodilator therapy, the patient is said to have improved with bronchodilation. Many patients benefit from a bronchodilator even if it does not produce a change in the above values: A positive response to a bronchodilator means the therapy is definitely helpful and the patient will also likely respond to steroid treatment. This is most often seen in patients with asthma and COPD.

Chest Radiography

Chest radiographs (x-rays) provide a view of the patient's internal thoracic anatomy as shadows of different shades of gray cast upon the x-ray image. Diseases of the chest that alter lung pathology are visible on chest x-rays, as they change the density of usual structures. The chest x-ray is also useful for identifying the position of tubes and catheters. For example, after intubation of the trachea, a chest x-ray is useful for determining whether the tube is in the correct position. The tip of the endotracheal tube is properly positioned if it is found to be 3 to 5 cm above the carina on the chest x-ray. Insertion of the endotracheal tube too far usually results in its passing into the right mainstem bronchus (Fig. 1.8). If the tube is not inserted into the trachea far enough, the tip will be seen near the larynx, where it is

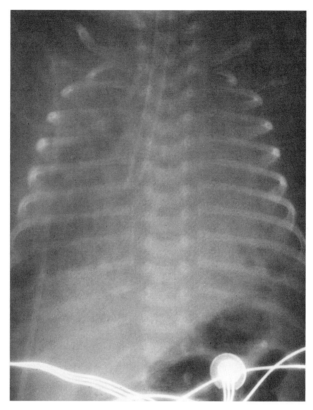

FIGURE 1.8 Chest radiograph showing endotracheal tube in the right mainstem bronchus.

prone to accidental extubation (Fig. 1.9). After placement of a chest tube to drain fluid out of the pleural cavity, a chest x-ray is used to see if the tube is in good position and if the lung has reexpanded. A chest x-ray following placement of a nasogastric tube is sometimes needed to ensure proper placement in the stomach (Fig. 1.10).

Interpreting chest x-rays requires many hours of supervised practice and cannot be taught in a book chapter. A few general guidelines, however, are presented in this section to help get you started. X-ray beams pass through the patient's chest and put different shades of gray shadows on the film according to the density of the tissue through which the beam passes. Four different densities can be detected by examining the shadows on a chest x-ray: bone, water, fat, and air. For example, x-rays passing through bony structures are absorbed by the dense material and leave a whitish shadow on the corresponding portion of the chest x-ray (**radiopaque**). Conversely, x-rays that pass through lung tissue (air) are not blocked and burn the corresponding portion of the chest x-ray black (**radiolucent**). Inspection of the shadows seen on the chest x-ray allows identification of the changes in chest anatomy that may be present with disease. A normal chest x-ray with the more prominent anatomical structures labeled is presented in Figure 1.11.

Diseases of the chest that cause the lung tissue to become more dense, such as pneumonia, cause the affected region to absorb more than a normal amount of the chest x-rays and leave a white shadow on the x-ray. Lung tumors also cause the corresponding portion of the chest x-ray to have a white shadow instead of the expected dark shadow seen in normal lung tissue.

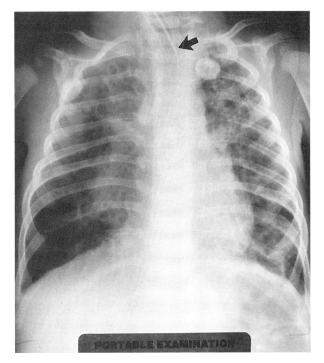

FIGURE 1.9 Chest radiograph showing endotracheal tube positioned too high in the trachea.

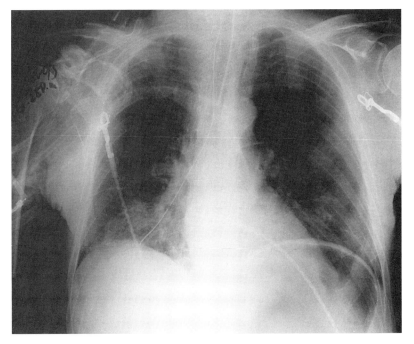

FIGURE 1.10 Chest radiograph showing the endotracheal tube in good position but the nasogastric tube accidentally placed in the right lung.

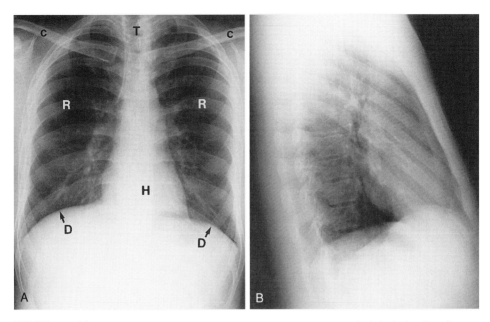

FIGURE 1.11 (A) Normal chest radiograph with normal structures labeled T = tracheal air shadow, R = ribs, C = clavicle, H = heart shadow, and D = diaphragm. (B) Normal lateral chest film.

Decreases in lung tissue density cause the chest x-ray to be abnormally dark in the corresponding regions. Emphysema and pneumothorax are examples of lung conditions that cause darker shadows on the chest x-ray. Examples of abnormal chest x-rays are presented throughout this text to help you learn the skill of interpreting x-rays.

The size of the heart is evaluated by examining the width of the cardiac shadow on the chest x-ray. Normally the heart shadow is less than half the width of the entire chest. Cardiomegaly causes the heart shadow to enlarge until it is larger than half the width of the chest on the chest x-ray. Cardiomegaly is most often seen in patients with left ventricular hypertrophy caused by ischemic heart disease.

Pulmonary edema is seen on the chest x-ray as diffuse, bilateral fluffy infiltrates, usually with an enlarged heart.

Computerized tomography (CT) is a specialized radiographic imaging procedure that provides more-detailed images of internal organs and possible pathology. While the conventional chest x-ray provides a two-dimensional image, CT provides a cross-sectional view (like slices) of the lungs and any abnormalities such as lung tumors. CT images are excellent for measuring the precise size and location of lung tumors. High-resolution CT provides even sharper images of the lung and is most useful for diagnosing interstitial lung disease.

Electrocardiography

The electrocardiogram (ECG) is a recording of electrical activity in the heart. It clearly shows cardiac rate and rhythm and gives some information about the status of the electrical conducting system in the heart, as well as the status of the heart muscle. It does not, however, reflect the pumping ability of the heart or predict the likelihood of myocardial infarction when done at rest.

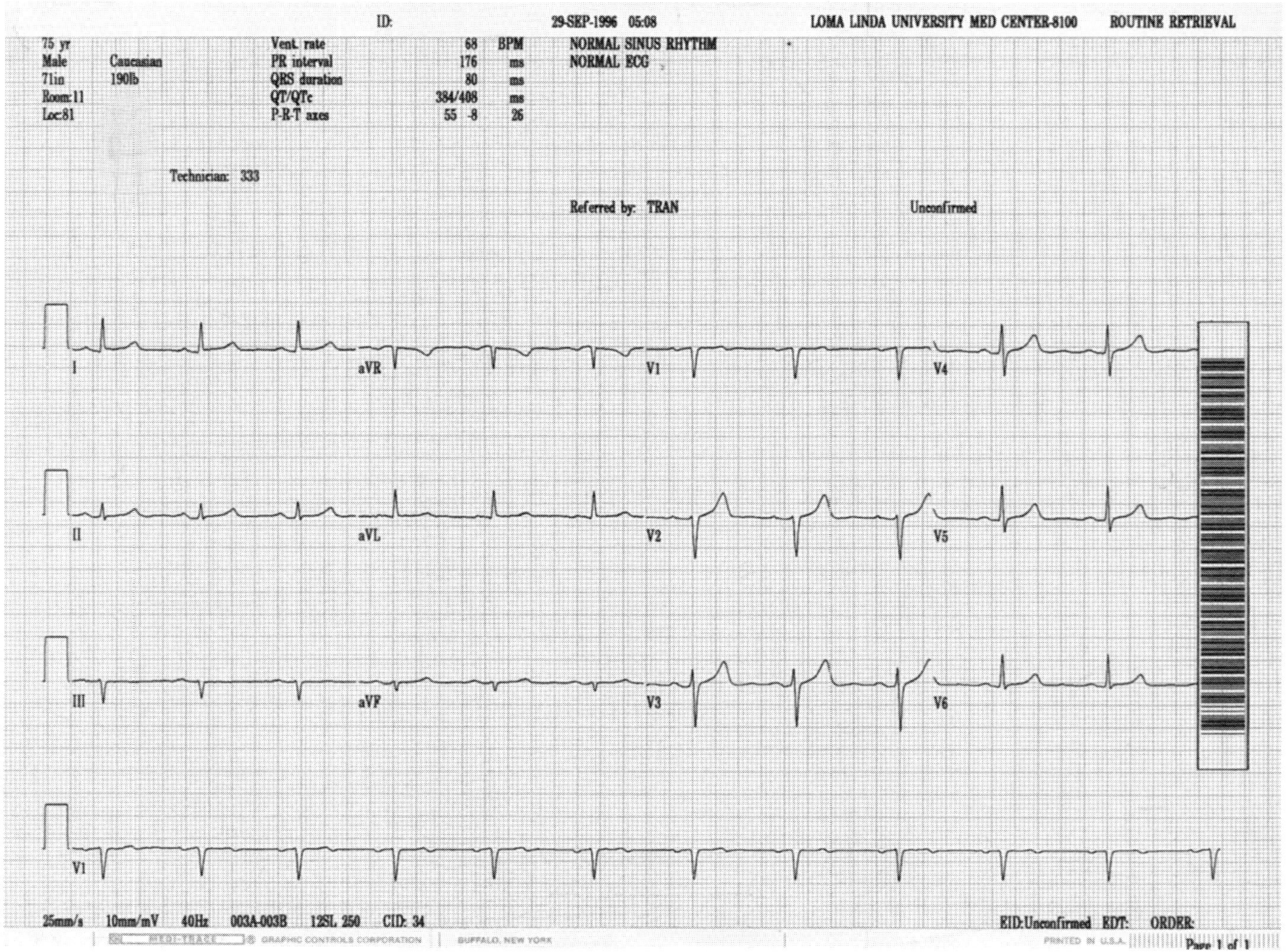

FIGURE 1.12 Normal ECG showing normal P, QRS, and T waves.

The SA node in the right atrium starts the heartbeat with an electrical impulse that causes the right and left atria to depolarize (P wave) and pump blood into the ventricles. Next, the impulse travels through the atrioventricular node to the ventricles, where it causes the ventricular muscles to depolarize (QRS wave), pumping blood into the arterial systems (Fig. 1.12). The muscle then returns to ready condition by repolarizing (T wave) in preparation for the next beat.

P waves are normally small, but may become larger if the atria hypertrophy. The QRS complex is divided into three waves. The Q wave is the first downward deflection of the QRS complex. It may not be present in some ECG recordings. The R wave is any upward movement following the Q wave, and the S wave is any subsequent downward deflection. The QRS complex is referred to as such even if not all three waves are present.

The normal ECG demonstrates an interval between the start of the P wave and the start of the QRS complex (known as the PR interval) of no longer than 0.20 seconds (five small boxes on the ECG grid), a QRS complex no wider than 0.12 seconds, and a flat (isoelectric) ST segment. A PR interval of longer than 0.20 seconds is known as heart block. A widened QRS interval is a sign of an internal conduction defect within the ventricles, and an elevated ST segment is consistent with myocardial ischemia.

Cardiac ischemia causes deep, inverted T waves, followed by ST-segment elevation and eventually large Q waves when the heart muscle cells have died. A lack of ECG abnormalities in the patient with chest pain provides evidence that the source of the discomfort may lie outside the heart. Please refer to the references at the end of this chapter for more detailed sources on ECG interpretation.

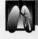

More on Mr. B

Mr. B is admitted to the coronary ICU with chest pain. He is started on oxygen therapy with a nasal cannula at 4 liters/minute. Venous blood is drawn to measure a CBC, which reveals the following: WBCs 14,000/mm^3, neutrophils 60%, bands 1%, lymphocytes 30%, and monocytes 2%.

Arterial blood is drawn for measuring ABGs. Results are as follows: pH 7.40, $Paco_2$ 30 mm Hg, Pao_2 55 mm Hg, HCO_3 15 mEq/liter, base excess -3, Fio_2 4 liters/minute by nasal cannula. A portable chest x-ray is taken to evaluate the heart and lungs (Fig. 1.13), and a 12-lead ECG is taken (Fig. 1.14).

QUESTIONS	ANSWERS
16. How would you interpret the CBC?	The WBC is elevated. This is common in response to stress and does not always indicate that infection is present. Since the bands are not elevated, infection is unlikely.
17. How would you interpret the ABGs?	The ABG results reveal respiratory alkalosis and metabolic acidosis with inadequate oxygenation despite administration of oxygen at a rate of 4 liters/minute.

18. What other test(s) should be done on the venous sample in this patient?

The venous blood should be analyzed for cardiac enzyme levels.

19. Do you see any significant abnormalities on the chest x-ray?

The chest x-ray demonstrates an enlarged heart. Notice that the width of the cardiac shadow is greater than one half the width of the chest. This is consistent with acute cardiac ischemia and heart failure. The chest x-ray also shows interstitial pulmonary edema, which is consistent with left ventricular failure.

20. What does the ECG show?

There are elevated ST segments in V1, V2, and V3.

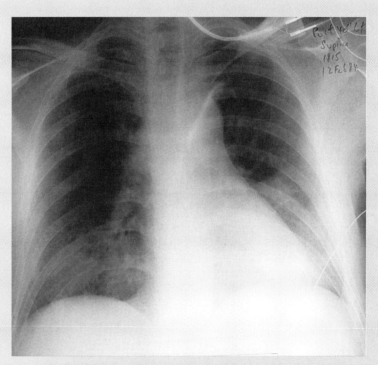

FIGURE 1.13 Mr. B's chest film showing an enlarged heart.

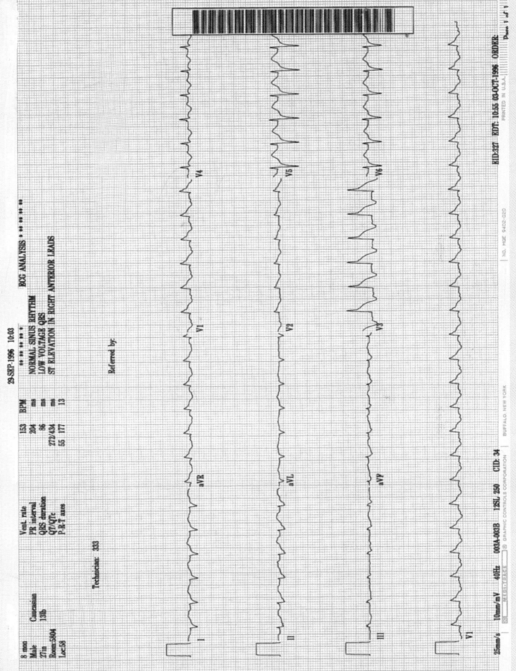

FIGURE 1.14 Mr. B's ECG showing elevated ST segments consistent with ischemia.

Mr. B Conclusion

Over the next 24 hours, Mr. B gradually improves. He is treated with furosemide (Lasix) to reduce the pulmonary edema, which allows better oxygenation on day 2. The cardiac enzymes are found to be elevated and confirm the diagnosis of myocardial infarction. Mr. B remains hospitalized for 10 days and is sent home and enrolled in a cardiac rehabilitation program. ■

KEY POINTS

- Whether in the emergency department, ICU, or home-care setting, patient assessment skills make the difference between inadequate and effective patient care.
- The therapist does not evaluate patients to make a diagnosis, but to assist the physician in determining the appropriate therapy and to monitor the effects of that therapy.
- Shortness of breath, as perceived by the patient, is known as **dyspnea.** Patients experiencing shortness of breath only in the reclining (supine) position are said to have **orthopnea.**
- Cough is often associated with airway disease. Common causes of cough include acute upper respiratory infections, asthma, gastroesophageal reflux, and bronchitis.
- Bacterial infections cause the sputum to increase in quantity and become purulent and colored, often green or yellow.
- **Hemoptysis** refers to the spitting up of blood from the tracheobronchial tree or lungs. When hemoptysis is caused by an infectious disease, the blood is often mixed with sputum.
- **Fever** is an abnormal increase in body temperature cause by disease. It is a nonspecific response to many problems, but most often occurs in response to an infection.
- All clinicians treating the patient should be familiar with his or her history of present illness as documented in the patient's chart.
- In general, the vital signs provide an index of the patient's acute condition. Most acute medical problems will be reflected by abnormal vital signs that will become more abnormal as the problem increases in severity.
- Tachycardia and tachypnea are often seen together and indicate stress on the cardiopulmonary system. Hypoxemia, fever, activity, and anxiety are common causes.
- **Hypertension** is present when the blood pressure exceeds 140/90 mm Hg. Hypertension is a very common problem in adults. The exact cause is often unknown, but it leads to numerous health problems including heart failure and stroke.
- **Sensorium** assessment is done by evaluating the patient's level of consciousness. It is an important parameter in monitoring the patient with cardiopulmonary disease because it reflects the adequacy of blood flow and oxygenation of the brain.
- Patients who breathe with a prolonged expiratory phase usually have narrowed intrathoracic airways. Common causes include asthma and COPD.

KEY POINTS (CONTINUED)

- Patients with restrictive lung disease (i.e., loss of lung volume) breathe with a rapid and shallow breathing pattern. The greater the loss of lung volume, the faster the respiratory rate.
- **Abdominal paradox** is an abnormal breathing pattern seen in patients who have diaphragm fatigue. It is recognized by observing the abdomen sink inward with each inspiratory effort.
- Peripheral atelectasis, pulmonary fibrosis, and pneumonia are examples of lung disorders that can cause harsh breath sounds over the affected region, which are termed **bronchial breath sounds**.
- Diminished breath sounds are heard in emphysema, pleural effusion, pneumothorax, and shallow breathing.
- **Wheezes** are produced by rapid airflow passing through narrowed airways that flutter between partially open and closed. They indicate intrathoracic airway obstruction and are most often heard on exhalation.
- **Stridor** is a monophonic wheeze heard over the upper airway. It is a serious sign of impending respiratory failure, and the patient with stridor must be monitored closely.
- **Crackles** are produced by the sudden opening of collapsed airways. Deep breathing in the patient with atelectasis or pulmonary fibrosis will result in fine, late-inspiratory crackles.
- Enlargement of the right ventricle usually results in an abnormal pulsation around the sternum, known as a right ventricular **heave**, which occurs with each systolic heart beat. Left ventricular enlargement causes an abnormal heave in the left anterior axillary region.
- S1 is produced by closure of the A-V valves during systole. S2 is produced by closure of the semilunar valves.
- **Murmurs** are adventitious heart sounds that may also be heard during auscultation over the heart. They are caused by turbulent blood flow through a narrow opening. Forward flow through and narrow valve or back flow through an incompetent valve will cause a murmur.
- **Hepatomegaly** (an enlarged liver) is a sign of right heart failure. This is common in patients with cor pulmonale.
- **Central cyanosis** is consistent with respiratory failure. **Peripheral cyanosis** suggests circulatory failure.
- **Leukocytosis** is defined as an abnormal elevation of the leukocyte count. **Leukopenia** is an abnormal decrease in the leukocyte count.
- **Polycythemia** refers to an abnormal increase in the red blood cell count. **Anemia** refers to an abnormal decrease in the red blood cell count.
- Measurement of cardiac enzymes in the blood is useful to evaluate the patient suspected of having a myocardial infarction.
- Hypoxemia is defined as an abnormal decrease in blood oxygen levels. This is measured by drawing an ABG sample.
- One of the most important measurements done during pulmonary function testing is the vital capacity. This is the total volume of gas the patient can exhale following maximal inspiration. The vital capacity indicates the patient's breathing capacity and ability to cough following surgery.

(key points continued on page 34)

KEY POINTS (CONTINUED)

- The chest radiograph provides details about the condition of the lungs and heart. The shadows that are dark (lung) result from the x-ray beam burning the film, while the shadows that are white (bone) result from most of the x-ray beam being absorbed.
- The electrical activity of the heart is summarized in the ECG recording. The P wave represents atrial contraction, the QRS represents ventricular contraction, and the T wave represents ventricular repolarization.

FURTHER READING

Wilkins, RL, Sheldon, RL, Krider SJ (eds): Clinical Assessment in Respiratory Care, ed 5, Mosby-Year Book, St. Louis, 2005.

2

Introduction to Respiratory Failure

Robert L. Wilkins, PhD, RRT, FAARC

James R. Dexter, MD, FACP, FCCP

CHAPTER OBJECTIVES:

After reading this chapter you will be able to state or identify the following:

- The definitions for respiratory failure, ventilatory failure, and oxygenation failure.
- The causes of respiratory failure.
- The effect of respiratory failure on the lung, heart, and other body systems.
- The clinical features associated with respiratory failure.
- The general treatment of respiratory failure.

INTRODUCTION

The production of energy in the body, which is necessary to maintain life, requires a constant supply of oxygen and nutrients to the tissues. Breathing provides a steady intake of oxygen to the lungs, where the oxygen diffuses through the alveolar capillary membrane into the blood **(external respiration)**. The circulatory system distributes the oxygenated blood to the various vascular beds, where oxygen is given up to the tissues **(internal respiration)**. In addition to oxygenation of the blood, the lungs also serve to rid the body of carbon dioxide (CO_2), a waste product of metabolism. The venous blood transports CO_2 to the lungs. The CO_2 diffuses into the alveoli and is subsequently exhaled into the atmosphere. This chapter is an introduction to the medical problems that can lead to inadequate gas exchange. Subsequent chapters provide specific examples of diseases that affect the heart and lungs.

  Respiratory failure is a general term that indicates failure of the lungs to provide adequate oxygenation or ventilation for the blood. **Oxygenation failure** is a more specific term indicating an arterial oxygen tension (PaO_2) of less than 60 mm Hg despite a fraction of inspired oxygen (FIO_2) of 0.50 or higher. **Ventilatory failure** refers to inadequate ventilation between the lungs and atmosphere that results in an inappropriate elevation of arterial carbon dioxide tension ($PaCO_2$) of greater than 45 mm Hg in the arterial blood.

  The term respiratory failure may be used in a more general fashion to describe failure of either external or internal respiration. For example, if the circulatory system fails to move the blood at a sufficient rate to meet metabolic demands, the transport of oxygen is inadequate and the tissues may become hypoxic. Although this is more accurately an example of circulatory failure, it does represent a breakdown in the system needed for respiration.

The amount of oxygen consumed and CO_2 produced each minute is dictated by the metabolic rate of the patient. Exercise and fever are examples of factors that increase the metabolic rate and place more demands on the cardiopulmonary system. When the cardiopulmonary reserve is limited by disease, fever may represent an added stress that precipitates respiratory failure and tissue hypoxia.

> **P**atients with acute respiratory failure have inadequate oxygention of the arterial blood or elevation of CO_2 levels or both.

This chapter provides an overview of the concepts important for managing respiratory failure and applies these concepts to a specific case of drug overdose. Drug overdose can often cause neuromuscular deficiency leading to ventilatory failure. This chapter provides specific information about drug overdose in addition to information about respiratory failure.

ETIOLOGY

Oxygenation Failure

Hypoxemia is present when the PaO_2 is below the predicted normal value for a given patient. Hypoxemia is classified as:

- Mild (PaO_2 60 to 79 mm Hg)
- Moderate (PaO_2 40 to 59 mm Hg)
- Severe (PaO_2 less than 40 mm Hg)

This classification is based on predicted normal values for a patient who is less than 60 years old and breathing room air. For older patients, subtract 1 mm Hg for every year over 60 years of age from the limits of mild and moderate hypoxemia. A PaO_2 of less than 40 mm Hg represents severe hypoxemia at any age.

Hypoxemia has potentially serious consequences because it can lead to inadequate tissue oxygenation (hypoxia). When hypoxemia is present, tissue oxygenation may be preserved by an increase in cardiac output. Patients with severe hypoxemia or marginal cardiac function may not be able to compensate adequately for the hypoxemia, resulting in tissue hypoxia. Tissue hypoxia of the heart complicates the problem by causing dysrhythmias and poor contractility, which add to the lack of oxygen delivery throughout the body.

The most common cause of hypoxemia is ventilation-perfusion ($\dot{V}/\dot{Q}$) mismatching, which occurs when some regions of the lung are poorly ventilated but remain perfused by pulmonary blood (low $\dot{V}/\dot{Q}$ (Fig. 2.1). Although regional vasoconstriction typically occurs in the pulmonary capillaries of the affected region, blood flow is not entirely stopped. As a result, some blood leaves the lungs without receiving adequate oxygenation and lowers the PaO_2. $\dot{V}/\dot{Q}$ mismatching also occurs when perfusion of a portion of the lung is reduced or absent despite adequate ventilation of the affected region (high $\dot{V}/\dot{Q}$).

Shunt is another cause of hypoxemia and refers to the movement of blood from the right side of the heart to the left side of the heart without coming into contact with ventilated alveoli. Shunt can be caused by a congenital heart defect (anatomical shunt), which allows the venous blood to bypass the pulmonary circulation through abnormal channels (e.g., ventricular septal defect). The most common cause of shunt, however, is pulmonary disease that results in collapsed or unventilated alveoli (physiologic shunt). In this

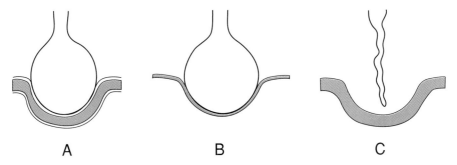

FIGURE 2.1 (A) Normal matching of ventilation to perfusion. (B) High $\dot{V}/\dot{Q}$, where ventilation is in excess of perfusion. (C) Low $\dot{V}/\dot{Q}$, where perfusion is in excess of ventilation (shunt).

situation, blood flow through the affected lung regions does not participate in gas exchange and may result in severe hypoxemia (PaO_2 less than 40 mm Hg) that does not respond well to oxygen therapy (see Fig. 2.1).

Hypoxemia can occur when an individual inhales a gas mixture that does not contain an adequate partial pressure of oxygen (low PIO_2). Breathing gas that lacks adequate oxygen results in a below-normal PaO_2 (arterial hypoxemia). This situation can occur at high altitude, during fires in an enclosed structure, and in cases of equipment failure while the patient is attached to a ventilator circuit.

Hypoventilation increases alveolar PCO_2 ($PaCO_2$) and decreases alveolar PO_2 (PaO_2). If the patient is breathing room air, hypoventilation can result in hypoxemia. Hypoxemia is less likely if the hypoventilating patient is breathing an elevated FIO_2.

> Oxygenation failure is a serious problem that can cause life-threatening organ dysfunction.

Ventilatory Failure

The ability to inhale requires a healthy neurological system that stimulates the respiratory muscles. Contraction of the diaphragm decreases the intrathoracic pressure and causes gas to flow into the lungs. Minimal effort is required if the chest cage is intact, airways are patent, and lungs are compliant.

The ability to exhale requires patent airways and a lung parenchyma with sufficient elastic recoil to hold the bronchioles open until exhalation is complete.

Causes of ventilatory failure include depression of the respiratory center by drugs, diseases of the brain, spinal cord abnormalities, muscular diseases (see Chapter 15), thoracic cage abnormalities (see Chapter 12), and upper and lower airway obstruction (Box 2.1). Upper airway obstruction may occur with acute infection and during sleep when muscle tone is reduced (see Chapter 18).

A number of factors can contribute to weakness of the inspiratory muscles and may tip the balance in favor of acute ventilatory failure. Malnutrition and electrolyte disturbances can weaken the ventilatory muscles, and pulmonary hyperinflation (e.g., emphysema) can make the diaphragm less efficient. Lung hyperinflation causes the diaphragm to assume an abnormally low position that results in a mechanical disadvantage (Fig. 2.2). These problems are common in patients with acute and chronic obstructive pulmonary disease (e.g., asthma, chronic bronchitis, emphysema; see Chapters 3 and 4).

PATHOPHYSIOLOGY

Oxygenation Failure

The severity of the hypoxemia and the patient's preexisting condition determine a patient's response to hypoxemia. A previously healthy patient will be unaffected by mild hypoxemia. A patient with severe cardiopulmonary disease, however, is likely to be in grave danger if oxygenation further deteriorates.

Patients usually respond to hypoxemia by increasing their rate of breathing (tachypnea). Tachypnea increases minute ventilation, decreases Pa_{CO_2}, and to some extent increases Pa_{O_2}. Since anatomical dead space (parts of the lung that are ventilated but not perfused) is fixed, tachypnea represents a major increase in the work of breathing. If the patient's respiratory system is unhealthy, as in obstructed airway disease, tachypnea may represent a serious increase in the work of breathing.

Hypoxemia stimulates the pulmonary capillaries to constrict in the affected regions. The pulmonary vasoconstriction will be widespread if the disease causing hypoxemia is prevalent throughout the lungs. Pulmonary vascular resistance (PVR) is markedly increased when widespread pulmonary vasoconstriction is present. This increases right heart workload and, if it continues for many months, can result in right ventricular failure. Right heart failure is characterized by increased pressure and dilation of the right heart chamber (as the heart pumps against the constricted capillaries). The combination of lung disease and right heart failure is known as **cor pulmonale**.

Cardiac rate and strength of contraction increase to compensate for hypoxemia. If coronary artery disease is present, the increased cardiac workload can lead to ischemia and irreversible damage (infarction). If the hypoxemia is severe or the heart cannot provide a sufficient increase in cardiac output to maintain adequate oxygen transport, the brain may be affected, resulting in a diminished sensorium and cognitive function. If the brain continues to be hypoxic, the patient will lose consciousness.

> **Box 2.1** Causes of Ventilatory and Respiratory Failure
>
> **VENTILATORY FAILURE**
> **Dysfunction of the Central Nervous System**
> - Drug overdose
> - Head trauma
> - Infection
> - Hemorrhage
> - Sleep-related apnea
>
> **Neuromuscular Dysfunction**
> - Myasthenia gravis
> - Guillain-Barré syndrome
> - Poliomyelitis
> - Amyotrophic lateral sclerosis
> - Spinal cord trauma
> - Long-term use of aminoglycosides
>
> **Musculoskeletal Dysfunction**
> - Chest trauma (flail chest)
> - Kyphoscoliosis
> - Malnutrition
>
> **Pulmonary Dysfunction**
> - Emphysema
> - Chronic bronchitis
> - Asthma
> - Cystic fibrosis
>
> **OXYGENATION FAILURE**
> - Pneumonia
> - Adult respiratory distress syndrome
> - Congestive heart failure
> - Obstructive lung diseases (e.g., asthma, bronchitis)
> - Pulmonary embolism
> - Restrictive lung diseases (e.g., pulmonary fibrosis, kyphoscoliosis)

> Oxygenation failure causes a large variety of pulmonary and cardiac changes designed to compensate for the lack of oxygen. Chronic oxygenation failure causes right heart failure resulting from long-term elevation of pulmonary vascular resistance.

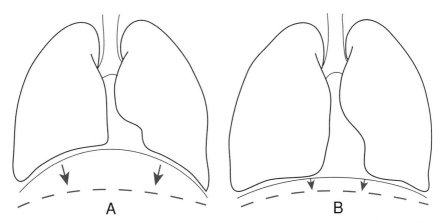

Figure 2.2 (A) Normal position of the diaphragm at end exhalation and end inhalation (dotted line). (B) Abnormal position of the diaphragm demonstrating the mechanical disadvantage associated with pulmonary hyperinflation.

Ventilatory Failure

Ventilatory failure is defined as a change in respiration resulting in an elevated Pa_{CO_2}. Since CO_2 is an acid substance in the blood, an acute increase in Pa_{CO_2} decreases arterial blood pH. The combination of an elevated Pa_{CO_2} and acidosis severe enough to drop the pH below 7.20 may have a profound effect on the body. Ventilatory failure with rising Pa_{CO_2} affects the brain much like an anesthetic and results in somnolence and eventually coma.

CLINICAL FEATURES

Oxygenation Failure

Inspection of the patient with severe hypoxemia typically reveals central cyanosis unless anemia is present and obscures the cyanosis. Central cyanosis is seen as a bluish discoloration of the tongue and mucous membranes. Anemia reduces the ability of clinicians to detect cyanosis because the bluish discoloration of tissues is due to desaturation of the hemoglobin. Vital signs are typically abnormal, revealing tachycardia, tachypnea, and hypertension. Severe acute hypoxemia may leave the patient confused, agitated, and slow to respond. Abnormal cardiac rhythms are common when severe hypoxemia is present. Premature ventricular contractions are an indication that the heart is hypoxic in patients who are hypoxemic. If the hypoxemia is chronic, cor pulmonale may develop causing hepatomegaly, JVD, and pedal edema. The hepatomegaly and pedal edema are the result of high venous pressure.

Laboratory abnormalities associated with hypoxemia include low Pa_{O_2}, Sa_{O_2}, and arterial oxygen content on arterial blood gas (ABG) analysis. If the hypoxemia is chronic, the bone marrow is stimulated to produce red blood cells, which results in polycythemia, (increased hemoglobin and hematocrit). When the hemoglobin increase is significant, the oxygen content of the arterial blood may be normal or near normal despite the presence of hypoxemia.

Diseases of the lung that cause oxygenation failure usually also cause abnormalities on the chest radiograph. Typical abnormalities include infiltrates consistent with pulmonary edema, adult respiratory distress syndrome (ARDS), atelectasis, or pneumonia (see Chapters 8, 11, 13, and 16). When the primary cause of the hypoxemia is outside the lung (e.g., shunting from a congenital heart defect), the chest radiograph is often normal unless a complicating respiratory problem is present.

Ventilatory Failure

There are few clinical findings specifically suggestive of an elevated Pa_{CO_2}. Clinical findings that suggest ventilatory failure include headache, diminished alertness, warm and flushed skin, and bounding peripheral pulses. These findings are very nonspecific, as they occur in a variety of conditions other than ventilatory failure. Since hypoxemia is often present in the patient with ventilatory failure, the clinical signs of inadequate oxygenation are often simultaneously present.

Hypothermia and loss of consciousness are common when the ventilatory failure is the result of an overdose of sedatives. Tricyclic antidepressants frequently increase heart rate and blood pressure and increase anticholinergic signs (such as hyperthermia, flushing, dilated pupils, intestinal ileus, and urinary retention). Breath sounds are often clear in the presence of drug overdose unless aspiration has occurred. Aspiration is more likely to occur when sedatives and alcohol are abused (because of a diminished gag reflex) and may result in crackles in the lower lobes, with a predominance in the right lower lobe.

The clinical signs of diaphragm fatigue provide an early warning of respiratory failure in the patient with respiratory distress. It strongly suggests that the patient is in need of ventilatory assistance (see Treatment section). Fatigue of the diaphragm initially results in tachypnea. This is followed by periods of respiratory alternans or abdominal paradox. Respiratory alternans is the short-term alternation between using the diaphragm for breathing and using the accessory muscles. Abdominal paradox is the inward movement of the abdomen with each inspiratory effort (Fig. 2.3). This is due to the flaccid status of the diaphragm, which results in its being drawn upward when the accessory muscles create a negative intrathoracic pressure (see Chapter 1).

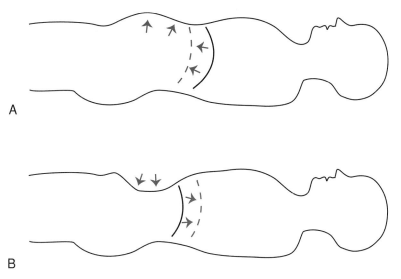

FIGURE 2.3 (A) Normal movement of the diaphragm and abdominal contents with breathing. (B) Abnormal, inward movement of the abdomen with each inspiratory effort as seen with diaphragm fatigue. This is known as abdominal paradox.

ABGs are very helpful for assessing the patient with ventilatory failure. The severity of ventilatory failure is indicated by the degree to which the $Paco_2$ increases. Measurement of arterial pH identifies the degree of respiratory acidosis present and suggests the level of urgency at which treatment needs to be implemented. The patient needs immediate care when the pH drops below 7.2, as is discussed in the next section.

TREATMENT

Oxygenation Failure

Elevation of Fio_2 is the initial treatment for hypoxemia. Oxygen supplementation rapidly corrects hypoxemia associated with $\dot{V}/\dot{Q}$ mismatching or hypoventilation. Oxygen therapy in this situation can be given by nasal cannula, simple mask, or entrainment mask. The entrainment mask delivers a specific Fio_2 regardless of the patient's breathing pattern. This is in contrast to the nasal cannula and simple mask, which allow the inhaled Fio_2 to vary with the patient's respiratory rate and tidal volume.

Hypoxemia caused by either anatomical or physiologic shunting is usually not responsive to increases in Fio_2 because blood traversing the shunt does not come into contact with ventilated alveoli. Treatment of anatomical shunt requires closure of the defect, if possible. Treatment of physiologic shunt requires reopening of alveoli. Shunt caused by collapse of alveoli often responds to positive pressure ventilation (PPV). PPV can decrease the patient's work of breathing and open collapsed alveoli to allow better gas exchange.

PPV is generally used to treat hypoxemia when the patient has a Pao_2 of less than 60 mm Hg despite an increase in the Fio_2 to 0.50 or higher (Table 2.1). The application of continuous positive airway pressure (CPAP) by mask is an acceptable temporary measure as long as ventilation is adequate and the patient's problem is likely to resolve quickly (e.g., postoperative atelectasis). Intubation and mechanical ventilation are needed if mask CPAP is not successful in correcting the hypoxemia and reducing the patient's work of breathing or when the problem is not likely to resolve quickly (e.g., ARDS). The application of positive end-expiratory pressure (PEEP) in conjunction with mechanical ventilation is usually needed to treat patients with severe hypoxemia caused by shunting. PEEP and CPAP allow adequate oxygenation at a lower Fio_2, thus reducing the risk of oxygen toxicity. The use of PEEP and its potential complications are described in more detail in Chapter 11.

Mechanical Ventilation

Conventional modes of mechanical ventilation are adequate for most patients. These include assist/control or intermittent mandatory ventilation (IMV). A ventilator set to assist/control delivers a preset tidal volume at a specified rate. The ventilator will also deliver a full mechanical breath each time the patient initiates an inspiratory effort. A ventilator set to IMV delivers preset tidal volumes at the preset rate but also allows the patient to take spontaneous breaths in between the mechanical breaths. As a result, the patient may receive the preset number of

Table 2.1 Clinical Guidelines for Initiation of Mechanical Ventilation (Adult Patients)

Respiratory rate	>30/minute
Vital capacity	<15 mL/kg
Minute ventilation	>10 liters/minute
Maximum inspiratory pressure	<20 cm H_2O
$Paco_2$ (acute change)	>50 mm Hg
Pao_2	<60 mm Hg on $F_iO_2 > 0.50$

mechanical breaths and as many spontaneous breaths each minute as desired. In most cases of using IMV a synchronized version is applied and is referred to as SIMV. The ventilator synchronizes the mechanical breaths with the spontaneous breaths to prevent stacking a mechanical breath on top of a spontaneous breath. Although IMV was popularized initially as a mode of weaning patients from mechanical ventilation, it is now also popular as a form of ventilator support. See the following discussion on treatment of ventilatory failure to become familiarized with setting tidal volume and rate during mechanical ventilation.

Mechanical ventilation is almost always initiated with inspiratory times much shorter than expiratory times. A long expiratory time allows adequate time for exhalation and reduces the chance of inadvertent air trapping. Prolonged inspiratory times with short expiratory times (inverse I:E) may improve oxygenation in some patients with low lung compliance and poor gas exchange. Inverse ratio ventilation (IRV) was first applied in neonates but is now also sometimes used in adult patients with refractory hypoxemia.

> Mild hypoxemia can be treated with simple oxygen therapy. Severe hypoxemia that responds poorly to oxygen therapy usually requires mechanical ventilation to keep the patient alive until the pulmonary problem resolves.

Most ventilators can be set to terminate the mechanical breath when a preset volume has been reached (volume control) or when a preset pressure has been reached (pressure control). Volume control ventilation has the advantage of ensuring that the patient will receive an adequate minute ventilation despite changes in the lung or chest wall compliance or airway resistance. The disadvantage of this mode is the high pressures that may be reached when compliance drops or airway resistance increases. Pressure control ventilation assures that high pressures will not be a problem, but minute ventilation may become dangerously low when lung compliance drops or airway resistance increases.

Ventilatory Failure

An acute elevation in $Paco_2$ indicates that the patient is unable to maintain adequate alveolar ventilation and may be in need of ventilatory assistance. The $Paco_2$ does not necessarily have to be above normal range to indicate the need for mechanical ventilation in all circumstances. For example, if an asthmatic patient is in acute respiratory distress and the $Paco_2$ increases from 30 to 40 mm Hg because of muscle fatigue, the patient would benefit from intubation and mechanical ventilation. This example illustrates how trends in the $Paco_2$ can be helpful in determining the need for mechanical ventilation.

Mechanical Ventilation

Once the patient is intubated, base the selected tidal volume on the presenting pathophysiology. Generally the tidal volume is set in the range of 5 to 10 mL/kg of ideal body weight (e.g., obese patients do not need enormous tidal volumes) Tidal volumes smaller than this tend to result in collapse of peripheral lung units. Tidal volumes larger than 10 mL/kg or large enough to produce plateau pressures of greater than 30 cm H_2O or peak airway pressure greater than 40 cm H_2O tend to overinflate the lungs and may result in barotrauma (e.g., pneumothorax, pneumomediastinum). This is especially true for patients with stiff lungs, such as those with ARDS.

The respiratory rate needed by the patient depends on his or her metabolic rate, but adults typically require 8 to 15 breaths per minute. Rates as low as 6 to 8 breaths per minute allow longer expiratory times and may be needed in patients with obstructive lung disease to minimize air trapping. Ventilation is adjusted in most patients to keep the $Paco_2$ between 35 and 45 mm Hg. One exception is the patient with a chronically elevated $Paco_2$ for whom the goal of mechanical ventilation is to return the pH to the normal range and the $Paco_2$ to the patient's baseline, rather than to the normal range. If patients with chronic hypoventilation and CO_2 retention are ventilated with enough vigor to achieve a normal $Paco_2$, respiratory alkalosis becomes a problem in the short term and ventilator weaning becomes a problem in the long term.

Initially the Fio_2 is set at 1.0 to ensure adequate oxygenation during this stressful period. An exception might be the patient in whom a recent ABG has demonstrated supranormal Pao_2 on an increased Fio_2. An Fio_2 of about 0.40 to 0.60 should be adequate in such cases. Once the patient stabilizes, the Fio_2 can be adjusted on the basis of pulse oximetry or ABGs.

Determine the cause of the ventilatory failure while initiating symptomatic treatment. In the case of drug overdose, attempt to identify the type of drug, the amount ingested, the length of time since ingestion, and whether trauma occurred. General goals in management of drug overdose are to prevent toxin absorption (e.g., stomach lavage, inducement of vomiting, use of charcoal), to enhance drug excretion (e.g., dialysis), or to prevent accumulation of toxic metabolic products (e.g., acetylcysteine as an antidote for acetaminophen overdose).

Weaning

Weaning the patient from mechanical ventilation can begin as soon as the cause of the respiratory failure has been corrected and the patient's medical problems are stable. Weaning parameters help determine when weaning is likely to be successful (Box 2.2), but traditional measures such as maximum inspiratory pressure or vital capacity are of limited value since they do not reflect the patient's endurance capabilities.

A useful weaning predictor may be the rapid shallow breathing index. This measure is determined by identifying the ratio of the breathing frequency (f) to the tidal volume (Vt) during spontaneous breathing without pressure support. Values below 105 breaths/min/L appear to be strong indicators that weaning will be successful.

Methods of weaning include IMV, pressure support (PS), and T-piece. Each method has advantages and disadvantages, but any one should effectively wean most patients when they are ready. Each method depends on decreasing the patient's ventilatory support under controlled circumstances while the patient is closely monitored. Extubation can occur when the patient's gag reflex is intact and the patient has demonstrated that the endotracheal tube is no longer needed.

IMV Weaning

IMV weaning decreases the number of mechanical breaths per minute every few hours until the patient no longer needs mechanical support or demonstrates poor tolerance of the weaning (e.g., 20% changes in pulse rate and blood pressure). The primary disadvantage of IMV is the potential increase in the work of breathing imposed on the patient by the ventilator circuit during

Box 2.2

Weaning Criteria
- Cause of respiratory or ventilatory failure is resolved
- Patient's condition is stable and improving
- Vital Capacity >10–15 mL/kg
- Resting minute volume is <10 liters/minute
- Maximum inspiratory pressure is >−20 cm H_2O
- Adequate oxygenation on FiO_2 <0.50
- Spontaneous respiratory rate <35 breaths/minute
- Spontaneous tidal volume >325 mL

spontaneous breaths. This increased workload is primarily due to excessive resistance at the demand valve and the endotracheal tube. Newer ventilators have improved this problem, but it remains a clinical issue in some patients. Adding PS to IMV can help overcome this problem.

Pressure Support

PS helps overcome the workload imposed by the resistance of the artificial airway and ventilator circuitry and assists ventilation by providing a set amount of positive airway pressure during inspiration. Weaning with PS begins by setting it at a level that results in an acceptable tidal volume and rate without use of accessory muscles. The respiratory therapist gradually lowers the preset PS on a regular basis (over a period of hours to days) while the patient is monitored. Mechanical ventilation can be discontinued once the patient is tolerating a low PS level (e.g., less than 5 cm H_2O), as evidenced by the patient's maintaining a normal pattern of breathing.

T-Piece Weaning

T-piece weaning is done by discontinuing mechanical ventilation for short periods of time and placing the patient on "blow-by" at an appropriate F_{IO_2}. The duration during which the patient is allowed to breathe spontaneously is gradually increased until the patient either shows signs of stress or no longer requires mechanical ventilation. This method of weaning has the advantage of giving the patient periods of rest when reconnected to the ventilator.

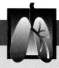

Ms. N

HISTORY

Ms. N is a 47-year-old white woman who was found unconscious on the floor of her apartment by a relative. Empty bottles of diazepam (Valium), effexor (antidepressant), and beer cans were nearby. The relative dialed 911, and the patient was transported to a local emergency room. During transportation, the patient had an adequate pulse rate but required ventilatory assistance with a bag-valve mask on oxygen. An ABG was obtained immediately, and a drug screen was ordered in the emergency room.

QUESTIONS	ANSWERS
1. What complications are likely to occur in this patient?	Common complications include respiratory depression, hypothermia or hyperthermia, cardiac irregularities, and vomiting and aspiration.
2. What information should the attending physician attempt to get from the relative or paramedics?	The physician should attempt to identify how much medication the patient swallowed and how much time has passed since ingestion. Some of the pertinent information could be obtained from the prescription labels on the bottles.
3. Is this patient most likely to be experiencing ventilatory or oxygenation failure?	The patient is most likely to experience ventilatory failure caused by depression of the central nervous system. Oxygenation failure would be expected only if gastric acid aspiration has occurred resulting in $\dot{V}/\dot{Q}$ mismatching.

4. Should the patient be intubated? If so, why?	Yes, the patient should be intubated to ensure adequate ventilation and to protect the airway from aspiration. The need for bag-valve-mask assistance demonstrates the need for intubation and mechanical ventilation.
5. What treatment should be provided?	The most urgent treatment needed after establishing an airway and ensuring adequate ventilation is to prevent further absorption of the overdose medication. This is accomplished with the use of charcoal to absorb and bind with the toxins. If the patient is awake and alert, vomiting is induced with syrup of ipecac; however, if the patient is lethargic or if mental status is rapidly deteriorating, stomach lavage is preferable. To protect the lungs, it is important to place an endotracheal tube before performing stomach lavage.

 ## More on Ms. N

PHYSICAL EXAMINATION

- **General.** An unconscious, slightly obese female with an 8.0-mm transoral endotracheal tube in place being ventilated with a hand resuscitator; Ewald tube in left nostril; gastric lavage fluid containing a large number of pill fragments; strong smell of alcohol; patient approximately 5 foot, 8 inches and 155 pounds

- **Vital Signs.** Pulse 124/minute, respiratory rate 12 to 16/minute with bag-valve mask, body temperature 35.3°C (95.6°F), blood pressure 120/75 mm Hg

- **HEENT.** No signs of trauma; pupils dilated with sluggish response to light

- **Heart.** Normal heart sounds with no murmurs

- **Lungs.** Breath sounds clear except in right lower lobe, where inspiratory crackles are heard

- **Abdomen.** Soft, obese, with no organomegaly or tenderness; bowel sounds present, but hypoactive

- **Extremities.** Warm to palpation with no edema, clubbing, or cyanosis

- **Initial ABG Findings.** (while patient is being ventilated with an F_{IO_2} of 1.0 via a bag-valve mask prior to intubation). pH 7.28, $Paco_2$ 54 mm Hg, Pao_2 135 mm Hg, Sao_2 99%, HCO_3 = 26 mEq/liter

QUESTIONS	ANSWERS
6. What accounts for the hypothermia?	Hypothermia is common in patients with an overdose of sedatives. Overdose with some antidepresents especially disrupts temperature regulation.
7. What accounts for the dilated and sluggishly reactive pupils?	Dilated and slowly reactive pupils are common in patients who overdose on sedatives and tricyclic antidepressants.

8. What could account for the crackles heard in the right lower lobe?	Crackles in the right lower lobe are most likely due to aspiration of stomach contents. Sedatives and alcohol cause decreased mental acuity and depressed pharyngeal muscle function, both of which contribute to a disturbed gag reflex and increase the chance of aspiration.
9. How would you interpret the ABG findings?	The ABG reveals an acute respiratory acidosis with adequate oxygenation. Respiratory acidosis is common in patients who overdose on sedatives, as sedatives depress the central nervous system and diminish the drive to breathe. Bag-valve-mask ventilation is often less effective than ventilation with a bag valve and a properly placed endotracheal tube because face masks can leak, causing some air to go down the esophagus (gastric inflation).
10. What is the significance of the pill fragments found in the contents of the stomach? Why was the charcoal given?	The presence of pill fragments in the stomach indicates that at least some of the pills were ingested somewhat recently. Gastric lavage and charcoal will probably prevent absorption of a large amount of the medication in the stomach.

More on Ms. N

Ms. N is transferred from the emergency room to the intensive care unit (ICU). While in the ICU, she is placed on continuous mechanical ventilation with a volume ventilator, and cardiac monitoring is continued.

QUESTIONS	ANSWERS
11. What laboratory and diagnostic tests would you suggest at this time?	To ensure adequate ventilation, it would be helpful to order a repeat ABG after initiation of mechanical ventilation. A chest x-ray would be helpful to investigate the crackles in the right lower lobe. A complete blood count (CBC) and electrolyte panel would be useful.
12. What ventilator settings would you recommend? Specifically suggest the mode of ventilation, tidal volume, rate, F_{IO_2}, and PEEP level.	The patient should be ventilated with the assist/control or IMV mode. The tidal volume should be in the range of 500 to 600 mL, since Ms. N's ideal body weight is approximately 60 kg. The mechanical rate should be about 10 to 14 per minute. The presence of inspiratory crackles indicates that the patient may have lung pathology that could lead to $\dot{V}/\dot{Q}$ mismatch or shunt. This suggests that an elevated F_{IO_2} will be needed to maintain adequate oxygenation. An F_{IO_2} in the range of 0.40 to 0.60 is a reasonable

place to start, since we know the patient has more than adequate oxygenation on an FIO_2 of 1.0. PEEP levels of greater than 5 cm H_2O should not be necessary unless the patient requires an FIO_2 of greater than 0.60 on mechanical ventilation.

More on Ms. N

The ventilator is set to deliver a tidal volume of 600 mL at a rate of 12 per minute with an FIO_2 of 0.45 in the assist/control mode. Twenty minutes after initiation of mechanical ventilation, an arterial blood sample is drawn and reveals the following: pH 7.51, $PaCO_2$ 32 mm Hg, PaO_2 88 mm Hg, and HCO_3 = 25 mEq. The chest x-ray shows patchy infiltrates in the right lower lobe, which is consistent with aspiration pneumonia (Fig. 2.4). The electrocardiogram monitor reveals a sinus rate of 115 to 120 per minute. Breath sounds are clear in all areas except the right lower lobe.

A drug screen indicates that the patient had also taken acetaminophen. Her blood alcohol level is 0.155, and the presence of antidepressant is confirmed via urinalysis.

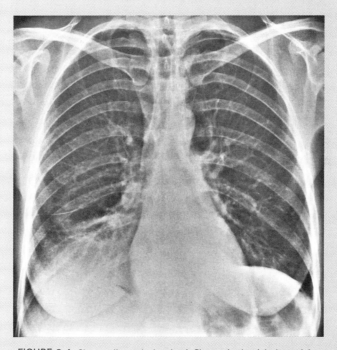

FIGURE 2.4 Chest radiograph showing infiltrates in the right lower lobe.

QUESTIONS	ANSWERS
13. How would you interpret the ABG results?	The ABG reveals an acute respiratory alkalosis with adequate oxygenation on an FIO_2 of 0.45. The respiratory alkalosis is the result of the mechanical ventilation with an excessive minute ventilation.
14. What changes in the ventilator settings would you suggest based on the ABG results?	The ventilator should be adjusted to deliver a lower minute volume. A reduction in the tidal volume or rate would reduce alveolar ventilation and allow the $PaCO_2$ to increase to a more normal range.
15. What is the treatment for acetaminophen overdose?	The antidote for acetaminophen overdose is acetylcysteine (Mucomyst). The need for treatment with the antidote is determined by the use of a nomogram to compare the amount of time passed since ingestion versus the acetaminophen plasma blood level. If the acetaminophen plasma level is at or above the minimum "treatment" level, the patient should be given an oral loading dose of N-acetylcysteine (140 mg/kg) followed by 17 maintenance doses of 70 mg/kg at 4-hour intervals. The N-acetylcysteine should be diluted with water, juice, or soda. N-acetylcysteine is also given when an acetaminophen plasma level is not available and the history of ingestion is greater than 7.5 g or 140 mg/kg.
16. What pulmonary complication is associated with aspiration pneumonia?	Aspiration pneumonia can lead to acute respiratory distress syndrome and severe respiratory failure (see Chapter 11).

 ## Ms. N Conclusion

The rate of the mechanical ventilator is reduced to 8 breaths per minute at the same tidal volume. Acetylcysteine is given to the patient to treat the acetaminophen overdose. Over the next 24 hours, the patient regains consciousness and is able to respond to commands and communicate by way of paper and pencil. She is weaned via T-piece and carefully observed. After 4 hours, her vital signs are normal and ABGs are as follows: pH 7.43, $PaCO_2$ 36 mm Hg, and PaO_2 79 mm Hg on an FIO_2 of 0.40. Based on these findings, Ms. N is extubated and placed on oxygen by mask with aerosol at an FIO_2 of 0.45. Over the next 24 hours, her pneumonia and general condition improve, and she is transferred to the psychiatric ward on day 3. The remainder of her hospital stay is uneventful. ■

KEY POINTS

- Breathing provides a steady intake of oxygen to the lungs, where the oxygen diffuses through the alveolar capillary membrane into the blood **(external respiration)**.
- The circulatory system distributes the oxygenated blood to the various vascular beds, where oxygen is given up to the tissues **(internal respiration)**.
- **Respiratory failure** is a general term that indicates failure of the lungs to provide adequate oxygenation or ventilation for the blood.
- **Oxygenation failure** is a more specific term indicating an arterial oxygen tension (Pao_2) of less than 60 mm Hg despite a fraction of inspired oxygen (Fio_2) of 0.50 or higher.
- **Ventilatory failure** refers to inadequate ventilation between the lungs and atmosphere that results in an inappropriate elevation of arterial carbon dioxide tension ($Paco_2$) of greater than 45 mm Hg in the arterial blood.
- The most common cause of hypoxemia is ventilation-perfusion ($\dot{V}/\dot{Q}$) mismatching. $\dot{V}/\dot{Q}$ mismatching occurs when some regions of the lung are poorly ventilated but remain perfused by pulmonary blood (low $\dot{V}/\dot{Q}$).
- $\dot{V}/\dot{Q}$ mismatching also occurs when perfusion of a portion of the lung is reduced or absent despite adequate ventilation of the affected region (high $\dot{V}/\dot{Q}$).
- Shunt is another cause of hypoxemia and refers to the movement of blood from the right side of the heart to the left side of the heart without coming into contact with ventilated alveoli.
- Causes of ventilatory failure include depression of the respiratory center by drugs, diseases of the brain, spinal cord abnormalities, muscular diseases (see Chapter 15), thoracic cage abnormalities (see Chapter 12), and upper and lower airway obstruction.
- Hypoxemia stimulates the pulmonary capillaries to constrict in the affected regions. The pulmonary vasoconstriction will be widespread if the disease causing hypoxemia is prevalent throughout the lungs. This can lead to cor pulmonale if the hypoxemia is chronic.
- Severe acute hypoxemia may leave the patient confused, agitated, and slow to respond. Abnormal cardiac rhythms are common when severe hypoxemia is present.
- Few clinical findings specifically suggest an elevated $Paco_2$. Clinical findings that suggest ventilatory failure include headache, diminished alertness, warm and flushed skin, and bounding peripheral pulses. These findings are nonspecific.
- Elevation of Fio_2 is the initial treatment for hypoxemia. Oxygen supplementation rapidly corrects hypoxemia associated with $\dot{V}/\dot{Q}$ mismatching or hypoventilation.
- PPV is generally used to treat hypoxemia when the patient has a Pao_2 of less than 60 mm Hg despite an increase in the Fio_2 to 0.50 or higher.
- The application of PEEP in conjunction with mechanical ventilation is usually needed to treat patients with severe hypoxemia caused by shunting. PEEP and CPAP allow adequate oxygenation at a lower Fio_2, thus reducing the risk of oxygen toxicity.
- An acute elevation in $Paco_2$ indicates that the patient is unable to maintain adequate alveolar ventilation and may be in need of ventilatory assistance. The $Paco_2$ does not necessarily have to be above normal range to indicate the need for mechanical ventilation in all circumstances.

(key ponts continued on page 50)

KEY POINTS (CONTINUED)

- Weaning the patient from mechanical ventilation can begin as soon as the cause of the respiratory failure has been corrected and the patient's medical problems are stable.
- A useful weaning predictor may be the rapid shallow breathing index. This measure is determined by identifying the ratio of the breathing frequency (f) to the tidal volume (Vt) during spontaneous breathing without pressure support. Values below 105 breaths/min/L appear to be strong indicators that weaning will be successful.

3

Asthma

Robert L. Wilkins, PhD, RRT, FAARC

Philip M. Gold, MD, MACP, FCCP

CHAPTER OBJECTIVES:

After reading this chapter you will be able to state or identify the following:

- The definition of asthma and status asthmaticus.
- The potential causes of asthma attacks.
- The effect of asthma attacks on lung function.
- The clinical features of patients having an asthma attack.
- The treatment of acute asthma including medications and indications for mechanical ventilation.
- The prognosis of patients with asthma.

INTRODUCTION

Asthma is an obstructive pulmonary disease characterized by diffuse airway inflammation and narrowing that occurs in response to various stimuli. An important feature of asthma is that the airway obstruction is entirely or partly reversible. In fact, between episodes patients often have no symptoms and their pulmonary function may be normal. In addition to the bronchospasm and airway inflammation, the asthmatic patient may also have excessive airway secretions. The combination of these features can lead to severe airway obstruction and death if appropriate treatment is not given.

A variety of terms are used in association with caring for the asthmatic patient. When the patient has an asthma attack that does not respond to conventional treatment, the condition is called **status asthmaticus**. **Occupational asthma** is the term used to describe bronchospasm that occurs in response to a provoking agent or agents in the work place. Typically individuals with occupational asthma are initially asymptomatic during periods of time away from work. With time, asthmatic symptoms persist away from the workplace. **Stable asthma** is present when a period of 4 weeks has passed during which an asthma-prone patient has had no increase in symptoms or no need for an increase in medication. Conversely, **unstable asthma** is present when a patient experiences increasing symptoms.

Because the definition of asthma is not standardized and the methods of diagnosing asthma

> Asthma is a chronic obstructive pulmonary disease characterized by attacks of diffuse airway inflammation and bronchospasm that occur in response to various stimuli. Between attacks, the asthmatic often has normal lung fuction.

often vary from one report to the next, the exact incidence of asthma in the United States and around the world is not known. In the United States the prevalence of asthma is believed to be between 3% and 5% and appears to be increasing, especially in young people, certain ethnic groups, and the poor.[1,2] The incidence appears to have been increasing in recent years for unknown reasons. In addition, the death rate from asthma is on the increase, particularly among African Americans.[3] The difference in death rates related to race and ethnicity may be related to access to health care and socioeconomic factors.

ETIOLOGY

The pathogenesis of asthma is incompletely understood. Why some patients develop asthma while others in the same family do not is a mystery. Genetics obviously plays an important role, and those born with atopy (allergic to specific allergens) are highly prone to develop asthma symptoms. Although the pathogenesis of asthma is not known, much is known about the triggers of asthma attacks.

> The most common trigger of asthma attacks is infection. Other triggers include exercise, dust, pollens, air pollution, and cold air. Identifying the triggers for each patient and the avoidance of these triggers are important features of the best treatment plan.

In many cases of asthma a specific provoking situation is linked to the onset of asthma attacks, and thus terms such as *exercise-induced* asthma or *pollen* asthma are frequently used. Patients with allergic asthma often have attacks provoked by many different allergens, including house dust mites, animal dander, and certain foods or food additives (e.g., sulfites). In addition to allergens, asthma attacks can be provoked by pharmacological agents (e.g., beta-adrenoceptor antagonists, aspirin), air pollutants (e.g., sulfur dioxide, oxidants), exercise, cigarette smoke, and airway infections. Viral infection of the respiratory tract is one of the most common triggers of asthma attacks.

PATHOPHYSIOLOGY

The combination of bronchospasm, mucus plugging, and mucosal edema leads to increased airways resistance (Fig. 3.1). Not all airways are affected to the same degree. The lack of uniform ventilation throughout the lung causes ventilation-perfusion ($\dot{V}/\dot{Q}$) mismatching, which results in hypoxemia. Pulmonary vascular resistance increases as a result of the hypoxemia.

> Asthmatics usually have mucus plugging and air trapping during attacks. This leads to a progressive increase in the work of breathing and fatigue of the breathing muscles if not reversed.

Initially airway obstruction primarily affects exhalation. This results in air trapping and progressive hyperinflation of the lungs. With air trapping residual volume increases at the expense of the vital capacity. The combination of increased airway resistance and lung hyperinflation significantly increases the work of breathing. Patients with a high work of breathing may experience respiratory muscle fatigue if the obstruction

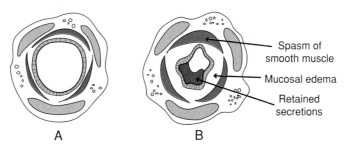

FIGURE 3.1 (A) Cross-sectional view of a normal airway. (B) Cross-sectional view of the airway of a patient with asthma. A combination of airway secretions, edema, and bronchospasm contribute to a reduction in the airway diameter.

persists. Patients with poor nutrition are more likely to experience fatigue of the breathing muscles and subsequent ventilatory failure.

CLINICAL FEATURES

History

Typically a patient having an acute asthma attack will complain of one or more of the following: chest tightness, difficulty breathing, wheezing, and coughing. The onset of these symptoms may be rapid or relatively slow. Often when the symptoms have a rapid onset, they may disappear rapidly with appropriate treatment. Although some idea of the seriousness of an asthma attack can be determined from the history, the degree of dyspnea is not a reliable predictor of severity. The interviewer should ask the patient about recent exacerbations, their severity, and their response to therapy.

Although dyspnea and wheezing are suggestive of asthma, disorders such as congestive heart failure, bronchitis, pulmonary embolism, and upper airway obstruction can cause similar symptoms. In most cases the patient's age, medical history, physical findings, radiographic studies, and laboratory tests will confirm the diagnosis.

Physical Examination

Physical examination of the asthmatic provides important objective information that will assist in confirming the diagnosis and identifying the severity of the obstruction. Inadequate assessment of the patient's status can be a fatal mistake because it can result in insufficient treatment and monitoring. Common findings associated with asthma include tachypnea, use of accessory muscles of breathing, prolonged exhalation, increased anteroposterior diameter of the chest, expiratory polyphonic wheezing, diaphoresis, and intercostal retractions. Severe asthma is suggested by pronounced use of accessory muscles, abnormal sensorium, paradoxical pulse, tachypnea, inability to speak, and wheezing on inhalation and exhalation. Additional signs of fatigue include decreasing peak flow, diaphoresis, and abdominal paradox. Abdominal paradox is seen as an inward movement of the abdominal wall during inspiration and is associated with fatigue of the diaphragm (see Chapter 1).

> A critical clinical finding to monitor in the patient having an asthma attack is the sensorium. When sensorium deteriorates, the patient is in trouble.

Accessory Muscle Use

Accessory muscles of breathing are used because of increased work of breathing. In addition, pulmonary hyperinflation causes the diaphragm to assume a flat position, placing that muscle at a mechanical disadvantage. A prolonged expiratory phase occurs as the intrapulmonary airways become obstructed and slow the movement of gas out of the lungs. Increased anteroposterior diameter occurs when air trapping and pulmonary hyperinflation are present. Polyphonic wheezing is produced as rapid airflow occurs through narrowed airways, resulting in vibration of the airway walls. Retractions are seen as intermittent depressions of the intercostal spaces with each inspiratory effort. Retractions result when a significant drop in intrapleural pressure causes the chest wall to sink inward. This suggests that the patient's work of breathing is markedly increased. The significant drop in intrapleural pressure is also responsible for the fall in pulse pressure during inspiration (paradoxical pulse).

It is not uncommon to see patients lean forward and brace their hands or elbows on a nearby table during an acute asthma attack. This is called the **tripod** position and it may improve the mechanical advantage of the accessory muscles.

Chest Radiograph

A chest radiograph is helpful for identifying the presence of complications such as pneumonia, atelectasis, or pneumothorax. The use of chest radiographs to evaluate routine asthma attacks, however, is not recommended. In the absence of complications, a chest radiograph is often normal or may demonstrate hyperinflation of the lung fields.

Pulmonary Function Studies

Complete pulmonary function studies should not be done when the patient is having an acute asthma attack. Simple bedside spirometry, however, is appropriate and very useful in determining the severity of obstruction and the response to therapy. Measurement of peak flow and forced expiratory volume in one second (FEV_1) are commonly used and easy to obtain unless the patient has severe dyspnea. A peak flow of less than 100 liters/minute or an FEV_1 of less than 1.0 liter in an adult suggests severe obstruction.

Bronchial provocation testing is useful in identifying the degree of airway reactivity in patients whose symptoms are typical of asthma but who have normal pulmonary function studies. Methacholine is most often used for bronchial provocation testing because it increases parasympathetic tone in the smooth muscles of the airways, resulting in bronchospasm. Asthmatics will have a greater than 20% decrease in FEV_1 in response to methacholine, whereas normal subjects have little or no response.

Arterial Blood Gases

Arterial blood gases (ABGs) are extremely useful for assessing the severity of an asthma attack, especially when the bronchospasm is severe enough to prevent the patient from performing a forced expiratory maneuver. The degree of hypoxemia and hypercapnia present are reliable indicators of the severity of the airway obstruction. Typically the $PaCO_2$ is decreased with the onset of an asthma attack. A normal or increased $PaCO_2$ suggests a more severe degree of obstruction and/or respiratory muscle fatigue.

An important goal of assessment in acute asthma is an efficient evaluation. Most asthmatic patients need immediate care, and an experienced clinician will perform an efficient yet effective assessment without delaying the onset of treatment. Avoiding unnecessary evaluation tools is an essential part of any assessment, especially when the patient is acutely ill.

> **A** rising $Paco_2$ is a sign of impending respiratory failure and suggests the potential need for ventilatory assistance.

TREATMENT

Initially the clinician should direct treatment toward achieving adequate oxygenation, providing bronchodilators, and decreasing airway inflammation. The majority of patients having an acute asthma attack become hypoxemic as a result of $\dot{V}/\dot{Q}$ mismatching. In some cases the hypoxemia will be severe enough to represent a serious threat to the patient's life, but it can almost always be corrected with appropriate oxygen therapy.

Pharmacological Agents

Numerous pharmacological agents are available to promote bronchodilation and reduce airway inflammation. These include beta-adrenergics, parasympatholytics, and corticosteroids. In the majority of mild cases, bronchospasm can be reversed by use of an aerosolized beta-adrenergic agent such as albuterol. Inhaled beta-agonist bronchodilators offer the following advantages over oral bronchodilators: a more rapid onset of action, lower dosage requirements, a lower incidence of systemic side effects, and better protection of the airways against provoking agents.

Albuterol is a popular bronchodilator used for the treatment of acute asthma attacks. It is available in a solution for small-volume nebulizer (SVN) treatments and as a metered-dose inhaler. The metered-dose inhaler (MDI) is a popular route for administering bronchodilators because it is simple for patients to use and it is an efficient way to deliver the medication. The MDI should be used with a spacer in place to reduce the deposition of medication in the oropharynx.[4] An MDI with a spacer has been shown to be effective in young children (<14 years) with asthma.[5]

Aerosolized bronchodilator treatments with an SVN are useful for patients who are unable to use MDIs and for administration during life-threatening episodes. The SVN treatments are usually given every 3 to 6 hours, but during severe bronchospasm they may be provided 20 minutes apart for three treatments as long

> **A** dministration of beta-adrenergics such as albuterol is the first step in the treatment of asthma attacks.

as the patient is monitored carefully. Continuous nebulization therapy for the administration of bronchodilator may prove useful when the asthmatic does not respond to conventional therapy. Continuous nebulization therapy is usually given in the intensive care unit (ICU) or emergency room. With this technique 10 mg of albuterol is nebulized over one hour.

During an acute, severe asthma attack, if the patient fails to respond adequately to inhaled beta-agonists, intravenous (IV) corticosteroids are added to the treatment plan. The anti-inflammatory effects of corticosteroids may take several hours to cause beneficial results when given intravenously. A large dose (500 mg) of methylprednisolone offers no advantage over a more conservative dose (100 mg) in the emergency department treatment of acute asthma. Use of corticosteroids early in the treatment of an acute episode may reduce the need for hospitalization. Oral prednisone (60 to 80 mg) provides therapeutic blood levels in about 1 hour and should be considered when a more rapid response is less critical.

IV aminophylline is not considered in the initial treatment of acute asthma in the emergency room or outpatient clinic due to the high incidence of adverse effects.

Anticholinergics such as ipratropium (Atrovent) have also been used in the management of bronchospasm. The combination of anticholinergic therapy and beta-agonists is safe and may be more effective than either drug alone. Research on this approach has shown mixed results.

> **P**atients having an asthma attack who do not respond promptly to beta agonists can be given corticosteroids and anticholinergics as second and third options.

Heliox, a low-density mixture of helium and oxygen, has been administered to patients with severe, acute asthma to lower the work of breathing. Current data do not suggest a clinical benefit to this mode of treatment.

Magnesium sulfate relaxes smooth muscle and has been shown to produce rapid reversal of bronchospasm in some patients with severe asthma. It is not considered standard care in the treatment of asthma.

Clinicians should avoid giving asthmatics certain medications during an acute asthma attack. Sedatives can induce ventilatory failure and should be given with caution unless the patient is intubated and being mechanically ventilated. Inhaled corticosteroids, acetylcysteine (Mucomyst), cromolyn sodium, and dense aerosols may increase bronchospasm, since these agents tend to be irritating to the airways.

Favorable prognostic signs include improvement in the vital signs, PaO_2, $PaCO_2$, breath sounds, sensorium, and breathing pattern. Since any one of these parameters can be misleading by itself, it is important to perform a thorough assessment to obtain a more accurate clinical picture of the patient's response to therapy.

Anti-IgE Antibodies

A new strategy for the treatment of asthma involves the use of Anti-IgE antibodies. Anti-IgE therapy shows promise because immunoglobulin E (IgE) plays a central role in the pathogenesis of allergic diseases such as asthma. An antibody (omalizumab) that binds IgE with high affinity appears useful in reducing allergic responses to inhaled allergens. Clinical trials examining the effectiveness of omalizumab (Xolair) have shown that subcutaneous injections reduce the number of exacerbations in steroid-dependent asthmatics.[6] Additionally, the use of Xolair allows patients to reduce their use of corticosteroids and improves their overall quality of life.[6,7] This medication does not appear to be effective when given via aerosol. The cost of Xolair exceeds that of other treatments and is estimated at $10,000 to $12,000 per year.

Mechanical Ventilation

If the patient becomes fatigued despite treatment, mechanical ventilation will be necessary. Although not every acute asthmatic patient with respiratory acidosis requires intubation and mechanical ventilation, a rising PCO_2 despite aggressive therapy is strong evidence that the patient is in serious respiratory distress and needs breathing assistance. The decision to intubate and mechanically ventilate the patient can be difficult, especially when the clinical findings are not convincing (Table 3.1). The physical findings, ABGs, and peak flow parameters provide the most reliable data for evaluating the need for mechanical ventilation. Patients with a history of steroid dependence and prior intubation are at greater risk for respiratory failure and the need for intubation.[8]

Once it is decided to intubate and begin mechanical ventilation, the patient must be sedated. Sedation improves patient comfort and reduces oxygen consumption during mechanical ventilation. Ventilator management of the severe asthmatic can be challenging

Table 3.1 Decision Making in Asthma

Admit Patient? Yes, if:	How to Recognize
The attack is severe	Use of accessory muscles at rest
	Paradoxic pulse present
	Inspiratory and expiratory wheezing present
	Peak flow is <100 L/min
	FEV_1 <1.0 L
	Significant hyperinflation noted on chest radiograph
The patient does not respond to initial therapy	Vital signs not improving
	Continued use of accessory muscles
	Pao_2 responds minimally to O_2 therapy

Intubate and Initiate CMV? Yes, if:	How to Recognize
The patient fatigues	$Paco_2$ rising
	Sensorium deteriorates
	Abdominal paradox present
	Peak flow decreasing
Respiratory failure present	Hypoxemia is present despite high Fio_2
	Severe respiratory acidemia (pH 7.25) occurs
	Central cyanosis
Cardiac arrest occurs	Pulse and respiratory effort absent
	Pallor
	Patient becomes unconscious

because of the high risk of air trapping and barotrauma. For this reason, choose ventilator settings that result in a low minute ventilation to allow maximum time for exhalation and minimize air trapping. This may result in $Paco_2$ elevation, but the benefit of avoiding barotrauma outweighs the risk of mild acidosis. This strategy of allowing the $Paco_2$ to increase above 45 mm Hg to avoid barotrauma during mechanical ventilation is called **permissive hypercapnia**.[9] In general, ventilate the asthmatic with a tidal volume <8 mL/kg, a rate of 8 to 12 breaths/minute, and an inspiratory flow of 80 to 100 mL/minute. In addition, keep the plateau pressure below 35 cm H_2O.[10] These strategies help reduce the incidence of air trapping and trauma to the lung.

Most asthmatics who are mechanically ventilated can be weaned within a few days. Weaning can begin when airway resistance returns to near-normal. Weaning is often quick in asthmatics because the airway obstruction is reversible.

> The use of mechanical ventilation in asthmatics is very challenging. Air trapping and auto–PEEP (positive end-expiratory pressure) are common complications that can lead to barotraumas, hypotension, and death. The use of small tidal volumes, low rates, and permissive hypercapnia is helpful.

Prevention

The ultimate goal in the management of asthma is to prevent or at least minimize future attacks by decreasing the level of airway responsiveness. Consequently, once the episode is over and the patient has recovered, assess the severity of the underlying asthma with a careful history, pulmonary function testing, and in selected cases, investigations of provoking agents

Box 3.1   Asthma Education

> Asthma education is a vital part of comprehensive management of asthmatic patients. Respiratory therapists (RTs) are excellent candidates to provide asthma education to individual patients or to groups of asthmatics as part of a community education program. RTs have a strong background in diseases of the chest such as asthma and are well trained in the equipment associated with asthma treatment. RTs can become certified by the national asthma education certification board (NAECB) by taking and passing a written test on asthma. An RT who passes the exam receives the AE-C credential, which indicates the person is certified in asthma education. The American Association for Respiratory Care provides education programs that prepare candidates for the NAECB examination.

(e.g., in suspected occupational asthma). Educate patients regarding the avoidance of provoking agents, use of medications, and medication side effects, thus enabling them to enjoy an active, independent lifestyle. Cromolyn sodium is helpful in stabilizing the mast cells to prevent the release of mediators, such as histamine, that can cause bronchospasm. Train the patient to use a peak flowmeter to monitor the degree of airway obstruction; such training allows patients to know when to increase their medication and when they need to seek medical attention (Box 3.1).

PROGNOSIS

The prognosis is excellent for the asthmatic who responds well to conventional treatment. It is not as good for the asthmatic patient who experiences respiratory failure and the need for mechanical ventilation. Long-term mortality rates are significantly higher for these patients.[11] The adverse prognosis for this subgroup of asthmatics is probably related to the greater severity of the disease. This group of asthmatics requires close follow-up and education to minimize the risk of future episodes of respiratory failure.

Adult patients with asthma appear to be at greater risk for developing chronic bronchitis and emphysema later in life.[12] This is true even after adjusting for smoking history and other potential associated risk factors.

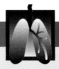 Ms. B

HISTORY

Ms. B is a 19-year-old bareback-bronco rider seen in the emergency department because of shortness of breath. Her dyspnea began during a particularly hard ride, which culminated in modest dust inhalation on the rodeo floor. She states that the tightness in her chest and shortness of breath were so severe that she had to eventually leave the rodeo and seek medical help. She is now very uncomfortable, even at rest. During the past week she has had a cough productive of greenish yellow sputum, mild fever, malaise, and fatigue, but she did not feel seriously ill until the onset of dyspnea at the rodeo earlier in the day. She denies previous lung problems except for mild "whistling" in her chest, which has occurred off and on during the past several years. She denies the use of any prescription medications and any previous episodes of dyspnea, chest pain, leg pain, hemoptysis, sinusitis, or allergies. Her family history is negative for lung disease.

QUESTIONS	ANSWERS
1. What is the key symptom to explore in greater detail?	The key symptom is dyspnea. Ms. B should be questioned to evaluate the severity of the dyspnea because this determines the urgency with which further evaluation and treatment should be pursued.
2. What are the differential diagnoses of this patient's problem, and what is the most likely diagnosis?	Asthma, acute bronchitis, congestive heart failure, flu syndrome, pneumothorax, pulmonary embolus, and psychogenic dyspnea are the differential diagnoses. Asthma exacerbated by acute bronchitis is the most likely diagnosis.
3. What details should the physical examination identify?	The physical examination should be directed toward identifying (1) signs that confirm or rule out the differential diagnoses and (2) the severity of the airway obstruction (see later in the chapter).
4. Why is Ms. B having trouble now rather than 2 months ago?	Ms. B is having trouble now because she has experienced the triple airway insults of respiratory tract infection, allergen (dust) inhalation, and recent severe exertion.

 ## More on Ms. B

PHYSICAL EXAMINATION

- **General.** Ms. B is alert but restless and in moderate respiratory distress. She is mildly diaphoretic, sitting up on the edge of the bed leaning forward with her arms braced on her knees; she has a frequent cough, productive of small amounts of greenish sputum

- **Vital Signs.** Temperature 37.5°C (99.5°F), respiratory rate 38/minute, blood pressure 170/95 mm Hg, heart rate 140/minute, paradoxical pulse 25 mm Hg

- **HEENT.** Sinuses are not tender to palpation; there are no nasal polyps; the alae nasii flare with inspiration

- **Heart.** Regular rhythm at 140/minute; no murmurs, gallops, or rubs; point of maximum impulse in normal position

- **Neck.** Trachea is midline and mobile to palpation; no stridor; carotid pulsations are normal and symmetrical bilaterally with no bruit; no lymphadenopathy, thyromegaly, or jugular venous distention; sternocleidomastoid muscles tensed during inspiration

- **Chest.** Increased anteroposterior diameter with decreased expansion during breathing; resonance to percussion moderately increased bilaterally; mild abdominal paradox with respiratory efforts

- **Lungs.** Rapid respiratory rate with prolonged expiratory phase and polyphonic wheezing heard over entire chest during inhalation and exhalation (Fig. 3.2)

- **Abdomen.** Soft, nontender; bowel sounds present; no masses or organomegaly

- **Extremities.** No clubbing, cyanosis, or edema; pulses normal and symmetrical in all areas

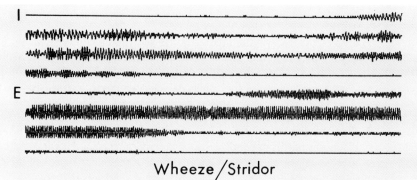

I

E

Wheeze/Stridor

FIGURE 3.2 Waveform analysis demonstrating an inspiratory and expiratory high-pitched wheeze. Time is represented on the horizontal axis and intensity (loudness) on the vertical axis. The pitch is indicated by the number of deflections per time period. Each horizontal line represents 0.34 second. (Reprinted from Respir Care 35:969, 1990, with permission.)

QUESTIONS	ANSWERS
5. What is causing Ms. B's wheezing?	Wheezing is caused by a decreased airway diameter, which is the result of bronchospasm, airway edema, and secretions. Rapid airflow through the partial obstruction causes the airway walls to "flutter," much like the reed in a musical instrument. It is important to note that relatively rapid airflow is needed to cause the flutter effect, and wheezing stops when a patient fatigues to the point where airflow is no longer rapid enough to vibrate the airway wall.
6. What is causing the paradoxical pulse, and what is the significance of this finding?	Paradoxical pulse (variation of the systolic pressure by greater than 10 mm Hg because of breathing efforts) can be caused by wide swings in intrathoracic pressure or by cardiac tamponade. In this case, the airway obstruction requires vigorous respiratory muscle effort that causes large changes in intrathoracic pressure. Although this finding has been shown to occur in more severe cases of asthma, its absence does not preclude severe airway obstruction.
7. What is the cause and significance of the accessory muscle use?	Accessory muscle use occurs when the lung hyperinflation associated with asthma causes the diaphragm to become flattened and therefore less effective. Retraction of the sternocleidomastoid is a reliable sign of severe airway obstruction.
8. What is the cause and significance of the paradoxical breathing pattern?	The paradoxical breathing pattern is a sign of diaphragmatic fatigue. It is recognized by noting inward movement of the abdomen during inspiration. Normally diaphragm contraction pushes the abdominal contents downward and the anterior abdominal wall out during inspiration. Fatigue of the diaphragm allows it to be "sucked" upward into the chest when the accessory muscles create a negative intrathoracic pressure during inspiration.

9. Why do patients in respiratory distress lean forward and brace their hands or elbows and what is this called?

Patients in respiratory distress who have developed diaphragmatic fatigue lean forward and brace their arms or elbows to stabilize the shoulder girdle and to provide a better mechanical advantage for the accessory respiratory muscles. This is called the tripod position.

10. What pathophysiology accounts for Ms. B's increased anteroposterior diameter?

The increased anteroposterior diameter is caused by air trapping that occurs when partial airway obstruction is present in the medium to small bronchi.

11. Does the physical examination provide evidence that hypoxemia is present, and if so what are the signs?

Although cyanosis is not present, clues that suggest hypoxemia include tachycardia, tachypnea, diaphoresis, and restlessness.

More on Ms. B

LABORATORY EVALUATION

Chest Radiograph. Moderate hyperexpansion with no evidence of infiltrates (Fig. 3.3)

ABGs. pH 7.38, $Paco_2$ 43 mm Hg, Pao_2 49 mm Hg on room air

Spirometry: FEV_1 = 1.5 liters (27% of predicted); Peak flow = 140 liters/minute; FVC = 2.1 liters (40% of predicted)

Hematology: Results pending

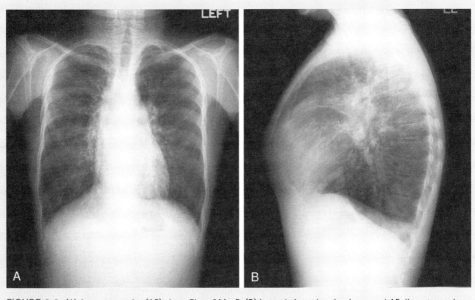

FIGURE 3.3 (A) Anteroposterior (AP) chest film of Ms. B. (B) Lateral view, showing increased AP diameter and low, flat diaphragm.

QUESTIONS	ANSWERS
12. How would you interpret the ABGs and spirometry results?	The ABG results suggest that Ms. B is tiring because the $Paco_2$ is now in the upper limits of normal. In most cases of asthma the $Paco_2$ is low until the patient becomes fatigued. The Pao_2 of 49 mm Hg indicates moderate hypoxemia on room air. These ABG results would strongly suggest the need for mechanical ventilation if Ms. B had been on maximum treatment before the arterial sample was obtained. The spirometry results are consistent with obstructive lung diseases such as asthma. The peak flow of 140 liters/minute and FEV_1 of 1.5 liters indicate moderate obstruction. The significant reduction in the forced vital capacity (FVC) indicates air trapping, which is most likely in this case (but could also indicate restrictive lung disease).
13. What treatment should be planned?	Treatment should include oxygen, aerosolized and IV bronchodilators, antibiotics, and hydration. Oxygen should be started at 4 to 6 liters/minute via nasal cannula or at 40% by entrainment mask and should be adjusted to keep the arterial oxygen saturation (Sao_2) greater than 90% (or the Pao_2 in the 60 to 80 mm Hg range). A $beta_2$-adrenergic bronchodilator should be administered. This is typically accomplished by administering aerosolized albuterol or other $beta_2$-specific bronchodilators by an MDI or SVN. High-dose parenteral corticosteroids should be started if the patient fails to respond promptly to $beta_2$-adrenergic bronchodilators. IV fluids are given to establish optimal thinning of airway secretions. Antibiotics may be needed to treat an upper respiratory tract infection if there is evidence of a bacterial infection (e.g., purulent sputum with numerous pus cells).
14. What are the possible medication side effects?	The bronchodilator can cause tachycardia, tremor, nausea, and dysrhythmias. Oxygen therapy is not likely to cause any side effects since most asthmatics are not CO_2 retainers and do not depend on their hypoxic drive.
15. Should you leave Ms. B to care for other patients while you are waiting for other test results?	This patient should not be left unattended for any reason. Ms. B needs close monitoring and evaluation, since respiratory failure could occur at any moment.

16. Should you admit Ms. B to the hospital?

Unless Ms. B improves dramatically with treatment in the emergency room, she should be admitted to the ICU. If she improves significantly in the emergency department, she could be admitted to a non-ICU service for treatment and observation (see Table 3.1).

17. How would you evaluate Ms. B's response to therapy?

The same techniques used for the initial assessment should be used to evaluate Ms. B's response to therapy. Sensorium is an important parameter to monitor because it will help evaluate the patient's condition and her ability to cooperate with treatment. Other physical examination findings, such as the degree of accessory muscle usage and the vital signs can be very useful. Simple spirometry tests such as the FEV_1, peak flow, or both can provide objective data regarding the course of recovery. ABGs should be obtained when the physical examination findings suggest a change in the patient's status.

18. What therapies should be avoided in this patient?

In this patient, sedatives, inhaled corticosteroids, cromolyn sodium, acetylcysteine, and dense aerosols should be avoided. In the presence of airway obstruction, cromolyn sodium can be added to the treatment plan once bronchodilator therapy has stabilized lung function. If this patient had presented with a history of hypertension, she might have been given a beta-adrenergic antagonist (e.g., Inderal), which increases bronchospasm. In such a case, a trial of calcium channel blockers to treat the hypertension would be better since they do not increase airway resistance.

19. If Ms. B fails to improve with conventional bronchodilators and corticosteroids, what other medication should be added to the treatment regimen?

Inhaled ipratropium bromide or atropine could be added to her treatment plan if the more conventional bronchodilators are not effective. The effects of atropine are additive to those of the adrenergic agonists.

20. When should mechanical ventilation be considered?

Mechanical ventilation should be considered if Ms. B's mental status deteriorates significantly, especially if this is associated with a rising $Paco_2$ (see Table 3.1) despite bronchodilator and oxygen therapy. Once mechanical ventilation is started, sedation can be used to make Ms. B more comfortable. Since she is alert and since treatment has not been initiated, mechanical ventilation is not yet mandatory.

More on Ms. B

In the emergency department Ms. B is started on oxygen via nasal cannula at 4 liters/minute. This results in an improvement in oxygen saturation from 87% to 97% as obtained by pulse oximetry. An IV line is established to deliver steroids, fluids, and antibiotics. Additionally, an SVN treatment with 0.3 to 0.5 mL albuterol diluted in 3 mL saline is provided.

Although this treatment results in improvement in Ms. B's dyspnea, her peak flow improves only slightly (150 liters/minute), and Ms. B continues to use her accessory muscles heavily to breathe. Based on the minimal improvement 1 hour after the initiation of bronchodilator therapy, it is decided to admit her for further care and close observation.

Ms. B is admitted to the respiratory ICU, where oxygen therapy, steroids, and fluids are given. The nebulized albuterol treatment is repeated. Ninety minutes after admission to the ICU, ABGs reveal the following: pH 7.43, $Paco_2$ 36 mm Hg, Pao_2 84 mm Hg, and HCO_3 25 mEq/liter. Peak flow measurement at this point is 145 liters/minute. The clinical examination reveals polyphonic wheezing throughout exhalation, normal sensorium, a respiratory rate of 32/minute, and a pulse rate of 126/minute. Because Ms. B is responding minimally to the aerosolized bronchodilator, the attending physician starts IV methylprednisolone with a bolus of 30 mg to be repeated every 4 to 6 hours. The Gram stain reveals numerous pus cells and gram-positive organisms.

QUESTIONS	ANSWERS
21. Should the use of methylprednisolone result in rapid improvement in Ms. B's airway obstruction?	The use of IV corticosteroids is not expected to result in rapid improvement in Ms. B's airway obstruction. In most cases, 4 to 6 hours is needed before significant improvement in peak flow or FEV_1 can be expected with the use of corticosteroids.
22. What are the potential side effects of steroids?	The potential systemic side effects of high-dose oral corticosteroids taken for prolonged periods of time are significant, including depletion of bone calcium, impairment of immunologic response, increased fat cell production and deposition in the subcutaneous tissues of the neck and trunk, weight gain, hypertension, and glucose intolerance. With the use of aerosolized corticosteroids, candidiasis (oral thrush) and dysphonia can occur. Since the patient in this case is expected to need only a short course of IV steroids these side effects are not a concern.

23. Is this patient a candidate for continuous nebulization of bronchodilator?

This patient could be a candidate for continuous nebulization therapy for the administration of aerosolized bronchodilator. This therapy has been shown to be safe and effective for the treatment of acute asthma in children and adults. Continuous bronchodilator nebulization has been suggested as a treatment alternative to intermittent therapy because the continuous administration could allow more optimal delivery of the nebulized medication. Prolonged inhalation should promote better distribution of the aerosolized drug and a more consistent topical administration of the bronchodilator to the bronchial smooth muscle. To avoid toxic side effects, a more dilute solution of the medication should be used such that the dose typically given in a 15-minute treatment is nebulized over a 1-hour period. Bronchodilators that have more specific b_2 response, such as terbutaline and salbutamol, are recommended to avoid cardiac side effects (e.g., tachycardia, palpitations). Continuous nebulization therapy may be initiated in asthmatics with impending respiratory failure who are not responding optimally to conventional therapy. More studies are needed to identify the role of this therapy in severe cases of asthma and the exact criteria for its use.

24. Are any favorable prognostic signs present at this point?

The improvement in Pao_2 and $Paco_2$ are favorable prognostic signs.

Ms. B Conclusion

Over the next 24 hours, Ms. B steadily improves. Peak flow improves to 220 liters/minute the next day and her vital signs return to near-normal. Wheezing improves and is heard only during the latter half of exhalation. The use of accessory muscles is minimal at this point. Ms. B is transferred to the general floor for maintenance therapy and evaluation of prophylactic therapy.

The remainder of Ms. B's hospital stay is uneventful, and she is discharged 3 days later with a follow-up outpatient appointment in 2 weeks. Ms. B is discharged on oral antibiotics and fluticosone/solmeterol diskus and with an albuterol MDI rescue inhaler. She is counseled on how to avoid dust inhalation, how to recognize and what to do in response to respiratory infections, and how to use the MDI. She is advised to use the MDI and diskus before performing any heavy exercise. ■

KEY POINTS

- **Asthma** is a chronic obstructive pulmonary disease characterized by diffuse airway inflammation and bronchospasm that occurs in response to various stimuli. A key feature of asthma is that the airway obstruction is entirely or partly reversible.
- When a patient has an asthma attack that does not respond to conventional treatment, the condition is called **status asthmaticus**.
- In addition to allergens, asthma attacks can be provoked by pharmacological agents (e.g., beta-adrenoceptor antagonists, aspirin), by air pollutants (e.g., sulfur dioxide, oxidants), exercise, cigarette smoke, and airway infections. Infection of the airways represents one of the most common triggers of asthma attacks.
- Asthma attacks cause a lack of uniform ventilation and $\dot{V}/\dot{Q}$ mismatching. In addition, the high airway resistance causes a high work of breathing and fatigue of the muscles of breathing.
- Clinical features of asthma include dyspnea, cough, tachypnea, wheezing, use of accessory muscles to breathe, and a prolonged expiratory time. Severe asthma causes inspiratory and expiratory wheezing, abnormal sensorium, heavy use of accessory muscles, and paradoxical pulse.
- ABGs reveal respiratory alkalosis with moderate hypoxemia in most cases. Respiratory acidosis occurs when fatigue of the inspiratory muscles is present.
- The chest radiograph in asthma shows hyperinflation. Pulmonary function tests show reduced expiratory flows that improve with bronchodilators.
- In the majority of mild cases, bronchospasm can be reversed by use of an aerosolized beta-adrenergic such as albuterol.
- During an acute, severe asthma attack, if the patient fails to respond adequately to inhaled beta-agonists, IV corticosteroids can be added to the treatment plan.
- Anticholinergics such as ipratropium (Atrovent) constitute a third therapeutic option after beta-agonists and corticosteroids.
- If the patient becomes fatigued despite treatment, mechanical ventilation will be necessary.
- In general, ventilate the asthmatic with a tidal volume <8 mL/kg, a rate of 8 to 12 breaths/minute, and an inspiratory flow of 80 to 100 mL/minute In addition, keep the plateau pressure below 35 cm H_2O.[10]
- The prognosis is excellent for the asthmatic who responds well to conventional treatment. It is not as good for the asthmatic patient who experiences respiratory failure and the need for mechanical ventilation. Long-term mortality rates are significantly higher for these patients.[11]

REFERENCES

1. CDC Asthma–United States, 1982–1992. MMWR Morb Wkly Rep 43:952, 1995.
2. Weiss, KB, Wagener, KD: Asthma surveillance in the United States. A review of current trends and knowledge gaps. Chest 98:179S, 1990.
3. Weiss, KB, Gergen, PJ, Crain, EF: Inner-city asthma: the epidemiology of an emerging US public health concern. Chest 101:362S, 1992.
4. Hess, D: Delivery of inhaled medication in adults. 2004 Up-to-date™

5. Benito-Fernandex, J, Gonzalez-Balenciaga, M, Capape-Zache, S, Vazquez Ronco, MA, Mintegi-Raso, S: Salbutamol via metered-dose inhaler with spacer versus nebulization for acute treatment of pediatric asthma in the emergency department. Pediat Emerg Care 20(10):656–659, 2004.
6. Soler, M, Matz, J, Townley, R, Buhl, R: The anti-IgE antibody omalizumab reduces exacerbations and steroid requirement in allergic asthmatics. Eur Respir J 18:254, 2001.

7. Finn, A, Casale, T, Deniz, Y, Ashby, M: Omalizumab improves asthma-related quality of life in patients with severe allergic asthma. J Allergy Clin Immunol 111:278, 2003.

8. Dhuper, S, Maggiore, D, Chung, V, Shim, C: Profile of near-fatal asthma in an inner-city hospital. Chest. 124:1880–1884, 2003.

9. Tuxen, DV. Permissive hypercapnic ventilation. Am J Respir Crit Care Med 150:870, 1994.

10. Boushey, HA, Venkayya, R: Mechanical ventilation in adults with status asthmaticus. 2004 Up-to-date.™

11. Marquette, CH, Saulnier, F, Leroy, O, et al: Long-term prognosis of near fatal asthma. A 6-year follow-up study of 145 asthmatic patients who underwent mechanical ventilation for a near-fatal attack of asthma. Am Rev Respir Dis 46:76, 1992.

12. Silva, GE, Sherrill, DL, Guerra, S, Barbee, RA: Asthma as a risk factor for COPD in a longitudinal study. Chest 126:59–65, 2004.

4

Chronic Obstructive Pulmonary Disease

Robert L. Wilkins, PhD, RRT, FAARC

Philip M. Gold, MD, MACP, FCCP

CHAPTER OBJECTIVES:

After reading this chapter you will be able to list or identify the following:

- A definition of COPD.
- The estimated incidence of COPD in the United States.
- The factors associated with the onset of COPD.
- The clinical features seen in patients with COPD.
- The criteria for mild, moderate, and severe COPD.
- How to manage the patient with mild, moderate, or severe COPD.
- The treatment usually needed to treat an acute exacerbation of COPD.

INTRODUCTION

Chronic obstructive pulmonary disease (COPD) is defined as a lung disease in which the patient has progressive airflow limitation that is not completely reversible.[1] The airflow limitation is most often associated with an inflammatory response in the lungs from exposure to noxious particles and gases over time. The progressive nature of COPD indicates that the airflow limitation gets significantly worse from one year to the next, especially if exposure to the offending agent continues. Initially the airflow limitation is not detected by the patient but becomes a problem when exercise tolerance decreases to the point that dyspnea interferes with daily activities. This usually occurs years after the initial decreases in expiratory flow identified by spirometry.

The terms **emphysema** and **chronic bronchitis** (CB) are often used when discussing COPD because these two lung disorders combine to cause the symptoms and other clinical features seen in patients with COPD. CB is characterized by excessive sputum production for at least three months of the year for at least two consecutive years. Emphysema is defined in pathological terms and refers to the destruction of gas exchange surfaces of the lung (alveoli). A significant number of patients with COPD have an element of reversible airway obstruction (asthma). Most patients with COPD have elements of CB, emphysema, and asthma, while some have a preponderance of one or the other (Fig. 4.1).

The exact incidence of COPD is not known, and estimates are dependent on the definition and criteria used. In 2000, a national survey estimated that about 10 million people (6% of the U.S. population) had COPD.[2] This survey asked participants if they have

FIGURE 4.1 Venn Diagram for COPD.

1 = CB patients with normal expiratory flows.
2 = Emphysema patients with normal flows.
3 = Patients with CB only.
4 = Patients with emphysema only.
5 = Patients with CB and emphysema.
6 = Patients with CB and asthma.
7 = Patients with emphysema and asthma.
8 = Patients with asthma, CB, and emphysema.
9 = Patients with asthma only.
10 = Patients with airway obstruction due to other causes.

From Murray, JF and Nadel, JA: Textbook of Respiratory Medicine. W.B. Saunders Company; Philadelphia, 1988.

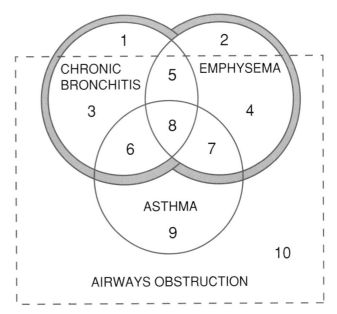

ever been told by a physician that they have chronic bronchitis or emphysema. The estimate of incidence rises to over 20 million in other surveys when the criteria for the diagnosis of COPD included patients with significant airflow limitation as seen on pulmonary function studies.[3] This discrepancy suggests that COPD is significantly underdiagnosed.

In 2000, about 730,000 patients were hospitalized because of COPD, and an additional 2.5 million hospitalized patients had COPD listed as a contributing factor.[2] In the same year, patients with COPD made more than 8 million visits to the doctor on an outpatient basis, and another 1.4 million sought care through the emergency department.[3] In addition, COPD is the fourth leading cause of death in the United States with more than 100,000 deaths occurring each year.[2] There is no doubt that COPD represents a major cause of morbidity and mortality in the United States and around the world and will continue to do so for some time. In addition, the economic burden of COPD on individuals and societies is substantial.[4]

> The exact incidence of COPD in the United States is not known but it is probably underestimated. Estimates that use measures of expiratory flow to define the presence of COPD suggest that more than 20 million people in the United States have COPD. The economic burden of this disease is large.

ETIOLOGY

Most cases of COPD are caused by a combination of exposure to noxious particles and fumes and host factors. Noxious particles and gases include cigarette smoke, smog, occupational dusts, and indoor pollutants. The risk of damage from any inhaled gas or particle depends on the degree of exposure over time, the composition of the inhaled substance, and the host's ability to tolerate the offending agent.

By far the most common noxious fumes and particles leading to COPD are those associated with cigarette smoke. Individuals who smoke have a much higher incidence of COPD, a larger decline in lung function over time, and a greater COPD mortality rate.[5] Cigarette smoke and exposure to occupational dusts and fumes act additively in increasing a person's risk of COPD.

The fact that some individuals smoke and do not develop COPD while others develop advanced disease is most likely related to genetic (host) factors. This is illustrated by the observation that COPD tends to run in families. Individuals with a parent who has been diagnosed with COPD are more likely to develop the disease, probably owing to a shared genetic risk.[6]

> The most common factor leading to the onset of COPD is cigarette smoking. Although only about 15% to 20% of smokers have been formally diagnosed with COPD, that figure is based on diagnosis by a physician and underestimates the true incidence. The percentage of smokers with lung function impairment is much greater.

Pulmonary emphysema develops in some patients with minimal or no smoking exposure as a result of an aPI deficiency. Normally the liver produces 200 to 400 mg/dL of alpha-protease inhibitor (aPI), which was previously called alpha$_1$-antitrypsin. aPI plays a role in inflammation and is mainly responsible for the inactivation of neutrophil elastase, an enzyme released from polymorphonuclear leukocytes (PMNs) that breaks down elastin during an inflammatory response. Therefore, a deficiency in aPI results in elastase-induced destruction of lung tissue, producing panlobular pulmonary emphysema. This occurs as a result of a genetically inherited homozygous trait that is present in approximately 1% of emphysema patients, who are initially symptomatic in the third to fourth decade of life. There is also evidence that cigarette smoking exacerbates the problem encountered in aPI deficiency. Homozygous aPI deficiency is also characterized by liver disease manifested as hepatomegaly, cholestasis, and elevated liver enzymes in infancy.

CLINICAL FEATURES

History

The patient with COPD usually complains of cough, sputum production, and exertional dsypnea. Cough and sputum production are especially common in the patient with a case of COPD dominated by chronic bronchitis pathology. The excessive sputum production and coughing is present owing to the hypertrophy and hyperactivity of the mucous glands lining the airways. Cough and sputum production increase with the onset of acute infection.

> Cough is the most common symptom in patients with COPD, but dyspnea is what causes them to seek medical help.

The dyspnea associated with emphysema usually progresses over time in such a way that increasingly less exertion causes increasing dyspnea. Eventually patients are unable to perform even simple activities such as walking to the bathroom without having to stop and catch their breath. In the rare patient with significant COPD who has no smoking history, aPI deficiency must be considered.

Physical Examination

The findings on physical examination vary widely and depend on the severity of the disease, the presence of acute exacerbations, and the degree to which CB or emphysema is present. Patients with mild disease and no acute problems (e.g., infection) have minimal abnormalities on physical examination. In contrast, the patient with severe COPD who is having an acute exacerbation has numerous abnormalities. The discussion below will focus on the findings associated with moderate to severe COPD.

Patients with stable disease have normal vital signs and sensorium at rest. Exacerbations usually cause an acute rise in heart rate and respiratory rate. If oxygenation is compromised significantly, the patient may be confused and disoriented. An abnormal sensorium is a sign of hypoxia and should alert the respiratory therapist (RT) to the need for aggressive therapy.

The breathing pattern of the patient with COPD is often helpful in determining the severity of the disease. Patients who breathe with a prolonged expiratory time and who use their accessory muscles to breathe at rest have more advanced COPD. Severe hyperinflation of the lung leads to a low, flat diaphragm and may result in **Hoover's sign**. This is seen as inward movement of the lower lateral chest wall with each inspiration and occurs when the diaphragm is pulling in from the sides rather than down from above. Hoover's sign indicates severe hyperinflation, and the patient is prone to diaphragm fatigue. Tripoding is also common when acute exacerbations are present (see Chapter 3).

Auscultation may reveal a large variety of abnormal lung and heart sounds. The patient with more severe emphysema will have diminished breath sounds throughout both lungs. Early-inspiratory crackles are heard with more severe COPD and are produced by the sudden opening of more proximal airways with each inspiratory effort. The crackles in such cases are scanty. Expiratory wheezing is common, especially in the patient with chronic bronchitis and during acute exacerbations.

Heart sounds may be difficult to hear, and the point of maximal impulse (PMI) may shift to the epigastric area when severe hyperinflation is present. Pulmonary hypertension may be present when chronic hypoxemia is a problem. This results in loud closure of the pulmonic valve and is known as a loud P_2. Chronic pulmonary hypertension leads to hypertrophy of the right ventricle. A heave may be felt at the lower right sternal border during systole in such cases.

The digits may reveal clubbing in some patients with COPD (Fig. 4.2). Why some patients develop this abnormality and others do not is not known. Its clinical significance is also unknown.

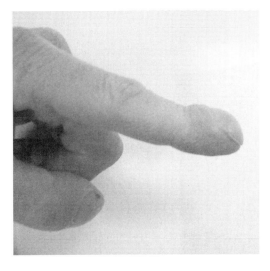

FIGURE 4.2 Digital clubbing.

> Signs of severe COPD on physical examination include heavy use of accessory muscles to breathe at rest, diminished breath sounds in all lung fields, and a prolonged expiratory time.

The onset of cor pulmonale causes numerous abnormalities that can be detected on the physical examination. The elevation of venous pressures leads to jugular venous distention (JVD), hepatomegaly, and pedal edema. If pressure in the neck veins appears to increase while the physician is pressing gently but firmly on the liver (right upper quadrant of the patient's abdomen), the hepatojugular reflex is present. The presence of this reflex is consistent with right heart failure.

Clinical Lab Data

The complete blood count may be normal or demonstrate leukocytosis when lung infection is complicating the COPD patient. Polycythemia is common in the patient with chronic hypoxemia, as this is the body's attempt to compensate for low oxygen levels in the blood.

The electrolyte panel often shows a low chloride concentration when the COPD patient has chronic respiratory acidosis. In addition, the total CO_2 is elevated in such cases, indicating an elevation of the bicarbonate level as compensation for respiratory acidosis. Sodium and potassium levels are often normal but can become abnormal when complicating heart failure and fluid retention are present and the patient is being treated with diuretics.

Arterial Blood Gases

Arterial blood gases (ABGs) are an important part of evaluating the patient suspected of having COPD. The results help determine the severity of the disease and guide treatment such as oxygen therapy and mechanical ventilation when needed. Initially the ABG shows mild to moderate hypoxemia with normal Pa_{CO_2} levels. As the disease progresses, the hypoxemia worsens and the patient often begins to retain carbon dioxide when severe disease is present. In most patients, the hypercarbia occurs gradually and is easily compensated for by renal elevation of bicarbonate. Acute exacerbations of COPD often cause more abrupt hypercarbia and result in respiratory acidosis. The acute respiratory acidosis is often reversed when appropriate treatment is applied.

> ABG results in the COPD patient at rest do not necessarily predict what changes will occur with exercise or sleep. It is not uncommon for hypoxemia to intensify during these two physiologic changes.

The onset of metabolic problems can make interpretation of the ABG difficult in the COPD patient and complicate treatment. For example, the onset of metabolic alkalosis superimposed on chronic respiratory acidosis can be difficult to recognize because the serum bicarb is already elevated. In addition, the metabolic alkalosis diminishes the patient's drive to breathe and may lead to worsening of the respiratory acidosis in the spontaneously breathing patient.

Chest Radiograph

The chest radiograph findings vary widely from one case of COPD to the next. Patients with minimal hyperinflation and mild to moderate disease often have a normal chest x-ray. Severe hyperinflation causes a large retrosternal airspace as seen on the lateral film and low flat diaphragm on the posterioanterior (PA) and lateral films (Fig. 4.3). A small narrow

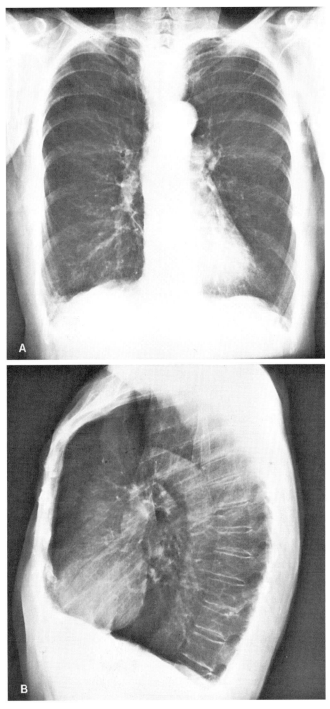

FIGURE 4.3 Chest radiograph of patient with COPD.

heart is also evidence of severe hyperinflation. The patient with significant hypertrophy of the airways may have "tram tracks" on the chest film. These are parallel, linear white shadows that result from thickening of the airways when chronic bronchitis is severe.

The chest radiograph is often used to document suspected complications such as pneumonia and pneumothorax in the COPD patient with severe shortness of breath. Some patients with COPD have heart failure and pulmonary edema complicating their condition. This may be seen as diffuse infiltrates and an enlarged heart on the chest film, but severe hyperinflation may make it difficult to recognize these findings.

Pulmonary Function Studies

The patient experiencing an acute exacerbation of COPD cannot perform a complete pulmonary function test (PFT). Simple peak flow and forced vital capacity measurements provide enough information to determine the status of the patient. A peak flow less than 100 L/min or forced expiratory volume in 1 second (FEV_1) of less than 1.0 L indicates severe obstruction and suggests that respiratory failure may occur soon if treatment is not given and successful. More complete tests can be done when the patient is stable.

The classic pattern seen on spirometry in the patient with COPD is reduced expiratory flows that are not responsive to bronchodilators. Vital capacity may be normal or reduced if severe hyperinflation is present. Severe hyperinflation is seen as elevation of the residual volume, functional residual volume, and the total lung capacity. Owing to loss of alveolar surface area, the Diffusion Capacity of the Lung for Carbon Monoxide (D_{LCO}) is reduced when emphysema is present.

Pulmonary function studies are used to stage the level of COPD in each patient and are also useful for following progression of the disease objectively over time. The American Thoracic Society criteria classify COPD in the following three stages based on pulmonary function results while the patient is stable:[7]

- **Stage 1.** FEV_1 >50% of predicted
- **Stage 2.** FEV_1 35% to 49% of predicted
- **Stage 3.** FEV_1 <35% of predicted

The GOLD criteria classify COPD into the following four stages:[8]

- **Stage 1.** FEV_1 >80% of predicted
- **Stage 2.** FEV_1 50% to <80% of predicted
- **Stage 3.** FEV_1 30% to 49% of predicted
- **Stage 4.** FEV_1 <30% of predicted

It has been recommended that routine spirometry be performed with all patients at risk for COPD (smokers over age 40) to detect asymptomatic airflow limitation.[9] In patients with established disease, spirometry, on a yearly basis, is useful to monitor clinical status and to assess the response to therapy. Patients presented with objective evidence of lung function abnormalities may be more likely to quit smoking.

Electrocardiogram

The electrocardiogram (ECG) may reveal right axis deviation when right ventricular hypertrophy is present. This is seen as a downward deflection of the QRS wave in lead I. Low voltage in the limb leads is often seen in the emphysematous patient when severe hyperinflation occurs.

TREATMENT

Management of Stable COPD

Treatment of the stable COPD patient depends on the severity of the disease. Those with mild disease (stage 1) who have minimal lung function impairment can be treated by their family physician. The primary goal for treatment of such patients is to remove the offending agent from the patient's environment. This usually consists of smoking cessation but may also include a change in employment or geographical location (if the patient lives near a major city with polluted air). The use of bronchodilators for patients with mild disease is on an as needed basis when dyspnea is present. Smoking cessation should be strongly recommended by the attending physician and RT in all cases of COPD but it provides the greatest benefit to those with mild disease.

Pharmacological Agents

Treatment of the COPD patient with moderate to severe disease (stages 2 and 3) usually centers around the use of pharmacological agents and should be directed by a pulmonologist when the patient has complex problems. Although bronchodilators do not change the long-term decline in lung function that is the hallmark of the disease, they play a key role in reducing symptoms such as dyspnea and improving the quality of life for COPD patients. They can be given on an as needed basis or on a regular basis to reduce symptoms.[10] The initial medication used is either a beta-agonist or an anticholnergic. A commonly used short-acting bronchodilator is albuterol, which has a rapid onset of action and is given via metered dose inhaler or medication nebulizer. The latter route is more expensive and requires more maintenance. The role of long-acting beta-agonists, such as salmeterol and formoterol, in the treatment of COPD is not well defined at this point. Some patients demonstrate improved dyspnea over time with their use, but more data is needed before strong recommendations can be made.[11]

The use of anticholinergics, such as inhaled ipratropium, are now considered an important part of the treatment plan for COPD patients with moderate to severe disease. A long-acting inhaled anticholenergic, tiotropium, was recently introduced and appears to be superior to ipratropium in causing bronchodilation for a longer period of time. This may be clinically useful in patients with treatment compliance issues (see Appendix B).

The combination of a beta-agonist and an anticholenergic is very popular for the treatment of COPD, and the effects of the two are additive.[12] This is a common strategy for treating the patient who does not respond to beta-agonists alone. A single metered-dose inhaler (MDI) is available that offers both medications in the same canister.

The use of methylxanthines, such as theophylline, in COPD is controversial.[13] The results of studies are mixed, with some showing benefit while others do not. The risk of toxicity is always a concern with theophylline because it has a narrow therapeutic index. Careful monitoring is essential if it is to be used in the long-term treatment of stable COPD. Starting the patient on methylxanthines are not recommended for the treatment of acute exacerbations.

> The primary goal of bronchodilators is to reduce dyspnea and improve the quality of life for the patient with COPD.

Corticosteroids may be useful on an intermittent basis when acute dyspnea does not respond to bronchodilators and oxygen therapy. Recent research has provided evidence that the combination of salmeterol and fluticosone produce greater improvement in FEV_1 than either agent alone. Inhaled corticosteroids have been shown to decrease the frequency of acute exacerbations.[13]

The preferred route of administration for steroids is the MDI, as it minimizes risk of systemic side effects. Long-term use of oral corticosteroids is considered only for COPD patients who have continued symptoms or severe airflow limitation despite maximal therapy with other agents.[14]

Oxygen therapy is an important part of treatment for the patient with more severe COPD. Patients with a PaO_2 below 55 or an SaO_2 below 88% while breathing room air at rest are candidates for long-term (>15 hrs/day) oxygen therapy. Patients with a PaO_2 of 55 to 60 mm Hg who have evidence of pulmonary hypertension (JVD, pedal edema) or polycythemia are also candidates for long-term oxygen therapy. The goal of oxygen therapy is to keep the PaO_2 above 60 mm Hg and/or the SaO_2 above 90%. Oxygen therapy has been shown to improve survival, exercise tolerance, and hemodynamics in COPD patients.[15]

Short-term oxygen therapy may be useful for treatment of the intermittent desaturations seen during exercise or sleep in selected COPD patients. Oxygen therapy is given on an as-needed basis in those cases. In most cases, oxygen therapy is given via nasal cannula at 1 to 4 L/min to achieve the desired oxygenation level.

Pulmonary Rehabilitation Programs

Pulmonary rehabilitation programs are beneficial for stable COPD patients, as they improve exercise tolerance and educate patients about their disease and how to manage it. Although lung function probably does not improve with pulmonary rehabilitation, the overall quality of life appears to improve, as evidenced by less dyspnea and improved mental health among patients who have participated in such programs. Patients with mild, moderate, and severe disease can benefit from a pulmonary rehabilitation program.

Surgery

Surgery may prove useful in treating the patient with severe COPD. Lung volume reduction surgery (LVRS) has been performed in selected patients to remove those the most diseased parts of the lung that are restricting function of more healthy lung tissue. Patients who have successfully undergone LVRS typically have severe upper lobe emphysema that has not responded to maximal conventional therapy. A multicenter study indicates that LVRS should be limited to patients with upper lobe disease and low exercise capacity.[10]

Management of the Acute Exacerbation

Treating the patient with COPD who is experiencing an acute exacerbation represents a major challenge. An important part of the initial management is determining the cause of the exacerbation. Possible causes include infection, bronchospasm, pulmonary edema, pneumothorax, and pulmonary embolism. It is important to distinguish the COPD patient with an acute exacerbation from one in whom the COPD has advanced to end-stage disease. In the latter case, treatment goals are strictly palliative.

Acute exacerbations are typically seen as a sudden increase in dyspnea and may be accompanied with increased cough, sputum production, and wheezing. Sputum may change color, consistency, and volume during an exacerbation, especially when infection is the precipitating cause. Fever is also common when infection is present, but its absence does not rule infection out. Wheezing is common when bronchospasm is adding to the patient's dyspnea.

The initial step in caring for the COPD patient experiencing an acute exacerbation is the assessment of the patient's condition. This is done by a combination of interview, physical examination, chest radiograph, blood tests, simple spirometry, and ECG. In all cases, the patient's current clinical condition and results of specific tests should be compared to previous results when the patient was stable. This comparison helps assess how sick the patient is and how far things have deteriorated since the last evaluation. For example, if the Pao_2 is now 56 mm Hg on room air but was only 64 mm Hg at the time of the last discharge, this would indicate that the current problem does not

> Evaluation of the COPD patient experiencing an acute exacerbation is vital but should not delay starting important treatment such as oxygen therapy.

represent a major change in lung function. If the previous ABG, however, revealed a stable Pao_2 of 75 mm Hg on room air, the current Pao_2 of 56 represents a significant change.

Pharmacological Agents

The first step in treating the patient with an acute exacerbation is to begin controlled oxygen therapy and determine if the problem is life threatening. If the threat is considered serious, the patient is admitted to the intensive care unit (ICU). Otherwise, the patient can be cared for in the emergency department and sent home for follow-up on an outpatient basis.

Provide oxygen therapy to keep the Pao_2 in the 60 to 80 mm Hg range and the Sao_2 above 90%. Entrainment masks provide a more controlled Fio_2 and may help avoid secondary hypercarbia but are not as well tolerated by the patient. The primary cause of death in the COPD patient with life-threatening disease is hypoxia, so oxygen therapy is vital to the survival of the patient.

Bronchodilators are given during acute exacerbations to reduce dyspnea and improve patient comfort. Beta-agonists are usually given first, and anticholinergics are added if the initial response is not optimal. Oral or IV glucocorticosteroids are recommended as an addition to the bronchodilators when dyspnea is severe and not responding well to bronchodilators. A short course of 30 to 40 mg of oral prednisolone daily is recommended.[16] Antibiotics are given when purulent sputum is present.

Mechanical Ventilation

Short-term ventilatory support may be needed when initial therapy with oxygen, bronchodilators, and corticosteroids does not stabilize the patient and return lung function to an acceptable level as seen on ABGs. Mechanical ventilation of the COPD patient experiencing an acute exacerbation is intended to improve survival and reduce dyspnea.

Recently, noninvasive positive pressure ventilation (NIPPV) has gained popularity since it avoids intubation and the complications associated with it. NIPPV has been shown to improve pH, $Paco_2$ and Pao_2 and reduces the length of hospital stays.[17] Typically NIPPV is applied using a tight-fitting face or nasal mask and allows adequate gas exchange while the acute problem causing the respiratory failure is resolving (e.g., congestive heart failure (CHF).) Once the patient improves and the cause of the acute problem begins to resolve, the patient can be easily weaned from NIPPV with a gradual decrease in positive pressure.

Mechanical ventilation via intubation is applied in the patient who responds poorly to initial therapy and when the cause of the respiratory failure is not expected to resolve quickly. Common modes of ventilation include assist control and pressure support alone or in combination with intermittent mandatory ventilation. The initial settings should attempt to return the $Paco_2$ to levels seen when the patient was stable and not necessarily to normal. The primary complication associated with PPV in COPD patients is auto-PEEP (see Chapter 3). This can be minimized by using small tidal volumes and long expiratory times.

> **W**eaning the patient with COPD from the ventilator can represent one of the most difficult tasks facing the RT. Asking the patient to resume the work of breathing should be done only when the patient's medical condition has been optimized.

Weaning from mechanical ventilation can be a major challenge, especially if the patient has been intubated for more that just a few days and has become dependent on the ventilator. There does not appear to be an advantage in using one method of weaning over another. T-piece, intermittent mandatory ventilation, or pressure support can be used, and each has its own advantages and disadvantages. NIPPV following extubation has been shown to expedite weaning in COPD patients while reducing the incidence of complications such as nosocomial pneumonia.[18]

 Mr. L

HISTORY

Mr. L is a 54-year-old white man currently employed as a machinist. He was seen in the pulmonary outpatient clinic for the first time complaining of shortness of breath with exertion and a productive cough. Mr. L stated that his coughing had recently increased and was producing thick, yellow sputum. He stated that his cough had been present for several years but was "usually not a problem." His cough has usually been productive of clear to white sputum in the morning. He had recently noticed more shortness of breath than usual and was now dyspneic at rest. Mr. L did admit to feeling warm at times during the past few days but had not taken his temperature with a thermometer. He denied chest pain, hemoptysis, sinusitis, weight loss, allergies, night sweats, or chills.

Mr. L admitted to smoking $2^1/_2$ packs of cigarettes per day for the past 30 years. He had attempted to stop on several occasions but was successful for no longer than 3 or 4 months. His machinist work had exposed him to many toxic fumes. His family history was positive for lung disease, as his father died of emphysema at the age of 64. His mother is alive and well at age 75. His sister is healthy at age 47, and his 51-year-old brother has diabetes.

QUESTIONS	ANSWERS
1. What medical problems are suggested by the medical history, and what are the key symptoms to explore?	The patient's medical history suggests chronic bronchitis exacerbated by a respiratory infection such as acute bronchitis, flu, bronchospasm, or pneumonia. The symptoms do not suggest congestive heart failure. Mr. L's cough and shortness of breath need evaluation. The interviewer should determine the severity of the dyspnea by asking about the degree to which it limits Mr. L's daily routine. The changes in Mr. L's dyspnea over the past years and factors that trigger the dyspnea are important in evaluating prognosis and avoiding exacerbation of the disease.

2. What is the significance of the patient's sputum color?	Uncomplicated chronic bronchitis most often causes clear or opaque sputum. Infection will most often cause the sputum to turn colored, but allergic reactions can also result in thick, yellow-green sputum.
3. What is Mr. L's smoking history in pack-years?	Mr. L's smoking history in pack-years is 75 pack-years (2.5 packs per day × 30 years = 75 pack-years).
4. What is the significance of the family and occupational history?	Mr. L's family history is significant, given that his father died of emphysema. It appears that the tendency for COPD is genetically transferable from parent to child, although the disease is not considered a hereditary disease. The occupational exposure to irritant gases as a machinist may have also increased his risk for lung disease.
5. What should the physical examination accomplish at this point in the assessment of the patient?	The physical examination should help determine the extent of Mr. L's pulmonary dysfunction (e.g., cyanosis, cor pulmonale, crackles, wheeze, pedal edema) and the cause of the symptoms. The clinician can accomplish this by assessing parameters such as vital signs, sensorium, breath sounds, respiratory pattern, heart sounds, and ankle edema.

 More on Mr. L

PHYSICAL EXAMINATION

- **General.** Patient alert and oriented, but in moderate respiratory distress; uses choppy sentences because of dyspnea and frequent coughing, which produces thick, yellow sputum

- **Vital Signs.** Temperature 38.1°C (100.6°F), respiratory rate 26/min, blood pressure 144/90 mm Hg; pulse 120/min

- **HEENT.** Tongue and mucous membranes slightly cyanotic; pupils equal, round, and reactive to light and accommodation (PERRLA); sinuses nontender to palpation

- **Neck.** Trachea midline and mobile; transmitted wheezes present, but no stridor present; carotids + + bilaterally with no bruits; JVD noted with head of bed elevated to a 45° angle; accessory muscles in neck tense with each inspiratory effort

- **Chest.** Anteroposterior diameter large, and chest wall excursion small; generalized hyperresonance but decreased resonance over right lower lobe noted on chest percussion; bilateral expiratory polyphonic wheezes, louder on right side, noted on auscultation of lungs; coarse crackles and bronchial breath sounds present over right lower lobe

- **Heart.** Regular rhythm with rate of 120/min; no murmurs or rubs noted; S_3 gallop and loud P_2 noted on auscultation of lungs; systolic heave noted at lower right sternal border; point of maximal impulse located in fifth intercostal space at midclavicular line on the left

- **Abdomen.** Soft and nontender; hepatomegaly present, and hepatojugular reflex positive; no evidence of paradoxical respiratory movement

- **Extremities.** No evidence of cyanosis or clubbing; pedal edema present and 2+ bilaterally in the lower extremities up to knee level; extremities dry and warm to touch

QUESTIONS	ANSWERS
6. How do you interpret the vital signs?	The patient's body temperature is elevated. Infections, either viral or bacterial, can cause fever. Fever increases the patient's oxygen consumption and places an increased demand on the cardiac and respiratory systems. The respiratory and heart rates are slightly elevated, which may be related to the fever or the hypoxemia, or both. Tachycardia and tachypnea help meet the increased need for oxygen consumption and CO_2 excretion associated with fever and help compensate for hypoxemia when present.
7. What is indicated by cyanosis of the tongue and mucous membranes?	Cyanosis of the tongue and mucous membranes of the mouth indicates central cyanosis. Central cyanosis is caused by hypoxemia, which turns the arterial blood dark. Polycythemia makes cyanosis more visible and anemia makes it difficult to recognize.
8. What are the possible causes of the expiratory polyphonic wheezes heard bilaterally and the bronchial breath sounds heard over the right lower lobe?	The expiratory polyphonic wheezes may be produced by one or more of the following: bronchospasm, mucosal edema, or excessive airway secretions. Intrathoracic airways tend to narrow slightly on exhalation owing to the additive effects of positive intrathoracic pressure and the decreased retractile forces of elastic fibers within the airway walls. When the airways are obstructed because of bronchospasm, edema, or secretions, exhalation can result in severe narrowing, resulting in vibration of the airway walls and therefore expiratory wheezes. Polyphonic wheezes suggest partial obstruction of many small airways, rather than one large upper airway. The bronchial breath sounds suggest consolidation in the right lower lobe. Normal lung tissue acts as a filter to sound, allowing only low-pitched sounds to pass. Consolidated lung allows the turbulent flow sounds of the larger airways to pass through the lung with little attenuation of the high-pitched sounds produced by turbulent flow in the larger airways. In such cases, the normal vesicular breath sound is replaced with a louder, higher-pitched, bronchial-type breath sound over the area of the consolidated lung.

9. What is suggested by the loud P_2?

The loud P_2 suggests pulmonary hypertension. Pulmonary circulation pressures increase as the capillary smooth muscle constricts in response to hypoxemia. Eventually, collagen tissue replaces the pulmonary arteriolar smooth muscle, causing irreversible pulmonary hypertension. The increase in pulmonary artery pressure causes the pulmonic valve to close more loudly than it would under normal conditions. A loud P_2 is best heard in the pulmonic area, which is located at the second left intercostal space near the sternal border.

10. What pathophysiology could be causing the JVD, hepatomegaly, hepatojugular reflex, and pedal edema?

JVD, hepatomegaly, pedal edema, and the hepatojugular reflex are typically caused by right heart failure which may be the result of left heart failure, acute severe pulmonary embolism, or chronic hypoxemia. Right heart failure allows filling pressures of the right heart to increase and all venous pressures to rise. High venous pressures result in distended neck veins; an engorged, swollen liver; and an accumulation of fluid in the lower extremities.

11. How is the hepatojugular reflex identified?

Right heart failure increases venous pressure and causes liver engorgement. If pressure in the neck veins appears to increase while the physician is pressing gently but firmly on the liver (right upper quadrant of the patient's abdomen), the hepatojugular reflex is present, which is consistent with right heart failure.

12. How is the severity of the pedal edema characterized?

The severity of the edema is graded on a scale of 1+ through 4+ on the basis of pitting produced by sustained, light pressure applied by the examiner over the tissue being examined. Minimal pitting edema is indicated as 1+, whereas 4+ suggests severe pitting edema that "weeps" when the examiner presses on the edematous tissue. In this case, 2+ pitting edema indicates a moderate degree of ankle edema. The level to which the edema extends up the lower extremities also indicates the severity of the right heart failure. In this case, the edema is at the level of the knees, which implies moderate disease. More severe heart failure causes the edema to extend higher.

13. What is the significance of the systolic heave located at the lower right sternal border?

A heave at the right sternal border is usually produced by contraction of an enlarged right ventricle. Right ventricular hypertrophy often occurs when the right heart pumps against high pressures for many months (much like the biceps of a compulsive weight lifter). The heave at the sternal border along with the JVD, hepatomegaly, loud P_2, and pedal edema are evidence of cor pulmonale. Right ventricular heave and a loud P_2 may be difficult to identify when the anteroposterior chest diameter is large. These findings of right heart failure suggest that the patient has had hypoxemia for many months or years.

14. What is indicated by the fact that Mr. L's accessory respiratory muscles of the neck are tensing with each inspiratory effort?

Use of the accessory muscles of respiration indicates that the patient has respiratory distress and the diaphragm is no longer able to provide adequate respiratory support. This is a common finding in patients with acute exacerbation of lung disease and provides an objective parameter for monitoring the patient's condition and response to therapy.

Box 4.1 Laboratory Evaluation

Chest Radiograph (Fig. 4.4)

ABGs

ABG	Value
pH	7.41
Pao_2	45 mm Hg on room air
$Paco_2$	44 mm Hg
HCO_3^-	28 mEq
$P(A-a)o_2$	53 mm Hg
O_2 content	16.4 mL

Complete Blood Count

	Observed	Normal
White Blood Cells (WBCs)	16 thousand/mm^3	4–11 thousand/mm^3
Red Blood Cells (RBCs)	5.7 million/mm^3	4.1–5.5 million/mm^3
Hemoglobin (g)	17.5	14–16.5
Hematocrit (%)	56	37–50
Segmented neutrophils (%)	77	38–79
Bands (%)	10	0–7
Lymphocytes (%)	10	12–51
Eosinophils (%)	1	0–8
Monocytes (%)	1	0–10

Chemistry: All within normal limits except for total CO_2 (slightly elevated at 34 mEq/L)

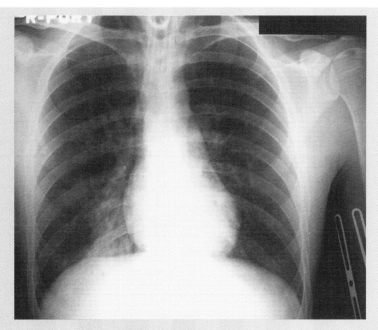

FIGURE 4.4 Mr. L's chest radiograph.

QUESTIONS	ANSWERS
15. How important is the chest radiograph in determining the cause of the patient's symptoms? What does it show to be the underlying condition of this patient's respiratory system?	The chest radiograph is very important, as it demonstrates an infiltrate typical of pneumonia in the right lower lobe. Respiratory infections are a common cause of exacerbation in patients with COPD.
16. How would you interpret the ABGs?	The ABG measurements reveal moderate hypoxemia on room air. This is a common finding in COPD patients, especially when an infection is present. The acid-base status shows both respiratory acidosis and metabolic alkalosis. Because the body never completely compensates for an acid-base disturbance and the pH is 7.41, there must be two simultaneous primary disturbances. It is possible that this patient's "normal" Pa_{CO_2} is greater than 45 mm Hg and is compensated for by an elevation of blood HCO_3^-. When an acute problem such as pneumonia occurs, significant hypoxemia can drive the patient's respiratory system to increase ventilation. This may result in relative hyperventilation, with the Pa_{CO_2} decreasing back to a more normal range, which causes acute respiratory alkalosis (even though the Pa_{CO_2} is normal) superimposed over chronic respiratory acidosis. If the patient had vomiting associated with his other symptoms, acute metabolic alkalosis might also have developed.

17. Should complete pulmonary function testing be done at this point?

This is not a good time to have the patient perform additional pulmonary function testing, as he is acutely ill. After his condition stabilizes, complete pulmonary function testing will provide a better indication of his underlying pulmonary disease.

18. How would you interpret the complete blood count (CBC)? What could be causing the elevated WBC count? What is the most likely cause of the elevated RBC count?

The CBC reveals elevated WBC and RBC counts. The leukocytosis is probably in response to the infiltrate seen on the chest radiograph. The elevation of the bands is known as a left shift, which indicates that immature WBCs are being released by the bone marrow in response to the acute infection. The elevated RBC count indicates that polycythemia is present. This abnormality may be secondary to a chronically low PaO_2. Polycythemia helps compensate for the hypoxemia by increasing the blood's oxygen-carrying capacity. Unfortunately, it also increases cardiac work load by increasing blood viscosity. Many pulmonary physicians phlebotomize patients to a hematocrit of less than 60% to decrease right heart work load and to prevent RBC slugging and arteriolar obstruction.

19. What is the tentative diagnosis, and should the patient be admitted to the hospital?

The tentative diagnosis is acute exacerbation of chronic bronchitis caused by pneumonia. The patient should be admitted for close monitoring, IV bronchodilators, steroids, antibiotics, and possible phlebotomy (see Appendix B).

20. What other diagnostic procedures should be ordered at this point?

Sputum analysis with a Gram stain and culture may help determine the cause of the pneumonia. An ECG may help rule out cardiac ischemia.

21. What therapy should the physician order for the patient?

Appropriate therapy for the patient at this point would include oxygen, antibiotics, bronchodilators, and steroids.

More on Mr. L

The patient is admitted to the pulmonary care unit. The physician writes orders for the following:

- Oxygen by nasal cannula 2 L/min titrated to achieve an arterial oxygen saturation (Sao_2) of greater than 90%

- Medication nebulizer with albuterol (Ventolin/Proventil) 0.5 mL and ipratropium 2.5 mL every 4 hours

- Methylprednisolone (Solu-Medrol) 125 mg IV every 6 hours × 3, and then 60 mg IV

- Cefuroxime 750 mg IV every 8 hours, and clarithromycin (Biaxin) 500 mg by mouth every 12 hours

- ECG

- Sputum Gram stain, culture, and sensitivity

QUESTIONS

ANSWERS

22. What is the goal of oxygen therapy in this case? What level of arterial oxygenation is appropriate? How should the oxygen therapy be evaluated? Once this patient is stable and ready to go home, should he be sent home on a regimen of oxygen therapy?

The goal of oxygen therapy is to correct the hypoxemia. A Pao_2 of 55 to 65 mm Hg is an appropriate level of oxygenation in this case. The hemoglobin is more than 90% saturated under most conditions at a partial pressure of about 60 mm Hg. Elevating the Pao_2 above 65 mm Hg does not add significant oxygen content to the arterial blood, but does slightly increase the risk of oxygen-induced hypoventilation.

The RT should evaluate the oxygen therapy by using a combination of parameters. Pulse oximetry is useful when changes in ventilation and therefore Pco_2 are not likely. The patient's mild hypoventilation makes it important to titrate the fraction of inspired oxygen (Fio_2) to result in an Sao_2 of 90% and to check ABGs to evaluate ventilatory and acid-base status.

The clinical findings of polycythemia and cor pulmonale strongly suggest that this patient would benefit from home oxygen therapy. If the patient's resting room air Pao_2 is less than 55 mm Hg at the time of discharge, home oxygen should be arranged. If the Pao_2 is 55 to 60 mm Hg, chronic home oxygen supplementation will be important, as the patient has both polycythemia and evidence of right heart failure. If the patient's resting Pao_2 is greater than 60 mm Hg, nocturnal desaturation may be demonstrated by nocturnal pulse oximetry monitoring and would indicate the need for oxygen during sleep.

23. What abnormalities on the ECG would demonstrate right-axis deviation? What does this abnormality indicate?

The negative deflection of the P and QRS waves in lead I is consistent with right-axis deviation. This finding is typical for patients with cor pulmonale. Normally, the mean axis of electrical activity for the heart is between 0 and +90. With pulmonary hypertension, enlargement of the right side of the heart causes the mean axis to shift to the right, somewhere between +90 and +180.

24. What type of bronchodilators are albuterol and ipratropium, and what are the possible side effects of these medications? Why give both bronchodilators together?

Albuterol is a sympathomimetic bronchodilator that has fewer side effects than isoproterenol. It is available in oral and aerosol forms. When administered by aerosol it produces significant bronchodilatation within 15 minutes and continues to cause bronchodilatation for 3 to 4 hours. Although tremors, nervousness, and cardiovascular side effects such as tachycardia and palpitations are possible with all beta-agonists, they are less common in patients using this medication. Ipratropium is an anticholinergic bronchodilator that is more effective in causing bronchodilation when combined with albuterol than either agent used alone.

25. What parameters should the RT monitor before, during, and after administration of the medication nebulizer treatments?

RTs should monitor the patient's vital signs, breath sounds, sensorium, and breathing pattern before, during, and after the treatment. Changes in these parameters will help assess the effectiveness of therapy and the onset of complications.

26. How should the overall effectiveness of the bronchodilators be evaluated?

The patient's dyspnea should improve if the bronchodilators are proving beneficial. Changes in breath sounds that indicate bronchodilatation include a decrease in the pitch, length, and intensity of the wheezing. Changes in the patient's breathing pattern with less use of accessory muscles and a shorter expiratory time also indicate improvement.

27. What should the RT do to improve the chances of obtaining an appropriate sputum sample for analysis?

The RT obtaining the sputum sample should explain the procedure to the patient, emphasizing that a true sample of phlegm from the lungs is needed. Asking the patient to rinse his mouth and brush his teeth just before obtaining the sample is a useful way of reducing sputum contamination by oral bacteria. The sample should be collected in a sterile sputum cup and then transported to the laboratory with the lid tightly in place. The patient's name and identification number must be secured to the container.

28. What is the most important advice this patient's physician could give him with regard to his long-term respiratory health?

The best advice health-care personnel can give to this patient is to stop smoking! This advice is easy to give, but not as easy for the patient to follow. Many patients will stop smoking upon the firm recommendation of the physician. The physician may also recommend nicotine gum, nicotine patches, or Welbutrin tablets. These are more effective in conjunction with a formal smoking cessation program. The American Lung Association and American Cancer Society have excellent smoking cessation programs.

 ## Mr. L Conclusion

Over the next several days, Mr. L steadily improves. His initial ABG reveals a PaO_2 of 66 mm Hg on 2 L/min of oxygen by nasal cannula. His dyspnea improves to the point where he can walk around the unit without significant difficulty by the third hospital day. On the fifth day, he is discharged on a regimen of oral antibiotics and oxygen. The attending physician requests a follow-up appointment with Mr. L at the pulmonary outpatient clinic in 1 week. ∎

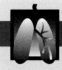

Mrs. G

HISTORY

Mrs. G, a 62-year-old white woman, was seen in the emergency department for complaints of increasing shortness of breath. She stated that she had the flu approximately 1$^1/_2$ weeks earlier and that her breathing has been more difficult since that time. Her ankles have been swollen for the first time, and sleeping during this time has required "two pillows to support her." She stated that occasionally she awakens in the middle of the night very short of breath. These episodes of nocturnal dyspnea are relieved by sitting up for several minutes. She has been producing $^1/_4$ cup of yellow sputum since the onset of the flu. Her exercise tolerance was 1 block but is now 20 feet. Mrs. G stated that 7 years ago her family physician told her she had pulmonary emphysema. Mrs. G started smoking at age 12 and smoked approximately 2 packs of cigarettes a day until she quit 2 years ago. Mrs. G took the following home medications: small-volume nebulizer (SVN) with metaproterenol four times a day, theophylline (Theo-Dur tablets) 200 mg two times a day, and oxygen via nasal cannula at 1 L/min.

QUESTIONS	ANSWERS
1. What symptoms should be explored in greater detail?	The key symptoms include increasing shortness of breath, exercise intolerance, orthopnea, PND, and sputum production. Because pulmonary emphysema is a progressive and chronic disease, gradual worsening of the pathology is expected. However, a sudden decline in respiratory status indicates an acute problem that is exacerbating the COPD. This patient should be questioned about her salt intake, including foods such as olives, pickles, and potato chips; exposure to known respiratory irritants; evidence of infection; and compliance with her treatment program. She should be questioned about subjective evidence of changes in her cardiac status to determine the presence of chest pain, palpitations, or fainting spells.
2. How many pack-years has this patient smoked, and how is this significant in terms of producing pulmonary symptoms?	A 96-pack-year smoking history is present (48 years $\times$ 2 packs per day). Generally a smoking history greater than 20 pack-years is required before symptoms of dyspnea and COPD begin to occur.
3. What is the most likely cause of the patient's pulmonary emphysema?	The most likely cause of the patient's pulmonary emphysema is cigarette smoking. Although men have historically outnumbered women in the development of smoking-related diseases, the increase in the number of female smokers since World War II has led to a related rise in the number of smoking-related diseases in women.

4. What is the most likely cause of the patient's exacerbation?

The patient's exacerbation is probably a result of her recent viral infection. Frequently, any acute illness will further compromise an already borderline respiratory status in COPD patients. Patients should be encouraged to get annual flu shots to minimize the chance of infection-induced exacerbations. This patient's dyspnea appears to be exacerbated by congestive heart failure (requiring several pillows for respiratory comfort at night).

5. What is the pathophysiological significance of the patient's orthopnea and paroxysmal nocturnal dyspnea (PND)?

Orthopnea and PND are generally caused by congestive heart failure. These symptoms occur as pulmonary vascular congestion increases in the reclining position. The congestive heart failure may be caused by ischemic heart disease or cardiomyopathy.

 More on Mrs. G

PHYSICAL EXAMINATION

- **General.** The patient is an alert, cachectic, white woman in moderate respiratory distress, sitting on the edge of her bed leaning forward with her elbows braced on the bedside table. She appears to have difficulty talking secondary to dyspnea and pursed-lip breathing.

- **Vital Signs.** Temperature is 37.0°C (98.6°F) orally; respiratory rate is 28/min; pulse is 108/min; and blood pressure is 142/80 mm Hg.

- **HEENT.** Unremarkable.

- **Neck.** Trachea is midline without stridor or masses. Carotid pulses are ++ without bruits; no lymphadenopathy or thyromegaly present; patient is using her sternocleidomastoid muscles during inspiration; no JVD is present.

- **Chest.** Increased anteroposterior diameter, large supraclavicular fossae, and mild abdominal paradox during respiratory efforts are present; significant protrusion of the ribs with moderate retractions is present during inspiration, with narrowing of the subcostal angle; there is chest expansion of 3 cm at the eighth thoracic vertebra and a diffuse reduction in tactile fremitus on palpation; PMI is not identified with palpation; increased resonance bilaterally on percussion.

- **Heart.** Heart sounds are very distant with a regular rate and rhythm of 108/min without murmurs.

- **Lungs.** There is bilateral reduction in breath sounds anteriorly and posteriorly with a prolonged expiratory phase on auscultation; occasional scattered expiratory wheezes are also present.

- **Abdomen.** Soft, nondistended, and nontender with bowel sounds present; no masses or organomegaly present. The abdomen sinks inward with each inspiratory effort (abdominal paradox).

- **Extremities.** No cyanosis, clubbing, or peripheral edema is present.

QUESTIONS	ANSWERS
6. Why is the patient pursed-lip breathing, and what physiological effect does it produce?	Pursed-lip breathing provides a positive intra-airway pressure that is thought to decrease airway closure and air trapping and to aid gas exchange. Patients often discover this maneuver on their own or learn it through formal instruction by health-care providers, although the exact benefit of this technique has not been established.
7. Why is the patient leaning forward on her elbows to breathe?	By leaning forward on her elbows (tripoding), the patient provides the accessory respiratory muscles with an optimal mechanical advantage by stabilizing the shoulder girdle to which they are attached. This makes the accessory muscles more efficient and may improve ventilation for patients with poor diaphragmatic function.
8. What is the significance of abdominal paradox during respiratory efforts?	Paradoxical abdominal movement during breathing is indicative of diaphragmatic muscle fatigue. When the diaphragm is fatigued, accessory muscles of respiration create a negative intrathoracic pressure, which pulls the fatigued diaphragm slightly upward and into the chest cage, causing the abdominal wall to sink inward rather than rise during inspiration.
9. What pathophysiology accounts for the patient's increased resonance, decreased tactile fremitus and decreased heart sounds?	The patient's increased resonance, decreased tactile fremitus, and decreased heart sounds are a result of the increased intrathoracic volume. The tissue destruction and hyperinflation caused by emphysema lead to poor sound transmission through the chest.
10. Why is the patient's PMI not felt? What is indicated when the PMI is in the epigastric area?	Normally the PMI is located along the left midclavicular line at the level of the fourth or fifth intercostal space. In emphysematous patients, the loss of lung recoil allows the natural tension of the diaphragm to go unopposed and results in flattening of the diaphragms. As a result, the mediastinal structures are elongated and the PMI assumes a more centrally located position lower in the chest or in the epigastric area. The lung hyperinflation in emphysema may reduce the examiner's ability to feel the PMI.
11. What is the significance of the chest expansion measurement?	Chest expansion as measured by palpation is normally 6 to 10 cm. In the case of emphysema, loss of elastic recoil causes chronic hyperinflation, which increases anteroposterior diameter to near maximum, resulting in the reduced ability of the chest cage to move with breathing.

12. What is the cause of the patient's decreased breath sounds?

Decreased breath sounds in patients with pulmonary emphysema result from both decreased sound production and decreased sound transmission. Loss of elastic recoil results in reduced expiratory flow rates, which minimizes turbulent flow sounds during exhalation. The inspiratory sounds are effectively filtered by the relatively large distal airspaces in emphysema, resulting in poor sound transmission to the chest wall.

13. What findings indicate the need for hospitalization?

The need for hospitalization of this patient is indicated by the signs of respiratory distress: (1) respiratory rate greater than 24/min, (2) paradoxical breathing pattern, and (3) use of accessory muscles. In addition, the peripheral edema (ankle swelling) indicates compromise of right heart function (see Appendix B).

Laboratory Evaluation

Chest Radiograph (Fig. 4.5)

ABGs on 1 L/min oxygen

ABG	Value
pH	7.32
$Paco_2$	62 mm Hg
Pao_2	50 mm Hg
HCO_3^-	30 mEq/L
Base Excess (BE)	+5
Hb	13.1 g/100 mL
Sao_2	85.5%
Oxygen-carrying capacity (Cao_2)	15.2 vol%

PFTs (From a previous admission when patient was stable)

	Value	% of Predicted
FVC	1.90 L	58
FEV_1	1.02 L	39
$FEF_{25-75\%}$	0.74 L	31
TLC	5.87 L	117
RV	3.97 L	226
FRC	4.33 L	120
D_{LCO}	6.4 mL/min/mm Hg	26

Complete Blood Count (CBC): Results pending
Chemistry: Results pending
Theophylline level: Results pending
ECG Findings: Sinus tachycardia with decreased voltage in the limb leads; tall, narrow P waves; occasional premature ventricular contractions

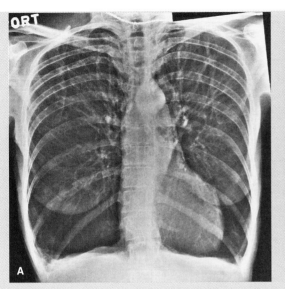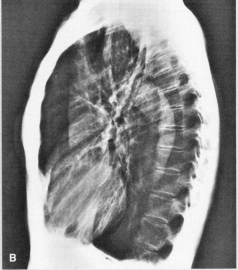

FIGURE 4.5 Mrs. G's chest radiograph.

QUESTIONS	ANSWERS
15. What chest radiograph findings suggest hyperexpansion in this patient?	Hyperexpansion can be assessed by counting the number of ribs seen above the diaphragm on the posteroanterior chest radiograph. More than 10 fully visualized posterior ribs, or 7 anterior ribs, indicates hyperexpansion. In addition, flattened diaphragms, increased intercostal spaces, and increased radiolucency indicate hyperexpansion. The lateral chest radiograph demonstrates flattened diaphragms and a large retrosternal airspace.
16. What is the significance of the decreased vascular markings on the chest radiograph?	Decreased vascular markings on the chest radiograph occur as a result of the pulmonary parenchymal destruction involving not only terminal airspaces, but also pulmonary capillary vasculature. Excessive vascular tapering suggests a more severe case of emphysema.
17. What is the patient's acid-base and oxygenation status?	The elevated $Paco_2$ and HCO_3^- indicate partially compensated respiratory acidosis. The patient has moderate hypoxemia on 1 L/min of oxygen, and other indices of oxygenation are abnormally low. Since Cao_2 takes into account saturation, hemoglobin level, and Pao_2, it can be used to assess oxygen-carrying capacity. The Cao_2 of 15.2 vol% (normally 16 to 20 vol%) is slightly reduced, primarily owing to the low Sao_2.

18. What is the cause of the decreased voltage and tall P waves in the limb leads, as noted on the ECG findings?

Lung hyperinflation and flattening of the diaphragms result in a more vertical position of the heart and a clockwise rotation along its longitudinal axis. This may cause a rightward shift of the QRS axis as measured by the limb leads. The mean QRS axis is also directed posteriorly and perpendicular to the frontal plane in emphysema. Electrical activity that is perpendicular to the frontal plane is not detected by the limb leads, which measure activity only in the frontal plane. As a result of the posterior shift of the mean QRS axis, the limb leads will reveal decreased amplitude. Hyperinflation also reduces the electrical conductivity of the lung, which adds to the decreased voltage seen in the limb leads of the ECG. Tall, narrow P waves (P pulmonale) indicate right atrial enlargement and are characteristic of severe pulmonary disease.

19. How do you interpret the PFT results?

The PFT results are consistent with pulmonary emphysema. The loss of airway elasticity results in collapsible airways and air trapping. The air trapping results in large lung volumes and capacities. The combination of a large intrathoracic volume, slow expiratory flow rates, and reduced diffusion capacity are typical of pulmonary emphysema.

20. What pathology accounts for the decreased D_{LCO}?

The decreased D_{LCO} is caused by the loss of pulmonary vascular bed resulting from tissue destruction and dilation of the terminal lung units. This results in a loss of alveolar/capillary surface area for diffusion.

21. What is your initial assessment of the patient's condition?

The initial assessment of this patient is acute exacerbation of pulmonary emphysema secondary to influenza and heart failure.

22. What treatment do you suggest?

Immediate treatment should consist of oxygen therapy at 2 to 3 L/min via nasal cannula in an attempt to increase the patient's Pa_{O_2} to approximately 60 to 65 mm Hg. Aerosolized adrenergic bronchodilators may prove beneficial to relieve any airway obstruction caused by reactive airways, thus reducing the patient's work of breathing. These can be administered with an MDI or SVN if the patient can take a deep breath spontaneously (greater than 15 mL/kg). IV corticosteroids may also prove useful if a reversible airway obstruction component is present. In this patient, the scattered wheezing suggests that bronchodilators may be beneficial. Sputum collection for Gram stain and culture and sensitivity is warranted in light of the yellow sputum and low-grade fever. Other measures that might prove beneficial should the patient have trouble clearing secretions include bland aerosol therapy and chest physical therapy. Heart failure should be treated with diuretics and vasodilators.

23. Should the patient be monitored for any special adverse reactions to therapy?

Yes, the caregivers should monitor the patient for certain side effects. The possible side effects of sympathomimetic bronchodilators include tachycardia, arrythmias, tremor, nervousness, and anxiety. Since the patient is a chronic CO_2 retainer, the RT should administer oxygen therapy carefully to avoid depressing the patient's hypoxic respiratory drive, thus inducing hypoventilation. Fixed-performance oxygen delivery devices that can administer precise oxygen percentages often can be used to carefully titrate oxygen delivery and minimize the chance of oxygen-induced hypoventilation.

24. Should high oxygen concentrations be administered to this patient if necessary?

High concentrations of oxygen may be lifesaving in certain situations. Oxygen should be administered judiciously to patients who are chronic CO_2 retainers; it should never be withheld for fear of dulling that drive at the expense of tissue oxygenation. Should the patient's drive to breathe diminish and result in an elevated Pa_{CO_2} to the point where the pH is less than 7.25 or the patient's sensorium is abnormal, mechanical ventilation should be used to support ventilation until the patient's respiratory status improves.

 More on Mrs. G

Mrs. G is admitted to the respiratory intensive care unit and started on the following medications: oxygen therapy at 2 L/min via nasal cannula; methylprednisolone (Solu-Medrol) 120 mg IV every 6 hours; SVN with 0.5 mL 0.5% albuterol; and 2.5 mL 0.9% saline every 4 hours and Fursemide 40 mg IV. Sputum for Gram stain and culture and sensitivity, theophylline level, and ABGs on 2 L/min are ordered.

Results of the sputum Gram stain show 2+ pus cells, no epithelial cells, and a few very small gram-negative rods; the culture eventually grows predominantly *Haemophilus influenzae* sensitive to ampicillin. Theophylline level is 8.1 mg/mL. ABG results on 2 L/min are: pH 7.33, Pa_{CO_2} 65 mm Hg, Pa_{O_2} 66 mm Hg, HCO_3^- 31 mEq/L, BE +4, Hb 13.0 g/100 mL, Sa_{O_2} 91.2%, Ca_{O_2} 16.2 vol%.

QUESTIONS	ANSWERS
25. What is the significance of the sputum Gram stain and culture?	The presence of pus cells in the sputum indicates inflammation or infection. The designations 1+, 2+, 3+, and 4+ are used to indicate the number of PMNs per oil immersion field (OIF), which the medical technologist determines in the following manner: 1+ = 1 to 5 PMNs per OIF; 2+ = 6 to 15 PMNs per OIF; 3+ = 16 to 50 PMNs per OIF; and 4+ = more than 50 PMNs per OIF. In addition, the absence of epithelial cells indicates a specimen that was not significantly contaminated by oral secretions. Gram stain and culture are used to identify specific microbe characteristics and to allow selective antimicrobial treatment. *H. influenzae* is a common cause of infection among patients with obstructive lung disease. The sensitivity to ampicillin means the infection should be easy to treat.
26. What antimicrobial agent is indicated?	Ampicillin is a broad-spectrum antibiotic commonly used for the treatment of sensitive strains of *H. influenzae*. It is inexpensive and has few side effects. Unfortunately, the incidence of penicillin-resistant *H. influenzae* infection is increasing.
27. What is the significance of the theophylline level?	The therapeutic theophylline level is 10 to 20 mg/mL of plasma, and a value of 8.1 mg/mL indicates that continuing oral Theo-Dur tablets may be helpful in relieving dyspnea. The serum level should be evaluated periodically. Since toxic side effects of theophylline, such as tremors, insomnia, nausea, seizures, and atrial and ventricular arrhythmias, can be manifested within the therapeutic range, levels should be maintained on the low end.
28. How do you interpret the patient's acid-base and oxygenation status on 2 L/min of O_2?	The patient's ABGs show a partially compensated respiratory acidosis. The administration of oxygen has improved the patient's plasma oxygenation and CaO_2 to an acceptable level, considering the patient's age and disease state. Further increases in PaO_2 can depress the patient's respiratory drive without improving the patient's CaO_2 significantly.

29. Are any other changes in the patient's therapy indicated?

The frequency of the patient's SVN treatments could be increased to every 2 to 3 hours to increase the bronchodilator effect if her pulse rate is not greater than 120/min. Another method of increasing the bronchodilator response would be the administration of an anticholinergic agent, such as ipratropium bromide, in conjunction with the sympathomimetic therapy.

30. By what mechanism other than bronchodilation might theophylline be beneficial in the treatment of emphysema?

In addition to bronchodilation, theophylline causes diaphragmatic stimulation and an increase in central respiratory drive, both of which increase ventilation.

31. If a patient's dyspnea was severe despite bronchodilator therapy, what other therapy might be beneficial?

Low-dose opiate drugs might decrease the subjective sensation of dyspnea. These agents can also increase exercise tolerance in some patients.

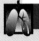 ## Mrs. G Conclusion

Mrs. G is started on ampicillin, and her Theo-Dur continued. The frequency of the SVN treatments is changed to every 3 hours and as needed, with an ipratropium bromide (Atrovent) MDI ordered to follow. During the day, the patient's respiratory status improves, and she feels more comfortable. SVN and MDI are changed to every 4 hours while awake and prn at night. Subsequent follow-up reveals a therapeutic serum theophylline level of 13.5 mg/mL. Over the next 2 days (days 2 and 3), the patient's oxygen is reduced to 1 L/min. At this time her breath sounds are clear, though decreased bilaterally, and her cough produces only opaque-white secretions. The patient is discharged to home on day 5 with the following medications: Theo-Dur 200 mg twice a day; oxygen via nasal cannula at 1 L/min; albuterol sulfate (Ventolin) via MDI 2 puffs every 4 hours and prn for dyspnea, with an Atrovent MDI to follow; and antibiotics. The patient is also encouraged to enter a pulmonary rehabilitation program to help manage her COPD optimally.

QUESTIONS	ANSWERS
32. How could the patient's disease progress and response to bronchodilator therapy be cost-effectively assessed at home?	A disposable peak-expiratory flowmeter can be used to assess therapy response as well as changes in function that may signify exacerbation of the disease process. ■

KEY POINTS

- Chronic obstructive pulmonary disease (COPD) is defined as a lung disease in which the patient has progressive airflow limitation that is not completely reversible. The terms *chronic bronchitis* and *emphysema* are frequently used when discussing COPD.
- The exact incidence of COPD is not known, and estimates are dependent on the definition and criteria used. The number of COPD patients in the United States is estimated to be somewhere between 10 and 22 million.
- There is no doubt that COPD represents a major cause of morbidity and mortality in the United States and around the world and will continue to do so for some time. In addition, the economic burden of COPD on individuals and societies is substantial.
- By far the most common noxious fumes and particles leading to COPD are those associated with cigarette smoke. People who smoke have a much higher incidence of COPD, a larger decline in lung function over time, and a greater COPD mortality rate.
- Cough is the most common symptom seen in patients with COPD, but dyspnea is what causes them to seek medical help.
- Patients with COPD often have diminished breath sounds, a barrel chest, and a prolonged expiratory time and use their accessory muscles to breathe at rest.
- Initially, the arterial blood gas shows mild to moderate hypoxemia with normal $Paco_2$ levels in the patient with COPD. As the disease progresses, the hypoxemia worsens and the patient often begins to retain carbon dioxide.
- The chest x-ray may show minimal changes with mild to moderate COPD. Severe disease causes significant hyperinflation and is seen as a low, flat diaphragm, a large retrostrernal airspace, and a small, narrow heart shadow.
- The classic pattern seen on spirometry in the patient with COPD is reduced expiratory flows that are not responsive to bronchodilators. Vital capacity may be normal or reduced if severe hyperinflation is present. Severe hyperinflation is seen as elevation of the residual volume, the functional residual volume, and the total lung capacity.
- The D_{LCO} is reduced when emphysema is present, owing to destruction of alveolar air spaces.
- The initial goal for treatment of COPD patients is to remove the offending agent from the patient's environment. This usually calls for smoking cessation,which slows the decline in lung function over time.
- Patients with mild to moderate COPD can be treated by their primary care physician with bronchodilators on a prn basis. Those with severe disease should be treated by a pulmonologist who has experience caring for patients with COPD.
- Although bronchodilators do not change the long-term decline in lung function that is the hallmark of the disease, they play a key role in reducing symptoms such as dyspnea and improving the quality of life for COPD patients.
- The initial bronchodilators given to the COPD patient include a beta-agonist, such as albuterol and/or an anticholenergic, such as inhaled ipratropium.

KEY POINTS (CONTINUED)

- Corticosteroids should be added to the treatment plan for patients with moderate to severe COPD.
- Oxygen therapy is needed when the PaO_2 falls below 55 mm Hg or when the SaO_2 falls below 88% at rest. The oxygenation levels of the COPD patient may deteriorate with exercise or sleep and cause polycythemia even though the PaO_2 is acceptable at rest.
- Pulmonary rehabilitation programs are beneficial for the stable COPD patient, as they can improve exercise tolerance and educate the patient about the disease and how to manage it.
- Treating the patient with COPD who is experiencing an acute exacerbation represents a major challenge. An important step in such cases is determining the cause of the exacerbation.
- The first step in treating the patient with an acute exacerbation is to begin controlled oxygen therapy and determine if the problem is life threatening. If the threat is considered serious, the patient is admitted to the ICU.
- Once oxygenation has been optimized, treatment with bronchodilators, corticosteroids, and antibiotics may be needed.
- Short-term ventilatory support may be needed when initial therapy with oxygen, bronchodilators, and corticosteroids does not stabilize the COPD patient and return lung function to an acceptable level as seen on ABGs.
- Noninvasive positive pressure ventilation (NIPPV) has gained popularity since it avoids intubation and the complications associated with it. NIPPV has been shown to improve pH, $PaCO_2$ and PaO_2 and reduces the length of hospital stays.
- Weaning the COPD patient from mechanical ventilation can be a major challenge, especially if the patient has been intubated for more that just a few days and has become dependent on the ventilator. There does not appear to be an advantage in using one method of weaning over another.

REFERENCES

1. Global Initiative for Chronic Obstructive Pulmonary Disease. I. Introduction and Definition. Available at: www.UpToDate.com (accessed 11-04).
2. Mannimo, DM, et al: Chronic obstructive pulmonary disease surveillance: United States, 1971–2000. MMWR Surveill Summ 51:1–16, 2002.
3. Mannino, DM: Epidemiology, prevalence, morbidity, and mortality, and disease heterogeneity. Chest 121:121S–125S, 2002.
4. Sullivan, SD: The economic burden of COPD. Chest 117:5S–9S, 2000.
5. Weiss, ST: Risk factors for COPD. Available at: www.UpToDate.com (accessed 11-04).
6. Global Initiative for Chronic Obstructive Pulmonary Disease. III. Risk Factors. Available at: www.UpToDate.com (accessed 11-04).
7. American Thoracic Society: Standards for the diagnosis and treatment of patients with COPD. Am J Respir Crit Care Med 152:S77, 1995.
8. World Health Organization: The GOLD global strategy for the management and prevention of COPD. Available at: www.goldcopd.com. (accessed 11-04)

9. Sutherland, ER, Cherniack, RM: Management of COPD. N Engl J Med 360L:2689–97, 2005.

10. Ferguson, GT: Overview of management of stable chronic obstructive pulmonary disease. Available at www.UpToDate.com (accessed 11-04).

11. Sin, DD, et al: Contemporary management of COPD. JAMA 290:2313, 2003.

12. In chronic obstructive pulmonary disease, a combination of ipratropium and albuterol is more effective than either agent alone. An 85-day multicenter trial. COMBIVENT Inhalation Aerosol Study Group. Chest 105:1411, 1994.

13. Hanania et al: Chest 124:834, 2003.

14. Global Initiative for COPD. VIII. Component 3: Manage Stable COPD. Available at: www.UpToDate.com (accessed 11-04).

15. Siafakas, NM, et al: Optimal assessment and management of COPD. The European Respiratory Society Task Force. Eur Respir J 8:1398, 1995.

16. Global initiative for COPD. IX. Component 4: Manage exacerbations. Available at: www.UpToDate.com (accessed 11-04).

17. Clinical indications for noninvasive positive pressure ventilation in chronic respiratory failure due to restrictive, COPD, and nocturnal hypoventilation: a consensus conference report. Chest 116:521, 1999.

18. Keenan, SP, et al: Effect of NIPPV on mortality in patients admitted with acute respiratory failure: a meta analysis. Crit Care Med 25:1685, 1997.

5

Cystic Fibrosis

N. Lennard Specht, MD, FACP

CHAPTER OBJECTIVES:

After reading this chapter you will be able to identify:

- The probability of a child being born with cystic fibrosis if both parents are carriers of the cystic fibrosis gene.
- The pathological changes in the lungs and pancreas associated with cystic fibrosis.
- The typical symptoms and physical examination findings associated with cystic fibrosis patients.
- The abnormalities seen on the chest radiograph in patients with cystic fibrosis.
- The typical pulmonary function study results seen in cystic fibrosis patients.
- The common results of sputum analysis from the patient with cystic fibrosis.
- The sweat chloride levels associated with cystic fibrosis in children and adults.
- The treatment of cystic fibrosis patients.
- The prognosis for patients with cystic fibrosis.

INTRODUCTION

Cystic fibrosis is the most common lethal genetic disease in the United States, affecting as many as 1 in 2000 Caucasian children.[1] The disease is typically diagnosed in infancy and causes many organs of the body to malfunction (Box 5.1). The principal problems associated with the disease are bronchiectasis (abnormal dilation of a bronchus), pancreatic exocrine insufficiency, and an elevated sweat electrolyte concentration. Patients with cystic fibrosis typically have more morbidity from pulmonary disease than any other aspect of the disease. Pulmonary disease is also the leading cause of death from cystic fibrosis.[2]

Cystic fibrosis was first formally portrayed in 1936, when Fanconi and colleagues[3] described two children with "cystic fibrosis of the pancreas and bronchiectasis." Cystic fibrosis was probably just as frequent and lethal centuries before Fanconi published his landmark article. In 18th- and 19th-century European literature, there are numerous references to children with abnormalities suggestive of cystic fibrosis. Most of these reports noted a correlation between a child's salty taste when kissed and the likelihood the child would die at a very young age.[4]

ETIOLOGY

Cystic fibrosis is an inherited disease that primarily affects Caucasians of European descent. The inheritance pattern is autosomal recessive, so patients affected by the disease have two genes for cystic fibrosis (one gene given by each parent). Those who have

Box 5.1 Organ Systems Involved in Cystic Fibrosis

Lungs

- Bronchiectasis
- Bronchitis
- Pneumonia
- Atelectasis
- Mucus plugging
- Respiratory failure

Pancreas

- Pancreatic exocrine insufficiency
- Recurrent pancreatitis
- Diabetes mellitus

Sweat Glands

- Increased electrolyte concentration in the sweat

Upper Airway

- Recurrent sinusitis
- Nasal polyps

Intestines

- Meconium plug
- Meconium ileus
- Intussusception

Liver

- Cirrhosis
- Neonatal jaundice

Gallbladder

- Cholelithiasis

Salivary Glands

- Altered electrolyte concentration of secretions

Reproductive System

- Obstructed vas deferens
- Decreased female fertility

only one gene for cystic fibrosis are called carriers. Carriers show no evidence of cystic fibrosis and live healthy lives. If two carriers have a child, however, chances are one in four that the child will have cystic fibrosis. It is estimated that between 1 in 16 to 1 in 35 Caucasians carry the cystic fibrosis gene.[5,6] The frequency of cystic fibrosis births among Asians (1:35, 100) and African Americans (1:15, 100) is much lower than among Caucasians.[5]

The gene responsible for the development of cystic fibrosis has been identified on chromosome 7.[7,8] The gene may be altered (mutated) in more than 1000 different ways; most of these mutations cause cystic fibrosis. The most common abnormality of the gene is deletion of three base pairs in the DNA. This three-base-pair deletion leads to the loss of one amino acid from the protein encoded by the gene. This mutation is known as ΔF508. The ΔF508 gene accounts for 70% to 75% of the genetic abnormalities responsible for cystic fibrosis. The severity of a patient's cystic fibrosis is partly related to the genetic form of the disease that he or she inherits.[9,10]

The cystic fibrosis gene (CFTR) contains the code for a large protein that regulates the flow of chloride ions (salt) through glands that secrete fluids (exocrine glands).[11,12] In addition to regulating chloride movement through the apical cell membrane, the chloride channel appears to have a tight spatial arrangement with many other membrane proteins. This entire complex regulates the flow of ions including chloride, sodium, and ATP across the cell membrane. Mutation of CFTR makes cystic fibrosis patients have a malregulation of the salt composition of their secretions, which is responsible for most, if not all, of the problems that these patients face.

PATHOPHYSIOLOGY

Cystic fibrosis is characterized as a generalized exocrinopathy. To some degree, the disease affects virtually all exocrine glands of the body. The classic triad of exocrine abnormalities consists of pancreatic insufficiency, chronic recurrent pulmonary infections, and an elevated sweat electrolyte concentration.[13]

The pancreas of patients with cystic fibrosis begins to show signs of disease before birth. As the disease progresses, the pancreas becomes smaller and fibrotic. Microscopic examination of the pancreas reveals obstruction of the pancreatic ducts and ductules. This is followed by dilation of the glandular lumen and, eventually, replacement of the exocrine glands with fibrous connective tissue.

Lung disease causes the greatest morbidity and mortality for patients with cystic fibrosis. The three most common pulmonary problems that these patients face are recurrent pulmonary infections, bronchiectasis, and bronchial hyperactivity. These problems may be mild in young children, but their frequency and severity increase as the disease progresses.

In the earliest stages of cystic fibrosis, the lungs often appear normal. As patients mature, however, the lungs show a progressive increase in the size and number of bronchial goblet cells (mucous glands) and inflammation in the peribronchial tissue. The airway mucosa changes from normal epithelium to stratified squamous epithelium in a process called *squamous metaplasia*. In patients who have had pulmonary symptoms for several years, these findings are more widespread and severe. Emphysematous changes are frequently seen, and hemorrhage can be found within the lung. Mucus plugging is seen in small airways, and bronchiectasis is a universal finding.

During the end stages of the disease, obstructive emphysema is frequent, but destruction rarely involves more than 10% of the lung.[14] Mucus plugging is pronounced, and abscesses are found distal to these plugs. Lymph nodes in the hilum of the lung are enlarged.[15]

> The pathological changes in the lungs associated with cystic fibrosis progress over time. Eventually, the lung becomes grossly abnormal owing to hyperinflation, fibrosis, and mucus plugging.

CLINICAL FEATURES

History

Cystic fibrosis is usually first recognized during infancy or childhood, but a small number of patients are diagnosed as young adults. Recurrent pulmonary infections are often the problem that first brings patients with cystic fibrosis to medical attention.[16] Children with cystic fibrosis have more frequent and more prolonged respiratory infections than normal children. Most infants with cystic fibrosis have a chronic cough and wheezing. As the disease progresses, symptoms of bronchiectasis become more prominent. Clubbing of the digits and dyspnea on exertion are also seen. Fevers are seldom present during exacerbations of bronchiectasis but may be very high during episodes of pneumonia. In advanced stages of the disease, complications of lung involvement include hemoptysis (which is occasionally massive), pneumothorax, atelectasis, cor pulmonale, and respiratory failure.

Pancreatic involvement with cystic fibrosis causes pancreatic exocrine insufficiency. The lack of pancreatic enzymes leads to maldigestion and malabsorption.

Pancreatic exocrine insufficiency is associated with diarrhea and stools that contain large amounts of fat. These symptoms are frequently associated with crampy abdominal pain, malnutrition, and failure to maintain a normal growth rate.[17] Other less common gastro-intestinal symptoms include meconium plug, intussusception (slipping of one part of the intestine into another part), rectal prolapse, intestinal obstruction, prolonged neonatal jaundice, hepatic cirrhosis, cholelithiasis (bile stones in gallbladder), recurrent pancreatitis, and diabetes mellitus.

Abnormalities of sweat production result in excessive concentrations of salt in the sweat. This increase in salt leads to a salty taste to the skin and the development of salt crystals on the skin or within clothing, particularly shoes. Loss of electrolytes during warm months of the year can lead to heat intolerance, heat prostration, electrolyte depletion, and dehydration.

Though the most severe respiratory problems occur in the lungs, the upper airway is also affected by cystic fibrosis. Cystic fibrosis patients frequently develop recurrent sinusitis and nasal polyps.

Almost all men and most women with cystic fibrosis are sterile. If a woman with cystic fibrosis becomes pregnant, she is not likely to carry the infant to term. If a woman with cystic fibrosis maintains the pregnancy to term, the infant will be a carrier of the cystic fibrosis gene or may have cystic fibrosis.

Physical Examination

The physical examination of affected patients is nearly always abnormal within a few years after the diagnosis is established. Cystic fibrosis patients are typically thin children or young adults. If respiratory distress is present, accessory muscles of respiration will be used. A productive cough is an almost universal finding. Examination of the extremities may disclose clubbing of the digits. The upper airway may reveal nasal polyps or tenderness over the sinuses. The chest may appear barrel shaped. The lungs usually have diffuse, coarse crackles and wheezes.

In advanced disease, cyanosis around the mouth is associated with hypoxemia. Auscultation of the heart may disclose a loud pulmonic component of the second heart sound (S_2), which is suggestive of pulmonary hypertension. Jugular venous distention and pedal edema are associated with the development of right heart failure (cor pulmonale).

Laboratory Evaluation

Arterial blood gases (ABGs) are nearly normal early in the disease, with an increase only in the alveolar-arterial oxygen gradient $P(A-a)O_2$. Hypoxemia on room air increases as the disease progresses. Hypercapnia and severe hypoxemia occur only with very advanced lung disease.

Serum chemistries and blood counts show no abnormalities unique to cystic fibrosis. With advanced disease, elevation of serum bicarbonate (HCO_3^-) is seen as a result of chronic respiratory failure, and elevations of the hematocrit may reflect chronic hypoxemia. Acute bronchopneumonia can lead to an elevation of the white blood cell (WBC) count, with an accompanying shift to more immature granulocytes. Serum protein and albumin concentrations may be low if malnutrition is present.

Patients with cystic fibrosis typically have pathogenic organisms in their sputum. The three organisms most commonly found are *Staphylococcus aureus*, *Haemophilus influenzae*, and *Pseudomonas aeruginosa*. The strain of *P. aeruginosa* found in patients with cystic fibrosis typically produces mucin. This mucoid form of *P. aeruginosa* is found almost exclusively in the airways of patients with cystic fibrosis. Severe exacerbations may be caused by several different strains of mucin-producing *P. aeruginosa*. A small number of patients with cystic fibrosis become infected with a group of bacteria called *Burkholderia cepacia* complex. Cystic fibrosis patient infected with *B. cepacia* complex have a more rapid loss of lung function[18] and have higher mortality rates if they undergo transplantation.[19] *B. cepacia* complex can be spread by direct contact between patients with cystic fibrosis. It is recommended to isolate patients infected with *B. cepacia* from other cystic fibrosis patients.

Chest Radiograph

The chest radiograph characteristically shows hyperinflation, seen as a flattening of the hemidiaphragms and an increase in the retrosternal airspace (Fig. 5.1). Bronchial wall thickening is commonly seen as parallel lines radiating outward from the hilum (**tram tracks**) (Fig. 5.2). Small, rounded opacities can be seen in the periphery of the lung, which may represent small abscesses distal to impacted airways. These areas of infection usually clear, leaving a residual of small cysts. Other abnormalities seen on chest radiographs include atelectasis, fibrosis, hilar adenopathy, acute bronchopneumonia, and pneumothorax (Fig. 5.3).

Pulmonary Function Studies

Pulmonary function testing is very useful to evaluate the extent of lung disease and follow the rate of disease progression. By following the rate of disease progression, the clinician

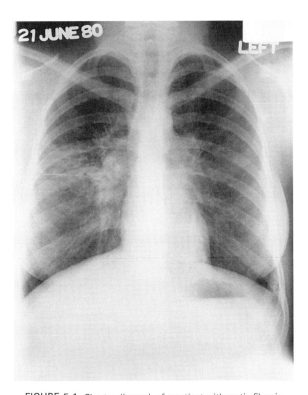

FIGURE 5.1 Chest radiograph of a patient with cystic fibrosis.

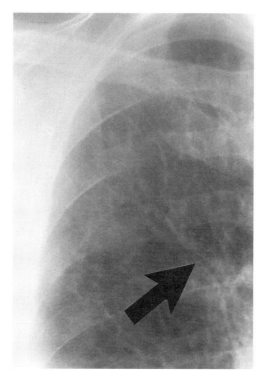

FIGURE 5.2 Close-up of bronchiectatic airway as seen on chest radiograph. Note that the thickened bronchial walls appear as parallel white lines, popularly called "tram tracks."

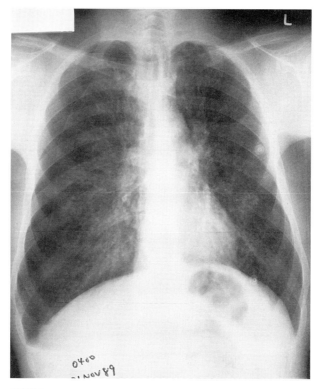

FIGURE 5.3 Chest radiograph of a patient with cystic fibrosis and a right pneumothorax. Note the pleural line visible in the right chest and the absence of lung markings beyond the line.

can increase therapy if lung function deteriorates unexpectedly. Spirometry typically reveals airway obstruction with a reduction in forced expiratory volume in 1 second (FEV_1). Loss of forced vital capacity (FVC) is seen in advanced disease. Both of these changes may improve after the administration of bronchodilators. Residual volume increases early in the course of the disease and can be best measured via body plethysmography.

> The signs of cor pulmonale (e.g., loud P_2 and jugular venous distention) in patients with CF suggest severe disease.

DIAGNOSIS

Sweat chloride measurement has been the standard technique for confirming the diagnosis of cystic fibrosis. Sweat secretion is stimulated, and sweat is collected under an airtight seal. After about 0.1 mL of sweat is collected, the electrolyte concentration is measured. In children, a sweat chloride concentration greater than 60 mEq/L is consistent with the diagnosis of cystic fibrosis.[20] A concentration greater than 80 mEq/L is usually required to confirm the diagnosis of cystic fibrosis in adults.[21] If the concentration is equivocal (50 to 80 mEq/L), a repeat measurement will usually resolve the question. Although the sweat electrolyte concentration is useful for confirming the diagnosis of cystic fibrosis, it must be performed with meticulous attention to detail, or the results may be misleading.[22] The diagnosis of cystic fibrosis can also be established through neonatal screening before symptoms develop.

Discovery of the cystic fibrosis gene has made it possible to perform diagnostic testing for some of the genetic abnormalities associated with cystic fibrosis. Testing for just the DF508 gene will identify about 70% of the abnormal genes or about 50% of affected patients. Testing for all currently known cystic fibrosis genes will identify the vast majority of the abnormal genes responsible for cystic fibrosis. Because routine genetic testing cannot identify 100% of the cystic fibrosis genes, it is best reserved for evaluation of patients with suspected cystic fibrosis who have equivocal results from sweat chloride testing and subjects who require genetic counseling because they are at high risk for having children with cystic fibrosis.[23] If it is likely that a couple will have a child with cystic fibrosis, the fetus can be checked with amniocentesis[24,25] or before implantation following in vitro fertilization.[26,27]

> The sweat chloride test for CF must be performed by experienced clinicians for the results to be most helpful in making the initial diagnosis.

TREATMENT

Initiating early treatment in patients with cystic fibrosis leads to a decreased rate of lung volume loss, improved weight gain, and improved survival rate.[28] The Cystic Fibrosis Foundation has a network of cystic fibrosis centers throughout the United States that monitor their patients frequently and aggressively treat disease flare-ups. Frequent monitoring and aggressive intervention results in improved outcome.[29]

Reversal of the Defect

Cystic fibrosis lung disease is caused by the dysfunction of a protein that regulates electrolyte movement. Several strategies are being attempted to reverse the defective electrolyte transport in the lungs of these patients.

Gene Therapy

Gene therapy holds great promise for patients with cystic fibrosis. If a normal gene for the chloride channel could be inserted into cells and these cells make a normal chloride channel, the molecular defect of the disease would be corrected. Correction of the molecular defect could cure cystic fibrosis. There are two problems gene therapy must overcome before its potential can be reached; first the cells that are most important to correct must be identified, and second, a reliable, safe way of placing a copy of the gene into those cells must be found.

Attempts at gene therapy thus far treat the surface of the airway, correcting only the epithelial cells on the surface. When the epithelial cells are corrected, chloride ions move normally across the airway. The reserve cells that generate future epithelial cells are not corrected, so the genetic correction is lost over a few days through the normal process of epithelial cell replacement. Submucosal glands that make mucous are also not corrected with surface treatments. It is not clear if cells in the submucosal glands need to be corrected to stop the progression of cystic fibrosis lung disease.

The normal gene is transferred to cells using two techniques. One technique uses specialized fat molecules called liposomes that form complexes with DNA. A mixture of liposomes is then applied to the surface of the nose or aerosolized into the airway. A small number of cells would then take up the normal gene from the liposomes and be corrected. A second technique is virally mediated gene transfer. For this technique, the normal chloride channel gene is inserted into a virus that has had its DNA inactivated. When the virus is placed on a respiratory epithelium, it injects the gene into epithelial cells. This technique is intermittently effective at transferring the gene for the normal chloride channel[30–32] but may cause an immune reaction that produces lung inflammation or makes future treatments less effective.[33]

Transplantation

Heart-lung transplantation and bilateral lung transplants have been used successfully to treat patients with end-stage lung disease caused by cystic fibrosis. Transplantation reverses the physiologic abnormalities that characterize cystic fibrosis lung disease[34] but requires immunosuppression, which can lead to opportunistic infections.[35] Indications for transplant include predicted five-year survival less than 30% and FEV_1 less than 30% predicted. Lung transplantation is available only at specialized transplant centers and costs $100,000 to $200,000 depending whether one or both lungs are transplanted.

Pharmacotherapy

Another approach to reversing the defect of cystic fibrosis is to give drugs that eliminate some or all of the abnormal electrolyte transport. Aerosolized amiloride,[36,37] nucleotides (for example adenosine[38,39] or INS37217[40]) may overcome some of the ion transport abnormalities associated with cystic fibrosis. Early trials of these substances have been promising, but it is not known whether these agents alter the course of cystic fibrosis.

Respiratory Secretions

The most significant health threat to cystic fibrosis patients is recurrent respiratory infections. These infections are associated with increased production of mucinous secretions and the tendency to obstruct small- and medium-sized bronchi with mucus plugs. Postural drainage and chest physiotherapy assist patients in clearing mucus plugs. Administration of chest physiotherapy results in an acute improvement in a number of pulmonary function measurements.[41,42] Autogenic drainage is a mechanism that patients use to clear their own pulmonary secretions;[43] it appears to be as effective as chest physiotherapy and postural drainage.[44]

The breakdown of neutrophils is an important cause of sputum viscosity in patients with cystic fibrosis. The DNA of dying neutrophils is released into the sputum, increasing its viscosity. Breaking up the DNA with the recombinant human deoxyribonuclease (DNase) improves sputum viscosity and clearance. The improved ability to clear secretions may be responsible for the reduction in the number of exacerbations patients on inhaled DNase experience. DNase inhalation also improves FEV_1 pulmonary function and reduces the need for antibiotic therapy.[45-47] Regular aerobic exercise also helps clear pulmonary secretions. Trampoline exercise has been recommended for cystic fibrosis patients,[48] but the risk of trampoline-related injuries suggests other forms of exercise are preferable.[49] Additional therapies to assist in bronchial clearance include airway oscillators,[50] voluntary coughing,[51] and the use of a positive expiratory pressure (PEP) mask.[52]

Most other treatments that have been used to help cystic fibrosis patients clear secretions have not been shown to be clearly beneficial and have not been widely adopted. These procedures include the following:

- Administration of mists and aerosols of saline or water to help hydrate secretions and make them easier to expectorate
- Administration of mucolytic aerosols to liquefy mucus plugs
- Bronchoscopy with bronchoalveolar lavage to clear mucus plugs from intermediate and small airways

> The most important management priorities for cystic fibrosis patients involve prevention of respiratory tract infections and early treatment of infections when they occur.

Respiratory Infections

Repeated lung infections are almost universal in patients with cystic fibrosis. These infections lead to destruction of lung tissue and therefore to loss of pulmonary function. Antibiotics are a critical component of the treatment of these infections and preservation of lung function. Although the exact timing for the initiation of antibiotics remains controversial, antibiotics are usually started when new symptoms develop that suggest respiratory infection. These symptoms may include change in cough, new onset of cough, change in character or consistency of sputum, sudden deterioration in pulmonary function, fever, chest radiograph changes, and lack of expected weight gain. The initial choice of antibiotics should be effective against organisms that commonly infect patients with cystic fibrosis. The antibiotic coverage is adjusted once the sputum culture discloses a predominant organism. Serious infections may require IV antibiotics. Prolonged courses of IV antibiotics usually begin in the hospital but may be continued at home after the patient or family has learned to administer the antibiotics.

Oral antibiotics are frequently used for less severe respiratory infections. Fluorinated quinolones belong to a potent class of oral antibiotics, many of which have acceptable activity against *P. aeruginosa*. These oral antibiotics are highly effective at controlling exacerbations of cystic fibrosis, but antibiotic-resistant strains may become a significant problem.[53]

Cystic fibrosis patients with significant pulmonary disease often need a variety of treatment modalities to clear mucus, reduce dyspnea, and treat infections.

Aerosolized tobramycin is well tolerated by children and adults with cystic fibrosis.[54] Tobramycin is typically nebulized twice daily every other month, which has been shown to reduce the frequency of exacerbations and to improve lung function in cystic fibrosis patients with stable disease.

Bronchial Hyperactivity

Many patients with cystic fibrosis have bronchial hyperactivity similar to asthma (see Chapter 3), so the symptoms of bronchial hyperactivity are usually treated with agents used to treat asthma. Treatment includes administration of inhaled or oral beta-agonists and theophylline. Anti-inflammatory agents (e.g., cromolyn sodium, inhaled or oral corticosteroids) have been helpful in some cases.

Airway Inflammation

Recurrent lung infections lead to an intense inflammatory response in the airways of cystic fibrosis patients. Controlling the inflammatory response may preserve lung function and help prolong the lives of these patients.

Giving the anti-inflammatory drug ibuprofen to result in a peak plasma concentration of 50 to 100 mcg/mL significantly slows the progression of lung disease.[55]

Giving the macrolide antibiotic azithromycin 250 mg per day to cystic fibrosis patients who have *P. aeruginosa* in their sputum improves their lung function and quality of life and reduces the frequency of bronchiactatic exacerbations. Because psuedomonas organisms are typically resistant to macrolides, the mechanism of action of azithromycin is unclear. Azithromycin may reduce airway inflammation or it may modify the pseudomonas to make it less pathogenic.[56]

Pancreatic Insufficiency

Patients with cystic fibrosis are frequently malnourished because of pancreatic exocrine insufficiency, inadequate food intake,[57] and the high metabolic demands associated with infection. Pancreatic enzyme replacement is standard therapy for relieving the symptoms of pancreatic exocrine insufficiency. The enzymes are usually given as capsules or pills before every meal and are adjusted to relieve steatorrhea (fatty stools). In addition, fat-soluble vitamins (A, D, E, and K) are routinely supplemented. Patients should be encouraged to eat a balanced diet and avoid excessive fat intake.[58]

PROGNOSIS

The prognosis for patients with cystic fibrosis is steadily improving. At one time, most patients would not live beyond their 10th birthday. Now, with aggressive treatment of this multisystem disease, most cystic fibrosis patients live past age 30.[59]

Ms. M

HISTORY

Ms. M is a 26-year-old woman who presented to the pulmonary clinic for the first time with complaints of dyspnea on exertion and a productive cough. She reports a productive cough for many years and periodically developed yellow or green sputum and occasional hemoptysis. These symptoms were attributed to bronchiectasis. When she was a child, her parents were told she had asthma. She also had many childhood respiratory infections requiring hospitalization. At age 11, she was told she had bronchiectasis. Since that time her therapy included inhaled albuterol and occasional antibiotic therapy. She had no regular pulmonary hygiene program.

Three weeks before admission, an increasingly severe cough producing greenish sputum developed. She also noticed increasing dyspnea on exertion and wheezing. Her family physician gave her a prescription for ciprofloxacin 750 mg twice daily, but her symptoms progressed despite this therapy. Her current symptoms increased to such a degree that she requested sick leave from her job as a secretary.

This is the third such episode Ms. M has experienced in the last year. Her previous episodes were successfully treated with oral ciprofloxacin. She chronically heard wheezing and crackles with breathing, particularly when she went to bed at night. She also had difficulty maintaining weight and felt she was far below her ideal weight. She did not have fever, chills, pharyngitis, cordon, or purulent nasal discharge. She had no problems with steatorrhea (fatty stools), nasal polyps, or sinus infections.

Ms. M never smoked. Her father had a chronic problem with bronchiectasis that began as a teenager. Ms. M had been tested for cystic fibrosis using a sweat chloride concentration when she was first diagnosed with bronchiectasis at age 11. Her sweat chloride concentration was 57 mEq/L.

QUESTIONS	ANSWERS
1. What features of this patient's history support the diagnosis of cystic fibrosis?	A number of features in the history support the suspicion that this woman has cystic fibrosis. The development of bronchiectasis at a young age, particularly in an area of the world where antibiotics are readily available, suggests cystic fibrosis. Children with cystic fibrosis are occasionally misdiagnosed in infancy as having asthma. Her weight loss and inability to maintain a normal body weight are indicative of cystic fibrosis, as are her symptoms of asthma and recurrent pulmonary infections in childhood.
2. Which parts of Ms. M's history suggest that she does not have cystic fibrosis?	This patient lacks certain classic characteristics of cystic fibrosis. She does not have diarrhea or symptoms of malabsorption that suggest pancreatic exocrine insufficiency and she lacks a history of sinus difficulties or nasal polyps.
3. Does her sweat chloride concentration help to clarify whether or not she has cystic fibrosis?	No, a sweat chloride value of between 50 and 80 mEq/L is considered equivocal.

4. What findings would you expect on physical examination if this patient has cystic fibrosis?

You would expect to find a thin, underweight woman with an increased anteroposterior (AP) chest dimension. Her fingers would show clubbing, and if the lung disease was very advanced, she would have some cyanosis. Auscultation of breath sounds would reveal inspiratory crackles and expiratory wheezing. If cor pulmonale was present, one would see distended neck veins and edema in the lower extremities and hear a loud P_2.

5. What additional testing would be appropriate to support or refute the diagnosis of cystic fibrosis?

Because the sweat chloride test done in childhood was equivocal, a repeat sweat chloride test should be performed. If the repeated sweat chloride concentrations are equivocal, then gene probes may be useful to determine whether she is homozygous for the cystic fibrosis genes.

 ## More on Ms. M

PHYSICAL EXAMINATION

- **General.** A thin, young, Caucasian woman with a productive cough; uses accessory muscles of respiration but appears to be breathing comfortably and can converse without apparent dyspnea.

- **Vital Signs.** Temperature 37.2°C; (99.0°F), pulse 71/min, respiratory rate 19/min; blood pressure 105/72 mm Hg.

- **HEENT.** Nasal polyp seen in left nares; no sinus tenderness noted; oral examination normal and mucous membranes moist; eye and ear examinations normal.

- **Neck.** Trachea in midline position; both carotid impulses normal in contour and intensity; no jugular venous distention.

- **Chest.** AP dimensions of chest increased; diffuse inspiratory and expiratory crackles with polyphonic expiratory wheezing heard over both lungs; hyperresonance noted with chest percussion.

- **Heart.** Regular rate with loud P_2 component of S_2 noted on cardiac auscultation; no murmurs or gallops noted; point of maximum impulse (PMI) difficult to appreciate but located in the fifth interspace 2 to 3 cm lateral to sternal border.

- **Abdomen.** Bowel sounds active, with no guarding or tenderness; liver 8 cm in the midclavicular line; no masses palpated.

- **Extremities.** Digital clubbing, but no cyanosis or edema; pulses equal and symmetrical.

QUESTIONS

ANSWERS

6. This patient does not have a fever at the time of examination or a history of fever before this visit. Does the lack of fever indicate that the patient does not have a significant exacerbation of her lung disease?

No. Patients with exacerbations of bronchiectasis typically complain of copious, grossly purulent secretions and dyspnea; however, fever is infrequent during bronchiectatic exacerbations. The best guide to determine the severity of a bronchiectatic exacerbation is the nature and severity of the symptoms. Fever is commonly found with pneumonia or viral respiratory infections; thus, if Ms. M had presented with a fever, pneumonia or viral illness would have been the most likely cause.

7. What is the significance of Ms. M's underweight appearance?

The underweight appearance is suggestive of cystic fibrosis in patients with symptoms such as these. Malnutrition develops in these patients as a result of (1) malabsorption owing to pancreatic exocrine insufficiency, (2) a lower than normal caloric intake, and (3) increased metabolic demands owing to respiratory effort and recurrent infections.

8. What is a nasal polyp, and what respiratory problems may it create?

A nasal polyp is an overgrowth of mucosa in the nose that leads to a fingerlike growth. These polyps tend to form in cystic fibrosis patients, and they may become so numerous or large that they completely block the nasal passages.

9. What is indicated by an increase in the AP dimension of the chest?

When the lungs become hyperexpanded because of air trapping, the chest enlarges, particularly in the AP dimension. This increase in chest diameter is associated with emphysema, chronic bronchitis, asthma, and cystic fibrosis.

10. What is the significance of the crackles heard over the lungs?

Crackles are associated with increased pulmonary secretions. In advanced cases of cystic fibrosis, the lung examination will almost always disclose crackles. The presence of crackles in this case does not necessarily represent pulmonary edema or pneumonia.

11. The S_2 has two components: an aortic sound (A_2) and a pulmonic sound (P_2). Describe the source of these heart sounds and the meaning of a loud P_2.

The S_2 has two components. One is created when the aortic valve closes (A_2) and the other is produced when the pulmonic valve closes (P_2). Normally, A_2 is louder than P_2; the reverse is suggestive of pulmonary hypertension.

12. Why does this patient have a cardiac PMI that is decreased in intensity and displaced from the normal position?

As the lungs hyperexpand because of obstructive lung disease, the heart is forced to assume a more vertical and central position in the chest. This change in position can be seen on physical examination by a movement of the PMI centrally and toward the epigastrium.

13. This patient has digital clubbing. What does clubbing of the fingers look like, and what it may indicate?

Clubbing is enlargement of the tips of the fingers and toes; it is convexity of the nails and is often seen in patients with chronic lung disease. It is unclear why clubbing develops in these patients.

14. What laboratory work should be ordered at this time?

Several questions should be clarified before the optimum treatment program can be initiated:

a. Does she have pneumonia or just an exacerbation of her bronchiectasis?
b. Is her dyspnea due, in part, to hypoxemia?
c. Is her nutrition adequate?

To evaluate for pneumonia, a chest radiograph plus a WBC count and differential should be ordered. Hypoxemia can be identified by ABG analysis. If chronic hypoxemia is present, there is usually an elevation of the hemoglobin concentration or the hematocrit. Malnutrition can be evaluated by measurements of serum proteins such as prealbumin, albumin, and total protein.

Box 5.2 Laboratory Evaluation

Chest Radiograph (Fig. 5.4)

ABGs (on room air)	
ABG	Value
pH	7.42
$Paco_2$	34 mm Hg
Pao_2	67 mm Hg
HCO_3^-	21 mEq/L
$P(A-a)O_2$	39 mm Hg
O_2 content	17.5 mL/dL

Complete Blood Count:		
	Observed	Normal
WBCs/mm^3	12,400	4,000–11,000
Red blood cells (M/mL)	4.7	4.1–5.5
Hemoglobin (g/dL)	14.2	14–16.5
Hematocrit (%)	43	37–50
Differential		
Segmented neutrophils (%)	72	38–79
Band neutrophils (%)	12	0–7
Lymphocytes (%)	13	12–51
Monocytes (%)	1	0–10
Eosinophils (%)	1	0–8
Basophils (%)	1	0–2

(box continued on page 113)

Chemistry:

	Observed	Normal
Na^+ (mEq/L)	138	136–146
K^+ (mEq/L)	4.6	3.5–5.1
Cl^- (mmol/dL)	106	98–106
HCO_3^- (mm/L)	20	22–29
BUN (mg/dL)	13	7–18
Creatinine (mg/dL)	0.7	0.5–11
Calcium (mmol/L)	2.1	2.1–255
Phosphate (mg/dL)	2.7	2.7–4.5
Uric acid (mg/dL)	3.4	4.5–8.2
Albumin (g/dL)	3.1	3.5–5.0
Protein (g/dL)	6.0	6.4–8.3

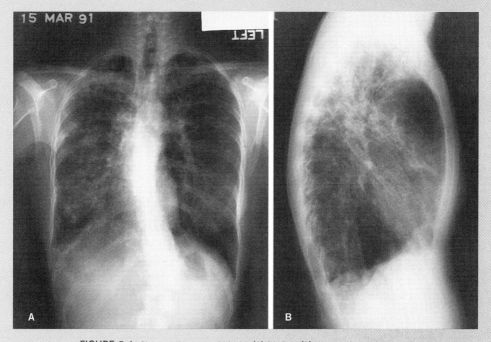

FIGURE 5.4 Chest radiograph of Ms. M. (A) PA film. (B) Lateral view.

QUESTIONS

15. How would you correlate Ms. M's chest radiograph with her condition?

ANSWERS

Scoliosis is noted in the thoracic and lumbar spine. The lungs are hyperexpanded with diffuse reticular nodular opacities throughout both lungs. Numerous cystic airspaces are seen, as are occasional thickened bronchial walls. This radiograph is consistent with a patient with bronchiectasis or cystic fibrosis. Although the disease is more pronounced in the right lung, no focal areas of pneumonia are seen. This woman appears very thin, with no excessive soft tissue shadows.

16. How would you interpret the ABGs?

Ms. M has a chronic respiratory alkalosis and a widened $P(A-a)o_2$. Mild hypoxemia is present.

17. Why are the WBC count and the number of band neutrophils elevated?

An acute infection of any type can elevate the WBC count and lead the bone marrow to release immature neutrophils (bands) into the blood to help fight the infection. In this case, the elevation is most likely due to either pneumonia or an exacerbation of bronchiectasis.

18. What do a low albumin and total protein level indicate?

Both of these serum proteins are likely to be depressed in the setting of malnutrition.

19. What additional diagnostic tests would be important to obtain?

With any infection, selection of the appropriate antibiotic is easiest if the physician knows the offending organism. It is important to culture the sputum to determine, if possible, what organism is causing her infection. Identifying the infecting organism in this case is very important, because Ms. M has already failed to respond to one course of antibiotics.

20. If the physician decides to admit this patient to the hospital, what respiratory therapy orders would you suggest?

Respiratory therapy should aim to reverse bronchospasm and assist in the clearance of secretions. Inhaled beta-agonists will help reverse bronchospasm. The optimum method of delivering beta-agonists is not clearly defined. Either a metered-dose inhaler (MDI) or a nebulized solution would be appropriate. To help clear secretions, chest physiotherapy and postural drainage should also be started. Other therapies, such as mist tents, bland aerosol therapy, and N-acetyl-L-cysteine, have been used to help patients clear pulmonary secretions, but they have not proved effective.

 More on Ms. M

Ms. M fails to improve on oral antibiotics, and her physician admits her to the medicine service for more aggressive treatment. The admitting orders include the following:

- Supplemental vitamins A, D, E, and K

- Aminophylline 1 g in 0.25 L normal saline: an initial IV infusion of 5 mg/kg over 30 minutes, then constant infusion at a rate of 0.5 mg/kg/hour

- Piperacillin IV 1 g every 6 hours

- Chest physiotherapy and postural drainage every 6 hours

- Theophylline level on the second hospital day

- Amikacin level before and after the third dose of amikacin

- Sputum Gram stain and culture

- Sweat chloride concentration

- Gene probe for the ΔF508 gene

QUESTIONS	ANSWERS
21. The admitting physician believes Ms. M may have cystic fibrosis. Why did the physician prescribe the supplemental A, D, E, and K vitamins?	Ms. M appears mildly malnourished on physical examination and on her admitting laboratory work-up. If she has cystic fibrosis she may have difficulty absorbing fat and the fat-soluble vitamins. To overcome the vitamin deficiency, these patients are generally given the supplemental fat-soluble vitamins A, D, E, and K.
22. What is albuterol? What are the potential side effects?	Albuterol is an inhaled beta-agonist. The purpose of giving it to this patient is to reverse bronchospasm, which is the cause of her wheezing and some of her dyspnea. The primary side effects of albuterol are tachycardia, tachyarrhythmias, and tremors.
23. Is the prescribed chest physiotherapy and postural drainage important for this patient, or should you recommend that it be discontinued? Why?	Chest physiotherapy is very important for patients with bronchiectasis and cystic fibrosis. Mucus plugs in the distal airways may obstruct these airways and cause right-to-left shunting, leading to small, distal abscesses. Therefore, clearance of mucus plugs is very important for patients with cystic fibrosis. Chest physiotherapy and postural drainage will help move these mucus plugs from the distal airways to the large central airways, from which they can be expectorated.
24. What is the most important thing that you as a respiratory care practitioner could teach this patient to help in her long-term health?	Ms. M has had no program of bronchial hygiene. She should be instructed in postural drainage, and a family member should be taught to perform chest physiotherapy. Other therapies that may assist bronchial hygiene include regular exercise and the use of PEP by mask or mouthpiece.
25. If this patient is found to have cystic fibrosis, what organisms would you expect to find on the sputum culture?	The three organisms most commonly found in the tracheal secretions of patients with cystic fibrosis include *H. influenzae*, *S. aureus*, and *P. aeruginosa*.
26. One of the microorganisms that patients with cystic fibrosis commonly have as a respiratory pathogen has a unique characteristic. What is unique about the *P. aeruginosa* found in cystic fibrosis patients?	The *P. aeruginosa* organism that infects patients with cystic fibrosis differs from the vast majority of *P. aeruginosa* isolates in that it produces mucin.
27. If Ms. M is found to have cystic fibrosis, what are the odds that she will have both copies of the ΔF508 gene?	The ΔF508 gene accounts for about 70% of the abnormal genes that cause cystic fibrosis. To have the disease, the affected individual must have two genes that cause cystic fibrosis. The chance that an individual with cystic fibrosis has both ΔF508 genes is $(0.7 \times 0.7 \times 100) = 49\%$.

More on Ms. M

The sputum culture grows a mucinous strain of *P. aeruginosa* that is resistant to ciprofloxacin. Ms. M's sweat chloride concentration is 103 mEq/L. The gene probe reveals only one copy of the ΔF508 gene.

QUESTIONS	ANSWERS
28. What effect does inhaled DNase have on the sputum of patients with cystic fibrosis?	DNase breaks up the DNA in the sputum of patients with cystic fibrosis. This effect decreases the viscosity of the sputum and makes it easier to expectorate. The administration of inhaled DNase in patients with cystic fibrosis has been shown to improve FEV_1, prolong the time between respiratory exacerbations, and improve survival.
29. Does Ms. M have cystic fibrosis?	Yes, the elevation of sweat chloride to 103 mEq/L confirms that Ms. M has cystic fibrosis. The gene probe found that Ms. M is heterozygous for the ΔF508 gene; however, there are several mutations of the gene other than ΔF508 that can lead to cystic fibrosis. The ΔF508 gene accounts for only 70% of the genes causing cystic fibrosis. Therefore, it is not surprising that Ms. M has only one of the ΔF508 genes yet still has cystic fibrosis.

Ms. M Conclusion

Ms. M. is hospitalized for 5 days. During this time she receives antibiotics, bronchodilators, inhaled DNase, and chest physiotherapy. Her symptoms improve greatly, showing marked reduction in coughing and dyspnea. She produces far less sputum, and the color is light yellow. She is trained to administer her own IV antibiotics and to perform postural drainage; her husband is trained to deliver chest percussion. Ms. M is discharged with a follow-up appointment with a pulmonary specialist.

Ms. M is a typical example of an older patient with cystic fibrosis. She has many classic features of the disease, but also lacks a significant number of common abnormalities. Pancreatic exocrine insufficiency is one classic finding that she does not have. Patients with normal pancreatic exocrine function have a better prognosis than those with pancreatic dysfunction.[60] ■

KEY POINTS

- Cystic fibrosis is the most common lethal genetic disease in the United States, affecting as many as 1 in 2000 Caucasian children.
- Cystic fibrosis is an inherited disease that primarily affects whites of European descent. The inheritance pattern is autosomal recessive, so patients affected by the disease have two genes for cystic fibrosis (one gene given by each parent).
- Those who have only one gene for cystic fibrosis are called carriers. Carriers show no evidence of cystic fibrosis and live healthy lives. If two carriers have a child, however, chances are one in four that the child will have cystic fibrosis.
- Cystic fibrosis is characterized as a generalized exocrinopathy. To some degree, the disease affects virtually all exocrine glands of the body. The classic triad of exocrine abnormalities consists of pancreatic insufficiency, chronic recurrent pulmonary infections, and an elevated sweat electrolyte concentration.
- Lung disease causes the greatest morbidity and mortality for patients with cystic fibrosis. The three most common pulmonary problems that these patients face are recurrent pulmonary infections, bronchiectasis, and bronchial hyperactivity.
- Recurrent pulmonary infections are often the problem that first brings patients with cystic fibrosis to medical attention.
- Pancreatic exocrine insufficiency is seen in cystic fibrosis patients and is associated with diarrhea and stools that contain large amounts of fat. These symptoms are frequently associated with crampy abdominal pain, malnutrition, and failure to maintain a normal growth rate.
- The chest radiograph characteristically shows hyperinflation, bronchial wall thickening (tram tracks), and small, rounded opacities in the periphery of the lung, which may represent small abscesses distal to impacted airways. These areas of infection usually clear, leaving a residual of small cysts.
- Other abnormalities seen on chest radiographs may include atelectasis, fibrosis, hilar adenopathy, acute bronchopneumonia, and pneumothorax.
- Spirometry typically reveals airway obstruction by demonstrating a reduction in forced expiratory volume in 1 second (FEV_1). Loss of forced vital capacity (FVC) is seen in advanced disease.
- Sweat chloride measurement has been the standard technique for confirming the diagnosis of cystic fibrosis. Sweat secretion is stimulated, and sweat is collected under an airtight seal. After about 0.1 mL of sweat is collected, the electrolyte concentration is measured.
- In children, a sweat chloride concentration greater than 60 mEq/L is consistent with the diagnosis of cystic fibrosis. A concentration greater than 80 mEq/L is usually required to confirm the diagnosis of cystic fibrosis in adults.
- Gene therapy is being developed to reverse the defective electrolyte transport in the lungs of cystic fibrosis patients.
- Heart-lung transplantation and bilateral lung transplants have been used successfully to treat patients with end-stage lung disease caused by cystic fibrosis.
- Postural drainage and chest physiotherapy assist cystic fibrosis patients in clearing mucus plugs. Chest physiotherapy results in an acute improvement in a number of pulmonary function measurements.

(key points continued on page 118)

KEY POINTS (CONTINUED)

- Antibiotics are a critical component of the treatment of respiratory infections and therefore preservation of lung function. Antibiotics are usually started when new symptoms develop that suggest respiratory infection. These symptoms may include change in cough, new onset of cough, change in character or consistency of sputum, sudden deterioration in pulmonary function, fever, chest radiograph changes, or lack of expected weight gain.
- The symptoms of bronchial hyperactivity are common in cystic fibrosis patients and are usually treated with agents used to treat asthma. Treatment includes the administration of inhaled or oral beta-agonists and theophylline.
- Giving the anti-inflammatory drug ibuprofen to result in a peak plasma concentration of 50 to 100 mcg/mL significantly slows the progression of lung disease.
- Pancreatic enzyme replacement is standard therapy for relieving the symptoms of pancreatic exocrine insufficiency in cystic fibrosis patients.
- The prognosis for patients with cystic fibrosis is steadily improving.

REFERENCES

1. Conneally, PM, et al: Cystic fibrosis: Population genetics. Tex Reprod Biol Med 31:639, 1973.
2. Levison, H, Tabachnik, E: Pulmonary physiology. In Hodson, ME, et al (eds): Cystic Fibrosis. Baillière Tindall, London, 1983, pp. 52–81.
3. Fanconi, G, et al: Das coeliakiesyndrom bei angeborener zysticher pankreasfibromatose und bronchiektasien. Wein Med Wochnschr 86:753, 1936.
4. Taussig, LM: Cystic Fibrosis. Thieme-Stratton, New York, 1984.
5. Palomaki GE: Clinical sensitivity of prenatal screening for cystic fibrosis via CFTR carrier testing in a United States panethnic population. Genet Med 6:405, 2004.
6. Castellani C, et al: Cystic fibrosis carriers have higher neonatal immunoreactive trypsinogen values than non-carriers. Am J Med Genet A 135:142, 2005.
7. Riordan, JR, et al: Identification of the cystic fibrosis gene: Cloning and characterization of the complementary DNA. Science 245:1066, 1989.
8. Rommens, JM, et al: Identification of the cystic fibrosis gene: Chromosome walking and jumping. Science 245:1059, 1989.
9. Kerem, E, et al: The relation between genotype and phenotype in cystic fibrosis of the most common mutation (delta F508). N Engl J Med 323:1517, 1990.
10. Garcia J, et al: Genotype-phenotype correlation for pulmonary function in cystic fibrosis. Thorax 60:558, 2004.
11. Rich, DP, et al: Expression of cystic fibrosis transmembrane conductance regulator corrects defective chloride channel regulation in cystic fibrosis airway epithelial cells. Nature 347:358, 1990.
12. Anderson, MP, et al: Generation of cAMP-activated chloride currents by expression of CFTR. Science 251:679, 1991.
13. Quinton, PM, Bijman, J: Higher bioelectric potentials due to decreased chloride absorption in the sweat glands of patients with cystic fibrosis. N Engl J Med 308:1185, 1983.
14. Esterly, JR, Oppenheimer, EH: Observations in cystic fibrosis of the pancreas. Part III. Pulmonary lesions. Johns Hopkins Med J 122:94, 1968.
15. Bedrossian, CWM, et al: The lung in cystic fibrosis: A quantitative study including prevalence of pathologic findings among different age groups. Hum Pathol 7:195, 1976.
16. Rosenstein, BJ, Langbaum, TS: Diagnosis. In Taussig, LM (ed): Cystic Fibrosis. Thieme Stratton, New York, 1984.
17. Schwachman, H: Gastrointestinal manifestations of cystic fibrosis. Pediatr Clin North Am 22:787, 1975.
18. Courtney JM, et al: Clinical outcome of Burkholderia cepacia complex infection in cystic fibrosis adults. J Cyst Fibros.3:93, 2004.
19. de Perrot, M, et al: Twenty-year experience of lung transplantation at a single center: Influence of recipient diagnosis on long-term survival. J Thorac Cardiovasc Surg 127:1493, 2004.
20. Gibson, LE, Cook, RE: A test of concentration of electrolytes in sweat in cystic fibrosis of the pancreas utilizing pilocarpine iontophoresis. Pediatrics 23:545, 1959.

21. Report of the Committee for a Study for Evaluation of Testing for Cystic Fibrosis. National Academy of Sciences, Washington, DC, 1975.

22. Rosenstein, BJ, et al: Cystic fibrosis: Problems encountered with sweat testing. JAMA 240:1987, 1978.

23. Statement from the National Institutes of Health Workshop in Population Screening for the Cystic Fibrosis Gene. N Engl J Med 323:70, 1990.

24. Jedlicka-Kohler, I, et al: Utilization of prenatal diagnosis for cystic fibrosis over the past seven years. Pediatrics 94:13, 1994.

25. Wertz, DC, et al: Attitudes toward the prenatal diagnosis of cystic fibrosis: Factors in decision making among affected families. Hum Genet 50:1077, 1992.

26. Cui, KH, et al: Optimal polymerase chain reaction amplification for preimplantation diagnosis in cystic fibrosis (delta F508). BMJ 311:536, 1995.

27. Storm, CM, et al: Reliability of polymerase chain reaction (PCR) analysis of single cells for preimplantation genetic diagnosis. J Assist Reprod Genet 11:55, 1994.

28. Dankert-Roelse, JE, te Meerman, GJ: Long term prognosis of patients with cystic fibrosis in relation to early detection by neonatal screening. Thorax 50:712, 1995.

29. Johnson, C, et al: Factors influencing outcomes in cystic fibrosis: A center-based analysis. Chest 123:20, 2003.

30. Drumm, ML, et al. Correction of cystic fibrosis defect in vitro by retrovirus mediated gene transfer. Cell 74:215, 1993.

31. Hay, JG, et al: Modification of nasal epithelial potential differences of individuals with cystic fibrosis consequent to local administration of normal CFTR cDNA adenovirus gene transfer vector. Hum Gene Ther 6:1487, 1995.

32. Knowles, MR, et al: A controlled study of adenoviral-vector-mediated gene transfer in the nasal epithelium of patients with cystic fibrosis. New Engl J Med 333:823, 1995.

33. Middelton, PG, et al: Gene therapy for cystic fibrosis: Which postman, which box? Thorax 53:197, 1998.

34. Alton, EW, et al: Effect of heart lung transplantation on airway potential difference in patients with and without cystic fibrosis. Eur Respir J 4:5, 1991.

35. Higenbottam, TW, et al: Mortality and morbidity following heart-lung transplantation for cystic fibrosis. Am Rev Respir Dis 141:605, 1990.

36. Knowles, MR, et al: A pilot study of aerosolized amiloride for treatment of lung disease in cystic fibrosis. N Engl J Med 322:1189, 1990.

37. Middleton, PG, Kidd, TJ, Williams, B: Combination aerosol therapy to treat Burkholderia cepacia complex. Eur Respir J 26:305, 2005.

38. Knowles, MR, et al: Activation by extracellular nucleotides of chloride secretion in the airway epithelia of patients with cystic fibrosis. N Engl J Med 325:533, 1991.

39. Jones, JR, et al: Extracellular zinc and ATP restore chloride secretion across cystic fibrosis airway epithelia by triggering calcium entry. J Biol Chem 12;279:10720, 2004.

40. Kunzelmann, K, et al. Pharmacotherapy of the ion transport defect in cystic fibrosis: Role of purinergic receptor agonists and other potential therapeutics. Am J Respir Med 2:299, 2003.

41. Desmond, KJ, et al: Immediate and long term effects of chest physiotherapy in patients with cystic fibrosis. J Pediatr 103:538, 1983.

42. Maxwell, M, Redmond, AO: Comparative trial of manual and mechanical percussion technique with gravity-assisted bronchial drainage in patients with cystic fibrosis. Arch Dis Child 54:542, 1979.

43. Partridge, C, et al: Characteristics of the forced expiration technique. Physiotherapy 75:193, 1989.

44. Giles, DR, et al: Short-term effects of postural drainage with clapping vs autogenic drainage on oxygen saturation and sputum recovery in patients with cystic fibrosis. Chest 108:952, 1995.

45. Hubbard, RC, et al: A preliminary study of aerosolized recombinant deoxyribonuclease I in the treatment of cystic fibrosis. N Engl J Med 326:812, 1992.

46. Aitken, ML, et al: Recombinant human DNase inhalation in normal subjects and patients with cystic fibrosis. JAMA 267:1947, 1992.

47. Fuchs, HJ, et al: Effect of aerosolized recombinant human DNase on exacerbations of respiratory symptoms and on pulmonary function in patients with cystic fibrosis: The Pulmozyme Study Group. N Engl J Med 331:637, 1994.

48. Stanghelle JK, et al: Effect of daily short bouts of trampoline exercise during 8 weeks on the pulmonary function and the maximal oxygen uptake of children with cystic fibrosis. Int J Sports Med 9(suppl 32), 1988.

49. Barak A, et al: Trampoline use as physiotherapy for cystic fibrosis patients. Pediatr Pulmonol 39:70, 2005.

50. Konstan, MW, et al: Efficacy of the Flutter device for mucous clearance in patients with cystic fibrosis. J Pediatr 124:689, 1994.

51. Zimman, R: Cough versus chest physiotherapy: A comparison of the acute effects on pulmonary function in patients with cystic fibrosis. Am Rev Respir Dis 129:182, 1984.

52. Steen, HJ, et al: Evaluation of the PEP mask in cystic fibrosis. Acta Paediatr Scand 51, 1991.

53. Radberg, G, et al: Development of quinolone-imipenem cross resistance in *Pseudomonas aeruginosa* during exposure to ciprofloxacin. Antimicrob Agents Chemother 34:2142, 1990.

54. Fiel, SB: Aerosol delivery of antibiotics to the lower airways of patients with cystic fibrosis. Chest 107:615, 1995.

55. Konstan MW, et al. Effect of high-dose ibuprofen in patients with cystic fibrosis. N Engl J Med 332:848, 1995.

56. Saiman L, et al: Azithromycin in patients with cystic fibrosis chronically infected with *Pseudomonas aeruginosa*: a randomized controlled trial. JAMA. 290:1749, 2003.

57. Hubbard, VS, Mangrum, PJ: Energy intake and nutritional counseling in cystic fibrosis. J Am Diet Assoc 80:127, 1982.

58. Dodge, JA: Nutrition. In Hodson, ME, et al (eds): Cystic Fibrosis. Baillière Tindall, London, 1983, pp. 132–141.

59. Patient Registry, Cystic Fibrosis Foundation.

60. Gaskin, K, et al: Improved respiratory prognosis in patients with cystic fibrosis with normal fat absorption. J Pediatr 100:857, 1982.

6

Hemodynamic Monitoring and Shock

Robert L. Wilkins, PhD, RRT, FAARC

James R. Dexter, MD, FACP, FCCP

CHAPTER OBJECTIVES:

After reading this chapter you will be able to state or identify the following:

- The definition of cardiac output, cardiac index, and circulatory shock.
- The factors that determine cardiac output.
- The three general causes of shock.
- The effects of shock on vital organ functions.
- The clinical features and hemodynamic findings typical for the different types of shock.
- The treatment for each type of shock.

INTRODUCTION

The circulatory system is composed of the heart, blood vessels, and blood. Each component plays a vital role in the process of circulation. The heart is the pump that provides the power to move blood throughout the blood vessels (perfusion). The blood vessels direct the blood from the heart to the tissues through arteries and capillaries and back to the heart through veins. The arteries are endowed with smooth muscle, which provides variable resistance to flow to help maintain the blood pressure (BP) needed for perfusion. Blood is the medium in which oxygen and other nutrients are carried to the tissues.

Supplementary organs involved in circulation include the lungs, which provide oxygen; the bone marrow, which provides red blood cells; the liver, which processes nutrients from the digestive tract; and the nervous system, which regulates muscle tone in the arteries.

The circulatory system can be divided into two major parts: the pulmonary system and the systemic system. The pulmonary system is made up of the right side of the heart (right atrium and right ventricle), pulmonary arteries, and pulmonary veins. The pulmonary arteries direct blood from the right ventricle to the lungs for gas exchange. The pulmonary veins conduct the oxygenated blood from the lungs back to the left side of the heart. The systemic system is made up of the left side of the heart (left atrium and left ventricle), the arteries, and the veins. The systemic arteries carry oxygenated blood from the left heart to the different organ systems, where oxygen and nutrients are given up to the tissues and metabolic waste products are removed. The veins return the partially deoxygenated blood back to the right side of the heart.

Because the purpose of circulation is to provide the organs of the body with oxygen and other vital nutrients, circulatory failure is defined in terms of vital organ system dysfunction. The patient is said to have circulatory failure, or **shock**, when circulation is not sufficient to meet the metabolic needs of vital organs such as the brain, heart, and kidneys. The primary problem associated with shock is the lack of adequate tissue oxygenation. Although the effects of inadequate tissue oxygenation are initially reversible, persistent hypoxia leads to complex changes that eventually cause irreversible tissue death.

WHAT IS CARDIAC OUTPUT?

The pumping function of the left ventricle is very important, since it moves the oxygenated blood to all areas of the body. The quantity of blood pumped out of the left ventricle each minute is known as the **cardiac output**. Normally, the adult cardiac output is 4 to 8 L/min. Since normal cardiac output is dependent on the size and metabolic rate of the patient, clinicians must interpret it in relation to the patient's body mass and metabolic rate. A cardiac output of 3.5 L/min might be acceptable for a petite, afebrile, resting woman, whereas this same value could represent a circulatory crisis for a large, male patient with a fever.

> The volume of blood pumped out of the left ventricle each minute is known as the cardiac output. The cardiac output divided by the body surface area (obtained from nomogram) is known as the cardiac index.

Cardiac index (cardiac output/body surface area) is a useful parameter because it accounts for variations in body size. The patient's body surface area in square meters can be determined from standard nomograms and is divided into the cardiac output to determine cardiac index. A normal cardiac index is 2.5 to 4.0 L/min/m^2.

WHAT DETERMINES CARDIAC OUTPUT?

Cardiac output is the product of heart rate and stroke volume (the volume of blood ejected by the ventricle with each contraction). Heart rate is strongly influenced by the sympathetic and parasympathetic nervous systems. Activation of the sympathetic nervous systems leads to tachycardia and usually increases cardiac output except at extremes. Stimulation of the parasympathetic nervous system promotes bradycardia, and profound bradycardia may reduce cardiac output.

Stroke volume is a function of three important factors: filling volume of the ventricle (**preload**), arterial resistance to flow out of the ventricle during contraction (**afterload**), and ventricular contractility (Fig. 6.1). Bedside clinicians must evaluate all three factors in patients with circulatory insufficiency.

Preload

The strength of myocardial muscle contraction is directly related (within limits) to the amount of stretch applied to the muscle prior to contraction. This precontraction stretch

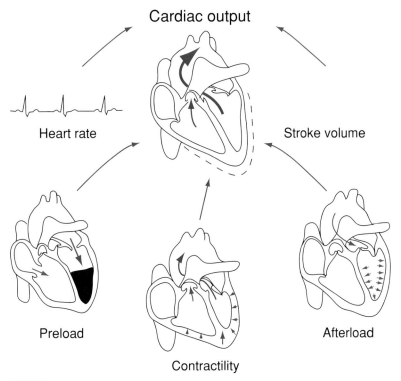

Cardiac output

Heart rate

Stroke volume

Preload

Contractility

Afterload

FIGURE 6.1 Factors determining cardiac output are stroke volume and heart rate. Stroke volume is determined by preload, afterload, and contractility. (From Wilkins, RL, Sheldon, RL, Krider, SJ: Clinical Assessment in Respiratory Care, Mosby–Year Book, St. Louis, 2005, with permission.)

is known as preload and is primarily a function of venous pressure, which determines the volume in the ventricle just prior to contraction. Up to a certain point, the more the ventricle is stretched during ventricular filling (diastole), the greater the force of the subsequent contraction and the greater the stroke volume (Fig. 6.2). If the filling of the ventricle is minimal (as in hypovolemia) the subsequent contraction results in a reduced stroke volume. Excessive overfilling of the ventricle also leads to a reduced stroke volume as a result of overstretching of the myocardium. The point at which optimal filling of the heart occurs varies from patient to patient, depending on the compliance and condition of the ventricles.

At the bedside, clinicians look at the patient's neck veins and measure central venous pressure (CVP) to evaluate right heart filling pressure. A CVP catheter is often placed through a major vein in the neck when accurate measurement of CVP is needed. Clinicians may also measure the pulmonary capillary wedge pressure (PCWP) to assess preload for the left ventricle. Physicians may place a balloon-tipped catheter into the pulmonary artery (PA) to obtain this measurement (Fig. 6.3). Indications for the use of a PA catheter are described below in the Treatment section. Normal CVP is 2 to 6 mm Hg, and normal PCWP is 4 to 12 mm Hg.

> The filling volume of the ventricles prior to contraction is one of the most important factors determining the subsequent volume of blood ejected during systole. Too little filling or too much filling leads to a reduced stroke volume.

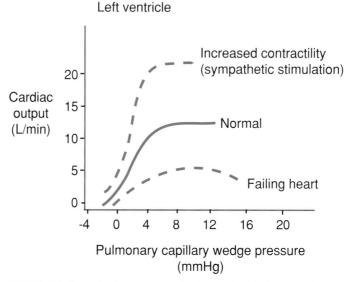

FIGURE 6.2 Ventricular function curves for the left ventricle. Note how the stroke volume increases with an increase in filling pressure, up to a certain point. Overfilling of the ventricle results in a decrease in stroke volume, especially in the failing heart. (From Wilkins, RL, Sheldon, RL, Krider, SJ: Clinical Assessment in Respiratory Care, Mosby–Year Book, St. Louis, 2005, with permission.)

Afterload

The tension created by the cardiac muscle fibers during contraction to overcome impedance to flow out of the ventricle (aortic blood pressure) is known as afterload. Since ventricular wall tension is very difficult to measure, other parameters are used to reflect afterload. Systemic vascular resistance (SVR) indicates afterload for the left ventricle; pulmonary vascular resistance (PVR) indicates afterload for the right ventricle (Table 6.1). Afterload for the left ventricle increases with systemic vasoconstriction and decreases with peripheral vasodilation. Afterload increases for the right ventricle with pulmonary vasoconstriction

Table 6.1 Hemodynamic Parameters

Parameter	Normal Range	Indication
CO	4–8 L/min	Total blood flow
CI	2.5–4.0 L/min/m^2	Blood flow for size of patient
CVP	0–6 mm Hg	Right ventricular preload
PCWP	6–12 mm Hg	Left ventricular preload
SVR	900–1400 dynes/sec/cm^5	Left ventricular afterload
PVR	200–450 dynes/sec/cm^5	Right ventricular afterload
MAP	80–100 mm Hg	Perfusion pressure
Pv$^-$O$_2$	35–45 mm Hg	Tissue oxygenation
PAP	20–30/6–15 mm Hg	Pulmonary artery pressure

CO = cardiac output; CI = cardiac index; CVP = central venous pressure; PCWP = pulmonary capillary wedge pressure; SVR = systemic vascular resistance; PVR = pulmonary vascular resistance; MAP = mean arterial pressure; Pv$^-$O$_2$ = mixed venous oxygen tension; PAP = pulmonary artery pressure.

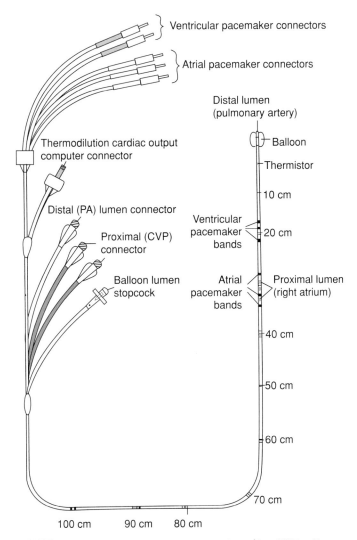

FIGURE 6.3 Illustration of a pulmonary artery catheter. (From Wilkins, RL, Sheldon, RL, Krider, SJ: Clinical Assessment in Respiratory Care, Mosby–Year Book, St. Louis, 2005, with permission.)

and decreases with pulmonary vasodilation. The interaction between cardiac output and afterload determines blood pressure.

The calculation of resistance requires measurement of the driving pressure across the circuit. For SVR this driving pressure is the difference between mean arterial pressure (MAP) and CVP; for PVR the driving pressure is the difference between mean pulmonary artery pressure (PAP) minus left atrial pressure (PCWP). Once the driving pressure is determined, the resistance can be calculated by dividing the cardiac output into the pressure difference:

$$SVR = \frac{MAP \text{ (mm Hg)} - CVP \text{ (mm Hg)} \times 80*}{Cardiac \text{ output (liters/minute)}}$$

$$PVR = \frac{PAP \text{ (mm Hg)} - PCWP \text{ (mm Hg)} \times 80*}{Cardiac \text{ output (liters/minute)}}$$

*Used to convert the units to dynes/sec/cm^5.

An appropriate level of afterload for the left ventricle is essential to maintain adequate perfusion pressures throughout the body. Decreases in afterload (peripheral vasodilation) will cause the BP to drop. The decrease in BP will stimulate the heart to increase cardiac output in an effort to maintain circulation. If the drop in afterload is excessive and the compensatory mechanisms are inadequate, BP may be inadequate for perfusion of vital organs (shock).

Contractility

The forcefulness of myocardial contraction is known as **contractility**. Even if the ventricle is adequately filled and resistance to outflow optimal, cardiac output will not be adequate if contractility is poor. Common vascular responses to decreased cardiac contractility include an increased afterload (elevated SVR) and increased preload (elevated CVP and PCWP). Factors that reduce cardiac contractility are called negative inotropes and include hypoxemia, acidosis, and medications such as beta-blockers. Damage to the myocardium as with myocardial infarction also reduces cardiac contractility. Factors that increase contractility are called positive inotropes and include certain beta-adrenergics (e.g., Isuprel) and parasympatholytics (e.g., Atropine).

> The most common cause of poor contractility in patients over age 55 is myocardial infarction. The use of beta-blockers also reduces contractility.

ETIOLOGY

Circulatory shock results from inadequate cardiac contractility (cardiogenic shock), failure of vascular tone (distributive shock), or inadequate circulating blood volume (hypovolemic shock). Cardiogenic shock is a common problem in the United States and is most often seen in the patient experiencing a myocardial infarction (MI). Approximately 6% to 7% of patients having an MI develop cardiogenic shock.[1-4] Cardiogenic shock is not limited to MI patients. It is also seen in those with dysrythmias, valve disease, and dilated cardiomyopathies.

Distributive shock is most often seen in the septic patient. Sepsis can lead to a complex biochemical response in the body that results in severe vasodilation with decreased afterload. Blood flow out of the heart (cardiac output) may be normal, but perfusion of the microvascular beds in the vital organs is not adequate owing to persistent hypotension. Maldistribution of blood flow is also seen in patients with anyphalactic shock and toxic shock and in some patients with brain injuries.

Bleeding from trauma or surgery and dehydration may result in significant hypovolemia (a decrease in circulating blood volume). This can precipitate hypovolemic shock when the circulating blood volume is inadequate to meet the metabolic needs of the body. This typically requires a loss of more than 20% to 25% of the circulating blood volume.[5]

> Septic shock causes a complex problem with maldistribution of blood flow and very low afterload. Cardiac output is often increased, but blood flow to vital organs is often inadequate owing to low perfusion pressures.

The role of metabolism in the evaluation of patients with circulatory failure is important to consider. Anything that increases the patient's metabolic rate can increase the incidence and severity of shock. For example, fever increases oxygen consumption and may result in shock in the patient with marginal cardiac function.

CLINICAL FEATURES

Shock typically produces a similar clinical picture in most patients, regardless of the cause. Patients in shock usually have hypotension, tachypnea, and tachycardia. The peripheral pulses are typically weak or "thready" as a result of the reduced stroke volume associated with shock. Signs of organ dysfunction are present and include oliguria (diminished urine output), altered sensorium, and hypoxemia. The skin often becomes cool and clammy in cardiogenic and hypovolemic shock as epinephrine is released, causing peripheral vaso-constriction in an attempt to compensate for the hypotension. An exception is early in the course of septic shock when peripheral vasodilation is caused by toxins, and the extremities are warm and dry. Inspiratory crackles are often heard during chest auscultation when the patient has excess fluid in the lungs because of heart failure (cardiogenic shock) or because of leaky blood capillaries (septic shock).

As shock becomes more severe and tissue perfusion decreases, the tissues switch to anaerobic metabolism and lactate builds up, causing metabolic acidosis. This is often (but not always) accompanied by a decrease in mixed venous oxygen tension (Pv^-O_2). The decrease in Pv^-O_2 occurs as tissues extract more than the usual amounts of oxygen from the slowly passing blood to compensate for the reduced cardiac output. Sepsis may paradoxically raise Pv^-O_2 by causing precapillary arterial-venous (AV) shunting and by disrupting the tissue's ability to use oxygen.

A reduced Pv^-O_2 in the shock patient is a sign that tissue oxygenation is inadequate. An elevated Pv^-O_2 may be an ominous sign that indicates tissue utilization of oxygen is faltering.

Laboratory Evaluation

Evaluation of serum electrolytes is useful in patients in shock because significant defects (e.g., low potassium) may contribute to the cardiovascular compromise and can be easily corrected. This evaluation is also useful in calculating the anion gap, which is used to detect the onset of lactic acidosis owing to lactic acid production from anaerobic metabolism. To calculate the anion gap, the Cl^- and HCO_3^- values are added, and the total is subtracted from the Na^+ value. Normal values are 8 to 16 mEq/L. An anion gap above 16 mEq/L in the patient with shock indicates that the shock is severe enough to cause lactic acidosis.

Physical Examination/Hemodynamic Monitoring

Patients with failure of vascular tone (e.g., septic shock, toxic shock) typically demonstrate fever or hypothermia and leukocytosis. Because the patient with septic shock often has peripheral vasodilation, the extremities may remain warm and pink despite poor circulation to the vital organs. Hemodynamic monitoring of the patient with septic shock reveals an increased cardiac output, reduced SVR, and a low to normal PCWP in the hyperdynamic phase of this syndrome. Pv^-O_2 may be normal despite inadequate tissue oxygenation. As mentioned above, the reason for the normal Pv^-O_2 in septic shock is probably due to decreased peripheral utilization of oxygen and peripheral precapillary AV shunts. Later the myocardium often becomes depressed and cardiac output decreases.

Patients in hypovolemic shock typically have poor perfusion to the extremities, which results in a slow capillary refill, peripheral cyanosis, and cool digits. Hemodynamic monitoring reveals reduced filling pressures of the heart (low CVP and PCWP), low cardiac

Table 6.2 Assessment of the Type of Shock

Parameter	Hypovolemic	Septic	Pump Failure
CO/CI	Decreased	Increased*	Decreased
CVP	Decreased	Normal to low	Increased
PCWP	Decreased	Normal to low	Increased
SVR	Increased	Decreased	Increased
MAP	Normal/low	Decreased	Decreased
Pv⁻O$_2$	Decreased	Normal	Decreased

*Cardiac output/index is often increased in the early phase of septic shock but may decrease later.

CO = cardiac output; CI = cardiac index; CVP = central venous pressure; PCWP = pulmonary capillary wedge pressure; SVR = systemic vascular resistance; MAP = mean arterial pressure; Pv⁻O$_2$ = mixed venous oxygen tension.

output, and high SVR. Urine output decreases in hypovolemic shock, as the kidneys try to conserve body fluids (Table 6.2).

Electrocardiogram

The electrocardiogram (ECG) usually shows tachycardia, although abnormal rhythms may be seen when coronary perfusion is inadequate. When coronary artery perfusion is inadequate, the ECG will show ST-segment elevation or depression or T-wave inversion or both (Fig. 6.4). When use of a vasopressor to correct hypotension is being considered, abnormal ST segments or T waves on the ECG suggest that the patient's heart may not tolerate the strain associated with an increased afterload from the vasopressor.

Chapter 8 reviews the clinical findings typical of cardiogenic shock resulting from left heart failure.

TREATMENT

A few general guidelines apply to treating all patients in shock. Oxygen therapy is needed to treat hypoxemia and maximize efficiency of circulation. Oxygen may be required in high concentrations (greater than 40%), especially if pulmonary edema is present. Endotracheal intubation is required when the patient's sensorium is depressed to the point where aspiration of gastric contents might occur when respiratory muscle fatigue requires mechanical ventilation or when hypoxemia requires positive end-expiratory pressure (PEEP).

Mechanical ventilation is often helpful in treating the patient in shock, as it reduces oxygen consumption of the respiratory muscles. Respiratory muscles use approximately 15% of the cardiac output, so when they rest, circulatory demands on the heart are reduced. The use of PEEP may be needed when the Pao$_2$ is less than 60 mm Hg on an Fio$_2$ greater than 0.50. This is most likely to occur in the patient with cardiogenic shock or in the septic patient who develops adult respiratory distress syndrome (ARDS).

Close monitoring of all patients diagnosed with shock in an intensive care unit (ICU) is important. A central venous catheter allows evaluation of central venous pressure and easy venous access for blood draws. Newer central venous catheters have oxygen saturation monitors at the tip for continuous monitoring of ScvO$_2$. A PA catheter allows accurate assessment of the cause of the circulatory problems and helps evaluate the patient's response to therapy (see Table 6.1). Its use, however, is typically limited to the more

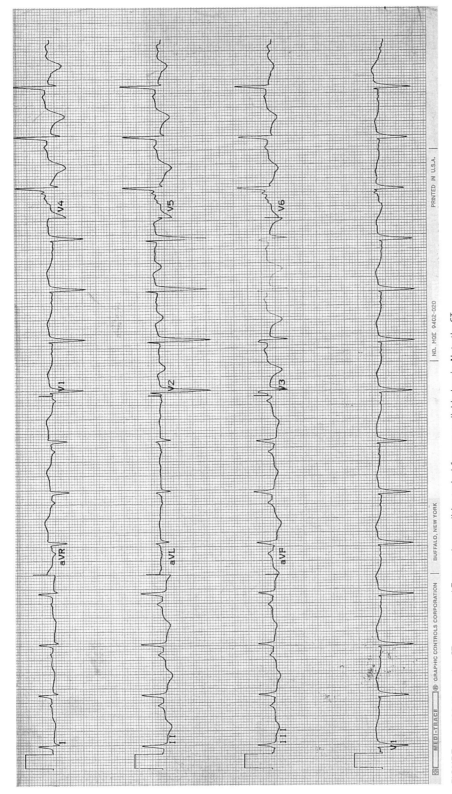

FIGURE 6.4 ECG illustrating ST segment and T wave abnormalities typical for myocardial ischemia. Note the ST segment depression and T wave inversion in leads V_3, V_4, V_5, and V_6. Also note the T wave inversion in leads I, II, III, and aVF. (Courtesy of Ken Jutzy, MD.)

complicated cases of shock and in those who do not respond to initial therapy. Clinical use of PA catheters has decreased since several studies have shown that complications associated with use of the catheters may offset the value of the information they provide.

Hypovolemic Shock

For patients in hypovolemic shock, rapid replacement of circulating blood volume is crucial. As a general rule, fluid resuscitation is needed whenever the systolic BP is below 90 mm Hg and there are signs of vital organ dysfunction (e.g., abnormal sensorium).[6] When the patient has lost large amounts of blood, it is ideal to use blood as the replacement. When there is no time to type and cross-match blood, rapid infusion of a volume expander (e.g., Ringer's lactate, normal saline, hetastarch) supports circulation until definitive treatment is available. In patients with hypovolemic shock not caused by bleeding, saline solutions are effective in expanding the circulating blood volume and are much less expensive than colloid-based solutions.[6-7]

Septic Shock

Antibiotics and volume expansion are essential for patients in septic shock. The source of the infection should be sought and may include surgical sites, wounds, indwelling catheters, and tubes, in addition to common infections such as pneumonia, urinary tract infection, and sinusitis. Volume expansion improves BP by filling the void created by the peripheral vasodilation associated with sepsis. Early and rapid fluid therapy has been shown to improve mortality in septic patients.[8] Maintaining CVP between 8 and 12 mm Hg is ideal for most patients, but a CVP of 12 to 15 mm Hg is needed for septic patients receiving mechanical ventilation.[9]

Vasopressors such as dopamine or norepinephrine improve hypotension by partially reversing the vasodilation caused by sepsis and by stimulating cardiac contractility and therefore improving cardiac output. They should be given when fluid therapy fails to restore adequate blood pressure and perfusion of vital organs.

Patients with severe septic shock often have severe depletion of protein C. Studies have shown that administration of recombinant human activated protein C (rhAPC) reduces mortality in high-risk patients (those with two or more organ system failures) with septic shock.[10] rhAPC has anticoagulant and anti-inflammatory properties that break the clotting cascade that is stimulated by infection and causes widespread tissue damage.

Since patients with septic shock often have problems with glucose metabolism, elevation of blood sugar levels are frequently seen. One large single-center study demonstrated that keeping the glucose level between 80 and 110 mg/dL by infusion of insulin improved survival in septic patients.[11] Since hypoglycemia is a possible result of insulin infusion, a continuous supply of glucose substrate (e.g., 5% dextrose by vein and/or high calorie enteral feeding) is usually given to prevent the blood sugar from dropping too low.

Cardiogenic Shock

Mechanical ventilation is most often needed in the patient with the type of shock that will not resolve quickly. Thus, those with septic shock or severe cardiogenic shock most often need mechanical ventilation.

Positive inotropics and vasopressors are the primary approach for treating most patients with cardiogenic shock. Inotropics, chronotropes, and vasoconstrictors, such as dopamine and norepinepherine, may be needed to improve blood pressure. Inotropics should not be used in the patient suspected of having acute myocardial infarction, as they may add to the stress on the heart and extend the infarction. Diuretics are needed when fluid retention is evident.

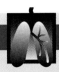

Mr. E

HISTORY

Mr. E is a 46-year-old white man brought to the emergency department by ambulance following a gunshot wound to the abdomen. The patient was found by the emergency medical technicians outside a local bar lying on his side in a pool of blood. At the scene of the shooting, the patient was found semiconscious with a pulse rate of 128/min, a breathing rate of 32/min, and a BP of 95/60 mm Hg. The single gunshot wound was stabilized by the ambulance crew and an IV infusion with normal saline was initiated prior to transfer to the hospital. At the emergency department, Mr. E's vitals were as follows: pulse thready at 130/min, respiratory rate 34/min, and BP 80/50 mm Hg. Mr. E was semiconscious and disoriented. His skin was cool and clammy to the touch, with peripheral cyanosis noted. Breath sounds and heart sounds were normal. His abdomen was distended and bowel sounds were absent. Neurologic status was grossly intact. Past medical and family history was not available.

QUESTIONS	ANSWERS
1. What is indicated by the cool, cyanotic extremities? What is suggested by the thready pulse?	Cool, cyanotic extremities indicate poor perfusion. Peripheral vasoconstriction is a compensatory mechanism in which the body attempts to preserve blood flow to the central, vital organs whenever BP decreases below a critical level. This results in the patient's feet and hands feeling cool to the touch. Peripheral cyanosis occurs when the tissues extract excessive amounts of oxygen from the slowly passing blood, leaving it very desaturated. The thready pulse indicates that this patient's stroke volume is abnormally low.
2. What is indicated by the abnormal sensorium?	The abnormal sensorium may indicate that the brain is not receiving optimal oxygenation. This is probably the result of inadequate perfusion to the brain, which occurs when the MAP drops below 90 mm Hg.
3. Is oxygen therapy indicated, and if so, at what FIO_2?	Oxygen therapy is useful whenever the patient demonstrates signs of circulatory or respiratory failure. An FIO_2 of 0.40 would be most appropriate.
4. What is your assessment of the patient's condition? Is shock present? If so, what is the most likely type of shock?	There is evidence of vital organ dysfunction (an abnormal sensorium), most likely as a result of poor circulation. The patient probably has hypovolemic shock owing to blood loss from the gunshot wound (see Table 6.2).
5. Should the patient be intubated and mechanically ventilated?	Mechanical ventilation is not indicated at this point, since there is no evidence of respiratory failure and the patient may respond rapidly to treatment. Intubation may be useful if the patient's mental status deteriorates to the point that he may aspirate if vomiting occurs.

6. What is the patient's most urgent need for care at this point?

The patient's most urgent needs are surgical repair of internal bleeding and replacement of the blood lost by hemorrhage. A blood sample should be obtained immediately for cross-matching so that the appropriate blood type can be given. A volume-expanding fluid must be given in large amounts until the cross-matching has been done. Additionally, the patient will need to be taken to the operating room to repair internal injuries related to the gunshot wound.

More on Mr. E

Mr. E is given oxygen via simple face mask. And a follow-up arterial blood gas (ABG) reveals: pH 7.41, Pco_2 34 mm Hg, Po_2 98 mm Hg. A CVP catheter is placed and gives a reading of 2 cm H_2O. Mr. E. is taken to the operating room, where the inferior vena cava and portions of the small bowel are repaired. A total of 4 units of whole blood and 3 L of normal saline are given to the patient.

Upon return to the ICU the patient assessment reveals: BP 125/75 mm Hg, pulse 96/min, respiratory rate 14/min via mechanical ventilation with a tidal volume of 800 mL, and an FiO_2 of 0.45. ABGs show a pH of 7.47, a Pco_2 of 33 mm Hg, and a PaO_2 of 110 mm Hg. CVP is 6 cm H_2O, and body temperature via rectal probe is 36.5°C (97.7°F). A urinary catheter is in place, and urine output was 50 mL for the 2 hours of surgery. The patient is nonresponsive because of the effects of general anesthesia. His peripheral pulses are normal, and his hands and feet are warmer than they had been before surgery.

QUESTIONS	ANSWERS
7. What is your assessment of Mr. E's circulatory status following the surgery?	Mr. E's circulatory status following surgery appears to be improved. This is based on the fact that his peripheral pulses, BP, CVP, and urine output are adequate and his extremities warmer.
8. Interpret the ABG findings following surgery. What changes in the ventilator settings do you recommend?	The ABGs reveal a respiratory alkalosis with a supernormal oxygenation on an FiO_2 of 0.45. This suggests that the FiO_2 and the minute volume could be decreased. A decrease in the minute volume can be accomplished by decreasing the tidal volume or decreasing the ventilator rate.
9. When should weaning from the mechanical ventilation begin?	Weaning from mechanical ventilation can begin as soon as the patient recovers from the effects of the general anesthesia. Evidence of recovery includes increased mental acuity, ability to follow commands, and a return of reflexes (e.g., gag reflex). Since there is no evidence of prior respiratory disease, the patient will probably not need the ventilator after he wakes up from the anesthesia.

10. What complications of circulatory shock might occur in this patient?	The patient is at risk for ARDS (see Chapter 11), disseminated intravascular coagulation (DIC), renal failure, sepsis, and postoperative atelectasis (see Chapter 13 for a discussion of postoperative atelectasis).

More on Mr. E

Mr. E is weaned from mechanical ventilation during the next 3 hours without difficulties. ABGs on an FIO_2 of 0.35 via entrainment mask show a pH of 7.43, PCO_2 of 36 mm Hg, and PO_2 of 88 mm Hg. Because of the injury to his intestinal tract, Mr. E is given IV feeding to meet his nutritional needs. Mr. E's only complaint at this time is abdominal pain related to the gunshot and subsequent surgery. The pain is controlled by IV morphine.

Over the next 3 days Mr. E continues to improve. His hemodynamic status is stable, with normal sensorium, BP, urine output, and vital signs. At the end of the third hospital day, Mr. E begins to complain of intermittent fever, chills, and general malaise. He subsequently becomes restless and somewhat confused. Physical examination at this time reveals the following findings.

PHYSICAL EXAMINATION

- **General.** Patient awake but slow to respond and confused; appears to be in mild respiratory distress.

- **Vital Signs.** Body temperature 38.5°C (101.3°F), respiratory rate 32/min, pulse rate 124/min, and BP 85/50 mm Hg.

- **HEENT.** Normal findings.

- **Neck.** Trachea midline, mobile, with no stridor; carotid pulses ++ with no bruits; no lymphadenopathy, thyromegaly, or jugular venous distention noted; accessory muscles of breathing not being used.

- **Chest.** Normal anteroposterior diameter and bilateral expansion noted with breathing; resonance to percussion normal bilaterally.

- **Lungs.** Rapid, shallow breathing noted; breath sounds normal in the mid and upper lung regions but diminished in the bases posteriorly with end-inspiratory crackles.

- **Heart.** Regular rhythm with a rate of 124/min; no murmurs or heaves noted; point of maximum impulse not palpable.

- **Abdomen.** Slightly distended, tender, and no bowel sounds noted; no masses or organomegaly noted.

- **Extremities.** No clubbing, cyanosis, or edema; pulses weak but present bilaterally; extremities warm to the touch.

Box 6.1 Addition Diagnostic Data

Because of the concern for Mr. E.'s hemodynamic status, a PA catheter is inserted. Hemodynamic and clinical measurements at this time reveal the following:

Measurement	Value
Cardiac output	6.0 L/min
Urine output	15 mL/hour
Plasma lactate	3.5 mmol/L (normal = 0.5 to 1.5 mmol/L)
Arterial pH	7.32
Pao_2	70 mm Hg on Fio_2 of 0.35
$Paco_2$	26 mm Hg
Plasma bicarbonate	16 mEq/L
SVR	675 dynes/sec/cm^5
PCWP	7 mm Hg
CVP	4 mm Hg

QUESTIONS	ANSWERS
11. Is there evidence of circulatory failure? If so, what is it?	Circulatory failure is present despite the normal cardiac output. Evidence to support this is found in the abnormal sensorium, low BP, reduced urine output, and elevated plasma lactate.
12. What do the ABG findings suggest? Are they consistent with the circulatory picture? If so, how? Does the acid-base status influence cardiac performance?	The ABGs suggest metabolic acidosis partially compensated for by hyperventilation. The patient also has mild hypoxemia on 35% oxygen. The metabolic acidosis and hypoxemia are consistent with circulatory failure. Lactic acidosis owing to anaerobic metabolism is common in circulatory failure and suggests a more severe case. Metabolic acidosis has a negative inotropic effect on the heart. Hypoxemia is common in patients in shock and in those who are bedridden following surgery. In this case, the hypoxia is probably the result of atelectasis and shunting.
13. How do you interpret the SVR? What could cause this finding?	The SVR is markedly reduced. The peripheral vasodilation is probably due to the release of chemical mediators (endotoxins) into the circulation from the infecting microorganism.
14. How do you interpret the PCWP?	The PCWP is at the lower end of normal limits. Most patients have a better stroke volume if the PCWP is in the range of 12 to 16 mm Hg.
15. How would you classify this type of circulatory problem?	This type of clinical picture suggests circulatory failure caused by sepsis or septic shock. This assessment is based on the fever, low SVR, and high cardiac output (see Table 6.2).

16. What therapy is indicated at this time?	Therapy should be aimed at improving the perfusion of vital organs. Even though the cardiac output is in the normal range, blood flow to many organs is insufficient as a result of the vasodilation and pre-capillary AV shunting. Giving IV fluids could help to increase the MAP and perfusion pressure by improving preload. Antibiotics are needed to treat the sepsis. Increasing the F_{IO_2} is needed to correct the hypoxemia. A vasopressor such as dopamine may be useful to increase the perfusion pressure if the patient does not respond adequately to fluid therapy. This patient will need close monitoring, since he is at high risk for respiratory failure and would then need intubation and positive pressure breathing.
17. What laboratory tests would you suggest be obtained at this time?	Laboratory tests that could be useful to assess this patient include an ECG, chest x-ray, complete blood count (CBC), blood cultures, and electrolytes. ABGs should be repeated if there is evidence of respiratory problems.
18. If Mr. E's body surface area is 1.7 m², what is his cardiac index? If cardiac output is 6.0 L/min and heart rate 124/min, what is the stroke volume?	Mr. E's cardiac index (CI) is 3.5 L/min/m². This is calculated by dividing the body surface area (BSA) into the cardiac output (CO), as follows: CI = CO/BSA = 6.0 liters/min ÷ 1.7 m² = 3.5 L/min/m² The stroke volume (SV) is calculated by dividing the heart rate into the cardiac output: SV = 6000 mL/min ÷ 124/min = 48 mL

 More on Mr. E

LABORATORY EVALUATION

- ECG. Sinus tachycardia with no evidence of ST-segment depression or elevation.

- Chest x-ray. Diminished lung volumes with normal heart size. No evidence of infiltrates or pulmonary edema.

- Electrolytes. Na^+ = 140 mEq/L; K^+ = 3.6 mEq/L; Total CO_2 = 17 mEq/L; Cl^- = 102 mEq mEq/L

- CBC. WBC = 18,500/mm³; 60% segmented neutrophils; 8% bands

Following the administration of fluids, the patient's PCWP increases to 12 cm H_2O, and cardiac output increases to 6.5 L/min. SVR is measured at 660 dynes/sec/cm⁵. Intravenous gentamicin and piperacillin are started. Pv^-O_2 is measured at 42 mm Hg. The patient remains semiconscious with a BP of 90/52 mm Hg, respiratory rate of 34/min, and a pulse rate of 130/min. His rectal temperature is 38.5°C (101.3°F).

QUESTIONS	ANSWERS
19. Calculate the anion gap for this patient and state what the results indicate.	The anion gap is calculated by subtracting the HCO_3^- and Cl^- from the Na^+ [140 − (102 + 17) = 21]. An anion gap of 21 is elevated above normal and indicates the presence of metabolic acidosis owing to (in this case) lactic acidosis.
20. What are the potential sources of the infection?	Potential sources of the infection include the abdominal wound and the IV feeding line.
21. Should the patient be intubated and mechanically ventilated?	Since this patient is not expected to recover quickly and oxygenation is marginal on supplemental oxygen, he could benefit from intubation and mechanical ventilation.
22. How is the effectiveness of the fluid therapy evaluated?	The fluid therapy is evaluated with a combination of hemodynamic parameters such as PCWP, BP, and cardiac output and by looking for evidence of improved organ perfusion (e.g., increased urine output). Evidence of better vital organ perfusion includes improved urine output and sensorium. In this case, it appears that the fluid therapy did not improve BP and vital organ perfusion despite an increase in cardiac output. This is typical for septic shock, in which maldistribution of circulation is prevalent.
23. What is indicated by the Pv^-O_2 of 42 mm Hg?	A Pv^-O_2 of 42 mm Hg is considered to be in the normal range and often indicates that tissue oxygenation is optimal. In this case, however, the normal Pv^-O_2 may be misleading because septic shock causes precapillary shunting and often results in an inappropriately increased Pv^-O_2. Since there is evidence that tissue oxygenation is less than optimal in this case, the Pv^-O_2 must be inappropriately elevated.
24. What is the significance of the patient having an elevated body temperature? How does this influence his clinical condition?	The elevated body temperature is significant because this results in an increased metabolic rate and adds to the problems created by circulatory failure.
25. What therapy is needed at this point?	Since volume expansion alone did not significantly improve BP, the use of a vasopressor is needed. Dopamine would be a good vasopressor at this time because it would also increase cardiac contractility and blood flow to the kidneys.

 ## Mr. E Conclusion

Over the next several days, the patient responds well to therapy despite the onset of respiratory failure due to ARDS (see Chapter 11). His hemodynamic status improves with the use of vasopressors and fluid therapy. He is eventually weaned from vasopressors and mechanical ventilation and transferred to the general care unit on the 12th hospital day. ■

Ms. T

HISTORY

Ms. T, an 18-year-old female from Missouri with cystic fibrosis, has been in southern California for 2 months. She was visiting Universal Studios in Los Angeles in January when she developed shaking chills, fever, and confusion and was brought to the hospital emergency department by her sister. She was hypotensive, dyspneic, tachypneic, and hypoxemic with an SpO_2 of 83% on room air. She denies cough or sputum production.

QUESTIONS	ANSWERS
1. What caused the shaking chills?	Chills are usually an indication that the set point of the body's thermostat has been adjusted upward. Shaking chills increase muscle activity, which increases heat production and helps the body achieve the higher temperature. Some forms of pneumonia classically start with rigors and chills. The shaking chills were probably caused by her body's response to an infection.
2. What is the significance of the confusion?	Confusion is very common in people with severe infections. It is evidence of inadequate cerebral perfusion, hypoxemia, and the direct effect of toxins produced by bacteria at the site of infection and carried via the blood to the brain. It may or may not be evidence of cerebral infection such as meningitis.
3. Is she in shock? If so, is it cardiogenic, hypovolemic, or septic shock?	The hypotension suggests that she is in shock, as does the confusion. She is young enough that it would be unlikely for her to have cardiogenic shock from a heart attack; she has not been fasting or bleeding, and Los Angeles in January is not likely to be hot enough to cause dehydration during a day trip to a theme park. The preexisting condition of cystic fibrosis makes infection likely, and the onset of shaking chills suggests infection, so the history strongly suggests that this is septic shock.
4. What are the first priorities for treatment?	Airway, breathing, circulation. She appears to be breathing adequately but needs oxygen supplementation. Fluid therapy may be adequate to correct the hypotension and should be used as the first choice, but if adequate fluid replacement does not resolve the hypotension, then vasopressors such as dopamine or norepinepherine could be added. Broad spectrum antibiotics would be important early in the course of treatment.

More on Ms. T

PHYSICAL EXAMINATION

- **General.** Withdrawn, confused, thin young woman in mild respiratory distress lying in bed in the emergency department. She nods yes and no to questions but does not make eye contact.

- **Vital Signs.** Pulse 125/min, respiratory rate 30/min breathing spontaneously, temp 38.8°C, BP 78/46; urine output since admission is negligible.

- **HEENT.** Pupils mid position with brisk response to light. Mucous membranes dry, no evidence of bruising or petechia

- **Neck.** Normal jugular venous pressure (JVP) and no lymphadenopathy.

- **Lungs.** Breath sounds on left greater than on right. Fine inspiratory crackles bilaterally with coarse airway crackles heard over the trachea.

- **Heart.** Rapid rhythm with a regular rate; no murmurs, gallops or rubs;

- **Abdomen.** Soft, scaphoid, with bowel sounds present. No organomegally, masses or tenderness.

- **Extremities.** Warm to palpation with no edema. There is cyanosis and clubbing.

QUESTIONS	ANSWERS
5. What caused the hypotension?	Hypotension is almost certainly caused by the bacterial toxins, resulting in decreased cardiac contractility and increased blood vessel dilation. This combination leaves the blood vessels relatively empty so that blood pressure drops.
6. What is causing the tachycardia?	The neurovascular response to low blood pressure is to increase cardiac output. If the heart has low contractility, then it can only increase output by increasing rate.
7. Why is the urine output so low?	Kidneys work by filtering fluid out of the blood. Filtration requires a pressure gradient across the blood vessel wall. Little filtration occurs when the mean arterial pressure is less than about 60 mm Hg. There may be several factors causing the low urine output including low blood pressure, direct bacterial toxic effects decreasing kidney effectiveness, and microvascular clotting caused by the bacterial toxins that also decreases function of all organs in the body but is often first seen in decreased kidney function.
8. What is the significance of fine crackles vs. coarse crackles?	Excess fluid in the small bronchi causes them to stick shut during exhalation. Surface forces of the fluid in the airways hold the airways shut during inspiration until the lungs are stretched enough to

overcome the surface forces and pop the airways open. This sounds a lot like Rice Krispies in milk and is called fine inspiratory crackles. It most commonly indicates excess fluid in the airways. It can also be caused by pulmonary fibrosis, which makes the lung stiff and allows the airways to stick shut on exhalation and pop open when the scarred areas are stretched. Coarse crackles usually suggest secretions retained in large airways.

9. What is the significance of the coarse crackles in a patient who denies cough and sputum production?

The presence of coarse crackles in a person who denies cough and sputum suggests that the person has poor awareness of the internal environment. Most people would cough and clear the secretions, but people with a weak cough or who do not notice secretions in their windpipe because of poor mentation may rattle with each breath. In a former era that was considered the "death rattle." It does not require immediate intubation and mechanical ventilation, but raises a concern that they might eventually be needed.

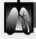

More on Ms. T

Box 6.2 Laboratory Data

Chest x-ray (see Fig. 6.5)

ABGs	
ABG	Value
pH	7.34
PaCO$_2$	57 mm Hg
PaO$_2$	127 mm Hg
HCO$_3$	29 mE/L
FIO$_2$	1.0

CBCs	
CBC	Value
WBC	24 k
Hgb	11 g/dL
Segs	63%
Bands	15%

Cocci comp fix (–)
Cortisol: 25 (within normal limits)
Hgb A1C: 5.8% (normal <7%)

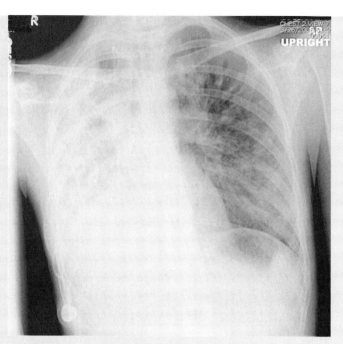

FIGURE 6.5 Chest x-ray from Ms. T.

QUESTIONS	ANSWERS
6. Interpret the chest x-ray.	The chest x-ray shows dense opacification of the right lung and patchy areas of opacification in the left lung. This is consistent with pneumonia filling the entire right lung and mildly affecting the left lung. It is not clear how much of the current findings are caused by the acute pneumonia and how much are caused by past infections associated with the cystic fibrosis.
7. Interpret the ABG.	The ABG shows acute and chronic hypoventilation. The elevated HCO_3 suggests that the $Paco_2$ is chronically elevated. The pH just below normal suggests that the $Paco_2$ is not usually this high. The oxygen level is in the normal range, but not for someone on 100% oxygen. Thus, there is relative hypoxemia, most likely caused by physiologic shunting of blood through alveolar capillaries that do not have air because of pus in the airways.

8. What is the significance of elevated WBC count and bands?

The elevated WBC count suggests stress, in this case caused by infection. The WBCs circulate in the blood but also are attached to the walls of the blood vessels (marginated) throughout the body, awaiting a call to action. Infection stimulates them to reenter the circulation and accumulate in the area of infection. Major infections use up all available mature WBCs (polys), and immature WBCs (bands) are released from the bone marrow to reinforce the mature polys.

9. Why check the cocci compliment fixation in this patient?

Cocci compliment fixation is the definitive test for Coccidoiodomycosis, which is common in southern California. Most people who get it are completely asymptomatic or have symptoms of only a mild cold. A few people become severely ill from "valley fever" and require hospitalization. It does not usually come on as dramatically as this case but should be ruled out in any visitor of more than 10 to 15 days duration who becomes ill with an infections disease. It can often be treated with oral medications.

10. Why was a cortisol level done on this patient?

Studies have shown that patients in septic shock severe enough to cause a low cortisol level survive more often with steroid supplementation.

11. The Hgb A1C was normal, suggesting that the patient did not have diabetes. Is it important to vigorously control blood sugar in this patient?

Studies have shown that patients in septic shock survive more often with careful control of blood sugar in the hospital even though they may not have been diabetic prior to the hospital admission.

12. Is Ms. T. in respiratory failure, and would it be appropriate to intubate and provide mechanical ventilation?

The patient is clearly in respiratory failure. She has no indicators demanding immediate intubation and mechanical ventilation, but the confusion and decreased mental acuity, poor cough and poor clearance of sputum, and extensive right pulmonary opacification on chest x-ray (CXR) suggest that it is just a matter of time before intubation and mechanical ventilation will be needed. A planned elective or semi-elective procedure is always preferable to an emergency or crash intubation.

13. Should Ms. T be intubated and placed on life support or should "palliative care" be provided? How would you decide?

There is always a question about the difference between what could be done and what should be done. Patients are not obligated to accept all known medical intervention. Most courts have ruled that the patient's wishes for intensity of care are the primary concern in determining whether to start or continue life support. If the patient is unable to understand the circumstances and make an informed decision, then the person designated as the medical decision maker by the durable power of attorney for health care (DPAHC) speaks for the patient. If there is no DPAHC, then the next of kin speaks for the patient based upon an understanding of what the patient would want under the circumstances. If the patient's wishes are not known, the family and health-care team should consider preexisting severity of illness, life expectancy prior to the acute illness, proportionality of pain and stress caused by the life support vs. potential for recovery, and quality and quantity expected in postrecovery life.

More on Ms. T

Volume expansion is accomplished with normal saline, and the BP stabilized at 118/60 mm Hg. Subsequent lactic acid level is 1.9, which is at the upper end of normal. Bronchoscopy is done to remove the airway secretions; the right bronchial tree is found packed with rust red pus and the left bronchial tree is packed with yellow pus. The airways remain full of pus after removal of 20 mL thick, tenacious secretions. An endotracheal tube is left in place at the end of the procedure because of the rapid reaccumulation of secretions during the procedure. Ms. T is started on mechanical ventilation so that she can be sedated for comfort. A CT scan of the chest is done (Fig. 6.6).

QUESTIONS	ANSWERS
14. What is the significance of the high-normal lactic acid level?	Shock means the tissues are starved for blood. With inadequate oxygen, the tissues will use the anaerobic pathway to generate energy. The end product of the anaerobic pathway is lactic acid. When oxygen is restored to the tissues, the lactic acid is metabolized. The high-normal value suggests that the lactic acid level had been elevated and that volume replacement restored tissue perfusion and that the lactic acid is being cleared.

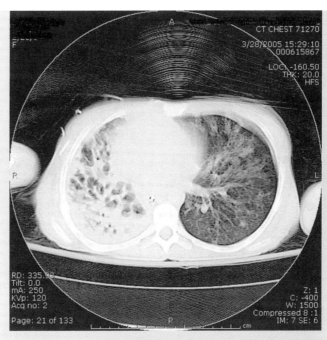

FIGURE 6.6 Chest CT of Ms. T.

15. What mode of mechanical ventilation should be used? What are the target SaO$_2$, pH, and airway pressures?

Volume-limited ventilation is safer given the large amount of airway secretions. Pressure-limited ventilation could lead to dangerously low tidal volumes in the event of mucus plugging. Target SaO$_2$ would be 90%. Target pH would be 7.35 to 7.40. Target peak airway pressure would be less than 40 cm H$_2$O. Target plateau pressure would be less than 30 cm H$_2$O. The right lung is likely to have very little compliance because of dense consolidation. Therefore, the ventilator tidal volumes will likely be very small. If the patient cannot be adequately ventilated with rapid respiratory rates and acceptable airway pressures, then hypercapnea should be permitted to a pH of approximately 7.20.

16. Should PEEP be used, and if so how much?

PEEP may be needed, but levels sufficient to keep airways open in the right lung would hyperexpand the left lung and cause barotrauma and poor ventilation-perfusion matching. The chest x-ray shows nearly complete opacification, suggesting the right lung is not functional at this time and is unlikely to be helped by PEEP, so PEEP levels should be used that are appropriate for the more compliant left lung. Starting the PEEP level at 5 cm H$_2$O seems reasonable.

17. What is the significance of the rust red right lung secretions and yellow left lung secretions.

Some pneumonias, most commonly klebsiella pneumonae, cause rust red secretions. People with cystic fibrosis are almost constantly infected with gram-negative rods and typically have copious thick yellow or green sputum. This patient may have a new klebsiella pneumonia in the right lung, causing the acute infection and shock in addition to the chronic gram negative rod (GNR) infection in the left lung.

18. Why would a CT scan be done in addition to the chest x-ray that was already done?

Chest x-rays show all chest structures superimposed upon one another. CT scans show the chest structures as if the chest were sliced like of loaf of bread. The CT scan pictures generally show slices of the chest about a half inch apart. The chest structures that are indistinct on the conventional chest x-ray are seen clearly on the CT scan. CT scans differentiate pleural fluid from consolidated lung tissue and will demonstrate the severity of lung destruction in this case.

19. Interpret the CT scan.

The CT scan shows dense consolidation of the right lung. Air bronchograms are visible in the lung tissue, and there is severe bronchiectasis with destruction of much of the lung.

20. Should a pulmonary artery catheter be placed at this time?

The measurements important to the management of this patient include central venous pressure (CVP), which indicates adequate volume replacement when the CVP is 4 to 12 cm H_2O, central venous oxygen saturation ($ScvO_2$), which indicates adequate tissue oxygenation when it is 70% or greater, and urine output, which indicates end organ function. Measuring cardiac output, cardiac index, and systemic vascular resistance are not needed at this time. A central line has been placed. It can be replaced with a pulmonary artery catheter in the future if needed. Although they provide theoretically important information, pulmonary artery catheters have not been shown to improve the mortality rate in patients with septic shock.

21. What are the chances for this patient's survival?

Septic shock is caused by a cascade of inflammatory events precipitated by infection. These include poor cardiac contraction and vasodilation, resulting in inadequate tissue perfusion. They also include diffuse intravascular clotting that can destroy organ tissue, with kidneys and lungs being most susceptible to injury. This patient appears to have a life-threatening infection but has responded well to initial therapy with improved blood pressure, urine output, and lactic acid clearance. In general, patients with septic shock have a mortality rate of around 40% to 50%. This case is complicated by the presence of severe cystic fibrosis. Patients with cystic fibrosis and pneumonia severe enough to cause respiratory failure have a much higher mortality rate.

Ms. T Conclusion

Ms. T is maintained on mechanical ventilation for the next three days. The infection worsens and Ms. T expires on the fourth hospital day. ■

KEY POINTS

- The quantity of blood pumped out of the left ventricle each minute is known as the **cardiac output**. Normal cardiac output is 4 to 8 L/min.
- Cardiac output is a function of stroke volume and heart rate. Normal stroke volume is 70 to 110 mL.
- Stroke volume is a function of three important factors: filling volume of the ventricle (preload), arterial resistance to flow out of the ventricle during contraction (afterload), and cardiac contractility.
- Circulatory shock results from inadequate cardiac contractility, failure of vascular tone (inadequate afterload), and hypovolemia (inadequate preload). Myocardial infarction is a common cause of poor contractility. Septic shock is a common cause of vascular tone failure. Surgery or hemorrhage are common causes of hypovolemic shock.
- Oxygen may be required in high concentrations (greater than 40%) to treat the patient in shock, especially if pulmonary edema is present.
- Mechanical ventilation is often helpful in treating the patient in shock, as it reduces oxygen consumption of the respiratory muscles and circulatory demands as well as treats the respiratory failure. It is most often needed in patients with septic shock or cardiogenic shock.
- For patients in hypovolemic shock, rapid replacement of circulating blood volume is crucial. Rapid infusion of saline solution is preferred in patients with hypovolemic shock not caused by blood loss.
- Antibiotics and volume expansion are essential for patients in septic shock.
- Positive inotropics and vasopressors are useful in treating most patients with cardiogenic shock.

REFERENCES

1. Goldberg, RJ, Gore, JM, Thompson, CA, Gurwitz, JH: Recent magnitude of and temporal trends (1994–1997) in the incidence and hospital death rates of cardiogenic shock complicating acute myocardial infarction: The second National Registry of Myocardial Infarction. Am Heart J 141:65, 2001.

2. Homes, DR Jr, Bates, ER, Kleiman, NS, et al: Contemporary reperfusion therapy for cardiogenic shock: the GUSTO-I trial experience. The GUSTO-I Investigators. Global Utilization of Streptokinase and Tissue Plasminogen Activator for Occluded Coronary Arteries. J Am Coll Cardiol 26:668, 1995.

3. Hand, Me, Rutherford, JD Muller, JE, et al: The in-hospital development of cardiogenic shock after myocardial infarction: Incidence, predictors of occurrence, outcome and prognostic factors. J Am Coll Cardiol 14:40, 1989.

4. Goldberg, RJ, Smad, NA, Yarzebski, J, et al: Temporal trends in cardiogenic shock complicating acute myocardial infarction. N Engl J Med 340:1162, 1999.

5. Gaieski, D, Manaker, S. General evaluation and differential diagnosis of shock in adults. Available at: www.up-to-date.com, accessed 11/5/06.

6. Rose, BD, Mandel, J: Treatment of severe hypovolemia or hypovolemic shock in adults. Available at: www.up-to-date.com, accessed 11/6/06.

7. Finfer, S, Bellomo, R, Boyce, N, et al: A comparison of albumin and saline for fluid resuscitation in the intensive care unit. N Engl J Med 350:2247, 2004.

8. Rivers, E, Nguyen, B, Havstad, S, et al: Early goal-directed therapy in the treatment of severe sepsis and septic shock. N Engl J Med 345:1368–1377, 2001.

9. Dellinger, RP, Carlet, JM, Masur, H, et al: Surviving sepsis campaign guidelines for management of severe sepsis and septic shock. Crit Care Med 32:858–873, 2004.

10. Bernard, GR, Vencent, JL, Laterre, PF, et al: Efficacy and safety of recombinant human activated protein C for severe sepsis. N Engl J Med 344:699–709, 2001.

11. van den Berghe, G, Wouters, P, Weekers, F, et al: Intensive insulin therapy in the critically ill patients. N Engl J Med 345:1359–1367, 2001.

7

Pulmonary Thromboembolic Disease

James R. Dexter, MD, FACP, FCCP

CHAPTER OBJECTIVES:

After reading this chapter you will be able to identify the:

- Frequency and mortality of venous thromboembolism.
- Predisposing factors for development of venous thromboembolism.
- Signs and symptoms of venous thromboembolism.
- Diagnostic studies used to confirm the presence of venous thromboembolism.
- Prevention and treatment strategies for venous thromboembolism.

INTRODUCTION

Pulmonary thromboembolism (PTE) refers to the vascular obstruction (embolization) of the pulmonary vessels by blood clots (**thrombi**) that have traveled through the venous system to the lungs. Other materials such as fat deposits, air, tumor fragments, and amniotic fluid can also produce an embolus but are much less common than venous thromboembolus. This chapter discusses the most common form of embolism, venous thromboembolism.

PTE is a relatively common disorder, with about 500,000 cases diagnosed each year in this country. PTE is believed to be responsible for killing 200,000 people a year.[1] For a variety of reasons, the exact number of patients developing PTE is not known.

ETIOLOGY AND PATHOLOGY

Three main factors (Virchow's Triad) are associated with the formation of deep venous thrombi (DVT): hypercoagulability, damage to the endothelial wall of the blood vessel, and venous stasis. Hypercoagulability is a factor in emboli caused by genetic deficiencies in antithrombin III, protein S, protein C, and lupus anticoagulant; in rare cases, it occurs in patients with homocystinuria and fibrinolytic abnormalities. Fractures and surgical procedures, along with trauma, are common causes of venous blood vessel damage. Stasis of venous blood flow (venous stasis) is common in many circumstances that promote physical immobilization, such as surgery, fractures, and prolonged illness.

Obesity, sedentary lifestyle, injuries/surgery, tumors, and genetic bad luck predispose to DVT.

Risk factors for DVT include age (greater than 70 years old), obesity, congestive heart failure, malignancy, burns, use of estrogen-containing drugs, and postoperative and postpartum states. These factors are additive in effect.

Although thromboemboli may form at almost any site, most originate in the deep veins of the lower extremities and pelvic region. Emboli rarely arise from the heart or upper extremities, and when they do they are often the result of an indwelling catheter. The embolic risk increases if thrombosis occurs in veins above the knee. Thrombi generally occur at the site of turbulent blood flow at the venous valves or at sites of endothelial (intimal) damage. With stasis, coagulation activity is localized and hence produces a red-fibrin thrombosis. This thrombus may then be dislodged and carried to the lungs. Risk of embolism appears highest within 72 hours after the development of DVT.

The pathological changes in the lung are related to both the magnitude of the occlusion and the subsequent degree of compromised pulmonary blood supply. Small thromboemboli may cause little or no injury to the distal lung tissue, whereas large thromboemboli may disrupt blood flow enough to injure lung parenchyma (infarction). About 10% of PTEs cause infarctions.[2] Most emboli cause more physiological disruption than would be expected from the extent of blood vessel obstruction. This is caused by the vasoactive mediators released by platelets contained in the clot.

PATHOPHYSIOLOGY

Pulmonary vascular obstruction owing to thromboembolism can affect both respiratory and hemodynamic systems. Vascular occlusion by a large **thrombus** decreases perfusion of the affected pulmonary vascular bed and initially leads to parenchymal areas with more ventilation than perfusion (alveolar dead space). Local bronchoconstriction also typically accompanies pulmonary embolism. The release of cellular mediators such as serotonin, histamine, and prostaglandins from platelets; local areas of alveolar hypocapnia; and hypoxemia are thought to be involved in causing the bronchoconstriction, although the exact etiology is unknown.

Bronchospasm may also cause hypoxemia during a pulmonary embolism by producing ventilation-perfusion ($\dot{V}/\dot{Q}$) mismatching. Although the entire cause of emboli-induced hypoxemia is unclear, many factors are probably involved, including venous shunting and reduced cardiac output resulting in an increased arterial-venous oxygen difference and worsened venous admixture. Obstruction of blood flow to the lung tissue results in a decrease in surfactant production about 24 hours after the embolization. This leads to decreased pulmonary compliance, atelectasis, and further $\dot{V}/\dot{Q}$ mismatching and hypoxemia.

Vascular occlusion and vasoconstriction cause an increase in pulmonary vascular resistance (PVR). Cardiac output is maintained only by increased right ventricular work and hence pulmonary artery pressures (PAPs). If the output of the right ventricle falls, filling of the left heart diminishes, resulting in systemic hypotension and eventual cardiovascular collapse. Approximately 50% or more occlusion of the pulmonary vasculature, however, must occur in previously healthy individuals before sustained pulmonary hypertension develops and cardiac output falls.

The severity of the hemodynamic compromise depends not only on the magnitude of the embolism but also on the patient's preexisting cardiovascular and pulmonary status. Pulmonary or cardiovascular diseases that limit the pulmonary vascular reserve, such as congestive heart failure, chronic obstructive pulmonary disease (COPD), and aortic or mitral valve disease, frequently result in greater than expected pulmonary hypertension compared to otherwise healthy patients.

Although pulmonary infarction is a potential consequence of thromboembolism, death of lung tissue owing to ischemia is uncommon because there is usually some perfusion past the embolus, collateral blood flow via bronchial arteries, and oxygenation from the airways. Pulmonary infarction is more likely in patients with left ventricular failure or COPD, probably because of reduced cardiac output or reduced collateral blood flow, respectively.

Natural resolution of the thromboembolus begins shortly after the clot lodges in the lung. Fibrinolysis is the process of clot destruction in which blood-borne and vascular endothelial factors, such as tissue plasminogen activator, act to dissolve the clot. Clot resolution involves organization of the thrombus, attachment to the vascular wall, and return of blood flow. Resolution usually results in complete or partial return of flow within 7 to 10 days. Perfusion can be restored with as little as 20% of the vessel diameter being patent.

CLINICAL FEATURES

History

The clinical symptoms of PTE are nonspecific, and emboli may occur without causing symptoms. Therefore, it is important to have a high index of suspicion, especially if risk factors are present.

The most common symptom associated with pulmonary embolism is transient acute dyspnea (Table 7.1).[3,4] Although less common, pleuritic chest pain and hemoptysis may indicate pulmonary infarction and pleural involvement. Syncope, although uncommon, suggests large clots and severe hemodynamic compromise. A sense of impending doom is a potential symptom and may be associated with large emboli and hypotension.

> Dyspnea is a very nonspecific symptom, but most patients with significant pulmonary embolus will have it. The diagnosis of pulmonary embolus should be considered in all patients with unexplained dyspnea.

Physical Examination

Physical examination of the patient with thromboembolism most commonly reveals tachypnea, tachycardia, and mild fever (Table 7.2).[3,4] Examination of the patient is most often normal, but if clots are large, there may be findings suggesting right ventricular strain (e.g., jugular venous distention). The lower extremities are often normal but may reveal swelling and tenderness associated with DVT. The patient's breath

Table 7.1 Common Symptoms in Pulmonary Thromboembolism

Symptom	% Occurrence
Dyspnea	73
Pleuritic pain	66
Cough	37
Leg swelling	28
Leg pain	26
Hemoptysis	13
Palpitations	10
Wheezing	9
Angina-like pain	4

SOURCE: Adapted from and used with permission of Stein, PD, et al: Clinical, laboratory, roentgenographic, and electrocardiographic findings in patients with acute pulmonary embolism and no pre-existing cardiac or pulmonary disease. Chest 100(3):598, 1991.

Table 7.2 Common Signs of Pulmonary Thromboembolism

Sign	% Occurrence
Tachypnea ($\geq$20 breaths/min)	70
Crackles	51
Tachycardia ($\geq$100 beats/min)	30
Increased P_2	23
Diaphoresis	11
Fever	7
Pleural friction rub	3
Cyanosis	1

SOURCE: Adapted from and used with permission of Stein, PD, et al: Clinical, laboratory, roentgenographic, and electrocardiographic findings in patients with acute pulmonary embolism and no pre-existing cardiac or pulmonary disease. Chest 100(3):598, 1991.

sounds may be normal or may reveal localized wheezing or crackles. A pleural friction rub may also be heard, particularly if infarction involving the pleura is present. Percussion of the chest wall is usually normal. Auscultation of the heart may identify loud pulmonic valve closure (P_2) as part of the second heart sound (S_2), S_2 splitting, and a possible S_3 or S_4.

Hemodynamic and Lab Evaluation

The insertion of a balloon-tipped, flow-directed catheter classically reveals an increased PAP and central venous pressure (CVP) and a normal or low pulmonary capillary wedge pressure (PCWP). A low PCWP occurs when significant occlusion of the pulmonary vasculature leads to inadequate filling of the left side of the heart. A pulmonary artery (PA) catheter is not commonly inserted to evaluate patients suspected of having PTE but may already be in place owing to hemodynamic abnormalities.

Arterial blood gases (ABGs) show an uncompensated respiratory alkalosis with mild to moderate hypoxemia on room air and an increased alveolar-arterial oxygen gradient when PTE is present.[2] ABGs do not play a major role in diagnosing the patient suspected of pulmonary embolism. The electrocardiogram is useful in determining the differential diagnosis, particularly in ruling out a myocardial infarction. It is normal in most cases but may show nonspecific ST and T wave abnormalities.[3]

Clot formation results in the release of a clot marker "D-dimer" that can be detected in the blood. Many inflammatory conditions result in an elevated level of D-dimer, but a negative result is relatively good evidence that no significant clot is being formed. Levels >500 ng/mL are consistent with PTE.

Radiography

The chest radiograph is often normal or may show only nonspecific abnormalities such as signs of volume loss, subsegmental atelectasis, or small pleural effusion (Fig. 7.1). Pulmonary vascular distention may be caused by pulmonary hypertension. A subtle, localized vascular narrowing in the area of decreased perfusion distal to the emboli may be evident ("Westermark's sign").

Most PTE originate in the leg veins, so a common diagnostic strategy is to use compression color flow Doppler ultrasound images of the leg veins. A negative study rules out significant residual clot in the leg as a threat for future emboli. A positive study reveals a reason to treat the patient with anticoagulant in a regimen equivalent to that required for pulmonary embolism.

> Pulmonary embolism can be difficult to diagnose because many of the signs and symptoms are nonspecific and routine chest x-rays are often normal.

$\dot{V}/\dot{Q}$ scans are frequently used to evaluate the patient suspected of having PTE. The scan demonstrates the difference between the alveolar distribution of inhaled

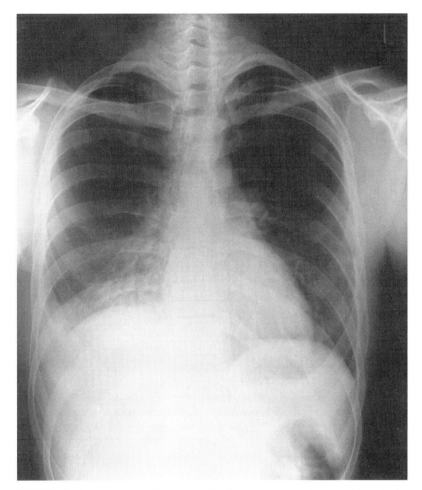

FIGURE 7.1 Chest radiograph of a patient with pulmonary embolism showing right hemi-diaphragm elevation and right lower lobe radiopacity as a result of atelectasis.

radioactive xenon-133 and pulmonary capillary distribution of albumin radioactively labeled with iodine or technetium. Healthy patients have an even distribution of ventilation and perfusion. Typical findings of a pulmonary embolus include normal ventilation but segmental or lobar defects in perfusion. Matching defects in ventilation and perfusion, such as those that occur with pneumonia, are nondiagnostic of pulmonary embolism. A normal perfusion scan effectively rules out thromboembolism. Normal ventilation in the presence of at least two segmental defects or one lobar defect in perfusion indicates a high probability that pulmonary embolism is present.

Pulmonary angiography is the diagnostic gold standard and also demonstrates the extent of vascular involvement.[2] A radiopaque contrast is introduced via catheter into the pulmonary artery (PA), and radiographs are taken as it circulates. Two signs are diagnostic of pulmonary emboli: (1) abrupt cut-off of a vessel and (2) intraluminal filling defects. Angiography requires catheterization of large veins and catheter manipulation through the right heart. Although complications such as dysrhythmias and hemorrhage are associated with these maneuvers, pulmonary angiography is generally safe.[5,6]

Most hospitals are now using pulmonary embolus protocol contrast injection computerized axial tomagraphy scans (CAT scan) to diagnose pulmonary embolus. These are much less invasive and require a smaller contrast load than traditional pulmonary angiography and are only moderately less diagnostic.

TREATMENT

Pulmonary thromboembolism therapy is aimed at treating the vascular occlusion and its pulmonary and hemodynamic consequences and preventing the reoccurrence of emboli.

Pharmacological Agents

Anticoagulant therapy using subcutaneous low-molecular-weight heparin (LMWH) or IV unfractionated heparin is the most common initial form of treatment.[7–9] Heparin inactivates thrombin and clotting factor X and inhibits platelet aggregation, thereby inhibiting the formation of new thrombi. Oral anticoagulants, such as the coumarin derivatives sodium warfarin (Coumadin) and dicumarol, inactivate the vitamin K–dependent clotting factors II, VII, IX, and X and are used for long-term therapy. **Anticoagulation** caused by unfractionated heparin therapy is monitored by the partial thromboplastin time (PTT); anticoagulation caused by the oral anticoagulants is monitored by the prothrombin time (PT). Heparin is almost always used initially and is usually continued for at least 5 days and until the PTT is stabilized in the therapeutic range. The duration of warfarin therapy varies, depending on the likelihood of clot recurrence. Patients with clots caused by easily identifiable insults and not associated with risk factors for recurrence are usually treated for 6 months, whereas recurrent clots or patients with scarred and distorted leg veins may require lifetime therapy.[10]

Although anticoagulants prevent new clot formation and the growth of already existing thrombi, they do relatively little to dissolve existing clots. Thrombolytic agents such as streptokinase, urokinase, and tissue plasminogen activator dissolve fresh clots and help restore vascular patency. Since these agents affect all recently formed clots and therefore increase the risk of bleeding, relative contraindications to their use include any bleeding risk such as recent surgical procedures, ulcers, stroke, and childbirth. Thrombolytic agents are most often used in patients with thrombi causing significant hemodynamic compromise. Thrombolytic treatment is most effective during the first 5 days after the clot formation and embolus because the clot cannot be lysed after it has stabilized, which requires about 5 days. Treatment with a thrombolytic agent is usually followed by heparin and warfarin therapy.

Surgery

Surgical removal of massive pulmonary emboli is probably not more effective than thrombolytic therapy. It is used only as a last resort because the mortality rate following this procedure is approximately 60%.

Since the advent of modern anticoagulant therapy, inferior vena caval interruption by surgical ligation, clips, or vena caval umbrella has been less frequently performed. These procedures limit the entry of clots into the pulmonary vasculature by blocking their path of entry from the lower extremities. Vena caval interruption is most often used if emboli recur after anticoagulation, in patients at such high risk of death that a subsequent embolus would probably be fatal, or when anticoagulant therapy is contraindicated. Vena cava filters often predispose the patient to eventually developing large collateral vessels that can act as a conduit allowing clots to bypass the filter and reach the lung.

Supportive Care

In addition to specific therapy, patients with pulmonary thromboembolism may need additional supportive treatment. Respiratory therapists administer oxygen when hypoxemia is present. The elimination of carbon dioxide is rarely a problem; however, the patient may benefit from intubation and mechanical ventilation if a massive embolus causes respiratory failure. If hypotension develops, volume expansion and dopamine can be used to maintain adequate perfusion pressure.

Prevention

Because pulmonary thromboembolism is a relatively common and potentially severe problem, prophylaxis is important for patients at high-risk for developing clots. There is no proven significant prophylactic benefit to wearing standard elastic stockings and ambulating early after surgical procedures. Three factors that have proved useful in preventing thromboembolism include low-dose heparin, sodium warfarin, and venous compression devices. Two to three doses of heparin each day administered subcutaneously is effective in many patients at risk because of surgical or medical immobilization and myocardial infarction. An equally effective regimen is LMWH once a day.

External venous compression devices, in which an air-filled cuff is alternately inflated and deflated, are effective in reducing thrombi formation in the lower legs. This modality is especially useful in patients who are at increased risk of bleeding if anticoagulant therapy were to be used.

> Strategies to prevent DVT and PTE are important, especially in high-risk patients, and probably save thousands of lives each year.

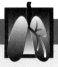

Mr. H

HISTORY

Mr. H is a 52-year-old Asian man who presents to the emergency department. His left leg is in a cast, and he states that 1 week ago he was in an automobile crash and broke his upper leg. Since that time he has had difficulty "getting around" and has mostly been lying on the couch watching television. On the evening of admission he noticed a sudden onset of dyspnea and chest pain. He denies having orthopnea, cough, hemoptysis, or wheezing. He routinely takes iron supplements and occasionally aspirin, but no other medications. He smoked two packs of cigarettes a day for 19 years but quit 3 years ago.

QUESTIONS	ANSWERS
1. What are the key pulmonary symptoms that the attending physician should explore in greater detail, and what problems do these symptoms suggest?	The key pulmonary symptoms in this case are dyspnea and chest pain. The sudden onset of the dyspnea and chest pain indicate an acute problem, rather than a chronic condition. Dyspnea and chest pain occur with pulmonary thromboemboli, pneumonia, myocardial infarction, and pneumothorax (Box 7.1). Differentiation among these medical problems is extremely important because they are all potentially fatal diseases with similar symptoms, yet they require different treatment.

2. What further questions should the physician ask of the patient to aid in the differential diagnosis?

Pertinent questions should attempt to differentiate between the problems that cause chest pain and those that cause dyspnea. The interviewer should identify the risk factors and other symptoms present in this patient for each of the diseases listed in the differential diagnosis. Risk factors for DVT include those that promote stasis, injury to blood vessels, or increased coagulability of the blood. Other symptoms associated with DVT include fever, leg tenderness, and hemoptysis. Risk factors for heart disease include hypertension, smoking, high cholesterol, a high-stress lifestyle, and lack of exercise. Other symptoms associated with heart disease include nausea, diaphoresis, radiation of the chest pain to the shoulder or jaw, and exercise-related pain. Risk factors for pneumonia include immune deficiency disorders, poor nutrition, chronic lung disease, head injuries, and chronic health problems. Other symptoms associated with pneumonia include cough, fever, and sputum production. Pneumothorax may present with only pleuritic chest pain and dyspnea.

3. Why is the diagnosis of pulmonary embolism most likely?

Two factors in the patient's history that favor the diagnosis of pulmonary embolism are trauma and immobilization. Trauma damages blood vessels and releases endothelial factors that promote clotting, whereas immobilization predisposes the patient to blood stasis.

Box 7.1 Differential Diagnosis of Pulmonary Thromboembolism

Pneumonia (bacterial or viral)
Pneumothorax
Aortic dissection
Tuberculosis
Acute pleuritis from:

• Collagen vascular disease
• Viral pleurisy

Myocardial infarction

More on Mr. H

PHYSICAL EXAMINATION

- **General.** A well-nourished Asian male who is alert and oriented, anxious, and in mild respiratory distress

- **Vital Signs.** Temperature 37.6°C (99.7°F) orally, respiratory rate 26/min, pulse 110/min, blood pressure 134/88 mm Hg

- **HEENT.** Unremarkable

- **Neck.** Supple with full active range of motion; trachea midline, mobile, and without stridor or wheezes; carotid pulses 3+, symmetric, and without bruits; no thryomegaly, jugular venous distention, or lymphadenopathy

- **Chest.** Normal configuration and expansion with breathing

- **Lungs.** Right middle lobe and right lower lobe late-inspiratory crackles revealed on auscultation

- **Heart.** Regular rhythm, with a rate of 110/min; a slightly increased S_2 (P_2) heard at the second intercostal space at the left sternal border; systolic heave located at the fourth intercostal space near the left border of the sternum

- **Abdomen.** Nondistended, soft, nontender with no masses or organomegaly

- **Extremities.** No cyanosis, digital clubbing, or peripheral edema; left leg in a cast

QUESTIONS	ANSWERS
4. What is the significance of Mr. H's anxiety?	Anxiety and apprehension may be produced by any medical condition. They are relatively common symptoms of pulmonary emboli and are usually displayed by restlessness and irritability. The etiology of these symptoms is unknown.
5. What is the significance of Mr. H's temperature?	Although the presence of a fever is common with infections such as pneumonia, a low-grade fever is also a common finding in pulmonary embolism and may help rule out other differential diagnoses, such as pneumothorax.
6. What is the significance of the systolic heave noted at the left sternal border?	A heave is an abnormal pulsation occurring on the precordium, and when palpated at the left sternal border, is often caused by right ventricular hypertrophy. A right ventricular heave is indicative of pulmonary hypertension. Many pulmonary vessels must be occluded before pulmonary hypertension develops. Therefore, a right ventricular heave indicates relatively severe disease.

7. What is the cause of the patient's crackles?	Crackles are a common finding in patients with pulmonary emboli. Atelectasis is a common result of pulmonary embolism and is most likely responsible for the inspiratory crackles. Atelectasis may also be the cause of the fever if infection is present.
8. What pathophysiology accounts for the louder P_2 component of the second heart sound?	The P_2 portion of the second heart sound (S_2) represents pulmonic valve closure. An increased intensity of the P_2 portion of that sound is indicative of more forceful valve closure caused by pulmonary vascular hypertension. Obstruction of the pulmonary vessels by thromboemboli causes an increase in PAP, which results in the valve's snapping shut with more force.
9. What findings, if any, indicate the presence of hypoxemia?	Although the patient is not cyanotic, more subtle signs of acute hypoxemia are present. Tachycardia and tachypnea are nonspecific cardiovascular and pulmonary responses to hypoxemia. The patient's anxiety might also indicate that he is hypoxemic.

 More on Mr. H

Box 7.2 Laboratory Evaluation

Chest Radiograph (see Fig. 7.2)

ABGs (on room air)

ABGs	Value
pH	7.51
$Paco_2$	30 mm Hg
Po_2	60 mm Hg
HCO_3^-	24 mEq/liter
Base excess (BE)	−1
Hb	13.1 g/100 mL
Sao_2	87.8%
Cao_2	15.6 vol%
$P(A-a)o_2$	52 mm Hg

• Complete blood count: Results pending
• Chemistry: Results pending
• Electrocardiogram (ECG): Sinus tachycardia

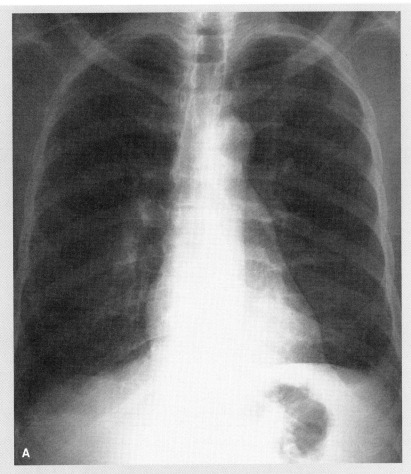

FIGURE 7.2 Chest radiograph on day of admission. (A) AP view.

QUESTIONS

10. What chest radiograph findings are consistent with pulmonary embolism? How do you interpret the chest radiographs?

ANSWERS

Although the findings on the chest radiographs are frequently nonspecific for thromboembolism, hemidiaphragm elevation is common and is probably indicative of atelectasis. The atelectasis is thought to occur as a result of bronchospasm, surfactant depletion, and underperfusion of alveolar spaces. Normally, most of the pulmonary perfusion is to the middle and lower lung fields. Most clots follow the perfusion to these areas, and as a result, atelectasis is most often found in the middle to lower lung fields. Mr. H's chest radiograph shows no significant abnormality, which is common for patients with pulmonary embolism.

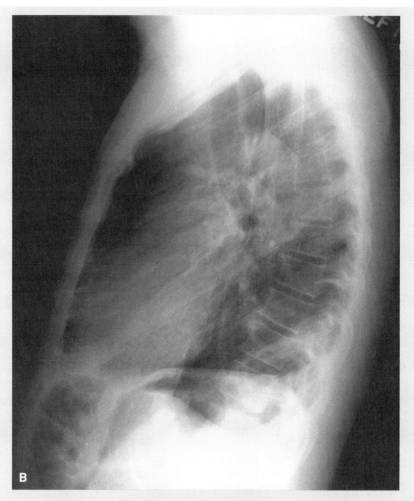

FIGURE 7.2 (B) Lateral view. (CONTINUED)

| 11. What is the patient's acid–base and oxygenation status? | The patient's acid–base status shows acute respiratory alkalosis. Moderate hypoxemia on room air is also present, which is common in patients with emboli. In addition, the arterial oxygen saturation (Sa_{O_2}) is low and the arterial oxygen content (Ca_{O_2}) slightly reduced. Because the calculation of Ca_{O_2} includes Sa_{O_2}, Pa_{O_2}, and hemoglobin, it reflects oxygen-carrying capacity, which in this case is mildly reduced, mostly owing to the low Sa_{O_2}. The alveolar-arterial oxygen gradient is increased as a result of the ventilated but underperfused regions of the lung affected by the embolus (dead space ventilation), resulting in $\dot{V}/\dot{Q}$ mismatch. |
| 12. What treatment would you suggest at this time? | Treatment at this time should consist of oxygen therapy administered via nasal cannula to increase the patient's Pa_{O_2} above 80 mm Hg. The physician |

should order IV anticoagulant therapy to prevent further thrombi. The use of thrombolytic agents is not indicated because of the relatively limited lung involvement and the absence of systemic hypotension. Should further embolization occur and cause hemodynamic compromise, the use of thrombolytic agents might be warranted.

13. What other diagnostic information would be useful?

The patient's history, physical, and diagnostic findings provide a presumptive diagnosis of pulmonary embolism. A V̇/Q̇ scan might be useful to confirm the diagnosis. Pulmonary angiography would better document the exact location and extent of the embolism, but is not necessary under these circumstances.

 ## More on Mr. H

A day later, after having a V̇/Q̇ scan (Fig. 7.3) and while ambulating around the unit, Mr. H states that he is feeling "worse" and having trouble breathing. He is acting very agitated and is slightly confused. There is no change in the physical examination findings, except that he is pale, his skin is cool and clammy, and his blood pressure is 88/45 mm Hg.

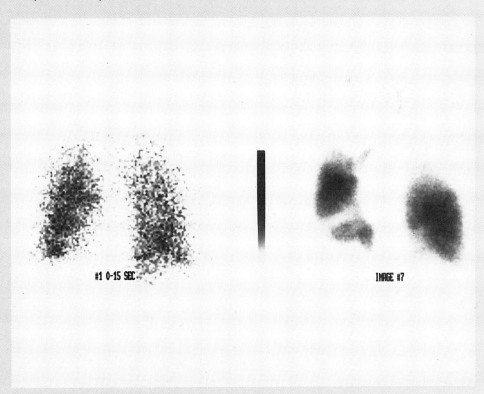

#1 0-15 SEC   IMAGE #7

FIGURE 7.3 Ventilation-perfusion (V̇/Q̇) scan (ventilation scan on left, perfusion scan on right) one day after admission, showing scattered reduced perfusion compared to ventilation on the right and left sides.

QUESTIONS	ANSWERS
14. What is the significance of the results of the $\dot{V}/\dot{Q}$ scan?	$\dot{V}/\dot{Q}$ scans depict the relative matching of ventilation to perfusion in the lung. In this case, segmental decrease in perfusion compared to ventilation in otherwise healthy lungs suggests vascular occlusion by pulmonary emboli. Unfortunately, other problems such as vasculitis, vasospasm, vessel destruction, and neoplastic vascular compression can reduce perfusion and result in similar findings during $\dot{V}/\dot{Q}$ scanning.
15. Of what significance is the change in Mr. H's mental status?	Agitation, confusion, anxiety, and restlessness are all nonspecific symptoms associated with severe diseases, including pulmonary embolism. The sudden change in mental status most likely indicates a deterioration in perfusion and oxygenation of the brain and in this case most likely represents the formation of another pulmonary embolus.
16. What pathophysiology accounts for Mr. H's hypotension?	Systemic hypotension in this case is a result of pulmonary vascular occlusion by thrombi. The vascular occlusion causes increased PVR, reduced right ventricular output, and corresponding decrease in left ventricular filling, cardiac output, and systemic blood pressure.
17. What therapy is indicated at this time?	Oxygen therapy and anticoagulant therapy are still indicated. An increased fraction of inspired oxygen (F_{IO_2}) is useful in this case because hemodynamics are marginal. In addition, thrombolytics may be necessary to induce rapid clot breakdown and aid the maintenance of cardiovascular hemodynamics.
18. Should Mr. H be admitted to the intensive care unit (ICU)?	The patient should be admitted to the ICU for close monitoring and definitive therapy. Massive pulmonary emboli are life threatening and require aggressive treatment.

More on Mr. H

Box 7.3 Additional Laboratory Evaluation

The attending physician inserts a PA catheter and orders another chest radiograph and ABG analysis. The results are as follows:

PA Catheter Data	
Measure	Value
CVP	16 mm Hg
PAP	45/32 mm Hg
PCWP	4 mm Hg
Cardiac output	2.7 liters/min
Cardiac index	1.6 liters/min/m^2

ABGs (on 6 liters/min O$_2$ by simple mask)	
ABG	Value
pH	7.37
Pa$_{CO_2}$	30 mm Hg
Pa$_{O_2}$	54 mm Hg
BE	−5
HCO$_3^-$	16 mEq/liter
Hb	13.5 g/100 mL
Sa$_{O_2}$	86%
Ca$_{O_2}$	15.8 vol%

QUESTIONS

19. What is the significance of the PA catheter measurements, and why is the cardiac output low?

20. What is the patient's prognosis?

21. What could explain the metabolic acidosis shown by the ABGs?

ANSWERS

The CVP and PAP are both elevated as a result of the pulmonary vascular obstruction that causes pulmonary hypertension. This causes an acute increase in right ventricular work and predisposes the patient to right ventricular failure. Cardiac output and cardiac index are reduced as a result of acute right ventricular failure, which reduces left ventricular filling (as evidenced by the low PCWP). These measurements indicate life-threatening disease with right heart failure.

Mr. H has a life-threatening problem that requires urgent treatment. Fatalities usually occur within the first hour after the embolus occurs. If the patient survives longer than 1 hour and appropriate treatment is initiated, there is a relatively good chance of survival.

The metabolic acidosis is most likely due to lactic acidosis. This is common in patients who have reduced cardiac output and tissue hypoxia, which leads to anaerobic metabolism and the production of lactic acid.

Mr. H Conclusion

Mr. H is admitted to the ICU and started on thrombolytic therapy, low-dose heparin therapy, and high-flow oxygen therapy. Within 24 hours of initiating thrombolytic therapy, his hemodynamic parameters normalize. Over the next several days Mr. H gradually improves, and on day 4 he is able to maintain adequate oxygenation via nasal cannula at 3 liters/min. The remainder of his hospital stay is uneventful, and on day 7 he is discharged on a regimen of sodium warfarin therapy. ■

KEY POINTS

- Pulmonary thromboembolism is a relatively common disorder affecting approximately 500,000 people and killing 200,000 people a year in the United States.
- Three main factors are associated with the formation of deep venous thrombi: hypercoagulability, damage to the endothelial wall of the blood vessel, and venous stasis.
- Although thromboemboli may form at almost any site, approximately 95% originate in the deep veins of the lower extremities, the remainder forming in pelvic veins.
- Pulmonary vascular obstruction caused by thromboembolism may affect both respiratory and hemodynamic systems. PTE leads to V̇/Q̇ mismatching and hypoxemia. Large PTE can cause decreased cardiac output owing to poor left ventricular filling.
- The most common symptom associated with pulmonary embolism is transient acute dyspnea.
- Physical examination of the patient with thromboembolism most commonly reveals tachypnea, tachycardia, and mild fever.
- The chest radiograph is often normal or may show only nonspecific abnormalities such as signs of volume loss, subsegmental atelectasis, or small pleural effusion.
- A common screening protocol includes an initial D-dimer followed by an ultrasound of the leg and/or V̇/Q̇ scan if the D-dimer is positive.
- Pulmonary angiography is the gold standard for diagnosing pulmonary embolism, but most hospitals are now using V̇/Q̇ scans and/or pulmonary embolus protocol contrast injection computerized axial tomagraphy scans (CAT scan) to diagnose pulmonary embolus. These are much less invasive, require a smaller contrast load than traditional pulmonary angiography, and are only moderately less diagnostic.
- Preventive strategies for venous thrombosis in high-risk patients may save thousands of lives a year.
- Treatment for venous thromboembolism typically consists of heparin/LMWH and warfarin for 6 months to life.

REFERENCES

1. Horlander, KT, Mannino, DM, Leeper, KV: Pulmonary embolism mortality in the United States, 1979–1998: An analysis using multiple-cause mortality data. *Arch Intern Med* 163:1711, 2003.

2. Thompson, BT, Hales, CA: Clinical manifestations of and diagnostic strategies for acute pulmonary embolism. Available at www.up-to-date.com 2005 (accessed 9-15-05).

3. Stein, PD, Terrin, ML, Hales, CA: Clinical, laboratory, roentgenographic and electrocardiographic findings in patients with acute pulmonary embolism and no pre-existing cardiac or pulmonary disease. Chest 100:598, 1991.

4. Stein, PD, Saltzman, HA, Weg, JG: Clinical characteristics of patients with acute pulmonary embolism. Am J Cardiol 68:1723, 1991.

5. Guidelines on diagnosis and management of acute pulmonary embolism. Task Force on Pulmonary Embolism, European Society of Cardiology. Eur Heart J 21:1301, 2000.

6. Hofmann, LV, Lee, DS, Gupta, A: Safety and hemodynamic effects of pulmonary angiography in patients with pulmonary hypertension: 10-year single-center experience. AJR Am J Roentgenol 183:779, 2004.

7. Hull, RD, Raskob, GE, Brant, RF, et al: Low-molecular-weight heparin vs heparin in the treatment of patients with pulmonary embolism. Arch Intern Med 160:229, 2000.

8. Buller, HR, Agnelli, G, Hull, RD, et al: Antithrombotic therapy for venous thromboembolic disease: The Seventh ACCP Conference on Antithrombotic and Thrombolytic Therapy. Chest 126:401S, 2004.

9. Wells, PS, Anderson, DR, Rodger, MA, et al: A randomized trial comparing 2 low-molecular-weight heparins for the outpatient treatment of deep vein thrombosis and pulmonary embolism. Arch Intern Med 165:733, 2005.

10. Agnelli, G, Prandoni, P, Becattni, C, et al: Extended oral anticoagulant therapy after a first episode of pulmonary embolism. Ann Intern Med 139:19, 2003.

Heart Failure

Arthur B. Marshak, MS, RRT, RPFT

George H. Hicks, MS, RRT

CHAPTER OBJECTIVES:

After reading this chapter you will be able to identify the following:

- The definition of heart failure and cor pulmonale.
- The risk factors for heart disease and failure.
- The three cardiac compensatory mechanisms involved when the heart begins to fail.
- The clinical features observed in both right and left heart failure.
- The clinical treatment of heart failure.
- The respiratory care management of cardiogenic pulmonary edema.

INTRODUCTION

Heart failure is a common complex clinical condition characterized by inability of the heart to maintain adequate blood circulation. In the United States about 4.9 million people have heart failure, with 550,000 new cases diagnosed annually. The disease is seen equally in men and women. Heart failure occurs in approximately 2.5% of white males, 1.9% of white females, 3.1% of black males, 3.5% of black females, 2.7% of Mexican-American males, and 1.6% of Mexican-American females.[1] In 2001 19,805 men and 33,023 women died of heart failure. One study showed a survival rate at 1, 2, 5, and 7 years after diagnosis of congestive heart failure of 74%, 65%, 45%, and 32%, compared with 97%, 94%, 80%, and 70% in a matched reference group without congestive heart failure.[2]

Physiologically, the failing heart is unable to maintain an adequate cardiac output despite appropriate venous return. As a consequence, hypoperfusion and pulmonary vascular congestion, known as cardiogenic pulmonary edema, occur. Clinical manifestations depend upon which side of the heart (left or right) fails and to what extent the cardiovascular system is able to compensate.

> Cor pulmonale occurs in patients with pulmonary disease when the right ventricle hypertrophies owing to pulmonary hypertension.

The term **congestive heart failure (CHF)** is frequently applied when making the diagnosis of heart failure. In general, CHF results in an accumulation of fluid in the lungs (pulmonary edema) and extremities (peripheral edema) as a consequence of left ventricular failure. **Cor pulmonale** is the term used to describe right ventricular enlargement and failure as a result of primary pulmonary disease.

ETIOLOGY

The factors that increase a person's risk for heart disease and failure include hypertension, diabetes, smoking, obesity, a high-fat diet, and family history of heart disease.[3] The Framingham Study has established that more than 60% of heart-failure cases are caused by hypertension and coronary artery disease.[4,5] Idiopathic dilated cardiomyopathy or primary myocardial disease causes 30% to 40% of cases;[1] valvular heart disease causes less than 20%.[4] Box 8.1 lists the various causes of heart failure.

Most acute episodes of heart failure occur in cardiogenic illness brought about by recognized risk factors. In addition to contributing to the etiology of heart disease, these factors may interfere with one or more of the compensatory mechanisms that support cardiovascular function. Knowledge of the various risk factors may greatly improve the recognition and treatment of heart failure. The more common factors and their prevalence in the U.S. population are listed in Table 8.1.

Acute cor pulmonale is frequently associated with an abrupt elevation of pulmonary artery pressure. This may be observed with massive pulmonary embolism, severe hypoxemic pulmonary vasoconstriction owing to acute respiratory failure, or mechanical constriction of the pulmonary vasculature secondary to bilateral pneumothoraces. Chronic cor pulmonale is responsible for 10% to 30% of admissions for presumed CHF and is primarily caused by chronic pulmonary diseases including chronic bronchitis, emphysema, and pulmonary fibrosis.

Box 8.1 The Etiologic Factors of Heart Failure*

Coronary artery disease
Hypertension
Primary or idiopathic dilated cardiomyopathy
Valvular abnormalities: regurgitation and stenosis
Congenital cardiac defects
Chronic pulmonary disease
Drugs: amphetamines, heroin, cocaine, anti-TB combinations, high-dose cancer chemotherapy combinations
Infectious myocardial inflammation
• Viral (e.g., influenza, mumps, and rabies)
• Bacterial (e.g., streptococcal–rheumatic heart disease)
• Mycotic (e.g., histoplasmosis)
Other causes
• Chronic alcohol ingestion
• Acute leukemia
• Metal poisonings (e.g., cobalt, iron, and lead)
• Metabolic defects (e.g., myxedema)
• Neurological disorders (e.g., Duchenne's muscular dystrophy)
• Trauma (e.g., cardiac tamponade)

*From: Chesebro, JH et al.: Cardiac failure: characteristics and clinical manifestations. In Brandenburg, RO (ed): Cardiology: Fundamentals and Practice, Chicago, Year Book, 1987.

Risk factors for heart failure include chronic heart disease, cardiac valve disease, hypertension, diabetes, smoking, obesity, and high-fat diet.

PATHOPHYSIOLOGY

The measurement of **cardiac output (CO)** is an indication of cardiac pump performance. CO is measured as the flow of blood from one ventricle in liters per minute. It is determined by heart rate (HR) and stroke volume (SV). The following equation describes this relationship:

$$CO = HR \times SV$$

Heart rate is regulated by the pacing system of the heart and influenced by the neurotransmitters (norepinephrine, epinephrine, and acetylcholine) released by the autonomic nervous system and adrenal glands. **Stroke volume** is influenced by venous return

Table 8.1 Population Attributable Risk Factor Ranking for Cardiac Failure[6-13]

Risk Factor	Prevalence in U.S. Population	Framingham Heart Study	NHANES-1 (Overall)
Hypertension	M 60%	M 39%	10%
	F 62%	F 59%	
Coronary artery disease			
Myocardial infarction	M 10%	M 34%	62%
	F 3%	F 13%	
Angina pectoris	M 11%	M 5%	
	F 9%	F 5%	
Obesity	M 22%	M 11%	8%
	F 21%	F 11%	
Diabetes	M 8%	M 6%	3%
	F 5%	F 12%	
Valvular heart disease	M 5%	M 7%	2%
	F 8%	F 8%	
Left ventricular hypertrophy (ECG)	M 4%	M 4%	NA
	F 3%	F 5%	
Current cigarette smoking	M 24%	N/A	17%
	F 19%		
Low physical activity	M 35%	N/A	9%
	F 40%		
Male gender	49%	NA	9%
<High school education	M 13%	N/A	9%
	F 11%		

(preload pressure), downstream resistance (afterload), myocardial contractility, and ventricular compliance. A more complete discussion of these factors and their interrelationships can be found in Chapter 6.

In the normal heart, there is an exceptional degree of autoregulation of cardiac output to meet metabolic demands and prevent an imbalance in output between the right heart and the left heart. A difference of as little as 1 mL/min can lead to venous congestion upstream from the failing ventricle. Left ventricular failure with congestion of the pulmonary circulation upstream from the left heart results in more disruptive symptoms than does a similar degree of right heart failure. The more muscular wall of the left ventricle is capable of performing much greater work than the less muscular right ventricle. The more limited functional capacity of the right ventricle predisposes it to failure when challenged with increasing preload or afterload or both. As a consequence, right heart failure commonly follows primary left heart failure. Interestingly, secondary right heart failure actually reduces the pulmonary congestion and the preload of the failing left ventricle, which provides a type of compensation. Rarely does primary right heart failure lead to left side failure.

A variety of functional changes occur in heart failure and influence myocardial performance, circulatory changes, fluid and electrolyte imbalance, and pulmonary dysfunction.

Myocardial Performance

The myocardial fibers in heart failure have decreased length-tension and force-velocity capabilities when stimulated to contract. This demonstrates the heart's reduced inotropic

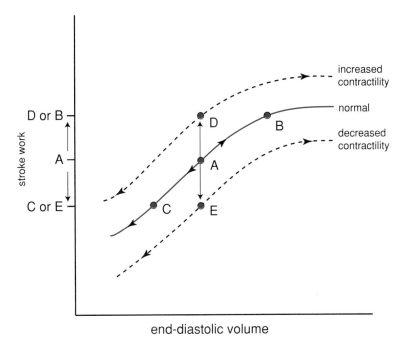

FIGURE 8.1 Frank-Starling ventricular function curves relating output (stroke work) and end-diastolic volume in three myocardial states of contractility. Output is varied along a single curve (e.g., A to B or A to C) as end-diastolic volume is altered by venous return. Output may also be changed by shifting from one curve to another (e.g., A to D or A to E) as the contractile or inotropic state of the ventricle is altered. Increased contractility can be brought about by hormonal or drug action, while decreased contractility is typical of heart failure.[58]

capacity and reduced ability to generate a normal stroke volume. The ejection fraction (the percentage of end diastolic volume pumped in one heart beat) can fall from a normal value of approximately 70% to as low as 10% in severe failure. These deficits result from reductions in contractility or alterations in the heart's preload and afterload.

Three cardiac compensatory mechanisms improve myocardial performance during the greater demands of exertion and in failure:

- **Autoregulation of the Heart.** As myocardial fibers are stretched by increasing end-diastolic ventricular pressure and volume, the fibers contract with greater force (**Frank-Starling response**). Figure 8.1 illustrates this relationship in both the normal and failing heart. In the normal heart, the increase in venous return and ventricular filling associated with exercise or other forms of stress is easily compensated for through this mechanism. Failure of a ventricle results in a progressive increase in end-diastolic volume and ventricular dilation. The Frank-Starling response improves myocardial performance in heart failure, but this improvement leads to vascular engorgement that backs up into the pulmonary or systemic venous systems in left or right heart failure, respectively. To complicate cardiac performance further, an overly elevated end-diastolic volume reduces the compliance of the ventricle, which reduces contractility and nullifies or greatly reduces the Frank-Starling response and further contributes to CHF.
- **Sympathetic Neural Responses.** During times of stress or hypotension, the sympathetic nervous system releases epinephrine and norepinephrine, which stimulate the beta and alpha receptors of the cardiac pacing system and myocardium. This results in increased heart rate and greater contraction, which improve cardiac output. During heart failure,

there is increased sympathetic activity and greater concentrations of epinephrine and norepinephrine in plasma during conditions of rest and exercise. This response improves cardiac performance initially, but it diminishes over time. Later, sympathetic stimulation can provoke ischemic symptoms if the myocardium's metabolic rate is stimulated beyond the coronary circulation's capacity to supply adequate blood flow to the myocardium. In chronic heart failure, persistent tachycardia develops, resulting in a reduction of the heart's ability to alter its rate from rest to exercise.

> When the heart begins to fail, it will try to compensate by an increase in force of contraction, increase in heart rate, and an increase in the muscle thickness of the ventricle.

• **Ventricular Hypertrophy.** Ventricular hypertrophy is an increase in myocardial muscle thickness and mass produced by chronic exposure to elevated vascular pressure, greater blood volume, and elevated sympathetic nervous system release of neurotransmitters (e.g., norepinephrine, dopamine). While the hypertrophy is beneficial for improving the strength of contraction in the early stages of heart failure, this benefit is eventually offset by a decreasing ventricular compliance. This condition is often further exacerbated by ischemic changes, which are brought about by inadequate oxygen delivery to an enlarged myocardium during conditions of increased myocardial work. Hypertrophy is not necessarily permanent if produced over a short period of time and then corrected. This reversal is common after surgical prosthetic replacement of a stenotic aortic valve.

Circulatory Changes

Significant systemic redistribution of blood flow occurs in heart failure as an important compensatory mechanism. This adjustment results in a diversion of the already reduced cardiac output away from renal and cutaneous tissues to the more important coronary and cerebral circulations. These adjustments occur during rest, but they are further intensified during exercise through the influence of the sympathetic nervous system.

In heart failure, the systemic vascular resistance is generally increased through the vasoactive effects of an elevated plasma norepinephrine concentration and vessel wall engorgement owing to sodium and water retention. This compromises the cardiovascular system's ability to undergo vasodilation, which limits its ability to increase oxygen transport and dissipate heat during exercise or other forms of stress. Thus, heart failure patients are often very sensitive to heat and have reduced exercise tolerance.

Right heart failure results in systemic venous and capillary congestion and hypertension. This leads to liver engorgement, portal hypertension, reduced lymph drainage back to the venous system, and fluid retention in various third spaces (e.g., dependent joint capsules, peritoneal cavity, pleural space).

Failure of the left heart produces pulmonary engorgement and hypertension. Initially, pulmonary artery diastolic pressure increases to around 12 to 18 mm Hg. This leads to increased blood flow to the upper lung or nondependent zones. Further failure results in greater pressures that can lead to pulmonary congestion and edema.

Fluid and Electrolyte Balance Imbalance

In heart failure, reduced cardiac output and generalized vasoconstriction result in renal hypoperfusion. This results in reduced glomerular filtration and subsequent sodium and water retention. Systemic venous congestion during right heart failure can lead to renal venous hypertension, which can cause reductions in glomerular filtration and increased tubular reabsorption of sodium. Thus, arterial hypoperfusion, venous hypertension, or both lead to renal responses that compound the congestive component of failure.

In addition to the renal vascular changes brought about by increased plasma concentrations of norepinephrine during heart failure, a variety of other hormonal adjustments induce further changes in renal function.[14] Reduced renal perfusion triggers the kidneys' production of renin, which stimulates the production of angiotensin I. Angiotensin I is converted to angiotensin II during transit through the pulmonary circulation. Angiotensin II stimulates renal tubular sodium reabsorption, causes vasoconstriction, which intensifies renal hypoperfusion, and stimulates adrenal gland secretion of aldosterone. Aldosterone induces further renal retention of sodium. Atrial natriuretic peptide (ANP), a small protein hormone produced by specialized stretch receptor cells in the atria, is secreted in greater quantities during heart failure.[15] Increasing levels of ANP stimulate the kidneys to excrete sodium. This effectively antagonizes the effects of aldosterone and helps limit the sodium and water retention common in heart failure.

As a result of these renal changes, patients in heart failure generally have increased blood volume, interstitial fluid volume, and total body sodium. This altered fluid and electrolyte balance, coupled with poor cardiac performance, can easily lead to the development of systemic and pulmonary edema.

Edema Formation

The movement of fluid back and forth between the vascular and interstitial spaces is a normal phenomenon. The movement of water is governed by the permeability of the capillary wall, capillary blood pressure, interstitial fluid pressure, and oncotic pressure (primarily the osmotic force generated by proteins) of blood and interstitial fluid. These forces are brought together in Starling's law of the capillary:

$$\text{Fluid movement} = \text{Kf} \left[(P_c - P_i) - (\pi_p - \pi_i) \right]$$

where Kf is the filtration constant for the capillary, P_c is the hydrostatic pressure within the capillary, π_p is the oncotic pressure exerted by interstitial fluid, P_i is the hydrostatic pressure of interstitial fluid, and π_i is the oncotic pressure exerted by interstitial fluid and is a reflection of the coefficient of protein. Normally these forces result in the net movement of about 150 mL of fluid into the interstitial space per hour. This fluid is absorbed by the lymphatics and returned to the systemic venous circulation and results in a stable interstitial fluid volume. When this natural drainage mechanism fails, excessive fluid collects in the interstitial space.

Edema is the term used to describe the clinical appearance of accumulated fluid in the interstitial spaces of the body. A variety of conditions can lead to the formation of edema:

- Increased capillary permeability (e.g., effects of sepsis)
- Increased capillary hydrostatic pressure
- Reduced blood protein concentration (e.g., hypoalbuminemia), which results in reduced oncotic pressure
- Lymphatic obstruction

Fluid retention and increased capillary blood pressure occur in CHF. Right heart failure causes systemic venous and capillary hypertension, which leads to systemic organ and dependent limb edema. In left heart failure, pulmonary circuit blood pressure increases as blood collects upstream from the failing left ventricle. Pulmonary capillary pressures begin to increase, and interstitial fluid accumulates along the vessel walls, around the small airways, and in the pleural space. This initially occurs in the dependent regions of the lung, where capillary pressures are the highest. As the severity of left heart failure increases, pulmonary edema occurs throughout the lung in those regions where pulmonary capillary pressures exceed 25 mm Hg.

Pulmonary Dysfunction

Pulmonary function is often disturbed during left ventricular failure (Table 8.2). Advanced left ventricular failure produces marked impairment in pulmonary function, whereas early left ventricular failure, with its attendant mild pulmonary hypertension (e.g., pulmonary artery wedge pressure [PAWP] of 15 to 20 mm Hg), actually improves gas exchange through an increased pulmonary blood volume and improved ventilation-perfusion ($\dot{V}/\dot{Q}$) matching. As left ventricular function deteriorates and increasing pulmonary congestion occurs, lung water increases. This causes decreases in lung volume and diffusion capacity and increases in airway resistance and $\dot{V}/\dot{Q}$ mismatching. Severe failure and frank alveolar flooding are often accompanied by a dramatic deterioration in forced vital capacity (FVC), forced expiratory volume in 1 second (FEV_1), lung compliance, and gas exchange, as well as a mixed respiratory and metabolic acidosis. These changes can cause further heart failure, which causes further pulmonary dysfunction, and thus a vicious circle of failure begins.

Table 8.2 Pulmonary Dysfunction During Left Heart Failure[25]

Severity	Pathophysiology	Pulmonary Abnormalities
Mild	Pulmonary vascular congestion	↑ D_{LCO} ↑ Pa_{O_2} Pa_{CO_2} and pH are normal
Moderate	Pulmonary interstitial edema	↓ FVC or unchanged ↓ FEV_1 or unchanged ↑ Closing volume ↑ V_D/V_T ↓ $\dot{V}/\dot{Q}$ matching ↓ D_{LCO} ↓ Pa_{O_2} ↓ Pa_{CO_2} and ↑ pH
Severe	Alveolar flooding	↓↓ FVC ↓↓ FEV_1 ↓↓ Compliance ↑↑ Closing volume ↑↑ V_D/V_T ↑↑ $\dot{V}/\dot{Q}$ matching ↓↓ D_{LCO} ↓↓ Pa_{O_2} ↑ Pa_{CO_2} and ↓ pH

D_{LCO} = carbon monoxide diffusing capacity of the lung; FVC = forced vital capacity; FEV_1 = forced expiratory volume in 1 second; V_D/V_T = ratio of volume of dead space to tidal volume; $\dot{V}/\dot{Q}$ = ventilation-perfusion ratio.

CLINICAL FEATURES AND LABORATORY FINDINGS

Clinical Features

The two major clinical manifestations of heart failure are (1) fluid retention and peripheral edema (associated with right ventricular failure) and (2) pulmonary vascular congestion (caused by left ventricular failure). This division is clinically useful but potentially misleading, since biventricular failure often occurs as one ventricle fails primarily and precipitates failure of the other. Cor pulmonale is difficult to recognize because the clinical picture is almost always dominated by chronic pulmonary disease. The clinical manifestations vary not only with the major form of heart failure present, but also with the patient's ability to compensate and his or her response to therapy.

The morbidity and mortality associated with heart failure necessitates early recognition and treatment. If the patient has a history of one or more risk factors (see Table 8.1), it is very useful to determine whether the heart failure is the primary or a contributing cause of the patient's complaints or condition.

The patient with left ventricular failure often presents with dyspnea, cough, reduced exercise tolerance, delirium, anxiety, and adventitious breath sounds (Table 8.3).[16] Cognitive impairment is not uncommon, owing to a decrease in cerebral blood flow, although it has been shown to improve with exercise training programs.[17,18] The increased sympathetic activity and release of norepinephrine combined with poor cardiac output leads to poor peripheral circulation. This often produces cool skin, diaphoresis, cyanosis of the digits, and peripheral pallor.

> The most common clinical signs of heart failure are dyspnea, cough, reduced exercise tolerance, abnormal breath sounds, tachycardia, and decreased sensorium.

Table 8.3 New York Heart Association Functional Classification of Heart Disease Correlated with Mortality

Functional Class	Definition	Manifestation	1–Year Mortality (%)
I	Patients with cardiac disease but without physical limitation	Ordinary activity does not cause undue fatigue, palpitations, dyspnea, or angina	0–5
II	Patients with cardiac disease that results in slight limitation; comfortable at rest	Ordinary physical activity results in fatigue, palpitations, dyspnea, or angina	10–20
III	Patients with cardiac disease resulting in marked limitation of physical activity; comfortable at rest	Less than ordinary physical activity results in fatigue, palpitations, dyspnea, and angina	35–45
IV	Patients with cardiac disease resulting in an inability to carry out any physical activity without discomfort	Symptoms of cardiac insufficiency or angina may be present, even at rest	85–95

Distended jugular veins, abdominal distention owing to ascites, hepatojugular reflux, and peripheral edema of the ankles are common findings of right ventricular failure.[16]

Dyspnea either at rest or with minimal exertion is frequently seen during significant failure.[19] It is also the most common sign of heart failure in the older population. The dyspnea commonly increases when the patient is lying flat (orthopnea) and abruptly after retiring at night (paroxysmal nocturnal dyspnea). This increase in dyspnea is caused by the addition to the lungs of about 1 liter of blood resulting in a threefold increase in the work of breathing when the patient is in the supine position. For this reason, these patients often report that their sleep is disturbed and that they sleep better with numerous pillows. Tachypnea is a compensatory breathing pattern that these patients often adopt.

Sleep disordered breathing is common in patients with CHF. Cheyne Stokes breathing with central sleep apnea has been found in 40% of patients with CHF, while obstructive sleep apnea/hypopnea was seen in 11%.[20] There is also evidence indicating that a history of obstructive sleep apnea may be an independent risk factor for CHF.[21]

Aerobic exercise capacity is frequently diminished in patients with chronic heart failure.[22] This impairment is associated with inadequate oxygen delivery to skeletal muscles, their subsequent shift to anaerobic metabolism, and consequent fatigue.[23,24] As heart failure increases and maximum cardiac output falls, exercise capacity and maximum oxygen utilization decrease. Patients with the poorest performance are at highest risk for complications, the need for hospitalization, and death.[25]

Physical Examination

Tachycardia is a common finding and represents a compensatory mechanism for maintaining cardiac output in the face of a poor stroke volume. Alterations in beat-to-beat blood pressure (pulsus alternans) may be detected, indicating severe myocardial disease. Tachycardia (heart rate greater than 100/min) and dysrhythmias may contribute to the degree of heart failure and may be secondary to associated electrolyte imbalance or drug toxicity. For these reasons, continuous electrocardiographic (ECG) monitoring is a standard of care during the acute phase of treatment.

Compensatory sympathetic vasoconstriction may maintain a normal blood pressure, but in severe failure the systolic and mean arterial pressures will be reduced (cardiogenic shock). The patient's peripheral skin temperature is frequently reduced, whereas core temperature may actually be elevated as a result of impaired heat dissipation.

Auscultation of the chest during left ventricular failure often reveals inspiratory crackles and polyphonic expiratory wheezes. Crackles occur as small airways of atelectatic regions "pop" open upon inspiration. Wheezes may be caused by reflex bronchoconstriction, a decrease in airway diameter caused by a decrease in overall lung volume, swelling of the bronchial mucosa, and obstruction by edema fluid in the airways.[26] Presence of an S_3 or S_4 or both and murmurs are common and may be more evident with exercise.

Peripheral edema, abdominal distention, and superficial abdominal vein distention are common findings of right and biventricular chronic heart failure. Liver congestion (hepatomegaly) and excessive peritoneal fluid retention (ascites) cause abdominal distention as a result of chronic venous hypertension and impaired lymphatic drainage. Hepatojugular reflux may also be present. In most adults, fluid retention of approximately 5 liters must occur before peripheral edema is detectable. Edema fluid collects in the most dependent regions of the body, such as the ankles in the upright patient (pedal edema). The edema formation may become so severe that the skin will pit upon pressing on it. Pitting is commonly evaluated on a scale of 1+ to 4+, where 1+ indicates slight edema and 4+ indicates severe edema often with seeping of fluid from beneath the skin, usually referred to as "weeping." Edema observed above the knee indicates more severe fluid retention than edema limited to the ankles. In bedridden patients edema rarely forms in the face but more often in the posterior parts of the arms, thighs, and legs.

Chest Radiography

Specific radiographic changes are associated with the three degrees of left heart failure, as follows:

- **Mild Failure.** Pulmonary venous congestion with widening of pulmonary arteries; redistribution of pulmonary blood flow to the upper lung fields.
- **Moderate Failure.** Cardiomegaly (heart greater than half the diameter of the thorax); pulmonary artery engorgement; interstitial pulmonary edema (presence of Kerley's A lines [1- to 2-cm lines of interstitial edema out from the hilum] and Kerley's B lines [short, thin, flattened streaks of interstitial edema outlining the subsegmental lymphatics that extend from the pleural surface]).
- **Severe Failure.** Cardiomegaly; pulmonary artery engorgement; interstitial pulmonary edema; fluffy, patchy alveolar edema (often in a "butterfly" pattern that radiates out from the perihilar region); and bilateral or unitlateral right-sided pleural effusion.

The progression of the density seen on the chest radiograph corresponds to the degree of failure. As the heart failure worsens, more and more fluid accumulates within the lungs and the "whiteness" on the chest radiograph intensifies and progresses from the more dependent regions toward the less dependent regions at the top of the lungs.

> The chest radiograph will show cardiomegaly, cephalization of blood flow, and Kerley's A and B lines when heart failure is present.

Electrocardiography

A variety of dysrhythmias occur during heart failure. Sinus tachycardia is the most common ECG abnormality. Frequent premature ventricular contractions and atrial fibrillation may contribute to failure or be a result of it. Bundle branch blocks and axis deviations are common in cardiac hypertrophy. QT-wave changes are frequently present and suggest myocardial hypoxia or infarction or both. Patients with chronic heart failure are at increased risk for sudden death with increasing QT dispersion and variation.[27] Changes in R wave magnitude, right axis, or right bundle branch block are more common during right heart failure.

Arterial Blood Gases

Arterial blood gas (ABG) analysis is useful for determining the degree of gas exchange derangement and the trend in the patient's pulmonary status. Reduced Pao_2, increased alveolar-arterial oxygen gradient ($P[A-a]o_2$), or reduced ratio of Pao_2 to fraction of inspired oxygen (Fio_2) are the most practical and sensitive signs of respiratory impairment during left heart failure. These changes indicate the magnitude of $\dot{V}/\dot{Q}$ mismatching and diffusion defects that occur as a result of pulmonary engorgement and edema. Respiratory alkalosis occurs frequently in the early period of failure and often continues until the patient is no longer able to compensate. With the onset of severe left ventricular failure and frank pulmonary edema, ventilatory failure is likely, and a combination of severe hypoxemia, carbon dioxide retention, and respiratory acidosis occurs. A mixed respiratory and metabolic acidosis is not uncommon in severe failure as the result of anaerobic metabolism caused by poor perfusion and hypoventilation.

Laboratory Studies

Routine laboratory studies are seldom useful in establishing heart failure as the cause of a patient's complaints, but some tests are useful. With chronic cor pulmonale, the hematocrit (Hct), hemoglobin (Hb) concentration, and erythrocyte count are frequently elevated 10% to 25% above normal values as the result of compensation for chronic hypoxia. Hyponatremia and hypokalemia are often seen in patients with CHF as a result of excessive fluid retention or diuretic therapy. In right ventricular failure with excessive liver engorgement, the bilirubin and liver enzymes (e.g., aspartate aminotransferase [AST]) may be elevated.[16]

An elevated atrial naturetic peptide (ANP) level is strongly associated with left ventricular failure. A finding of levels greater than 54 pmol/liter is highly sensitive and specific in detecting individuals with asymptomatic heart failure.[15] A bedside test of the plasma natriuretic peptide (BNP) can distinguish heart failure–related dyspnea from that caused by lung disease. A BNP value of >100 pg/mL has a sensitivity of 90%, specificity of 74%, and predictive accuracy of 81% in diagnosing dyspnea caused by heart failure.[28]

Hemodynamic Monitoring

Pulmonary artery catheterization can be used to evaluate the degree of pulmonary hypertension and the cardiac output. It has been use to guide therapy in patients with severe heart failure.[29] Table 8.4 lists the combinations of physical findings and hemodynamic data that predict the severity of heart failure and patient outcome after a myocardial infarction (MI). The echocardiogram, Doppler flow, and radionuclide studies are useful in establishing the anatomic changes in heart structure and motion typically found in failure. Often the findings include dilated end-diastolic ventricular dimensions, hypertrophic myocardial changes, valvular dysfunction, and reduced ventricular motion and ejection fraction.

The combination of physical assessment, chest radiography, ABG analysis, ECG, and hemodynamic monitoring forms the core of early detection and management.

Table 8.4 Hemodynamic and Physical Finding Subsets After Heart Failure from Acute Myocardial Infarction (125)

Subset	PAWP (mm Hg)	Cardiac Index (liters/minute/m²)	Mortality (%)
I. No pulmonary congestion and no peripheral hypoperfusion	≤18	>2.2	3
II. Pulmonary congestion and no peripheral hypoperfusion	>18	>2.2	9
III. Peripheral hypoperfusion and no pulmonary congestion	≤18	≤2.2	23
IV. Pulmonary congestion and peripheral hypoperfusion	>18	≤2.2	51

PAWP = pulmonary artery wedge pressure

TREATMENT

Therapy for heart failure is based upon the cause of failure, its severity, and the secondary complications. Therefore, treatment focuses on eliminating the cause of failure, reducing cardiac workload, and supporting the function of other organs.

Reduction of Cardiac Workload

Cardiac function can be improved by reducing myocardial workload and enhancing contractility. The most effective approach to reducing cardiac work is reduction of afterload. This can be achieved with lifestyle changes and medications. Lifestyle changes that reduce cardiac work include engaging in appropriate physical activity, reducing emotional stress, losing weight (if patient is overweight), and eating a low-salt diet. Bed rest and sedation with appropriate drugs (e.g., morphine, midazolam [Versed]) may be necessary to reduce anxiety and agitation, which cause cardiac stimulation. Afterload reduction can be induced with direct-acting vasodilators (e.g., nitroglycerin, nitroprusside, isosorbide, hydralazine, minoxidil). Decreasing the vasoconstrictive effects of norepinephrine with an alpha-adrenergic receptor–blocking agent (e.g., prazosin, trimazosin) is also useful to achieve indirect vasodilation. Vasodilation and afterload reduction occur with the suppression of angiotensin II production. Angiotensin II is a powerful vasoconstrictive hormone produced from angiotensin I by angiotensin-converting enzyme (ACE). Use of an ACE inhibitor (e.g., captopril) results in generalized vasodilation and reduced blood pressure. Another approach to vasodilation and afterload reduction is the use of calcium channel blockers (e.g., verapamil, nifedipine). Calcium channel blockers inhibit the action of vasoconstrictive mechanisms and are also useful in controlling tachydysrhythmias.

> Pharmacological treatment of heart failure focuses on decreasing afterload, increasing contractility, and decreasing fluid overload.

Despite drug therapy, the mortality rate for patients with severe heart failure and cardiogenic shock ranges from 80% to 90% or higher. This has emphasized the need for other ways of reducing cardiac work and improving the basic problem of poor blood flow. Circulatory assistance devices provide a mechanical approach to improving blood flow and reducing cardiac work. Such devices include the intra-aortic balloon pump, ventricular assist devices, and a total artificial heart. These devices can correct the acute problem of poor blood flow and give the patient time to respond to drug therapy or survive long enough for a heart transplant.

Improvement of Cardiac Pump Performance

Inotropes (e.g., digitalis, dopamine, dobutamine, amrinone) are used to improve ventricular function by increasing contractility. This action, improves cardiac output and reduces congestion. Digitalis remains the most frequently prescribed inotropic agent for heart failure and is the drug of choice. Patients with chronic heart failure owing to systolic dysfunction are the most responsive. Digitalis intoxication can occur. The classic signs and symptoms include nausea, vomiting, insomnia, altered color vision, and irregular cardiac rhythm (e.g., frequent premature ventricular contractions).

Myocardial contraction is a highly aerobic process that requires an ample and stable supply of oxygen. Frequently the patient with heart failure has a compromised coronary circulation. This defect may be the primary trigger for failure or will limit the ability of the heart to compensate, or both. Supplemental oxygen is frequently employed to improve oxygen delivery to the myocardium.

Prevention of Dysrhythmia

Cardiac dysrhythmias can cause or exacerbate heart failure. The use of antidysrhythmic drugs to control bradycardia (e.g., atropine) and tachycardia (e.g., procainamide, metoprolol, bretylium) is frequently necessary.

Control of Sodium and Fluid Retention

Sodium and water retention can be improved with bed rest, which induces a natural diuresis by the kidneys. Upright positions decrease sodium and water excretion and should be restricted until fluid and electrolyte balance is more acceptable. Dietary restriction of sodium and water and diuretics are useful in controlling water retention.

High-dose diuretic therapy is usually started at the beginning of severe CHF and then tapered off as the patient responds. The endpoint of diuretic therapy is frequently the fluid volume status that gives maximal cardiac output without causing pulmonary congestion. This usually results in a targeted PAWP (preload pressure) of 15 to 18 mm Hg. It frequently takes as long as 24 hours after the optimal preload pressure is achieved for the inspiratory crackles and radiographic signs of pulmonary edema to disappear. Careful use of these agents is necessary to avoid overdiuresis, which could lead to electrolyte imbalance and rebound hypotension. Careful fluid replacement and potassium therapy is almost always necessary to avoid hypokalemia and fluid imbalance.

Prevention of Thromboembolism

Patients in heart failure are at high risk for clotting disorders and development of emboli. The potential for devastating systemic or pulmonary embolization necessitates the use of prophylactic anticoagulants (e.g., heparin). Long-term anticoagulant therapy reduces the risk of embolization by reducing the viscosity of blood, which reduces the myocardial workload.

In cases of severe CHF, patients require most, if not all, of the above measures. The actions of these agents can be seen in Figure 8.2, which shows a family of Frank-Starling cardiac output and left ventricular filling pressure (preload) curves. The diuretics reduce preload and venous congestion but do not directly improve cardiac output. Vasodilators reduce afterload and improve cardiac output. Inotropic agents improve contractility and reduce preload when used with vasodilators. This results in improved cardiac performance and reduced venous congestion.

Surgical treatment of heart failure is directed toward specific repair of the cause. This includes valvular repair or replacement and coronary artery bypass grafting for coronary artery disease. For younger patients with refractory myopathy, cardiac transplantation offers the best hope for long-term treatment of severe CHF.

Respiratory Care for Cardiogenic Pulmonary Edema

Initial treatment with high levels of oxygen is necessary to improve arterial oxygenation, which will improve cardiac function. Unless contraindicated, patients should initially receive 100% oxygen by face mask to return arterial oxygenation saturation levels above 90%. A nonrebreathing mask with adequate flow may also be used if a high-flow system is not available.

High-flow continuous positive airway pressure via mask (mask CPAP) can be useful in treating the heart failure patient with significant pulmonary edema and dyspnea. It

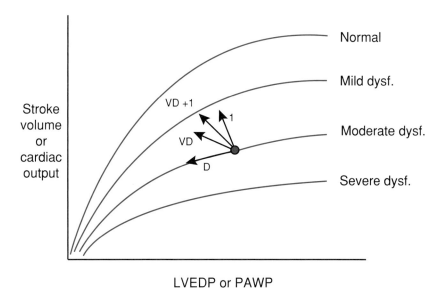

FIGURE 8.2 Frank-Starling left ventricular function curves relating preload pressure (left ventricular end-diastolic pressure [LVEDP] or pulmonary artery wedge pressure [PAWP] and stroke volume or cardiac output. Curves showing normal and various degrees of dysfunction (dysf) are shown. Diuretics (D) are shown to reduce preload and venous congestion without acutely improving cardiac output. Inotropic drugs (1) or vasodilators (VD) and especially the combination of these two (VD + 1) shift heart function toward better cardiac output with reduced preload.[16]

can result in rapid improvement in oxygenation and reductions in respiratory and heart rate. Although hypoventilation and subsequent hypercapnia are potential contraindications to the use of mask CPAP, they have not detracted from its effective use in treating hypoxemia induced by heart failure. The suggested mechanism behind the effectiveness of mask CPAP in this setting is improved lung compliance, reduced work of breathing, improved gas exchange, and reduced vascular congestion. Mask CPAP should be used with a nasogastric tube in place.

> Oxygen therapy is the most important respiratory care treatment option in heart failure patients.

It should be avoided if the patient is at high risk for vomiting or has severe respiratory acidosis (pH less than 7.20).

If patients on CPAP develop progressive respiratory acidosis, bilevel noninvasive positive pressure ventilation (BiPAP) should be considered. Greater control over the inspiratory and expiratory cycles is available and may prolong the time before invasive mechanical ventilation in necessary. Both CPAP and BiPAP have been shown to be effective in treating heart failure and the associated Cheyne Stokes respirations.[30–32]

Intubation and ventilatory support are necessary when a patient exhibits a grave clinical picture of poor respiratory function (e.g., cyanosis and periodic breathing pattern) or evidence of severe respiratory failure (pH less than 7.20, $Paco_2$ greater than 50, Pao_2 less than 50) while receiving oxygen therapy. Typical initial ventilator settings are assist/control mode, Fio_2 of 1.0, V_T 5 to 10 mL/kg (ideal body weight), respiratory rate >10 to 15/min, and sensitivity of −2 cm H_2O. The addition of positive end-expiratory pressure (PEEP; 5 to 15 cm H_2O) is appropriate if the oxygenation and lung mechanics remain poor despite ventilatory support with an elevated Fio_2 (e.g., greater than 50%).

Special attention to airway care is necessary after intubation in patients with frank pulmonary edema. Edema foam must be cleared rapidly to improve the effectiveness of the oxygen therapy and ventilatory support. In the past, aerosolized ethyl alcohol (20% to 40%) was used to reduce the pulmonary edema foam, but this has been abandoned because of its bronchial irritation and the more direct response to airway suctioning and application of high-dose diuretics.

Aerosolized bronchodilators (e.g., albuterol) should be used in patients who have a component of asthma or bronchitis or both. Iprotropium bromide has been shown to produce bronchodilation in patients who have chronic CHF.[33] Incentive spirometry is also useful during the recovery phase to promote lung expansion and airway clearance.

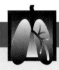

Mr. P

HISTORY

Mr. P, a 69-year-old Hispanic man, is a retired supervisor at a building cleaning service. He has a history of coronary artery disease, dysrhythmia, chronic obstructive pulmonary disease (COPD), and a recent episode of pneumonia and a small anterior wall MI, which required a 1-month hospitalization at the local county hospital. He was discharged 3 days ago with an extensive assortment of medications to control his cardiac, renal, and pulmonary function. While at home he experienced a coughing spell that led to increasing shortness of breath and mild substernal pressure. He became increasingly anxious and requested that the paramedics be called and that he be taken to the hospital immediately because he could not "catch his breath" and that his "heart would not slow down." He was brought to the hospital and treated with oxygen via face mask at 9 liters/min.

QUESTIONS	ANSWERS
1. What signs and symptoms should you evaluate immediately upon Mr. P's arrival?	You should evaluate level of consciousness, signs of delirium, signs of a patent airway, spontaneous breathing and chest motion, quality of breath sounds and their symmetry, pulse rate, blood pressure, and temperature. You should also look for symptoms of respiratory distress, shock, and mental impairment. You should carefully monitor the effect of the administered oxygen on his COPD status.
2. What diagnostic techniques could you use to help determine the cause of Mr. P's shortness of breath?	You could evaluate the severity and origin of his shortness of breath by taking a rapid history to determine the triggering factors that led to the sudden exacerbation. After you perform a careful and rapid physical evaluation followed by appropriate laboratory studies, you should sort out the source of the dyspnea (pulmonary versus cardiac).
3. What therapeutic techniques should be readily available upon Mr. P's arrival?	Oxygen therapy (via non-rebreathing mask, high-flow/high FIO_2 device), intubation equipment, manual resuscitation bag with proper mask, oxygen reservoir, venous and arterial line placement equipment, various fluids for vascular support, appropriate resuscitation drugs, and medications for pain and agitation should be readily available.

More on Mr. P

PHYSICAL EXAMINATION

- **General:** An obese, elderly male with an approximate weight of 115 kg (250 lbs) who is alert and in obvious respiratory distress while sitting up despite oxygen therapy via face mask at 9 liters/min; spouse states, and patient confirms, history of moderate smoking for 20 years and cessation 10 years ago; history of MI 10 years ago, multiple hernia operations 10 years ago, chronic lung disease; recently hospitalized for pneumonia and heart disease; indicates compliance with medications and low-salt, low-fat diet

- **Vital Signs.** Temperature 37.5°C (99.5°F); respiratory rate 31/min, blood pressure 100/70 mm Hg; heart rate 160/min, nail bed refill 5 seconds

- **HEENT.** Pupils equal and reactive to light; some nasal flaring; normal oral structures

- **Neck.** Trachea in midline; no signs of inspiratory stridor or laryngeal abnormality; carotid pulses + + bilaterally without bruit; no signs of lymphadenopathy or thyroidomegaly; noticeable jugular venous distention; some tensing of sternocleidomastoid and scalene muscles during inspiration

- **Chest.** Normal chest configuration; no scars; some diminished motion noted; bilateral inspiratory crackles from bases midway up chest, with some scattered expiratory wheezes

- **Heart.** Heart tones diminished; point of maximal impulse not palpable; no murmurs, rub, or gallop

- **Abdomen.** Obese and soft; no hepatomegaly; bowel sounds not heard clearly

- **Extremities.** Moving all extremities; +2 pulses felt throughout; 2+ pitting edema in both ankles; no clubbing; skin cool and clammy with some digital cyanosis

QUESTIONS	ANSWERS
4. What are the possible causes of Mr. P's respiratory distress?	Mr. P's respiratory distress may be caused by pulmonary edema owing to left ventricular failure, exacerbation of his COPD, MI, or pulmonary infection.
5. What signs and symptoms indicate heart failure?	His signs and symptoms of heart failure include rapid onset of dyspnea, anxiety, disproportionate tachycardia and relatively low blood pressure, inspiratory crackles in the dependent lung regions, jugular venous distention, cool, diaphoretic skin and poor peripheral circulation, and ankle edema.
6. How will left ventricular failure influence respiratory function?	Left ventricular failure can induce pulmonary hypertension, increased lung water, increased airway resistance, alveolar edema, increased work of breathing, decreasing pulmonary compliance, $\dot{V}/\dot{Q}$ mismatching, diffusion defect, hypoxemia, and ventilatory failure.

7. What diagnostic techniques should you use to further evaluate Mr. P's cardiorespiratory distress?

For further evaluation of his cardiorespiratory distress, ABGs, chest radiograph, and a 12-lead ECG with subsequent ECG monitoring are needed immediately. Continuous noninvasive monitoring of his oxyhemoglobin saturation and blood pressure will further help guide his cardiopulmonary care. Laboratory assessment of the complete blood count, electrolytes, and standard blood chemistry are indicated. Assessment of his cardiac enzymes (creatinine kinase [CK]) and digitalis levels would help rule out an MI and help guide digitalis therapy.

More on Mr. P

Box 8.2 Bedside and Laboratory Evaluations

ECG: Supraventricular tachycardia of 158/min, normal axis, first-degree atrioventricular (AV) block, and left bundle branch block
Chest Radiograph (see Fig. 8.3)

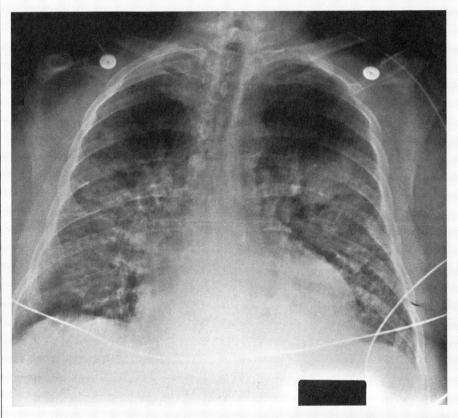

FIGURE 8.3 Portable AP chest radiograph taken at admission in the emergency department.

(box continued on page 181)

ABGs	
ABG	Value
pH	7.24
$Paco_2$	51 mm Hg
Pao_2	44 mm Hg
HCO_3^-	22 mEq/liter while breathing oxygen via face mask at 9 liters/min

Hematology	
Measure	Value
Hct	45%
Hb	15 g/dL
RBC	$5.2 \times 10^6/mm^3$
White blood cell (WBC) count	15.2×10^3
Platelets	262×10^3

Chemistry: Results pending

QUESTIONS	ANSWERS
8. What does the ECG indicate?	The ECG indicates severe tachycardia as well as other cardiac conduction disturbances. This rate is out of proportion with the resulting blood pressure and is probably contributing to or causing acute CHF.
9. What does the chest radiograph indicate?	The chest radiograph reveals cardiomegaly, bilateral pulmonary vascular engorgement, interstitial and alveolar edema, and atelectasis bilaterally; some Kerley's B lines in both bases; and no signs of pleural effusion or hemopneumothorax. The trachea is seen in the midline. Some scoliosis is seen in the cervical and thoracic vertebral column, but the rib cage looks normal. No mediastinal masses are noted.
10. How would you interpret the ABG data?	The ABG shows severe hypoxemia owing to one or more of the following: hypoventilation, diffusion defect, shunting, and $\dot{V}/\dot{Q}$ mismatching. Hypoventilation, despite significant tachypnea, indicates a ventilatory decompensation that is producing uncompensated respiratory acidosis. Considering this patient's history of COPD, you should consider applying an alternate acid-base classification: an acute-on-chronic respiratory acidosis accompanying a loss of accumulated base owing to a metabolic acidosis; however, no other data presented support such a classification. These findings are consistent with severe cardiogenic pulmonary edema.

11. What do the hematological data indicate?	The hematological data are relatively normal with the exception of the slight-to-moderate elevation of the WBC count, which may be caused by an infection or induced by stress.
12. What respiratory care is indicated at this time?	The oxygen therapy currently in use is inadequate to support oxygenation. Although the patient has significant hypoxemia and moderate ventilatory failure, intubation and ventilatory support is not indicated at this time because of the strength of the respiratory efforts and the lucid state of the patient. BiPAP or mask CPAP may be attempted to improve ventilatory mechanics and improve oxygenation. If the patient's clinical status or the ABGs were to deteriorate, intubation and mechanical ventilatory support would be necessary. Aerosolized bronchodilator therapy (e.g., albuterol, ipratropium bromide) should be continued to optimize airway resistance, given the clinical findings of wheezes and the history of COPD.
13. What cardiac care is indicated at this time?	Supraventricular tachycardia of this magnitude is a dangerous condition requiring immediate treatment and continuous ECG and blood pressure monitoring. IV lines should be placed in case it becomes necessary to give resuscitative drugs. Drug therapy (e.g., verapamil) should be administered to induce rapid reduction of the heart rate. If this is unsuccessful, electrocardioversion should be attempted. Fluid retention should be relieved with high-dose diuretics (e.g., furosemide). Reduction of afterload and improvement of myocardial contractility should be carried out carefully with vasodilators (e.g., hydralazine, captopril) and inotropic agents (e.g., digitalis).

 More on Mr. P

In the emergency department, continuous ECG and pulse oximetry are started, two peripheral IV lines are placed, and oxygen therapy is switched to a non-rebreathing mask supplied with oxygen at a rate of 18 liters/min. Two cardioversion attempts are made (100 watt-sec followed by 150 watt-sec), but both are unsuccessful. A single dose of slowly administered verapamil is given with a prompt decline in heart rate to 130/min. Furosemide, isosorbide, captopril, digitalis, morphine sulfate, and erythromycin are started. Mr. P is transferred to the coronary care unit (CCU) with the diagnosis of heart failure secondary to one or more of the following: supraventricular tachycardia, possible MI, possible dietary indiscretion, possible noncompliance in taking his medication, and possible underlying pulmonary infection. Upon admission to the unit, an arterial line is placed and continuous ECG and pulse oximetry monitoring are continued.

BEDSIDE FINDINGS

Mr. P is alert, sitting up in bed, in obvious respiratory distress despite receiving high-concentration oxygen via non-rebreathing mask, and somewhat anxious. Occasionally he coughs up thick, brown sputum. He stated, "I'm afraid to be taken off the oxygen." He is being given a combination of 500 mcg of ipratropium bromide and 2.5 mg of aerosolized albuterol diluted in 3 mL of saline every 2 hours, and he indicates that these treatments help reduce his dyspnea.

Box 8.3 Laboratory Evaluation

Vital Signs, Hemodynamics, and Urine Output	
Measure	Value
Rectal temperature	37.2° (99.0 F)
Respiratory rate	33/min
Heart rate	132/min
Systemic arterial blood pressure	143/97 mm Hg
SpO_2	81%
Breath sounds	Bilateral inspiratory crackles expiratoy wheezes
Urine output	500 mL over the past hour since hospital admission and furosemide administration

ECG Findings

Sinus tachycardia of 130/minute, first-degree AV block, and left bundle branch block

ABGs	
ABG	Value
pH	7.26
$Paco_2$	51 mm Hg
Pao_2	49 mm Hg
HCO_3^-	24 mEq/liter
$P(A - a)o_2$	660 mm Hg
Pao_2/Fio_2	49 (assumes Fio_2 1.0)
SaO_2	79% (calculated)

Electrolytes and Chemistry	
Measure	Value
Na^+	137 mEq/liter
K^+	3.7 mEq/liter
Ca^{++} (ionized)	8.2 mg/dL
Cl^-	101 mEq/liter
Glucose	239 mg/dL
Blood urea nitrogen	13 mg/dL
Creatinine	1.3 mg/dL

Cardiac Enzymes: Pending
Microbiology: Sputum smear and cultures pending

QUESTIONS	ANSWERS
14. What do the bedside findings and vital signs indicate about Mr. P's response to treatment?	Mr. P's bedside findings indicate that his heart rate, blood pressure, and urine output have responded, but that his respiratory status has not improved.
15. What do the laboratory findings indicate about Mr. P's status?	The ECG changes are very encouraging, and Mr. P's chemistry panel is acceptable; however, the ABG and acid-base balance indicate severe hypoxemia despite very high concentrations of oxygen and continued hypoventilation with respiratory acidosis in the face of significant tachypnea.
16. What changes, if any, in Mr. P's respiratory care would you recommend?	Mr. P is now a candidate for a mask-CPAP trial or BiPAP. Clinicians who take a more aggressive approach may consider mechanical ventilation. Continuation of aerosolized bronchodilators to help reduce his work of breathing is appropriate. Leaving him in a state of significant dyspnea and in respiratory failure while waiting for the diuresis to reduce the pulmonary edema borders on cruelty.

 ## More on Mr. P

Following assessment of Mr. P's condition, he is placed on a continuous high-flow mask-CPAP system, and a nasogastric tube set to suction is inserted. The initial settings are as follows: flow = 60 liters/min, FiO_2 = 1.0, and CPAP = 5 cm H_2O. Initially Mr. P. is apprehensive but becomes less dyspneic and his respiratory rate decreases to 28/min, heart rate decreases to 103/min, blood pressure remains stable at 140/96, and SpO_2 increases to 89% after 30 minutes of CPAP and continued diuresis. CPAP is increased to 7.5 cm H_2O to achieve further improvement in gas exchange and respiratory mechanics and to attempt reduction of his FiO_2. After another 30 minutes of treatment, the following observations and data were collected.

Box 8.4 Bedside Findings

Mr. P is sitting up in bed, wearing a clear plastic CPAP mask. He is alert, communicative, and appears more comfortable with less dyspnea. He continues to use his accessory muscles with some thoracoabdominal asynchrony. The FiO_2 is reduced to 0.80 with orders to keep his SpO_2 greater than 92%. Chest auscultation reveals improved aeration throughout the lower lung zones with scattered inspiratory crackles and occasional expiratory wheezes and rhonchi.

Vital Signs and Laboratory Evaluation	
Measure	Value
Temperature	37.3°C (99.1°F)
Respiratory rate	23/min
Heart rate	98/min
Systemic arterial blood pressure	138/98 mm Hg
SpO_2	96%
Urine output total of 1.9 liters over the past 4 hours since admission	

ECG Findings: sinus tachycardia, first-degree AV block, and left bundle branch block

ABGs ($F_{IO_2} = 0.80$)	
Measure	Value
pH	7.39
Pa_{CO_2}	50 mm Hg
Pa_{O_2}	96 mm Hg
HCO_3^-	30 mEq/liter
$P(A - a)O_2$	465 mm Hg
Pa_{O_2}/F_{IO_2}	120
Sa_{O_2}	97% (calculated)
Sp_{O_2}	= 96% (pulse oximeter)

QUESTIONS

ANSWERS

17. How would you interpret Mr. P's bedside findings and vital signs?

Mr. P's bedside findings and vital signs indicate mild-to-moderate respiratory distress, reduced work of breathing, enhanced oxygenation, an improving cardiovascular response, and a continued brisk diuresis.

18. What do the ABGs indicate?

ABGs reveal improving oxygenation, although his F_{IO_2} requirement remains elevated with a declining $P(A - a)O_2$. Hypoventilation and a compensated respiratory acidosis persist, which are common in patients with a history of COPD.

19. What respiratory care would you recommend at this time?

Mr. P continues to respond well to the mask CPAP, diuretic, vasodilators, and inotropic therapy. His treatment is on the right course and should allow continued reduction of the F_{IO_2} by 10% increments until 40% is reached. If his respiratory and cardio-vascular status are stable or improving at that point for 1 hour or more and the tachypnea decreases to less than 22/min, the CPAP levels can be reduced to 5 and then 0 cm H_2O. He could then be placed on oxygen therapy via nasal cannula. Continued car-diopulmonary monitoring remains necessary.

Mr. P Conclusion

Mr. P's respiratory status continues to improve over the next 8 hours as the F_{IO_2} is gradually reduced to 0.40. His respiratory rate remains less than 20/min, heart rate is in the 85 to 95/min range, blood pressure drops to 125/75 mm Hg, and Sp_{O_2} is maintained at greater than 95%. Breath sounds reveal better aeration with scattered expiratory wheezing. A chest radiograph (Fig. 8.4) at this time shows almost complete interval clearing with some scattered atelectasis in the right perihilar region and basal zones of the right and left lungs. Heart size is reduced, and all other anatomic structures appear to be unchanged. Digitalis levels are found to be in the therapeutic range. The ABG results are as follows: pH = 7.37, Pa_{CO_2} = 49 mm Hg, Pa_{O_2} = 105 mm Hg, and HCO_3^- = 29 mEq/liter. The CPAP level is gradually reduced to 0 cm H_2O over the next hour. Mr. P tolerates this change and exhibits no noticeable changes in clinical state or pulse oximetry. He is placed on a nasal cannula at 4 liters/min, which is later reduced to 2 liters/min. Cardiac enzyme levels (CK and lactate dehydrogenase) are found to be in the high-normal range, suggesting that he did not have an MI. Therapy with diuretics, vasodilators, inotropic agents, aerosolized bronchodilators, and oxygen are continued upon Mr. P's transfer to the post-CCU, and he begins to ambulate. He is discharged 2 days later in stable condition with an assortment of medications to support him at home. ■

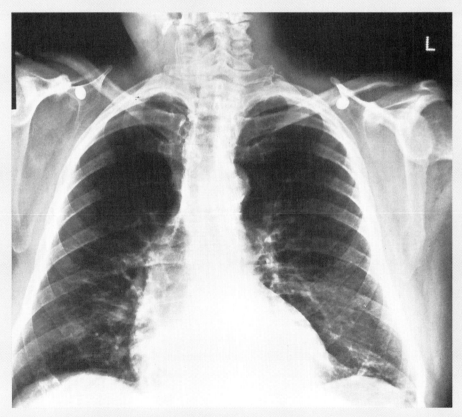

FIGURE 8.4 Portable AP chest radiograph taken 12 hours after admission to the hospital.

KEY POINTS

- Heart failure occurs when the heart is unable to pump adequate amounts of blood to the lungs and the peripheral tissues.
- Congestive heart failure results in fluid accumulating in the lungs (pulmonary edema) and dependent extremities (peripheral edema).
- Cor pulmonale describes right heart enlargement and failure as a result of pulmonary disease.
- The two most common causes of heart failure are hypertension and coronary artery disease.
- To compensate for heart failure the heart will attempt to increase rate, contractility, and ventricular muscle thickness.
- When the right heart fails, fluid backs up in the venous and capillary circulation, leading to peripheral edema and hypertension.
- Left heart failure produces pulmonary engorgement, flooding of the alveoli, and pulmonary hypertension.
- Edema occurs when the lymphatic system cannot drain the interstitial space of the accumulated fluid.
- Clinical presentation of heart failure includes dyspnea, cough, decreased sensorium, abnormal breath sounds, and tachycardia.
- Sleep disordered breathing is common in heart failure patients.
- Breath sounds heard include inspiratory crackles and wheezes.
- Chest radiography in left heart failure shows cardiomegaly and Kerley's A and B lines.
- Right heart failure on chest radiographs presents as enlarged systemic veins and right-sided chambers and pulmonary hypovolemia.
- ABGs show an all-round decrease in oxygenation levels in left heart failure.
- Laboratory values are not usually significant except in cor pulmonale, where the hematocrit, hemoglobin concentration, and erythrocyte count are frequently elevated 10% to 25% above normal.
- A combination of a thorough history, physical assessment, chest radiography, ECG, and hemodynamic monitoring forms the core of early detection and management.
- Treatment focuses on eliminating the cause of failure, reducing cardiac workload, and supporting the function of other organs.
- Patients with heart failure are at high risk for developing systemic and pulmonary emboli. Prophylactic anticoagulants are used to minimize these risks.
- Initial treatment with high levels of oxygen is necessary to improve arterial oxygenation, which will improve cardiac function.
- High-flow continuous positive airway pressure via mask (mask CPAP) and BiPAP are two additional therapies that can be used if supplemental oxygen delivery by itself is not sufficient.
- Intubation and ventilatory support are needed if the patient's respiratory failure is not reversed with less invasive techniques.
- Aerosolized bronchodilators (e.g., albuterol) should be used in patients who have a compounding component of asthma, bronchitis, or both.

REFERENCES

1. American Heart Association, Heart Disease and Stroke Statistics–2005 Update.
2. van Jaarsveld, CHM, Ranchor, AV, Kempen, GIJM, et al: Epidemiology of heart failure in a community-based study of subjects aged ≥57 years: incidence and long-term survival. Eur J Heart Failure. 8(1): 23–30, 2006.
3. Alexander, M, et al: Hospitalization for congestive heart failure: explaining racial differences. JAMA 274:1037–1042, 1995.
4. Killip, T: Epidemiology of congestive heart failure. Am J Cardiol 56:2A, 1985.
5. Kannel, WB, et al: Cardiac failure in the Framingham Study: twenty-year follow-up. In Braunwald, E, et al (eds): Congestive Heart Failure: Current Research and Clinical Applications. Grune & Stratton, New York, 1982, pp. 15–30.
6. Kannel, WB: Incidence and epidemiology of heart failure. Heart Fail Rev 5, 167–173, 2000.
7. Kenchaiah S, Narula, J, Vasan, RS: Risk factors for heart failure. Med Clin N Am 88:1145–1172, 2004.
8. He, J, Ogden, LG, Bazzano, LA, et al: Risk Factors for Congestive Heart Failure in US Men and Women: NHANES I follow-up study. Arch Intern Med 161:996–1002, 2001.
9. Macera, CA, Ham, SA, Yore, MM, et al : Prevalence of physical activity in the United States: Behavioral Risk Factor Surveillance System, 2001. Prev Chronic Dis 2005. Available at: http://www.cdc.gov/pcd/issues/2005/apr/04_0114.htm.
10. _____ Percentage of smoking prevalence among US adults, 18 years of age and older, 1955–2003. Available at: http://www.cdc.gov/tobacco/research_data/adults_prev/prevali.htm.
11. _____ National Center for Health Statistics. Health United States, 2004, With Chartbook on Trends in the Health of Americans. Hyattsville, MD, 2004.
12. _____ Profile of General Demographic Characteristics: 2000, US Census Bureau, Census 2000. Available at: http://www.census.gov/Press-Release/www/2001/demoprofile.html.
13. _____ The Graduates: Educational Attainment, 2000. In Population Profile of the United States: 2000 (Internet Release), US Census Bureau, Census 2000. Available at: http://www.census.gov/population/www/pop-profile/profile2000.html.
14. Dzau, VJ, et al: Relation of the renin-angiotensin-aldosterone system to clinical state in congestive heart failure. Circulation 63:645–651, 1981.
15. Lerman, A, et al: Circulating N-terminal atrial natriuretic peptide as a marker for symptomless left-ventricular dysfunction. Lancet 341:1105–1109, 1993.
16. Amsterdam, EA, et al: Today's workup for heart failure. Patient Care 29:58–71, 1995.
17. Lackey, J: Cognitive impairment and congestive heart failure. Nurs Stand 18(44):33–36, 2004.
18. Tanne, D, Freimark D, Poreh, A, et al: Cognitive functions in severe congestive heart failure before and after an exercise training program. Int J Cardiol 103:145–149, 2005.
19. Ahmed, A, Allman, RM, Aronow, WS, et al: Diagnosis of heart failure in older adults: predictive value of dyspnea at rest. Arch Gerontol Geriatr 38:297–307, 2004.
20. Cormican, LJ, Williams, A: Sleep disordered breathing and its treatment in congestive heart failure. Heart 91:1265–1270, 2005.
21. Shahar E, Whitney CW, Redline S, et al: Sleep-disordered breathing and cardiovascular disease: cross-sectional results of the Sleep Heart Health Study. Am J Respir Crit Care Med 163:19–25, 2001.
22. Weber, KT, et al: Oxygen utilization and ventilation during exercise in patients with chronic cardiac failure. Circulation 65:1213–1223, 1982.
23. Zelis, R, et al: A comparison of regional blood flow and oxygen utilization during dynamic forearm exercise in normal subjects and patients with congestive heart failure. Circulation 50:137–143, 1974.
24. Litchfield, RL, et al: Normal exercise capacity in patients with severe left ventricular dysfunction: compensatory mechanisms. Circulation 66:129–134, 1982.
25. Bittner, V, et al: Prediction of mortality and morbidity with a 6-minute walk test in patients with left ventricular dysfunction. JAMA 270:1702–1707, 1993.
26. Snashall, PD, Chung, KF: Airway obstruction and bronchial hyperresponsiveness in left ventricular failure and mitral stenosis. Am Rev Respir Dis 144:945–956. 1991.
27. Abelmann, WH, Gilbert, EM: QT dispersion and sudden unexpected death in chronic heart failure. Lancet 343:327–329, 1994.
28. Morrison LK, Harrison, A, Krishnaswamy, P, et al: Utility of a rapid B-natriuretic peptide assay in differentiating congestive heart failure from lung disease in patients with dyspnea. J Am Coll Cardiol 39:202, 2002.
29. Forrester, JS, Diamond, G, Chatterjee, K, et al: Medical therapy of acute myocardial infarction by application of hemodynamic subsets. N Engl J Med 295:1356–1362, 1976.
30. Kohnlein, T, Welte, T, Tan, L, et al: Assisted ventilation for heart failure patients with Cheyne-Stokes respiration. Eur Respir J 20:934–941, 2002.
31. Krachman, SL, D'Alonzo, GE, Berger, TJ, et al: Comparison of oxygen therapy with nasal continuous positive airway pressure on Cheyne-Stokes respiration during sleep in congestive heart failure. Chest 116:1550–1557, 1999.
32. Willson, GN, Wilcox, I, Piper, AJ, et al: Noninvasive pressure preset ventilation for the treatment of Cheyne-Stokes respiration during sleep. Eur Respir J 17:1250–1257, 2001.
33. Rolla, G, Bucca, C, Brussino, L, et al: Bronchodilator effect of ipratropium bromide in heart failure. Eur Respir J 6:1492–1495, 1993.

9

Smoke Inhalation Injury and Burns

George H. Hicks, MS, RRT

Carl A. Eckrode, MPH, RRT

> ## CHAPTER OBJECTIVES:
>
> After reading this chapter you will be able to state or identify the following:
>
> - The factors that influence the mortality rate from burn injury.
> - The toxic nature of smoke inhalation and the fire environment.
> - The pulmonary and systemic changes that occur following smoke inhalation and burn injury.
> - The effects of smoke inhalation injury on the upper and lower airways.
> - The diagnosis of smoke inhalation injury and CO poisoning.
> - The methods used to determine the type and extent of burn injury.
> - The emergent treatment for smoke inhalation injury and CO poisoning.
> - The airway and ventilatory support strategies for smoke inhalation and burn injury.
> - The fluid, antibiotic, surgical, and nutritional support used in the treatment of burn injuries.

INTRODUCTION

The catastrophic loss of 491 people in the Coconut Grove nightclub fire in 1942 and other significant fires stimulated the need for a better understanding of burn and smoke inhalation injury, their treatment, and fire prevention in general. Despite advanced understanding and remarkable improvements in treatment and prevention, fire continues to be a major source of injury, death, and economic loss in this country. In 2003, fire departments responded to 1.6 million fires, 470,000 people were injured, 45,000 people were hospitalized, 4,000 people died, and there was over $14.3 billion in property damage and burn-related medical care.[1,2] Burns rank as the third most common cause of serious injury and death for all ages and races and both sexes. Residential fires are the most common setting for burn-related injuries and the site of 80% of the deaths on scene.[1] The overall mortality rate has steadily declined for the past 50 years and is currently about 5% to 10% for those with burns that require hospitalization.[3–6] With increasing total body-surface area (TBSA) burns and age, the mortality rates increase (Fig. 9.1). Women between the ages of 30 and 59 appear to have a twofold higher risk of mortality when compared to men of the same age.[4] Currently, the victim of fire-related injuries who has an 80% TBSA burn and is treated in a burn center has a 50% chance of survival.

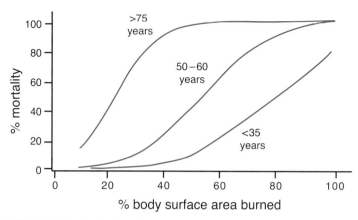

FIGURE 9.1 The distribution of mortality in burn victims for different age groups and size of burn. (Adapted from data presented in Tompkins, RG, et al: Prompt eschar excision: a treatment system contributing to reduced burn mortality: a statistical evaluation of burn care at Massachusetts General Hospital (1974–1984). Ann Surg 204:272, 1986).

Asphyxiation, systemic poisoning, and respiratory tract injury from smoke inhalation cause 50% to 90% of deaths in victims at the scene of a fire or shortly afterward.[7,8] The prevalence of smoke inhalation injury among burn victims admitted to burn centers ranges from 10% to 35%.[4–10] The mortality rate among burn victims with significant smoke inhalation injury is much higher. The mortality rate for a large burn (>40% TBSA) is reported at 3%. This climbs to 27% when combined with inhalation injury and it increases to 95% in those with large burns and smoke inhalation injury and for those who are more than 60 years old (Fig. 9.2).[5]

> The overall mortality rate for a 65-year-old person who has a 20% TBSA burn and significant smoke inhalation injury is approximately 40%.

Burn injuries are highly complex. They are not confined to the integumentary and respiratory systems. Although it is convenient to categorize post-burn injuries into various periods or phases, in reality they often present in an overlapping pattern. Pulmonary complications are frequently found in the burn victim and are found in various time frames after the burn.[10–12] The early or resuscitative phase (first 24 hours) is usually associated with respiratory complications arising from inhalation of toxic or hot gases, fluid loss, and heavy sedation. In the intermediate, or post-resuscitative, phase (2 to 7 days), analgesic-related respiratory dysfunction, secretion retention, airway obstruction, atelectasis, acute respiratory distress syndrome (ARDS), and hypermetabolic-induced ventilatory failure can all occur or in varying combinations. During the late phase (beyond 7 days), infectious pneumonia, sepsis syndrome, multiple organ dysfunction, pulmonary embolism, and chronic pulmonary disease are the more frequent types of respiratory dysfunction.

The pulmonary problems listed above, coupled with the other pathophysiological changes, make the burn victim one of the most challenging patients to care for. These problems are complex but predictable. This allows a more successful approach through the principles of support and prevention. This chapter focuses on the pulmonary changes and required treatment for smoke inhalation and burn injuries.

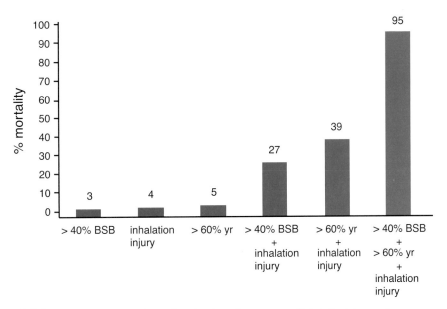

FIGURE 9.2 The distribution of mortality when burn size, presence of inhalation injury, and age are considered. BSB, body surface area burn. (Adapted from data presented in Ryan, CM, et al: Objective estimates of the probability of death from burn injuries. N Engl J Med 338:362, 1998.)

ETIOLOGY

Burn injuries can be caused by exposure to fire, superheated gases, scalding liquids, chemicals, and electrical currents (e.g., lightening or high-voltage conductors). Most injuries occur in residential fires. Analysis of the fire environment reveals highly complex and variable conditions. Heat production, and the chemical and physical nature of the smoke produced in a fire, must be taken into account. The factors that make the fire environment complex include the types and amounts of fuels being burned, the availability of fresh air, and the proximity of the victim to the heat and combustion by-products. The nature and extent of injuries can be calculated as the product of exposure to heat and smoke over time.

Air temperatures can rapidly climb to 1000°F in less than 10 minutes in a fuel-rich environment such as a home, office, or vehicle. As the heat builds, spontaneous combustion of other fuel sources (e.g., carpet, furniture, wall coverings, appliances, flammable liquids and gases) can occur, developing dense smoke and providing conditions ideal for a **flash over**. Flash over is usually seen as a wall of fire extending down from the ceiling and billowing out of openings in doorways or windows. Industrial or shipboard fires can produce much higher temperatures, as well as steam. Steam has a significantly higher heat energy content than dry gases at the same temperature and can scald greater areas of skin and cause a deeper respiratory tract thermal injury if inhaled. Scalding of the skin is more common in the very young and elderly when the temperature of bath water is misjudged and excessive.

> The heat content of steam is 540 times as much as that of dry air.

The burning of various fuels found in modern residential, office, and industrial settings produces a large number of combustion products.[13,14] Some of the more common

Table 9.1 Toxic Gases Found in House Fire Smoke

Substance	Source	Effect
Ammonia	Melamine resins	Inflammation
Aldehydes (acrolein, acetaldehyde, formaldehyde)	Wood, cotton, paper	Inflammation
Benzene	Petroleum products	Irritation and coma
Carbon dioxide	Organic materials	Asphyxiation and coma
Carbon monoxide	Organic materials	Asphyxiation and coma
Hydrogen chloride	Polyvinyl chloride	Inflammation
Hydrogen cyanide	Polyurethanes	Cellular asphyxia
Isocyanate	Polyurethanes	Inflammation and bronchospasm
Organic acids (acetic and formic acid)	Wood, cotton, paper	Inflammation
Oxides of nitrogen and sulfur	Nitrocellulose film	Pulmonary edema
Phosgene	Polyvinyl chloride	Inflammation

toxic chemicals produced are listed in Table 9.1. A variety of aldehydes (e.g., acrolein), organic acids (e.g., acetic acid), and products of oxidation (e.g., SO_2, NO_2) are all potent respiratory tract irritants. They are produced from burning wood, cotton, paper, and many plastics. As the fire continues, carbon dioxide is produced and can increase beyond 5%, while the oxygen concentration can drop below 10%.[16] With the decreased oxygen availability, incomplete combustion results in the production of carbon monoxide (CO) and hydrogen cyanide (HCN).[13–15] When plastics (e.g., polyvinyl chloride) are burned, they can produce hundreds of toxic chemicals, including hydrogen chloride, phosgene, chlorine, perfluoroisobutylene, and CO.[13,17] The burning of polyurethane-rich materials, such as nylon and various types of upholsteries, can produce isocyanates and hydrogen cyanide (HCN).[13,15]

Smoke is composed of both gas molecules and soot particles. Soot particles are produced with various diameters, including those in the 0.1 to 10 μm range that can penetrate into and be deposited all along the respiratory tract and cause injury.[14,18] The soot particles can behave as vehicles for the transport of various noxious chemicals into the respiratory tract.

> The inhalation of smoke can result in rapid asphyxiation and inflammatory changes in the upper and lower airways.

The chemical products of combustion can be divided into two categories: those that produce toxic effects systemically upon absorption and those that produce inflammatory changes upon contact with the mucosa. An additional factor that contributes to the severity of smoke inhalation injuries is being trapped in an enclosed space (e.g., closed rooms or vehicles) and breathing hypoxic gas mixtures that result from the rapid depletion of oxygen during the fire.

In summary, the nature and severity of injury is a function of many factors. The size and depth or degree of the skin burn, the heat and chemical composition of the gases inhaled, the extent and duration of exposure, and the age and preexisting health status of the victim are all important factor to assess.

PATHOPHYSIOLOGY

Early Pulmonary and Systemic Changes: Within 24 Hours Post-Burn

Exposure to the hypoxic and poisonous environment of a fire can cause rapid and severe organ dysfunction. The mechanism of this type of dysfunction involves reductions in both oxygen transport and its utilization, as well as altered tissue metabolism. The tissues of the central nervous system and myocardium are particularly at risk.

Carbon Monoxide

CO is readily produced in the fire environment, especially if oxygen levels are low and combustion is incomplete. The CO produced is easily absorbed into the blood from the inhaled gas and is highly toxic.[19] It rapidly converts oxyhemoglobin (HbO$_2$) to **carboxyhemoglobin** (HbCO). This conversion is driven by CO's higher affinity for the ferrous binding sites in hemoglobin (more than 200 times that of O$_2$). HbCO levels in nonsmokers are normally less than 3%. In minor smoke inhalation it can increase to 15% and climb to more than 60% in severe smoke inhalation. Conversion of HbO$_2$ to HbCO compromises oxygen transport, primarily through HbCO's inability to carry O$_2$. The presence of CO also retards oxygen release from hemoglobin's remaining ferrous binding sites by a chemically induced increase in HbO$_2$ affinity. The hemoglobin conversion and inhibition of oxygen release results in a functional form of anemia that causes reduced oxygen transport and hypoxia despite the presence of a normal PaO$_2$ in the plasma.

CO is also capable of binding to other heme-containing proteins such as cytochrome oxidase within mitochondria, myoglobin in skeletal and cardiac muscle, and guanylyl cyclase that catalyses that production of cycGMP.[19] When CO binds to these proteins, it disables or modifies their normal functions. CO poisoning of cytochromes in the mitochondria results in reduced ATP synthesis and an anaerobic metabolic acidosis, as well as the formation of

> CO poisoning can rapidly lead to fatigue, dysrhythmias, heart failure, seizure, and coma. It may also result in delayed neuropsychological deficits.

highly toxic free radicals of oxygen.[20] Skeletal muscle and cardiac muscle dysfunction occur as a result of the inability of myoglobin to store and release sufficient oxygen. This can rapidly lead to fatigue, dysrhythmias, and possibly heart failure.[21] CO binding to guanylyl cyclase results in the production of excessive levels of intracellular messenger cycGMP; this disrupts autonomic organ regulation and can cause cerebral vasodilation.[22] Rapid loss of consciousness and cerebral edema owing to CO poisoning is also associated with the production of nitric oxide (NO) and other oxygen free radicals that cause vasodilation and hypoperfusion of the brain.[23,24] Some patients appear to recover from CO poisoning and then demonstrate personality changes, movement disorders, and cognitive deficits. Collectively, this is known as delayed neuropsychologic sequelae (DNS). DNS can occur days to months after significant CO poisoning and is more often associated with unconsciousness at the time of admission.[25] Lethal CO poisoning generally occurs with HbCO concentrations greater than 50% to 60%.

Hydrogen Cyanide

Inhaled hydrogen cyanide (HCN) has also been linked to early and late death in burned patients.[15,26,27] HCN is easily transported to the tissues through the circulatory system and binds to the cytochrome oxidase enzymes of the mitochondria. This also results in inhibition of oxidative cellular metabolism and a shift to **anaerobic metabolism** and elevated lactic acid production. Fatal exposure to HCN is generally associated with blood levels that exceed 1 mg/liter and is frequently associated with severe CO poisoning.[27]

Other Considerations

The reduced oxygen transport, cellular metabolic dysfunction, release of inflammatory mediators, and altered vascular changes that rapidly develop following the inhalation of toxic gases and the thermal injury of the skin can compromise the nervous system, cardiovascular, and skeletal muscle functions. These are the primary causes of death during the immediate period after severe smoke inhalation.

Thermal injury to the respiratory tract is frequently confined to the face, oral and nasal cavities, pharynx, and trachea.[10] The lower respiratory tract is spared because of the upper airway's efficient cooling of hot dry gases and reflex laryngospasm and glottic closure.[28,29] Thermal injury to the upper airway results in blistering, edema, accumulation of thick saliva, and glottic closure in severe cases.[30] These changes usually develop in the first 8 hours and can lead to partial or total airway obstruction.

Chemical injury to the respiratory tract, brought about by inhalation of toxic gases and irritant-laden soot particles, extends the injuries further into the lung. This can cause acute tracheobronchitis, bronchospasm, bronchorrhea, mucosal sloughing, airway obstruction and, in severe cases, rapid onset of pulmonary edema.[31–33] After chemical exposure, the ciliary transport mechanism of the mucosa is often inactivated or destroyed. This can lead to further mucus retention, alveolar de-recruitment, and regional atelectasis and sets the stage for respiratory tract infection.

Large skin burns and smoke inhalation injury have been shown to cause the following within minutes to hours post-injury: increased pulmonary and bronchial blood flow, increased pulmonary vascular pressures, increased systemic and pulmonary capillary permeability, pulmonary and systemic edema, cardiac failure (myocardial depression), surfactant dysfunction, and increased apoptosis (programmed cell death) of respiratory tract cells.[34–39] These can result in decreased lung compliance and increased airway resistance.[40] Gas exchange is altered by ventilation-perfusion ($\dot{V}/\dot{Q}$) mismatching and increased dead space ventilation (V_D/V_T).[37,41] These changes lead to decreased Pa_{O_2}, a decreased Pa_{O_2}/Fi_{O_2} ratio, and an increase in the necessary minute ventilation to normalize the Pa_{CO_2}. The initial arterial blood gas (ABG) changes include hypoxemia and respiratory alkalosis in most cases and mixed respiratory and metabolic acidosis in more severe cases of asphyxiation. The pulmonary response to burn and smoke inhalation injury are summarized in Table 9.2.

Early systemic changes are associated with the degree of decline in oxygen transport, metabolic derangement, the release of inflammatory mediators, and fluid loss. Organ dysfunction, induced by hypovolemic and cardiogenic shock, is one of the primary systemic insults in the early period after a major full-thickness burn of the skin. Early hypovolemia occurs following massive fluid shifts out of the vascular compartment as a result of an injured and hyper-permeable microvasculature. This massive fluid shift results in a generalized edema that peaks within eight to 24 hours and is dependent on the magnitude of the burn and the adequacy of the fluid resuscitation.

> Circumferential burns of the chest can result in reduced chest wall compliance and increased work of breathing.

Burned skin also loses its elasticity, becomes less compliant with the edema formation, and contracts. In circumferential burns of the extremities, the tightening skin can further impair circulation and can result in distal limb tissue necrosis. When there are circumferential burns of the chest and abdomen, it can

Table 9.2 Pulmonary and Gas Exchange Response to Moderate-to-Severe Burn and Smoke Inhalation Injury in a Laboratory Animal Model*

Response	Hours Post-Injury			
	6	12	24	48
Static compliance	−25%	−30%	−40%	−60%
Airway resistance	+20%	+85%	+125%	+200%
$\dot{V}/\dot{Q}$ mismatching	+7%	+15%	+18%	+25%
Pao_2/Flo_2	−11%	−23%	−32%	−40%
Oxygen consumption	+15%	+20%	+35%	+50%
Dead space ventilation	−15%	−5%	+20%	+30%
$Paco_2$	−10%	−5%	−2%	+10%
pH	7.35	7.45	7.42	7.38

*Adapted from: Shimazu, T, et al: Ventilation-perfusion alterations after smoke inhalation injury in an ovine model. J Appl Physiol 81:2250, 1996 and Soejima, K, et al: Pathophysiology and analysis of combined burn and smoke inhalation injuries in sheep. Am J Physiol Cell Mol Physiol 280:L1233, 2001.

result in reduced chest wall compliance,[42] which results in an increase in the work of breathing and may lead to severe ventilatory compromise.

Cardiovascular and hematological instability (Table 9.3) occur from the loss of fluid volume and the release of various mediators. Fluid loss can exceed 4 mL/kg of body weight per hour in major burns.[43,44] Cardiac output is frequently decreased as a result of hypovolemia, the production of myocardial depressant factors (e.g., NO, pro-inflammatory cytokines, and macrophage migration inhibitory factor), hypoxia, and increased systemic and pulmonary vascular resistance.[45–48] CO may not play a strong role in the depression of cardiac function in mild to moderate poisoning.[49] Systemic blood pressure may be low to normal, and heart rate is usually increased.[44] Older patients may not tolerate massive fluid

Table 9.3 Changes in Systemic Hemodynamics, Blood, and Oxygen Kinetics after Severe Burns in Humans*

	Period		
	Early	Intermediate	Late
Heart rate	+50%	+75%	+25%
Blood pressure (mean)	Normal	+10%	+30%
Cardiac index	−15%	+65%	−15%
Left ventricular stroke work	−50%	Normal	−55%
Vascular resistance	+30%	−30%	−20%
Blood volume	−20%	+15%	−30%
Hematocrit	+3%	−30%	−30%
Oxygen transport	−15%	+25%	−60%
Oxygen consumption	+35%	+70%	−40%

*From six patients (35% to 60% of BSA third-degree burns). The early period was the first 25% of their course, the late period was the last 25% of their course, and the intermediate period was the time between early and late periods. Values are expressed as percent change from data taken from 17 healthy control subjects.

SOURCE: Adapted from Shoemaker, WC, et al: Burn pathophysiology in man. I. Sequential hemodynamic alterations. J Surg Res 14:64, 1973.

resuscitation and are thus at risk for congestive heart failure. Immune suppression and alterations in leukocyte and macrophage function commonly occur during this period. Hemolysis and the development of disseminated intravascular coagulation can occur and further compromise the microcirculation.

The metabolic rate is often depressed in the very early period as a result of asphyxiation from severe hypoxia and abnormal circulation. After a massive release of catecholamines, in response to the stress, metabolism quickly increases and may produce metabolic acidosis if the oxygen demand exceeds the delivery rates.

Intermediate Pulmonary and Systemic Changes: 2 to 7 Days Post-Burn

Signs of respiratory distress are often seen in burn victims after 24 to 48 hours. In those with severe burns (>40% TBSA) but no inhalation injury, lung function is often stable but can be complicated by burn and fluid resuscitation-induced pulmonary edema and reduced chest wall compliance. The early increase in pulmonary blood flow (largely driven by increased bronchial blood flow) and increased pulmonary vascular resistance often returns to normal during this period.[37,38] The hypermetabolic state often continues during this period and results in increased CO_2 production and O_2 consumption, which can further tax a patient's marginal respiratory function to the point of failure.

In patients with inhalation injury, the upper airway edema usually begins to resolve between days 2 and 4. Mucosal inflammation secondary to chemical injury results in increased mucus production and decreased clearance secondary to ciliary dysfunction. Smaller airway injury, manifested as a lingering bronchitis with or without bronchospasm, usually peaks on day 2 or 3. With more severe mucosal injury, the mucosal tissue often becomes necrotic and sloughs, usually on days 2 through 4. The necrotic debris and mucus retention often result in airway plugging, alveolar de-recruitment and atelectasis.[31,32] The atelectasis is further promoted by the victim's inability to breathe deeply and cough effectively as a result of reduced chest and lung compliance, increased airway resistance, pain, use of narcotics, immobility, and inadequate airway care. The impaired secretion clearance, atelectasis, and burn-induced immune suppression set the stage for bacterial colonization, infectious bronchitis, and pneumonia.

During the intermediate period, the major pulmonary complications that can occur include atelectasis, pleural effusion, acute lung injury (ALI) and acute respiratory distress syndrome (ARDS; see Chapter 11). ARDS occurs in approximately 50% of burn victims who require ventilatory support.[50–53] It can be classified as being caused by either direct pulmonary injury (smoke inhalation or pneumonia) or extra-pulmonary causes (burned skin or septecemia). A large variety of mechanisms have been implicated:

- Surfactant dysfunction
- Increased pulmonary blood flow and capillary hyperpermeability that are induced by pro-inflammatory mediator release from neutrophils, macrophages, and injured tissues (e.g., lipid peroxides, NO, cytokines, endothelin, bradykinin, and possibly thromboxane and substance P)
- Compliment-activated leukocytes that migrate to the lung and release toxins (e.g., proteolytic enzymes, oxygen free radicals)
- Bacterial translocation from the gut to the circulation
- Coagulation defects[54–63]

> **A**RDS occurs in 50% of burn patients who require ventilatory support.

Patients who have had careful fluid resuscitation and have resolved cardiac failure are usually hemodynamically stable during this period. Cardiac output and systemic blood pressure improve, and a persistent tachycardia, secondary to the elevated catecholamine release, typically occurs during this period (see Table 9.3). Systemic vascular resistance declines and an adequate urine output is frequently seen if sufficient fluid is given. The erythrocyte damage, secondary to the cutaneous thermal injury, usually levels off during this period and the hematocrit stablizes.[44]

The metabolic rate during this phase continues to be 30% to 100% elevated above the predicted basal metabolic rate and, if not supported with sufficient calories, can lead to a catabolic state and poor wound healing.[29] A negative nitrogen balance resulting from catabolism of blood and muscle proteins is common, and stress-induced diabetes can also occur.

Late Pulmonary and Systemic Changes: Beyond 7 Days Post-Burn

In this later period, the hypermetabolic state can persist for 1 to 3 weeks, and the resting CO_2 production rates can exceed 400 mL/min. This added load on the respiratory system significantly increases the work of breathing and, compounded by a possible muscle catabolism, can result in respiratory muscle fatigue and ventilatory insufficiency.

Infection is the most common and serious problem in this period. Most burned patients become colonized with Staphylococcus bacteria within a week of admission, many acquire methicillin-resistant *S. aureus* (MRSA), and some are colonized with *Pseudomonas aeruginosa*.[64] Current techniques of burn wound care, however, have significantly reduced the incidence of invasive infections, cellulitis, and overall mortality. Infectious pneumonia is the most common organ after the skin to be infected and the most common cause of severe sepsis in those with major burns.[65] Significant sepsis occurs in about 30% of burned patients and remains an important cause of morbidity and mortality.

Multiple organ dysfunction syndrome (MODS) occurs when two or more organs begin to function abnormally. It is thought to be most often the result of sepsis that triggers an imbalance in the release of mediators that up- and down-regulate inflammation and coagulation. This imbalance brings about widespread inflammation and microcirculatory disruption that leads to the dysfunction of numerous organs. MODS occurs in about 25% of these patients, is typically caused by pulmonary infection, occurs about a week to 10 days after the burn injury, and is the most common cause of death.[65]

Pulmonary embolism can develop in some burn patients as a result of coagulation abnormalities and venous stasis from long periods of little or no mobility.[66] It generally occurs within 2 weeks of the burn injury but in some cases may develop months after the injury. Tachypnea, increasing minute ventilation and a marked decrease in the $P_{O_2}/F_{I_{O_2}}$ ratio or an increase in the $P(a - {\rm ET})_{CO_2}$ indicate that significant embolization may have occurred.

After several months of recovery from severe inhalation injury and burns, some patients continue to experience dyspnea, chronic cough, and increased reactive airway disease.[67–71] Those who develop severe cases of ARDS can develop persistent diffusion impairment, restrictive pulmonary function, and decreased exercise tolerance.[72] In some with inhalation injury and prolonged intubation or tracheostomy tube placement, there is increased risk of developing subglottic or tracheal stenosis from granuloma formation weeks to months after the initial injury and airway care.[73,74] However, many smoke inhalation victims have few or no long-term symptoms and have normal pulmonary function.[75] These discrepancies may be

> Many of the survivors of smoke inhalation injury have normal pulmonary function one year after their injuries.

the result of the "dose" of smoke inhalation they received, the number and degree of complications, and their underlying health condition.

CLINICAL FEATURES

The increased morbidity and mortality associated with inhalation injury in the burn victim necessitates early recognition and treatment. The primary survey of the burn patient, like other trauma patients, should include evaluation of the ABCs: airway, breathing, circulation, and the cervical spine.

The secondary survey of the burn patient is a more detailed evaluation that should include the evaluation of the circumstances of the burn injury and determine if there is history of exposure to a smoke-filled or enclosed environment. In the absence of clinical findings, if the history suggests exposure to smoke, there should be a high index of suspicion for inhalation injury.

Organs that are more oxygen dependent (e.g., brain and heart) are the first to show dysfunction and indicate inhalation injury. It should be assumed that burn patients presenting in an unconscious state were exposed to asphyxiating conditions (low FIO_2) or to toxic gases (e.g., CO, HCN) or both. This requires immediate and aggressive treatment. Tables 9.4 and 9.5 list the major signs and symptoms associated with various levels of CO and HCN poisoning. The classic description of CO poisoning, a cherry-red skin color, is an unreliable sign, especially in the hypotensive victim. Electrocardiograms (ECGs) often show tachycardia and may show signs of ischemic heart disease. In some, CO poisoning can resemble the classic clinical and ECG findings of heart attack.[76] The sampling of arterial blood for direct determination of Hbco content is the most important diagnostic indicator of CO poisoning. Hbco content is also a potential indicator of the dose of smoke inhaled. Low levels of Hbco, however, do not rule out significant pulmonary injury in the intermediate or later post-burn periods.

> **P**ulse oximetry will indicate a falsely elevated oxyhemoglobin saturation in a patient who has significant CO poisoning.

Pulse oximetry should not be used to indicate the level of HbO_2 concentration in the patient who is known or suspected to have been poisoned by CO. Oxyhemoglobin and Hbco have similar light-absorption spectra in the two regions that are used by the pulse oximeter.

Table 9.4 Clinical Manifestations of Carbon Monoxide Poisoning

Degree of Poisoning	Blood Hbco Concentration (%)	Signs and Symptoms
Mild	3–10	None; angina in patients with coronary artery disease
	10–20	Mild headache, exercise-induced angina, and dyspnea
Moderate	20–40	Headache, dyspnea, vomiting, muscular weakness, dizziness, visual disturbance, impaired judgment
Severe	40–60	Syncope, increasing tachypnea and tachycardia, chest pain, hypotension, coma, convulsion, irregular breathing pattern, and rhabdomyolysis
Life threatening	>60	Coma, shock, apnea, and death

Hbco = carboxyhemoglobin

As a result, pulse oximeters give a falsely high value for the total (fractional) HbO_2 concentration when $Hbco$ concentrations are elevated.[77,78] Blood HbO_2 and $Hbco$ can be properly determined by analyzing an arterial sample in a bench-top oximeter that uses multiple wavelengths (five or more) of light.

Facial burns, singed nasal hair, oral and laryngeal edema, and carbonaceous deposits in the airway and sputum suggest inhalation injury, but the presence or absence of these findings is not considered a reliable indication of the degree of inhalation injury.[10] Carbonaceous sputum, while considered to be a very sensitive sign of smoke inhalation, may not be seen for 8 to 24 hours or more and may occur only in about 40% of victims with significant pulmonary injury.[79] Stridor, hoarseness, difficulty speaking, and chest retractions suggest upper airway injury and the need for careful evaluation. Cough, dyspnea, tachypnea, cyanosis, wheezing, crackles, and rhonchi are indicators of a more severe form of inhalation injury.

Fiberoptic laryngoscopy and bronchoscopy have been found very useful to evaluate the presence of upper airway injury and remove excess saliva, sputum, and carbonaceous debris.[80,81] The only clinical situation where bronchoscopy may fail to identify an inhalation injury is in the immediate post-burn period if the patient is in severe hypovolemic shock.

Table 9.5 Clinical Manifestations of Hydrogen Cyanide (HCN) Poisoning

Blood HCN Concentrations (mg/liter)	Signs and Symptoms
0.2–0.3	Tachycardia
	Tachypnea
	Dizziness
	Stupor
0.3–1.0	Progressive stupor
	Cardiac dysrhythmias
	Seizures
>1.0	Coma
	Apnea
	Death

Chest Radiograph

Chest radiographs frequently do not show signs of the severity of inhalation injury in the early period and lag behind the pulmonary changes. The chest x-ray is useful in the initial assessment of the burn victim to determine if other pathological conditions exist and to locate the position of the endotracheal tube after intubation. CT scans of the chest of a victim of smoke inhalation injury may be more useful to detect and determine the severity of the pulmonary injury.[82]

Pulmonary Function Studies

Spirometry has been found useful in detecting small and upper airway injury.[83] Peak expiratory flow and forced expiratory flow rates at 50% of the forced vital capacity (FVC) are both markedly decreased and correlate well with xenon-133 lung scan results in victims of smoke inhalation.[84] The utility of spirometry, however, is limited to patients who can follow commands and perform an acceptable FVC effort.

Arterial Blood Gases

ABG analysis is useful in diagnosing and trending the patient's pulmonary insult. Reduced PaO_2 and a decreased PaO_2/FIO_2 may be the most practical and sensitive signs of respiratory impairment (e.g., <300 mm Hg indicates ALI and <200 indicates ARDS). Reduced PaO_2 is most often the result of $\dot{V}/\dot{Q}$ mismatching. Respiratory alkalosis may also be found in the early post-burn period and often continues during the hypermetabolic phase. Metabolic aci-

> Maintaining a burn patient's base deficit above −6 mEq/L during the resuscitative phase of care improves the patient's survival.

dosis and ventilatory failure are signs of life-threatening injuries. The presence of an excessive base deficit (BD) of less than −6 mEq/L and/or an elevated serum lactate are important markers of a poor perfusion state during the resuscitation and follow-up care of the burn patient. A persistent BD of less than −6 mEq/L in the first 24 hours is associated with a higher incidence of ARDS, MODS, and death.[85,86]

ECG and Hemodynamic Monitoring

ECG and hemodynamic monitoring are essential in patients with burns of greater than 10% TBSA, regardless of whether or not they have concomitant smoke inhalation injury. Central venous or pulmonary artery pressure, cardiac output, and urine output must be monitored to optimize fluid resuscitation to avoid hypotension, renal failure, and fluid overload in the severely burned patient.

Physical assessment, fiberoptic bronchoscopy, chest radiography, ABG analysis, ECG, and hemodynamic monitoring form the core of cardiopulmonary assessment. Repeated evaluation of the burn victim with these techniques will enable the clinician to detect cardiopulmonary changes and intervene appropriately.

The secondary survey of the burn patient should include a head-to-toe evaluation of their injuries and pain, further attention to their fluid resuscitation, and assessment of their past medical history. To assess the cutaneous injury, a complete physical examination, weight determination (for trending fluid balance), and calculation of TBSA burned are performed. The rule of nines (Fig. 9.3) can be used to estimate the total size of the injured area by determining the amount of injury to each extremity, the head, and the anterior and posterior trunk. Each of these anatomic areas represents approximately 9% to 18% of the TBSA in adults. A computerized body-surface mapping program (Sage 2) has been developed to better determine the burn size and to map the response to treatment.[87] The burn depth is determined by its clinical appearance:

- **Partial thickness-superficial (first degree):** A burn to the epithelium that is manifested by erythema and pain
- **Partial thickness-deep (second degree):** A burn of the epithelium and dermis that is manifested by erythema, blisters, and pain
- **Full thickness (third degree):** A burn that destroys the skin through or into the hypodermis, manifested by pale or gray-brown, leather-like skin. There is no pain in this area because all sensory organs in the skin are completely destroyed.

TREATMENT

The goals of respiratory care for the burn patient include:

- Achievement of a patent airway
- Secretion removal
- Maintenance of effective ventilation
- Preservation of lung volume
- Adequate oxygenation
- Maintenance of acid-base balance

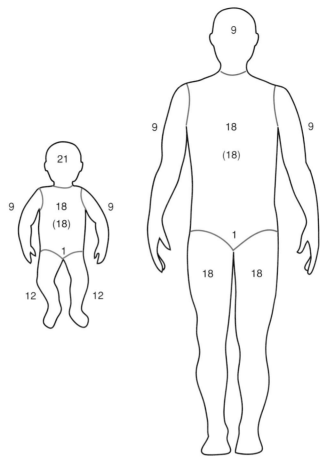

FIGURE 9.3 The percentage of surface area covered by skin in various body regions of the infant and adult.

- Cardiovascular stability
- Cervical spine protection
- Support of metabolism
- Suppression of infection
- Prevention of pulmonary embolism
- Control of pain
- Appropriate monitoring

Most burn victims are initially stabilized in a community hospital and are then transported to a burn center for treatment. The American Burn Association's recommendation criteria for referral to a burn center is summarized in Box 9.1.

Airway

As stated earlier, the immediate signs of inhalation injury are characterized by facial burns, soot in the mouth, and partial airway obstruction. Burn victims with minor upper airway injury should be closely monitored for airway closure or other signs of pulmonary involvement.

Box 9.1 American Burn Association Burn Unit Referral Criteria

Burn injuries that should be referred to a burn unit include the following:

1. Partial thickness burns greater than 10% total body surface area (TBSA)
2. Burns that involve the face, hands, feet, genitalia, perineum, or major joints
3. Third-degree burns in any age group
4. Electrical burns, including lightning injury
5. Chemical burns
6. Inhalation injury
7. Burn injury in patients with preexisting medical disorders that could complicate management, prolong recovery, or affect mortality
8. Any patient with burns and concomitant trauma (such as fractures) in which the burn injury poses the greatest risk of morbidity or mortality
9. Burned children in hospitals without qualified personnel or equipment for the care of children
10. Burn injury in patients who will require special social, emotional, or long-term rehabilitative intervention

They should be given supplementary oxygen via non-rebreathing mask until the Hbco is less than 10% and placed in a high Fowler's position to reduce the work of breathing. Bronchospasm should be treated aggressively with aerosolized beta-agonists (e.g., albuterol).

Airway maintenance with an oral endotracheal tube of the largest size that can be placed is needed in cases where upper airway closure is anticipated or significant inhalation injury is found.[73,88] The swelling of the upper airway will make it difficult to impossible for successful intubation if the situation is allowed to progress to complete airway closure. Leave the endotracheal tube uncut to accommodate facial swelling. Secure the tube with cotton ties over the ears so that adjustments can be made as the face swells rather than using adhesive tape under the ears, which will not adhere well following the application topical antibiotics and the sloughing of facial skin. Extubation should only be done if the patient is improving, can maintain his or her own airway and secretions, can ventilate without difficulty, and can demonstrate a cuff-leak when 30 cm H_2O of pressure is delivered at peak airway pressure when the cuff is deflated. The absence of a cuff-leak indicates that substantial airway edema or tracheal stenosis exists. This will necessitate further evaluation and treatment. Systemic corticosteroid treatment prior to extubation and aerosolization of racemic epinephrine post-extubation to treat lingering airway edema are commonly used.[89]

> Unconscious burn victims should be given 100% oxygen until their Hbco is less than 10%.

Early tracheostomy in this setting remains controversial.[73] It has been found to be effective in blunt force trauma patients and helps in secretion clearance and early weaning from the ventilatory support and reduces the incidence of nosocomial pneumonias.[89] However, in a recent study of burn patients it was not found to reduce length of time on ventilatory support, the incidence of pneumonia, length of stay in the hospital, or survival.[90,91] Placement of a tracheostomy is appropriate for the patient who will require ventilatory support for more than 10 days or who has ongoing secretion clearance problems.

Clearance of Secretions

Clearance of secretions becomes an increasingly important issue as the injured mucosal lining of the airways sloughs and forms plugs. The delivery of heated and humidified gas is essential along with adequate hydration and airway suctioning to mobilize and remove secretions. Chest physical therapy, while important, may not be tolerated by patients if they have burn injuries on their chest and back. Fiberoptic bronchoscopy for visual clearance of the airway is frequently needed for patients who develop airway plugging and for the collection of sputum specimens for microbial surveillance.

Carbon Monoxide Poisoning

The burn victim who is found in a coma must be assumed to have sustained severe asphyxia and/or CO poisoning. Basic and advanced life support are needed immediately to provide a patent airway and cardiorespiratory support. Oxygen therapy forms the cornerstone for the emergent treatment of hypoxia and CO poisoning. Elimination of CO is accelerated when supplemental O_2 is administered (Table 9.6). For burn victims in whom smoke inhalation is suspected and who have moderately elevated Hbco (less than 30%) and stable cardiopulmonary function, 100% O_2 at a rate of 15 liters/min from a tight-fitting nonrebreathing mask is the method of choice. Oxygen therapy should continue until the Hbco is reduced to less than 10%. High-flow mask CPAP at 5 to 10 cm H_2O pressure and 70% to 100% O_2 may be useful in patients who have minimal thermal injuries to the face and upper airway and have increasing dyspnea and hypoxemia that is not relieved by the use of a nonrebreathing mask.[92] For those with a more severe form of CO poisoning (Hbco greater than 30%) that results in coma, intubation and ventilatory support with 100% O_2 is needed. Rapid referral for hyperbaric O_2 therapy at 3 atm for 30 minutes to 1 hour is useful to improve patient outcomes in severe CO poisonings.[19]

Mechanical Ventilation

Conventional ventilatory support with positive end-expiratory pressure (PEEP) is needed for patients who develop respiratory failure, pneumonia, or ALI/ARDS or who require sedation and paralysis. Ventilatory support is needed when the patient's ABGs indicate respiratory failure (Pao_2 less than 50 mm Hg, $Paco_2$ greater than 50 mm Hg, and pH less than 7.20) or when the clinical picture indicates impending respiratory failure (respiratory rate greater than 35/min and significant use of accessory muscles). The initial settings would be assist-control ventilation, rate 15/min, V_T 6 to 8 mL/kg, T_I 1 second, sufficient inspiratory flow to meet patient demand, Fio_2 100%, PEEP 5 cm H_2O. Titrate the Fio_2 to maintain a Pao_2 of 100 mm Hg unless the Hbco is greater than 10%. PEEP is used to preserve lung volume and may need to be increased to higher levels when the patient's Fio_2 requirement climbs above 40% and/or the patient develops atelectasis. As the pulmonary insult resolves, the need for ventilatory support may continue in patients who maintain high metabolic rates and minute volume requirements.

Because of the spectrum of pulmonary dysfunctions that may be encountered, the ventilator of choice should be able to provide a variety of modes and monitoring features that will facilitate safe and effective ventilation. Pressure-controlled modes of ventilation that automatically adjusted to deliver a targeted V_T at the lowest pressure (e.g., pressure-regulated volume control,

Table 9.6 **Half-Life of Carboxyhemoglobin (Hbco) While Breathing Different Oxygen Concentrations**

Hbco Half-Life (min)	Inhaled O_2 and Atmospheric Pressure
280–320	21% @ 1 Atmosphere (air)
80–90	100% @ 1 Atmosphere
20–30	100% @ 3 Atmospheres (hyperbaric chamber)

autoflow or pc+) are popular and offer the added advantage of higher initial flow to meet the patient's inspiratory effort. The ventilator should be able to deliver stable tidal ventilation with peak pressures below 35 cm H_2O as the respiratory mechanics change and be able to provide pressure support ventilation to facilitate spontaneous breathing. Adjust tidal volume (V_T) to the 6 mL/kg range to avoid further lung injury and reduce mortality if the patient develops ALI or ARDS.[93] In cases where there is an increased risk of further lung injury and barotrauma from over-inflation, the V_T and minute ventilation can be adjusted down and permissive hypercapnia allowed ($Paco_2$ of 55 mm Hg and pH $\geq$7.30) to reduce further lung injury.[93,94]

Tracheal Gas Insufflation

Another novel approach to reduce V_T, airway pressure, and the potential of lung injury while maintaining $Paco_2$ during severe ARDS is the use of tracheal gas insufflation (TGI).[95] TGI helps wash out CO_2 in the anatomic dead space and airway by the delivery of oxygen at 5 to 10 L/min through a small bore catheter that is placed in the endotracheal tube down to a point just above the carina.[95] Another issue that can arise in these patients during conventional ventilation at elevated respiratory rates and minute ventilation is the development of insufficient time to exhale, gas trapping, and auto-PEEP. Regular efforts should be made to determine the level of auto-PEEP and reduce it to acceptable levels through reduction of respiratory rate and sedation in order to avoid lung injury, barotrauma, or reduced cardiac output.

High-Frequency Ventilation

A growing body of evidence has shown that high-frequency ventilation delivered by the volumetric diffusive respirator (VDR) or oscillator is useful in supporting and improving gas exchange in the burn patient with significant inhalation injury.[96–101] The use of the VDR in these patients has resulted in improved oxygenation, lower airway pressures, reduced barotraumas, improved secretion mobilization, and improved survival when compared to conventional ventilatory support. It should be noted that these studies have not compared high-frequency ventilation with low tidal-volume conventional ventilation that follows the ARDSnet protocol. High-frequency ventilation is used primarily as a rescue mode of ventilation in some burn centers for patients who are refractory to conventional ventilation. In other centers it is the primary mode of ventilation for patients with large TBSA burns and inhalation injury. The VDR delivers high-frequency percussive pulse breaths and intermittent pressure-controlled convective breaths and can be adjusted to allow spontaneous breathing with PEEP.

> The use of high-frequency ventilation for the burn patient with significant smoke inhalation injury has been shown to improve oxygenation, reduce barotrauma, improve secretion mobilization, and improve survival.

Fluid Balance

Careful maintenance of fluid balance is necessary to minimize the development of shock, renal failure, and pulmonary edema. Hemodynamic stability can often be maintained through IV fluid resuscitation of the patient according to the Parkland formula of 4 mL of isotonic crystalloids per kilogram per percentage TBSA burn over a 24-hour period (half of the fluid volume is given during the first 8 hours and the other half is given over the next 16 hours) to maintenance a urine output of 30 to 60 mL/hour.[102] Often, the burn patient with significant inhalation injury requires greater amounts of fluid. The fluid administration is then tapered down as the patient stabilizes and the swelling subsides. However, the large volumes of fluid given to these patients can result in the development of pulmonary edema. Monitoring pulmonary artery pressures in addition to urine output can be a better guide to the adequacy of fluid replacement and the need for vasopressor therapy.[103] Frequent analysis of the electrolyte panel and acid-base status is required to avoid potential imbalances. The IV administration of high-dose ascorbic acid in the first 24 hours is recommended and has been shown to reduce resuscitation fluid volume requirements, edema formation, and the severity of respiratory dysfunction.[104] The use of systemic corticosteroids for the treatment of pulmonary edema during the first several weeks following the burn and smoke inhalation injury is contraindicated because of an increased risk of infection.[12]

Escharatomy

In cases where circumferential burns of the thorax occur, the burned skin will need to be cut (escharotomy). This is done by making lateral incisions in the anterior axillary line extending from 2 cm below the clavicle to the ninth or tenth rib and transverse incisions across the chest at the top and bottom to form a square. Escharotomy of the chest will relieve the compressive effect of the burned skin.

Feeding

Feeding the burn patient appropriately is an important form of support. Because burn patients are often hypermetabolic, careful evaluation is needed for appropriate feeding to avoid catabolic wasting of muscle tissue and poor burn wound healing. Predictive formulas such as the Harris-Benedict and Curreri have been used to estimate the metabolic rate of the burn patient; however, the use of commercially developed portable analyzers for serial measurements of indirect calorimetry have been found to be more accurate.[105,106] With very large burns (greater than 50% TBSA), patients are often given a diet with caloric content that is 110% or more of their resting energy expenditure to facilitate wound healing and avoid catabolism. As the wounds close and heal, feedings are tapered back to the patient's resting energy expenditure to avoid overfeeding. In addition, enteral feeding with the amino acid glutamine supplements has been shown to improve gut wall integrity, reduce bacteremia, and decrease overall mortality.[107,108]

Pain Control

During the course of care for burn patients, adequate control of pain and agitation is essential. Opioids, anxiolytics, and muscle blocking agents are commonly used to manage the severely burned patient in the acute critical care period. Often, pain control by standard regimens (IV or IM bolus) is inadequate. Consideration should be given to the use of patient-controlled analgesia for burn patients when they stabilize.[109]

Prevention of Burn Complications

Isolation technique, room pressurization, air filtration, and wound covering form the front lines of infection defense. Infections should be treated with specific antibiotics. Topical treatment of the wound with cream-base antibiotics (e.g., silver sulfadiazine [Silvadene]) is commonly employed to prevent wound infection. The appropriate systemic antibiotics are found through serial wound, blood, urine, and sputum cultures. Prophylactic antibiotics are not

> Early burn wound excision and covering reduces infection and improves survival.

commonly used in these patients because resistant bacterial strains can develop and produce a pneumonia that is more refractory to treatment. Early dead skin excision and wound covering with different types of barriers and grafts has become commonplace in the treatment of the burn patient to prevent infection and speed recovery.

To prevent disseminated intravascular coagulation and pulmonary embolism, heparin therapy may be needed, especially in patients who remain immobile.

Clearly, the prevention and early detection of fires remains the most important actions to be taken to reduce the morbidity and mortality rates associated with the burn victim.

Mr. S

HISORY

Mr. S, a 45-year-old man, was using a propane-powered camp heating unit in his house trailer when it exploded and caught the trailer contents on fire. He sustained flash and flame burns and smoke inhalation. After a minute or two, he stumbled out of the burning trailer and collapsed on the ground. A neighbor called the paramedics, and they arrived on scene within 5 minutes and began trauma life support and transported him to a nearby community hospital approximately 30 minutes following the injury. Mr. S is a manual laborer with a history of 32 pack years of smoking, ethyl alcohol abuse, remote IV drug abuse, and one incidence of aspirin abuse and GI bleed that resulted in treatment in the emergency department.

QUESTIONS	ANSWERS
1. What signs and symptoms should be evaluated immediately upon Mr. S's arrival?	The following signs should be evaluated: patency of the airway, breathing status, quality of breath sounds, pulse rate, blood pressure (BP), level of consciousness (Glasgow coma scale), and cervical spine protection until spinal injuries are ruled out. Symptoms of respiratory distress, shock, and mental impairment should be noted.
2. What facts should be gathered to help determine the severity of Mr. S's injuries?	The severity of Mr. S's injuries can be evaluated by determining whether he was burned in an enclosed space; whether there is evidence of inhalation injury; how long he was exposed to flame and smoke; the approximate percentage of TBSA burned and the degree or thickness of the burn, the length of time since his injury; his age, height, and weight; and any underlying medical conditions that may complicate his injuries.
3. What therapeutic techniques should be readily available upon Mr. S's arrival?	Oxygen therapy (cannula or non-rebreathing mask), intubation equipment, manual resuscitation bag with proper mask, ventilatory support equipment, venous and arterial line placement equipment, crystalloid fluids for vascular support, appropriate resuscitation drugs, and medications for pain and agitation should be ready upon his arrival.

More on Mr. S

PHYSICAL EXAMINATION

- **General.** Mr. S is a thin-appearing man who weighs approximately 75 kg and is 194 cm tall. He has burns of his face, neck, arms, and legs; he is lying supine on an emergency department bed, restless, moaning, somewhat responsive to questions with a hoarse voice and in apparent respiratory distress while breathing with the aid of supplementary oxygen from a non-rebreathing mask and reservoir being supplied with oxygen at 15 L/min; Glasgow coma scale 14

- **Vital Signs.** Temperature 36.5°C, respiratory rate 26/min, BP 138/86 mm Hg, heart rate 134/min, nail-bed refill 2 seconds

- **HEENT.** Anterior part of face received partial and full-thickness burns; corneas were not burned, pupils equal and reactive to light; nasal flaring, nasal hairs singed; some erythema and soot seen in the oral cavity

- **Neck.** Burns down to the clavicles; trachea is midline; some inspiratory stridor; carotid pulses +++ bilaterally without bruit; no signs of lymphadenopathy, thyroidomegaly, or jugular venous distention; obvious tensing of sternocleidomastoid and scalene muscles during inspiration

- **Chest.** No burns observed; some scattered expiratory wheezes bilaterally; occasional thoracoabdominal paradoxical motion

- **Heart.** Regular rhythm at 130 to 140/min; normal first and second heart sounds without murmurs, gallops, or rubs

- **Abdomen.** Slender, no burns observed; soft, non-tender; bowel sounds indistinct; no masses or organomegaly

- **Extremities.** Moving all extremities; circumferential partial and full thickness burns on all extremities with exception of feet and axillary areas; no digital clubbing; no obvious cyanosis; some signs of swelling

QUESTIONS	ANSWERS
4. Which of Mr. S's signs and symptoms indicate inhalation injury?	Inhalation injury is indicated by the presence of tachypnea, stridor, voice changes, accessory muscle tensing, erythema about the face and presence of soot in the mouth, nasal flaring, singed nasal hair, wheezing, and thoracoabdominal wall paradoxical motion.
5. If Mr. S had circumferential burns of his thorax, what influence would this have on his respiratory function?	If circumferential burns of his thorax had occurred, it could result in decreased thoracic compliance and increased work of breathing.
6. What are the possible causes of Mr. S's respiratory distress?	His respiratory distress is probably due to some inhalation of hot gas and smoke, which can cause upper airway edema, bronchospasm, and possibly chemically induced acute tracheobronchitis.

Increasing lung water, secondary to the inhalation injury and a large cutaneous burn, may be accumulating and inducing increased airway resistance, decreased pulmonary compliance, V̇/Q̇ mismatching, and hypoxemia.

7. What diagnostic techniques should be used to evaluate Mr. S's respiratory distress?

To evaluate his respiratory distress further, the following tests may be useful: chest radiograph, fiberoptic laryngoscopy, and bronchoscopy; a CT lung scan would be helpful in making the diagnosis of inhalation injury but it may not be practical in this setting.

8. What laboratory tests and other determinations are now needed to make a more complete evaluation?

Laboratory assessment should include a complete blood count, electrolytes, ABG, Hbco, standard blood chemistry, hepatitis C status, and a screening for alcohol and illegal drugs.

9. What techniques are needed to monitor Mr. S's cardiovascular status?

A more precise estimation of the burn size should be determined through careful physical examination and the use of a Lund-Browder burn chart to help guide fluid therapy. ECG monitoring and placement of peripheral venous, central venous, and arterial lines are needed to guide the maintenance of hemodynamic stability.

 ## More on Mr. S

BEDSIDE AND LABORATORY FINDINGS IN THE COMMUNITY HOSPITAL

Burn Depth and Size. Partial and some full thickness, approximately 50% of TBSA

ECG. Sinus tachycardia of 134/min without any other abnormalities

Arterial BP. 138/82 mm Hg

Chest Radiograph. Normal thoracic, diaphragmatic, cardiac, anatomy; hyperinflated lung fields and no signs of infiltrate, atelectasis, pulmonary edema, masses, or foreign bodies at this time

ABGs. pH 7.30, $Paco_2$ 32 mm Hg, Pao_2 186 mm Hg, Hbo_2 saturation (Sao_2) 91%, Hbco 18%, HCO_3^- 15 mEq/liter, base deficit −5 while breathing 100% O_2 from a non-rebreathing mask

Hematology. Hct 43%, red blood cells (RBCs) 4.3 × 106/mm³, white blood cells (WBCs) 8.1 × 10³, platelets 361 × 10³

Chemistry and toxicology. Results pending

QUESTIONS	ANSWERS
10. How would you evaluate the ECG and hemodynamic findings?	The ECG and hemodynamic measurements indicate tachycardia and borderline hypertension are acceptable, given the pain and the extent of his injuries. Placement of a central venous catheter is indicated to facilitate fluid resuscitation and drug administration.

11. What does the chest radiograph indicate?

The chest radiograph suggests hyperaeration and is otherwise normal.

12. How would you interpret the ABG data?

The ABG shows partially compensated metabolic acidosis, hyperventilation, hypoxemia, minor-to-moderate CO poisoning, and a PaO_2/FIO_2 of 186, which indicate $\dot{V}/\dot{Q}$ abnormality, diffusion defect, and/or intrapulmonary shunting.

13. What do the hematological data indicate?

The hematological data are normal and do not indicate loss of blood.

14. What respiratory care is indicated at this time, and how should it be evaluated?

The patient should be intubated with a cuffed 8.0-mm internal diameter endotracheal tube. The endotracheal tube could be placed with the aid of a bronchoscope. After intubation, visual inspection of the depth of the airway, chest motion, and breath sounds are needed to determine appropriate airway placement. Mr. S will need mechanical ventilatory support to help avoid and manage further gas exchange derangement if they occur. Initial ventilator settings should be as follows: assist/control mode, set V_T at 700 mL, set rate at 16/min, adequate inspiratory flow to maintain an inspiratory-expiratory ratio (I:E) greater than 1:2, PEEP 5, and 100% FIO_2. Oxygen therapy is primarily directed toward treating the CO poisoning. In-line aerosolized bronchodilator treatment (e.g., six puffs of albuterol via metered dose inhaler) should be given for the apparent bronchospasm. Physical examination of the chest, vital signs, ABG, and chest radiograph should be done to determine Mr. S's response. Escharotomy of his arms and legs may be needed to prevent constriction of the blood flow to his hands and feet if the swelling and contracture becomes excessive.

15. What hemodynamic support is indicated at this time, and how should it be evaluated?

Fluid resuscitation with crystalloid IV infusion according to the Parkland formula (i.e., 4 mL/kg/TBSA burn over 24 hours) must be started. Placement of a central venous pressure (CVP) catheter is needed to facilitate fluid resuscitation, and renal output must be monitored for proper hydration.

16. What complications may occur in the next 24 to 48 hours, and should the patient be transported to a burn center?

Over the next 24 to 48 hours and beyond, Mr. S is at continuing risk for the development of circulatory and respiratory failure, airway edema, acute lung injury, acid-base and electrolyte imbalance, and infection of his wounds. This patient meets the burn unit referral criteria of the American Burn Association and should be transported to a regional burn center; he has a burn of more than 10% TBSA, some full thickness (3rd degree) burns, burns of his face, and inhalation injury.

More on Mr. S

In the emergency department of the community hospital, Mr. S has a peripheral IV catheter placed, he is sedated, orally intubated with an 8.0 cuffed endotracheal tube, and placed on mechanical ventilation with 100% O_2. A jugular central venous catheter is placed and fluid resuscitation started. A nasogastric tube is inserted, along with a urinary catheter with a closed-collection system. A chest radiograph is obtained, and the airway is in satisfactory position, but the CVP catheter is found to extend into the right shoulder region. Mr. S is further stabilized at the community hospital and then transferred by air ambulance to a regional burn center for intensive burn care. Upon arrival at the burn center, approximately 5 hours after the incident, he is fully evaluated and found to have received partial and full-thickness burns to 45.7% of his body and probable inhalation injury. His initial treatment includes continued ventilatory support with pressure controlled assist/control mode, V_T 0.7 liter, rate 16/min, 100% O_2 and 5 cm H_2O of PEEP, fluid resuscitation at 1000 mL/hour $\times$ 8 hours followed by 500 mL/hour over next 16 hours, sedation and paralysis with morphine, ativan and vecuronium, wound care with topical antibiotics and dressings, ascorbic acid, acetaminophen, H2 blockers for stomach acid, bowel clearing, 12 lead ECG, chest radiograph, radial artery catheter placement, ABG, electrolytes, and CBC determination. The chest radiograph (Fig. 9.4) shows the endotracheal tube in an acceptable position, a right pneumothorax, and a poorly placed central venous line. The pneumothorax is thought to have been caused by either lung puncture from the placement of the CVP catheter or rupture of the lung during ventilatory support. A chest tube is placed in the right hemithorax and attached to a three-chamber chest tube drainage system with -20 cm H_2O suction, and the CVP catheter is replaced. Mr. S's Hbco is found to be 8%.

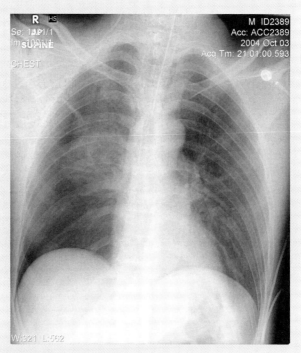

FIGURE 9.4 Chest radiograph shortly after admission to the burn center.

During the first 48 hours following admission, Mr. S receives 27.2 liters of fluid and has a total urine output of 5.1 liters. Over the next several days, the aggressive fluid resuscitation and sedation are tapered down, and edema of the face and extremities develop and begin to subside. His FIO_2 is adjusted down to 0.40, while pulse oximetry and ECG are monitored. His wheezing increases, and the bronchodilator therapy is changed to 10 puffs of the Combivent (albuterol and ipatropium) via in-line delivery with a chamber in the inspiratory limb of the ventilator circuit at a frequency of q2h and prn.

On the third day post-injury, Mr. S's sputum becomes more copious, and his FIO_2 requirements increase to 0.60 to maintain his oxyhemoglobin saturation above 92%. On the fourth day after injury the decision to begin the surgical removal of the burned skin and grafting is put on hold as Mr. S continues to deteriorate. His bedside findings, vital signs, chest radiograph, ventilator settings, and laboratory data are as follows.

BEDSIDE FINDINGS

Mr. S is lying supine with bacitracin and polymyxin B ointment on his face, silver sulfadiazine cream and bandages covering all other burned areas. Generalized edema of the burn areas has decreased somewhat. He is being kept sedated and paralyzed with morphine, ativan, and vecuronium. He is being turned and repositioned every 2 hours and he is passively following the support being supplied by the ventilator. The endotracheal tube has 25 cm H_2O pressure in the cuff, and no gas leakage is heard over the cuff site. The airway is secured with cloth ties and shows the 24-cm mark at the teeth. His breath sounds reveal scattered expiratory wheezes and rhonchi bilaterally. On suctioning his airway, moderate amounts of tan sputum flecked with soot are removed. In-line ventilator circuit delivery of 10 puffs of Combivent continues every 2 to 4 hours and as needed.

Box 9.2 Physical Examination

Vital Signs	
Measure	Value
Temperature 37.5°C; Respiratory rate	22/min
Heart rate	105/min, sinus rhythm
Hemodynamics	
Measure	Value
Systemic arterial BP	105/55 mm Hg
CVP	7 mm Hg
Urine output averaging 100 mL/hour	
Chest Radiograph. See Figure 9.5	
Ventilator Settings and Findings	
Measure	Value
Assist/control	
Pressure control mode	
V_T	0.7 L
Set and total rate	20/min

(box continued on page 212)

Box 9.2 Physical Examination (CONTINUED)

T_I of 1.0 seconds, I:E 1:2

V_E	15.9 liters/min
Peak inspiratory pressure	38 cm H_2O
Plateau pressure	31 cm H_2O
FIO_2	90%
PEEP set at 7 cm H_2O	
Auto-PEEP	14 cm H_2O
Static compliance (C_{st})	25 mL/cm H_2O
Effective airway resistance (R_{aw})	8 cm H_2O/liter/second

Laboratory Evaluation

ABGs	Value
pH	7.36
$Paco_2$	46 mm Hg
Pao_2	91 mm Hg
HCO_3^-	25 mEq/liter
Base deficit	0
Pao_2/FIO_2	101
Sao_2	96% (co-oximeter)
Spo_2	97% (pulse oximeter)

Hematology

Measure	Value
Hct	42%
RBC	$4.58 \times 10^6/mm^3$
WBC	$10.2 \times 10^3/mm^3$
platelets	$253 \times 10^3/mm^3$

Electrolytes and Chemistry

Measure	Value
Na^+	141 mEq/liter
K^+	3.8 mEq/liter
Cl^-	102 mEq/liter
Glucose	135 mg/dL
BUN	21 mg/dL
Creatinine	1.1 mg/dL

Microbiology. Blood, sputum, and wound smear cultures pending

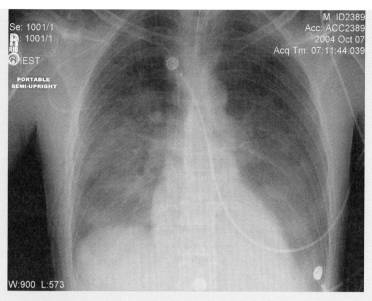

Se: 1001/1
1001/1
RIO
CHEST

PORTABLE
SEMI-UPRIGHT

M ID2389
Acc: ACC2389
2004 Oct 07
Acq Tm: 07:11:44.039

W:900 L:573

FIGURE 9.5 Chest radiograph 4 days after admission to the burn center.

QUESTIONS

17. What do Mr. S's airway care and breath sounds indicate? What would you recommend at this time?

ANSWERS

His airway is of an appropriate size and position. His breath sounds indicate proper placement. Cuff pressure is effectively sealing the trachea at a safe pressure that is high enough to help avoid silent aspiration of saliva around the cuff. Placement of a tracheostomy tube is not indicated at this time. His breath sounds indicate retained secretions, continuing bronchospasm, and little or no resumption of a significant pneumothorax. The in-line aerosolization of Combivent via metered-dose inhaler is appropriate and should be evaluated for effectiveness by evaluating the ventilator graphic display (e.g., pressure-volume curve) and by comparing the ventilator peak inspiratory pressure and peak plateau pressure difference before and after treatments. The copious amounts of tan and soot-flecked sputum removed from the airway indicates inhalation injury and the possibility of ventilator-associated pneumonia. They do not appear to be grossly consistent with airway plugging or hemorrhage at this time. Special attention to the airway, its maintenance, keeping the patient's head up at 45°, frequent hand washing, and sterile technique is necessary to help avoid or reduce the incidence of ventilator-associated pneumonia.

18. How would you describe his hemodynamics? What effects could these hemodynamics have on lung function?

The hemodynamics are acceptable when considering his injury. The filling pressures (CVP) indicate that Mr. S is adequately hydrated and will need the infusion rate to be adjusted to maintain an acceptable urine output. If fluids are tapered too much, however, renal function and other organ functions could be jeopardized as a result of hypovolemic shock.

19. How would you describe the radiographic changes since the initial chest film taken shortly after admission to the burn center?

This portable anterior-posterior chest radiograph taken on the fourth day after his injury shows normal bony structures, normal heart size, scattered flitrates in both lung fields with greater involvement of both lung basal lobes, and that the endotracheal tube, chest tube, CVP catheter, and nasogastric tube are all in appropriate positions. These findings are consistent with pneumonia and/or ARDS. It would be appropriate to start antibiotics and perform a bronchoscopy to clear the airways and to obtain a sputum specimen with a protected brush to assess him for infection and ventilator-associated pneumonia.

20. How would you describe the ventilator settings, breathing pattern, pulmonary mechanics, and ABG findings? What would you recommended at this time?

Mr. S's ventilator settings indicate that he is receiving a V_T of 9.3 mL/kg, his FIO_2 setting is excessive, he is following the set rate of the ventilator, and he is generating unacceptable levels of auto-PEEP as a result of gas trapping produced by his respiratory pattern combined with the increased effective airway resistance. It is important to track the auto-PEEP in order to evaluate its effects on lung distention, lung mechanics, and hemodynamics. The auto-PEEP can be reduced by lowering the respiratory rate, increasing the expiratory time, continuing the bronchodilator treatments and airway care, and maintaining his sedation to avoid patient overtriggering. The very low compliance and elevated resistance measurements are consistent with the chest radiograph and bedside findings of secretion retention, bronchospasm, pneumonia, ARDS, and probable underlying COPD. His PaO_2 is adequate, but the measures to maintain it are dangerously excessive and need reevaluation and adjustment. The acid-base balance is normal and indicates effective resuscitation. At this point it would be appropriate to consider reduction of his V_T to 6 mL/kg, higher PEEP to recruit atelectatic regions of his lungs, and reduction of the FIO_2 in accord with the ARDSnet protocol. In addition, it would be appropriate to consider permissive hypercapnia by reducing his V_T and rate if the initial adjustments do not reduce the auto-PEEP and elevated plateau pressure.

21. What do his other laboratory findings indicate?

The hematological data indicate an acceptable RBC mass and count. The mildly elevated WBC is consistent with this type of trauma or early sepsis or both. Because of the elevated risk for ventilator-associated pneumonia and the current clinical picture, sputum and blood specimens should be collected for microbiological analysis. The electrolytes, hemodynamics, and renal function are remarkably normal considering the amount of fluid that he has received. A slight hyperglycemia is noted and may be a result of glucocorticoid and catecholamine release secondary to the trauma or the IV fluids being given or both and may need to be managed with insulin.

Mr. S Conclusion

After Mr. S's cardiopulmonary status is assessed, his sedation is increased, he is started on ceftazidime and vancomycin, a broncoscopy is performed, and sputum samples are collected. The V_T is reduced to 500 mL to yield a delivered V_T of 6.7 mL/kg, the respiratory rate is reduced to 18/min, the T_I is reduced to 0.6 s to yield an I:E of 1:4.5, and the set PEEP is increased through a series of steps to 14 cm H_2O. This allows his FIO_2 to be titrated down to 60% as his status is monitored with continuous end-tidal CO_2, pulse oximetry, and serial ABG analysis. At this point his auto-PEEP is 16 cm H_2O, the plateau pressure is 28 cm H_2O, the compliance increases to 33 mL/cm H_2O, end-tidal CO_2 is 49 mm Hg, and SaO_2 is 94%. An arterial blood sample is collected, and the following results are found: pH 7.31, $PaCO_2$ 54 mm Hg, PaO_2 79 mm Hg, PaO_2/FIO_2 131, HCO_3 26 mEq/liter, and a base deficit of −4.

Improved oxygenation is noted by the increased PaO_2/FIO_2 and acceptable PaO_2 and SaO_2. The reduction of the V_T and rate settings results in an acceptable auto-PEEP, airway pressures, and compliance and an acceptable permissive hypercapnia. The use of prone position to recruit atelectatic lung segments is tried, but he develops significant oxyhemoglobin desaturations to 70% and it is decided not to prone him. On this day a metabolic study is done to evaluate his condition. It shows that his VO_2 is 366 mL/min, VCO_2 is 299 mL/min, and his resting energy expenditure is 2556 Kcal/day, which is 164% of his predicted basal metabolic rate. His feeding and caloric intake are adjusted so that he is receiving 110% of his resting energy expenditure to meet his energy needs and to avoid over feeding him. This is repeated several more times during his course to adjust his feeding.

Over the next 7 days, Mr. S's condition oscillates between improvement and setback. The bronchoscopy is tolerated without complication and shows that he has moderate inflammation of his airways and moderate amounts of thick sputum with small plugs. The sputum cultures found more than 100,000 bacteria/mL and grew out *Streptococcus pneumoniae* and *Haemophilus influenzae*. The ceftazidime and vancomycin are stopped and he is started on levofloxacin. Episodes of coarse and wheezy breath sounds, sputum retention, and infiltrates and atelectasis reoccur several times and require elevated levels of FIO_2 and adjustment of his PEEP and bronchoscopy. During this period the chest tube is removed without incident, the CVP line is replaced, a Dobbhoff feeding tube is placed, and the arterial catheter removed. He is started on two puffs of fluticasone bid for his persistent wheezing. Ten days post-burn, it is decided to place an 8-mm tracheostomy tube because of the ongoing secretion problems and ventilatory support requirements.

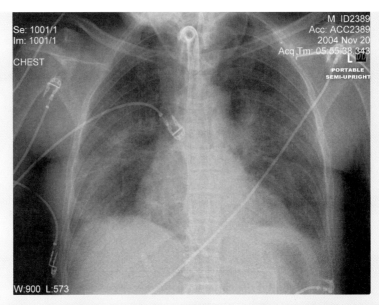

FIGURE 9.6 Chest radiograph 35 days after admission to the burn center.

Gradually over the next several weeks, Mr. S's pulmonary status improves. His Fio_2 and PEEP requirements decline, the bronchodilator treatments are reduced to q4h and prn, he completes an 8-day course of antibiotics, his secretion production decreases, and his sedation is tapered over the next week. On the 13th and 16th days post-burn it is decided that he is stable enough to tolerate two surgical procedures to remove burned skin and to graft skin from the unburned areas to the excised areas. Mr. S tolerates these procedures with modest increases in his metabolic rate and minute ventilation requirements. On the 35th day after admission to the burn center, his chest radiograph shows acceptable placement of a tracheostomy tube and improvement in the infiltrates (Fig. 9.6).

On the 40th day post-burn, the sedation is tapered, his metabolic rate reduced, his anxiety well controlled, and his pulmonary insult resolved enough that it is felt that he can begin a gradual process of weaning ventilatory support. He is switched from assist-control mode to mandatory minute ventilation with the following settings: V_T 600 mL, rate 10/min, pressure support 10 cm H_2O, Fio_2 40%, and PEEP 10 cm H_2O. After several minutes he stabilizes with a sinus tachycardia of 105/min, respiratory rate of 22/min, pressure support V_T is 688 mL, and oxyhemoglobin saturation is 96%. Mr. S tolerates this for 35 minutes until his respiratory rate increases to 35/min and V_T drops to less than 0.3 liter. At this point the pressure support is increased to 18 cm H_2O to reduce his tachypnea and increase his V_T. Over the next several days his respiratory strength and stamina increase. On the 43rd day after his burn injury he is able to tolerate breathing spontaneously through his tracheostomy tube with supplemental oxygen being supplied by a tracheostomy mask delivering 40% oxygen and cool aerosol. He continues to receive tracheostomy care, regular suctioning, two puffs of Combivent q4h and two puffs of fluticasone bid for his persistent wheezing. Two weeks later his tracheostomy is successfully removed. Sixty-one days after his admission to the burn center Mr. S is discharged to a skilled nursing facility for follow-up care in his community. ∎

KEY POINTS

- The mortality rate for a large burn climbs when combined with inhalation injury and increases to 95% in those with large burns and smoke inhalation injury and who are more than 60 years old.
- Low oxygen and elevated CO and HCN are produced in fires and can cause asphyxiation and rapid CNS dysfunction.
- Smoke is an aerosol that contains particles laden with irritating aldehydes, organic acids, and products of oxidation that can penetrate deep into the respiratory tract.
- Thermal injury to the respiratory tract is frequently confined to the face, oral and nasal cavities, pharynx, and trachea.
- Chemical injury to the respiratory tract can be brought about by inhalation of toxic gases and irritant-laden soot particles that can cause acute tracheobronchitis, bronchospasm, bronchorrhea, mucosal sloughing, airway obstruction, and rapid onset pulmonary edema.
- Large skin burns and smoke inhalation injury can cause the release of various mediators that result in increased pulmonary blood flow, increased capillary permeability, pulmonary and systemic edema, cardiac failure, and surfactant dysfunction.
- Pulmonary physiological changes following burn and inhalation injury include decreased lung and chest wall compliance, increased airway resistance, $\dot{V}/\dot{Q}$ mismatching, and increased V_D/V_T.
- Massive fluid shift and generalized edema usually peak within 8 to 24 hours.
- Respiratory mucosal inflammation, increased mucus production, mucosal sloughing, decreased mucus clearance, and airway plugging usually follow inhalation injury for 3 to 4 days.
- Most burn patients become colonized with Staphylococcus bacteria, methicillin-resistant *S. aureus* (MRSA), and *P. aeruginosa*.
- Respiratory tract infection, ARDS, MODS, and pulmonary embolism are complications of burn and inhalation injury.
- Hypermetabolism is a frequent occurrence following burn injury and can lead to elevated minute ventilation and catabolism of muscle and blood proteins.
- Some patients may, following prolonged intubation or tracheostomy, develop subglottic or tracheal stenosis weeks to months after the initial inhalation injury.
- Patients who present in an unconscious state may have been exposed to asphyxiating conditions, low F_{IO_2}, CO, and/or HCN.
- Pulse oximetry should not be used to indicate the level of HbO_2 concentration in the patient who is known or suspected to have been poisoned by CO.
- Facial burns, singed nasal hair, oral and laryngeal edema, carbonaceous deposits in the airway and sputum, cough, wheezing, stridor, and dyspnea all suggest inhalation injury.
- The chest x-ray is frequently normal in the first 24 hours following inhalation injury.
- The presence of a persistent base deficit of less than -6 mEq/liter and/or an elevated serum lactate indicate poor perfusion and prognosis.
- The rule of nines can be used to estimate the total size of a burn injury. Each extremity and the head are approximately 9%, and the anterior and posterior trunk are each 18% of the TBSA in adults.
- A burn injury of the skin can be classified as partial thickness or full thickness.

(key points continued on page 218)

KEY POINTS (CONTINUED)

- The goals of respiratory care include patent airway, secretion removal, maintenance of effective ventilation, preservation of lung volume, adequate oxygenation, maintenance of acid-base balance, cardiovascular stability, cervical spine protection, support of metabolism, suppression of infection, prevention of pulmonary embolism, and appropriate monitoring.
- An oral endotracheal tube should be placed when upper airway closure is anticipated or significant inhalation injury is found.
- Secretion clearance is important, as the injured mucosal lining of the airways sloughs and forms plugs.
- Elimination of CO is accelerated when supplemental 100% O_2 is administered and should continue until the Hbco is less than 10%.
- Conventional ventilatory support settings are assist-control ventilation, rate 15/minute, V_T 6 to 8 mL/kg, T_I 1 second, sufficient inspiratory flow to meet patient demand, FIO_2 100%, and PEEP 5 cm H_2O.
- High-frequency ventilation delivered by a VDR or oscillator is useful in supporting and improving gas exchange in the burn patient with significant inhalation injury.
- IV fluid resuscitation with the Parkland formula (4 mL/kg/% TBSA burn over a 24-hours) should be given to maintain a urine output of 30 to 60 mL/hour.
- IV administration of high-dose ascorbic acid should be given to reduce resuscitation fluid volume requirements, edema formation, and the severity of respiratory dysfunction.
- In cases where circumferential burns of the thorax occur, chest escharotomy will improve chest wall elasticity and compliance.
- The isolation technique, dead skin excision, wound covering, and topical antibiotics reduce the incidence of severe infection and improve survival.
- Careful feeding of the burn patient is necessary to support metabolism and wound healing.

REFERENCES

1. National Center for Injury Prevention and Control, Centers for Disease Control and Prevention, Atlanta, GA. Available at: www.cdc.gov/ncipc.
2. Karter, MJ: Fire Loss in the United States during 2003. National Fire Protection Association, Fire Analysis and Research Division, Quincy, 2004.
3. Tompkins, RG, et al: Prompt eschar excision: a treatment system contributing to reduced burn mortality: a statistical evaluation of burn care at Massachusetts General Hospital (1974–1984). Ann Surg 204:272, 1986.
4. O'Keefe, GE, et al: An evaluation of risk factors for mortality after burn trauma and the identification of gender-dependent differences in outcomes. J Am Coll Surg 192(2):153, 2001.
5. Ryan, CM, et al: Objective estimates of the probability of death from burn injuries. N Engl J Med 338:362, 1998.
6. Santaniello, JM, et al: Ten year experience of burn, trauma, and combined burn/trauma injuries comparing outcomes. J Trauma 57:696, 2004.
7. Herndon, DN, et al: Incidence, mortality, pathogenesis and treatment of pulmonary injury. J Burn Care Rehabil 7:184, 1986.
8. Moylan, JA: Inhalation injury. J Trauma (suppl) 21:720, 1981.
9. Nishimura, N, Hiranuma, N: Respiratory changes after major burn injury. Crit Care Med 10:25, 1982.
10. Cahalane, M, Demling, RH: Early respiratory abnormalities from smoke inhalation. JAMA 251:771, 1984.
11. Zawacki, B, et al: Smoke, burns and the natural history of inhalation injury in fire victims. Ann Surg 185:100, 1977.
12. Demling, RH, LaLonde, C: Burn Trauma. Thieme Medical Publishers, New York, 1989.

13. Alarie, Y: Toxicity of fire smoke. Crit Rev Toxicol 32(4):259, 2002.
14. Cohen, MA, Guzzardi, LJ: Inhalation of products of combustion. Ann Emerg Med 12:628, 1983.
15. Symington, IS, et al: Cyanide exposure in fires. Lancet 1:91, 1978.
16. Crapo, RO: Smoke-inhalation injuries. JAMA 246:1694, 1981.
17. Dyer, RF, Esch, VH: Polyvinyl chloride toxicity in fires. JAMA 26;235(4):393,1976.
18. Stone, JP, et al: The transport of hydrogen chloride by soot from burning polyvinyl chloride. J Fire Flamm 4:42, 1973.
19. Kao, LW, Nanagas, KA: Carbon monoxide poisoning. Emerg Med Clin N Am 22:985, 2004.
20. Zhang, J, Piantadosi, CA: Mitochondrial oxidative stress after carbon monoxide hypoxia in the rat brain. J Clin Invest 90:1193, 1992.
21. DeBias, DA, et al: Effects of carbon monoxide inhalation on ventricular fibrillation. Arch Environ Health 31:42, 1976.
22. Verma, A, et al: Carbon monoxide: a putative neural messenger. Science 259:381, 1993.
23. Meyer-Witting, M, et al: Acute carbon monoxide exposure and cerebral blood flow in rabbits. Anaesth Intensive Care 19:373, 1991.
24. Ischiropopoulos, H, et al: Nitric oxide production and perivascular tyrosine nitration in brain after carbon monoxide poisoning in the rat. J Clin Invest 97:2260, 1996.
25. Thom, SR, et al: Delayed neuropsychologic sequelae after carbon monoxide poisoning: prevention by treatment with hyperbaric oxygen. Ann Emerg Med 25:474, 1995.
26. Baud, FJ, et al: Elevated blood cyanide concentrations in victims of smoke inhalation. N Engl J Med 325:1761, 1991.
27. Barillo, DJ, et al: Cyanide poisoning in victims of fire: analysis of 364 cases and review of the literature. J Burn Care Rehabil 15:46, 1994.
28. Moritz, AR, et al: The effects of inhaled heat on the air passages and lungs: an experimental investigation. Am J Pathol 21:311, 1945.
29. Demling, HR: Management of the burn patient. In Shoemaker, WC, et al (eds): Textbook of Critical Care. ed 2. WB Saunders, Philadelphia, 1990.
30. Haponik, EF, Lykens, MG: Acute upper airway obstruction in burned patients. Crit Care Report 2:28, 1990.
31. Hubbard, GB, et al: The morphology of smoke inhalation injury in sheep. J Trauma 31:1477, 1991.
32. Matthew, E, et al: A murine model of smoke inhalation. Am J Physiol Lung Cell Mol Physiol 280:L716, 2001.
33. Cox, RA, et al: Airway obstruction in sheep with burn and smoke inhalation injuries. Am J Respir Cell Mol Biol 29(3 pt 1):295, 2003.
34. Peitzman, AB, et al: Measurement of lung water in inhalation injury. Surgery 90:305, 1981.
35. Robinson, NB, et al: Ventilation and perfusion alterations after smoke inhalation injury. Surgery 90:352, 1980.
36. Demling, R, et al: Effect of graded increases in smoke inhalation injury on the early systemic response to a body burn. Crit Care Med 23:171, 1995.
37. Shimazu, T, et al: Ventilation-perfusion alterations after smoke inhalation injury in an ovine model. J Appl Physiol 81:2250, 1996.
38. Soejima, K, et al: Pathophysiology and analysis of combined burn and smoke inhalation injuries in sheep. Am J Physiol Cell Mol Physiol 280: L1233, 2001.
39. Li, W, et al: The change in apoptosis and proliferation of pulmonary tissue cells in rats with smoke inhalation injury. Zhonghua Shao Shang Za Zhi 18(3):139, 2002.
40. Zheng, HF, et al: The changes in the pulmonary surface tension and the tissue content of surfactant substance protein B during early post-injury stage in rabbits inflicted with smoke inhalation injury. Zhonghua Shao Shang Za Zhi 20:141, 2004.
41. Stollery, DE, et al: Dead space ventilation: a significant factor in respiratory failure after thermal inhalation. Crit Care Med 15:260, 1987.
42. Demling, RH, et al: Early pulmonary and hemodynamic effects of a chest wall burn (effect of ibuprofen). Surgery 104(1):10, 1988.
43. Mason, AD, et al: Hemodynamic changes in the early post-burn period: the influence of fluid administration and a vasodilator. J Trauma 11:36, 1971.
44. Shoemaker, WC, et al: Burn pathophysiology in man. I. Sequential hemodynamic alterations. J Surg Res 14:64, 1973.
45. Soejima, K, et al: Role of nitric oxide in myocardial dysfunction after combined burn and smoke inhalation injury. Burns 27:809, 2001.
46. White, J, et al: Cardiac effects of burn injury complicated by aspiration pneumonia-induced sepsis. Am J Physiol Heart Circ Physiol 285:H47, 2003.
47. Willis, MS, et al: Macrophage migration inhibitory factor (MIF) mediates late cardiac dysfunction following burn injury. Am J Physiol Heart Circ Physiol Sep, 2004.
48. Warden, GD: Burn Shock Resuscitation. World J Surg. 16:16, 1992.
49. Westphal, M, et al: Acute effects of combined burn and smoke inhalation injury on carboxyhemoglobin formation, tissue oxygenation, and cardiac performance. Biochem Biophys Res Commmun 7:945, 2004.
50. McArdle, CS, Finlay, W: Pulmonary complications following smoke inhalation. Br J Anaesth 47:618, 1975.
51. Pruitt, BA, et al: Progressive pulmonary insufficiency and other pulmonary complications of thermal injury. J Trauma 15:369, 1975.

52. Dancey, DR, et al: ARDS in patients with thermal injury. Intensive Care Med 25:11235, 1999.

53. Hudson, LD, et al: Clinical risks for development of the acute respiratory distress syndrome. Am J Respir Crit Care Med 151:293, 1995.

54. Demling, RH, et al: The lung inflammatory response to thermal injury: relationship between physiologic and histologic changes. Surgery 106:52, 1989.

55. Ravage, ZB, et al: Mediators of microvascular injury in dermal burn wounds. Inflammation 22:619, 1998.

56. Jin, LJ, et al: Lung dysfunction after thermal injury in relation to prostanoid and oxygen radical release. J Appl Physiol 6:103, 1986.

57. Oldham, KT, et al: Activation of complement by hydroxyl radicals in thermal injury. Surgery 104:272, 1988.

58. Basadre, JO, et al. The effect of leukocyte depletion on smoke inhalation injury in sheep. Surgery 104:208, 1988.

59. Laffon, M, et al: Interleukin-8 mediates injury from smoke inhalation to both the lung endothelial and alveolar epithelial barriers in rabbits. Am J Resp Crit Care Med 160:1443, 1999.

60. Cox, RA, et al: Enhanced pulmonary expression of endothelin-1 in an ovine model of smoke inhalation injury. J Burn Care Rehabil 22:375, 2001.

61. Soejima, K, et al. Role of nitric oxide in vascular permeability after combined burns and smoke inhalation injury. Am J Respir Crit Care Med 163:745, 2001.

62. Murakami, K, Traber, DL: Pathophysiological basis of smoke inhalation injury. News Physiol Sci 18:125, 2003.

63. Wong, SS, et al: Substance P and neutral endopeptidase in development of acute respiratory distress syndrome following smoke inhalation. Am J Physiol Lung Cell Mol Physiol 287:L859, 2004.

64. Erol, S, et al: Changes of microbial flora and wound colonization in burned patients. Burns 30:357, 2004.

65. Fitzwater, J, et al: The risk factors and time course of sepsis and organ dysfunction after burn trauma. Trauma 54:959, 2003.

66. Coleman, JB, Chang, FC: Pulmonary embolism: an unrecognized event in severely burned patients. Am J Surg 130:697, 1975.

67. Chu, C, et al: Early and late pathological changes in severe chemical burns to the respiratory tract complicated with acute respiratory failure. Burns 8:387, 1982.

68. Brooks, SM, et al: Reactive airways dysfunction syndrome (RADS). Persistent asthma syndrome after high level irritant exposure. Chest 88:376, 1988.

69. Kinsella, J, et al: Increased airways reactivity after smoke inhalation. Lancet 337:595, 1991.

70. Fogarty, PW, et al: Long term effects of smoke inhalation in survivors of the King's Cross underground station fire. Thorax 46:914, 1991.

71. Park, GY, et al: Prolonged airway and systemic inflammatory reactions after smoke inhalation. Chest 123:475, 2003

72. Orme, J Jr, et al: Pulmonary function and health-related quality of life in survivors of acute respiratory distress syndrome. Am J Respir Crit Care Med 167:690, 2003.

73. Lund, T, et al: Upper airway sequelae in burn patients requiring endotracheal intubation or tracheostomy. Ann Surg 201:374, 1985.

74. Yang, JY, et al: Symptomatic tracheal stenosis in burns. Burns 25:72, 1999.

75. Bourbeau, J, et al: Combined smoke inhalation and body surface burns injury does not necessarily imply long-term respiratory health consequences. Eur Respir J 9:1470, 1996.

76. Mevorach, D, Heyman, SN: Pain in the marriage (husband and wife have heart-attack symptoms caused by carbon monoxide poisoning). N Engl J Med 332:48, 1995.

77. Buckley, RG, et al: The pulse oximetry gap in carbon monoxide intoxication. Ann Emerg Med 24:252, 1994.

78. Hampson, NB: Pulse oximetry in severe carbon monoxide poisoning. Chest 114:1036, 1998.

79. DiVencenti, FC, et al: Inhalation injuries. J Trauma 11:109, 1971.

80. Hunt, JL, et al: Fiberoptic bronchoscopy in acute inhalation injury. J Trauma 15:641, 1975.

81. Masanes, MJ, et al: Fiberoptic bronchoscopy for the early diagnosis of subglottal inhalation injury: comparative value in the assessment of prognosis. J Trauma 36:59, 1994.

82. Park, MS, et al: Assessment of severity of ovine smoke inhalation injury by analysis of computed tomographic scans. J Trauma 55:417, 2003.

83. Haponik, EF, et al: Acute upper airway injury in burn patients. Serial changes of flow-volume curves and nasopharyngoscopy. Am Rev Respir Dis 135:360, 1987.

84. Petroff, PA, et al: Pulmonary function studies after smoke inhalation. Am J Surg 132:346, 1976.

85. Choi, J, et al: The 2000 Moyer Award. The relevance of base deficits after burn injuries. J Burn Care Rehabil 21:499, 2000.

86. Cartotto, R, et al: A prospective study on the implications of a base deficit during fluid resuscitation. J Burn Care Rehabil 24:75, 2003.

87. Sage 2 Burn Diagramming, SageDiagram, LLC. Available at: www.sagediagram.com.

88. Venus, B, et al: Prophylactic intubation and continuous positive airway pressure in the management of inhalation injury in burn victims. Crit Care Med 9:519, 1981.

89. Silver, GM, et al: A survey of airway and ventilator management strategies in North American

pediatric burn units. J Burn Care Rehabil 25:435, 2004.

90. Lesnik, I, et al: The role of early tracheostomy in blunt, multiple organ trauma. Am Surg 58:346, 1992.

91. Saffle, JR, et al: Early tracheostomy does not improve outcome in burn patients. J Burn Care Rehabil 23:431, 2002.

92. Haponik, EF: Smoke inhalation injury: Some priorities for the respiratory care professional. Respir Care 37:609, 1992.

93. ARDS Network: Ventilation with lower tidal volumes as compared with traditional tidal volumes for acute lung injury and the acute respiratory distress syndrome. The Acute Respiratory Distress Syndrome Network. N Engl J Med 342:1301, 2000.

94. Reynolds, EM, et al: Permissive hypercapnia and pressure-controlled ventilation as treatment of severe adult respiratory distress syndrome in a pediatric burn patient. Crit Care Med 21:944, 1993.

95. Hoffman, LA, et al: Tracheal gas insufflation. Limits of efficacy in adults with acute respiratory distress syndrome. Am J Respir Crit Care Med 162:387, 200.

96. Cioffi, WG, et al: High-frequency percussive ventilation in patients with inhalation injury. J Trauma 29:350, 1989.

97. Rodeberg, DA, et al: Decreased pulmonary barotrauma with the use of volumetric diffusive respiration in pediatric patients with burns: the 1992 Moyer Award. J Burn Care Rehabil 13:506, 1992.

98. Rodeberg, DA, et al: Improved ventilatory function in burn patients using volumetric diffusive respiration. J Am Coll Surg 179:518, 1994.

99. Carman, B, et al: A prospective, randomized comparison of the Volume Diffusive Respirator vs conventional ventilation for ventilation of burned children. 2001 ABA paper. J Burn Care Rehabil 23:444, 2002.

100. Reper, P, et al: High frequency percussive ventilation and conventional ventilation after smoke inhalation: a randomised study. Burns 28:503, 2002.

101. Cartotto, R, et al: High frequency oscillatory ventilation in burn patients with the acute respiratory distress syndrome. Burns 30:453, 2004.

102. Scheulenm, JJ, Munster, AM: The Parkland formula in patients with burns and inhalation injury. J Trauma 22:869, 1982.

103. Kim, KM, et al: Comparison of cardiac outputs of major burn patients undergoing extensive early escharectomy: esophageal doppler monitor versus thermodilution pulmonary artery catheter. J Trauma 57:1013, 2004.

104. Tanaka, H, et al: Reduction of resuscitation fluid volumes in severely burned patients using ascorbic acid administration: a randomized, prospective study. Arch Surg 135:326, 2000.

105. Turner, WW, et al: Predicting energy expenditures in burned patients. J Trauma 25:11, 1985.

106. Saffle, JR, et al: Use of indirect calorimetry in the nutritional management of burned patients. J Trauma 25:32, 1985.

107. Wischmeyer, PE, et al: Glutamine administration reduces gram-negative bacteremia in severely burned patients: a prospective, randomized, double-blind trial versus isonitrogenous control. Crit Care Med 29:2075, 2001.

108. Garrel, D, et al: Decreased mortality and infectious morbidity in adult burn patients given enteral glutamine supplements: a prospective, controlled, randomized clinical trial. Crit Care Med 31:2444, 2003.

109. Prakash, S, et al: Patient-controlled analgesia with fentanyl for burn dressing changes. Anesth Analg 99:552, 2004.

10

Near Drowning

William F. Galvin, MSEd, RRT, CPFT, FAARC

CHAPTER OBJECTIVES:

After reading this chapter you will be able to identify:

- The role played by the respiratory therapist in the assessment and management of near-drowning victims.
- A definition of drowning, near drowning, and related nomenclature.
- The epidemiology and demographics associated with drowning.
- The risk factors that contribute to drowning.
- The pathology and pathophysiology of drowning; to include the neurological insult, pulmonary insult, and hemodynamic and electrolyte effects.
- The drowning sequence and priorities in initial rescue.
- The clinical features and initial assessment of near-drowning victims.
- The clinical outcomes for near drowning.
- The treatment of near-drowning victims.
- The prognostic indicators for near drowning.
- Strategies to prevent drowning.

INTRODUCTION

Whether it be an unsupervised infant found face down in a bath tub, an adolescent found submerged in a neighbor's unfenced pool, or the still and lifeless bodies of two buddies discovered on the beach after partaking of an alcohol-related weekend fishing trip, drowning is a catastrophic and horrific event. Respiratory therapists are often called on to care for the near-drowning victim. Since the acute phase of near drowning primarily entails resuscitation efforts and the late phase potentially involves congestive heart failure, pneumonia, and/or acute respiratory distress syndrome (ARDS) and with it the concomitant use of mechanical ventilation, the role of respiratory therapists in treating near-drowning victims is important. Knowing how to diagnose and effectively manage near-drowning patients is a critical responsibility of the respiratory therapist. This chapter discusses current information related to drowning and near drowning. It focuses on the definitions and related nomenclature, epidemiology, causes and risk factors, pathophysiology, drowning sequence and initial rescue, clinical features and initial assessment, treatment, prognosis and outcomes, and preventative measures associated with drowning.

> Drowning can occur in a bathtub, bucket, toilet, or swimming pool and has a high association with alcohol use and abuse.

DEFINITIONS

The literature contains many definitions associated with drowning and near drowning.[1–3] Early literature refers to drowning as death by suffocation resulting from submersion.[4–10] Some definitions specify a time frame, for example, death within 24 hours of rescue,[1,5,11,12] while others allude to the pathophysiological state and use terms such as *wet drowning* or *dry drowning*.[1,13] **Wet drowning** and **dry drowning** simply refer to the presence or absence of liquid in the lungs. Other terms refer to the condition of the victim when first observed during the incident such as active drowning or passive or silent drowning.[1,13] Active drowning refers to a witnessed drowning in which the victim is making some motion, while passive or silent drowning refers to an unobserved event in which the person is discovered motionless in the water. Frequently, the adjectives *fatal* or *nonfatal* will be inserted that simply refer to the outcome, and *intentional* or *unintentional* may be employed to describe causality. Cold water drowning refers to drowning in an outside body of water, usually during the autumn, winter, or early spring months with a patient core temperature of less than or equal to 32°C on arrival to the emergency department. Warm water drowning describes higher temperatures (greater than 32°C).[14] Finally, secondary drowning is a term used to describe an unrelated event such as a heart attack, seizure, or cervical spine injury that results in the victim's submersion and subsequent death.

The classic and most widely used definition of drowning is that proposed by Model in 1981: **Drowning** is defined as suffocation by immersion, especially in water. In addition, Model[15] proposed the following nomenclature and definitions: Drowning *without aspiration* refers to dying from respiratory obstruction and asphyxia while submerged in a fluid medium; drowning *with aspiration*, refers to dying from the combined effects of asphyxia and changes secondary to aspiration of fluid while submerged; near drowning without aspiration, entails survival, at least temporarily, following asphyxia owing to submergence in a fluid medium; near drowning with aspiration, is survival, at least temporarily, following aspiration of fluid while submerged.

Additionally, the term **near drowning** has been applied to those who are successfully resuscitated and survive at least 24 hours.[4–7,9,16] If death occurs within the first 24 hours, drowning is listed as the primary cause. Should the victim survive the initial 24 hours but die later of complications, the primary cause of death is attributed to the complications (e.g., brain death, renal failure, sepsis, ARDS), and the secondary cause listed as near drowning. Box 10.1 provides a compilation of definitions and nomenclature associated with drowning.

Regrettably, these varied definitions and related terms have created considerable ambiguity in terms of clarity of definition as well as an inability to gather data, perform statistical studies, and report results. In an attempt to provide clarity and uniformity, a Task Force of the World Congress on Drowning suggested that previous terms be abandoned and the medical and scientific community adopt the following definition: *Drowning is the process of experiencing respiratory impairment from submersion/immersion in liquid*.[1,3,17,18] This definition suggests that the drowning process[13] is a continuum that begins when the victim's airway lies below the surface of the liquid, usually water, and the victim voluntarily holds his or her breath. The Task Force recommends that the terms *immersion* and *submersion* be included in the definition, as immersion connotes partial coverage with a liquid (head out of water) and submersion entails total coverage (head submerged in water). Regardless of the definition employed, drowning is a fatal condition and its prevention requires a thorough understanding of the epidemiology, contributing factors, pathophysiology, and management.

> Regardless of the definition employed, drowning is fatal.

EPIDEMIOLOGY

The World Health Organization estimates the annual death rate from drowning at nearly half a million people worldwide,[1,2] making drowning the second leading cause of unintentional death globally.[1,19] Experts suggest that this number is grossly underestimated because of a lack of a standardized definition of drowning and a lack of consistency in reporting of the data. Data from the World Health Organization identifies the Western Pacific, South-East Asian, and African Regions as representing the largest percentages of worldwide drowning, with 33.4%, 22.4%, and 22.3%, respectively. The Americas represent the lowest percentage of the worldwide problem, with 6% of drowning deaths.

In 2002 the Centers for Disease Control (CDC) reported 3,482 accidental drowning deaths in the United States.[20] Drowning represented the seventh leading cause of unintentional injury deaths for all ages,[21] was the leading cause of death among toddlers 12 to 23 months of age in 2000,[12] and was the second leading cause of injury-related death for the 1 to 14 year old age group.[22] Another source estimates that for every child who drowns, there are one to four nonfatal submersions serious enough to result in hospitalization.[2,23–27] Another source estimated a rate of three emergency department care visits per drowning, with more than 40% requiring hospitalization.[28] The CDC also reports that males account for 78% of drowning deaths in the United States.[22] Brenner and associates[29] examined the location of drowning in infants, children, and adolescents in the United States and reported that 55% of infant drowning deaths were in bathtubs. In 2001 the overall age-adjusted drowning rate for African Americans was 1.4 times higher than for Caucasians, and the Centers for Disease Control and Prevention noted that after the age of 5 years, the risk of drowning in a swimming pool was greater among

Box 10.1 Terms Related to Drowning

Active drowning. A witnessed drowning in which the victim is making some motion.

Cold water drowning. A drowning in an outside body of water during the autumn, winter, or early spring months with a patient core temperature of less than or equal to 32°C on arrival to the emergency department. Some use water temperature less than 20°C.

Drowning. Suffocation by immersion, especially in water.

Drowning with aspiration. Dying from the combined effects of asphyxia and changes secondary to aspiration of fluid while submerged.

Drowning without aspiration. Dying from respiratory obstruction and asphyxia while submerged in a fluid medium.

Dry drowning. The absence of liquid in the lungs.

Fatal or nonfatal. Refers to the outcome.

Iceberg phenomenon. People who have been submerged but have subsequently not died from drowning.

Immersion. Partial coverage with a liquid (head out of water).

Immersion syndrome. Development of asystole or ventricular fibrillation resulting from sudden immersion in very cold water.

Intentional or unintentional. Describes causality.

Near drowning. A critical aquatic predicament resolved by successful water rescue. It has also been applied to those who are successfully resuscitated and survive at least 24 hours.

Passive or silent drowning. An unobserved event after which the person is discovered motionless in the water.

Postimmersion syndrome. The development of ARDS after a near drowning incident.

Secondary drowning. An unrelated event such as a heart attack, seizure, or cervical spine injury that results in the victim's submersion and subsequent death.

Submersion. Total coverage (head submerged in water).

Wet drowning. The presence of liquid in the lung.

African-American males compared with Caucasian males. In 2002 statistics provided by the Consumer Protection Safety Council[30] indicated that 67% of all drowning deaths occurred in backyard pools, spas, and hot tubs; the majority of drowning incidents occurred while the child's supervisor assumed the child was safely indoors, and the event occurred in less time that it takes to answer the phone. Finally, data on nonfatal and fatal drowning deaths in recreational settings indicate that the nonfatal drowning rate for males is nearly twice that for females, and the fatal rate for males is almost five times that of females.[21]

Near drowning takes a tremendous toll on affected families and society as a whole. Typical medical costs can range from $75,000 for initial treatment to $180,000 a year for long-term care. Additionally, the total cost of a single nonfatal drowning victim who sustains brain injury can be more than $4.5 million, and the annual lifetime costs of drowning among children ages 14 and under is approximately $6.8 billion, with children ages 4 and under accounting for $3.4 billion, or half of these costs.[31]

> Toddlers between the ages 1 and 4 and adolescents and young adults between the ages of 15 and 24 are at significantly greater risk for death from drowning.

ETIOLOGY

Drowning and near drowning are major causes of morbidity and mortality, and numerous factors contribute to the actual event. A technical report provided by Benner and associates[12] provides one of the more thorough and comprehensive list of contributing factors associated with drowning and near drowning. Benner's risk factors are identified in Box 10.2 and include sociodemographic factors, temporal and geographic variables, location and circumstances, lapses in adult supervision, alcohol, swimming ability, and underlying medical conditions.

With regard to socioeconomic status, drowning rates were inversely related to per capita income for all age groups.[32] However, studies have demonstrated that affluence has resulted in an increase in the number of residential pools (approximately 10,000 pools in 1950 to 3.4 million in-ground pools and 3.2 million above-ground pools today), and this increase may explain an increase in drowning deaths.[33]

Temporal and geographic variations profoundly affect the incidence of drowning. One study[34] indicates that two thirds of drowning victims under the age of 15 died during the months of May through August and that drowning shows the greatest seasonal variation of all causes of unintentional injury death. The consistency of these patterns is not fully understood, but speculation is that it may be due to the school year.

Location and circumstances surrounding drowning incidents are addressed in a national study of childhood drowning[31] that indicated that 39% of all drowning deaths occurred in pools (14% residential pools, 7% community pools, and 18% unknown), 37% occurred in open bodies of water (lakes, rivers, and ponds), 18% occurred in and around home (bathtubs, buckets, and spas), and the remaining 6% were listed as other. Ironically, 90% of all drowning deaths occur within 10 meters of safety.[35]

Box 10.2 Factors Associated with Drowning and Near Drowning

- Sociodemographic factors
- Temporal and geographic variables
- Location and circumstances
- Lapses in adult supervision
- Alcohol
- Swimming ability
- Underlying medical conditions.

One of the more compelling claims regarding the issue of supervision of infants and toddlers in and around sources of water[23] indicates that inadequate supervision is the most common factor associated with submersions. A sobering statistic cited in a study[31] reveals that 88% of children are under some form of supervision when they drowned. According to the American Red Cross, a child can drown in fewer than 2 inches of water and in less than 5 minutes.[33]

Alcohol is estimated to be involved in 30% to 50% of adolescent and adult drowning deaths[24,36] and appears to be the overwhelming cause of drowning associated with recreational aquatic activity.[37] Data provided by the U.S. Coast Guard indicate that 705 people were killed in boating incidents in 2002. Of the boating fatalities, 70% were attributed to drowning, and alcohol was involved in 39% of the reported boating fatalities.[38]

While a high percentage of people who drown are nonswimmers or poor swimmers (as many as two-thirds),[10] there are conflicting opinions as to the role of swimming skill and ability in preventing drowning and near drowning.[39,40] It has been suggested that a daily swimmer will obviously have increased exposure to the water and, coupled with a high degree of confidence, be exposed to increased risk and greater likelihood of a drowning event.[41] Swimming with a friend, in the presence of a lifeguard, and using a flotation device are all reasonable strategies to employ. Swimming instruction along with water-safety training and dealing with hazardous aquatic environments, such as rip tides, strong currents, waves, underwater obstacles, depth and temperature of the water, can better prepare an individual to deal with the risk of drowning. The American Academy of Pediatrics recommends that children are generally not developmentally ready for formal swimming lessons until after their fourth birthday.[42]

Underlying medical conditions can also expose an individual to greater risk for drowning. Individuals with known seizure disorders are especially at high risk for drowning. Children with epilepsy are estimated to be at 4 to 14 times greater risk for drowning than children without epilepsy.[24] It has been recommended that children with epilepsy should shower rather than bathe in a tub. Additionally, the literature indicates that the physically and mentally handicapped are at greater risk as are those with other illnesses, such as cerebrovascular accidents, myocardial infarctions, and cardiac arrhythmias. SCUBA diving and head or spinal cord injury are also associated with drowning.

> Turning your attention away from an infant or toddler for just a brief moment can result in a drowning incident. That means pouring a cup of coffee, answering the phone, a knock at the door, or stirring the spaghetti sauce all can result in disaster. Complete and total surveillance and vigilant supervision is essential.

PATHOPHYSIOLOGY

Drowning can occur in freshwater, which is most frequent, in salt water (sea, brackish), or in any fluid. The majority (85% to 90%) of drowning victims aspirate fluid into their lungs, referred to as wet drowning. The volume aspirated is usually small (less than 22 mL/kg) and often may include vomit, bacteria, and other debris present in the fluid. Victims usually swallow large amounts of water (liquid) during their struggle to remain afloat, and vomiting with aspiration is a frequent occurrence, especially during resuscitation. The remaining 10% to 15% of drowning victims do not aspirate fluid into their lungs and as noted previously experience dry drowning. Death without aspiration results from acute asphyxia thought to be brought about by laryngospasm or prolonged breath holding and subsequent hypoxia. Laryngospasm can result when a small amount of fluid enters the region of the larynx as the victim gasps for air while fully or partially submerged.

Neurological Insult

The hallmark neurological events found in drowning are hypoxia and ischemia. **Hypoxia** is an insufficient oxygen supply to a particular tissue of the body. **Ischemia** results when blood flow to a tissue or organ system is diminished or when the blood oxygen content is markedly diminished. In near-drowning incidents the brain may become hypoxic before cardiac arrest occurs. Blood flow may continue under anaerobic conditions for a period even after the oxygen supply has been depleted. Most people lose consciousness after 2 minutes of anoxia, and brain damage may occur after 4 to 6 minutes.[43]

Submersion times as long as 40 minutes[44] have been reported with full recovery. These unique incidents are more common in frigid water. The brain-protective effects of a rapidly induced hypothermia are more likely to occur in children less than 5 years of age than adults because they have a greater body surface area to body weight (mass) ratio and can lose body heat more rapidly. This, combined with ingestion of frigid water, may protect the brain by decreasing brain metabolism and reducing oxygen requirements before cardiac arrest. An intact diving reflex[4,7,8] (i.e., breath holding, bradycardia, and peripheral vasoconstriction when the face is immersed in cold water) is another possible factor contributing to full recovery.

Energy in the form of adenosine triphosphate (ATP) is produced by metabolic pathways including glycolysis, the tricarboxylic acid (TCA) cycle, and oxidative phosphorylation[45] under aerobic conditions (Figure 10.1). Glycolysis occurs in the cell cytoplasm, whereas the TCA cycle and oxidative phosphorylation take place in the mitochondria of the cell. ATP provides energy for many active transport mechanisms that maintain homeostasis (e.g., sodium-potassium pumps, calcium pumps), which are found in cellular membranes.[46] Under anaerobic conditions (inadequate oxygenation), the TCA cycle and oxidative phosphorylation no longer function, leaving glycolysis as the major ATP producer.[45] Glycolysis under anaerobic conditions is rapid; however, for a new supply of glucose to be provided, tissue perfusion must continue. The anaerobic metabolism of each glucose molecule produces a net of 2 ATP compared to 36 ATP produced when aerobic conditions exist.

Brain cells are strictly aerobic, and during hypoxic conditions, injury can rapidly occur as oxygen and energy supplies diminish. Active transport mechanisms begin to slow down or quit working altogether as a result of the diminished supply of energy. Cellular integrity becomes jeopardized as potassium is lost from within the cell and sodium and calcium flood into it.

Pulmonary Insult

Aspiration occurs in 85% to 90% of near-drowning patients. Pulmonary injury is more frequent in this group than in those who do not aspirate. The volume, type of fluid aspirated, and components found in the aspirated fluid (e.g., bacteria, emesis) determine the extent of pulmonary injury.

Fresh water is hypotonic to the blood and is rapidly absorbed into the blood stream when aspirated. It destroys pulmonary surfactant, thereby increasing surface tension properties within the lung, which results in atelectasis.[47–51] Seawater is hypertonic to the blood (approximately 3% saline) and upon aspiration, causes fluid from the blood to flood into the alveoli. Alveolar collapse occurs as surfactant is washed out and surface tension forces increase. In either fresh- or saltwater aspiration, the end result is usually a combination of pulmonary edema and atelectasis.

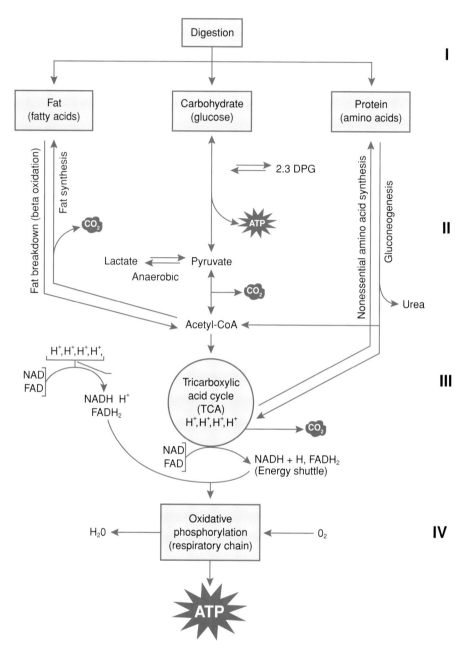

FIGURE 10.1 Four major phases of metabolism are schematically illustrated. Phase I: Digestion and nutrient absorption of fat, carbohydrate, and protein. Phase II: Breakdown of fatty acids, glucose, and amino acids to acetylcoenzyme A (acetyl5CoA), which can either synthesize—directly or indirectly—fat, carbohydrate, or amino acids as needed or go on to have more energy extracted from it in phases III and IV. Phase III: Tricarboxylic acid cycle, where most of the body's carbon dioxide (CO_2) is produced, as well as where most of the molecular energy shuttles (nicotinamide-adenine dinucleotide [NAD], flavin adenine dinucleotide [FAD]) receive their energy supply (in the form of hydrogen atoms). Shuttles transport energy to the respiratory chain. Phase IV: Inner mitochondrial membrane, where oxidative phosphorylation occurs (production of adenosine triphosphate [ATP] in the presence of oxygen) and oxygen is the final acceptor of the now energy-depleted electrons and hydrogen ions.

Pulmonary edema and atelectasis both result in ventilation-perfusion ($\dot{V}/\dot{Q}$) mismatching, intrapulmonary shunting ($\dot{Q}s/\dot{Q}t$), a decrease in functional residual capacity, and a decrease in lung compliance. These abnormalities often lead to refractory hypoxemia.[52]

Aspirated substances may include mud, sand, bacteria, and gastric contents. Such substances create inflammatory processes throughout the respiratory tract, resulting in alveolitis, bronchitis, and pneumonitis when aspirated.

ARDS is a common complication of near drowning and probably results from pulmonary and microvascular injury associated with aspiration or an inflammatory response or both. Activated granulocytes can cause alveolar-capillary membrane injury by releasing lysosomal enzymes and oxygen free radicals. As the alveolar-capillary membrane is damaged, protein-rich fluid can flood the interstitial space, overwhelming the ability of the pulmonary lymphatics to remove it. If not removed, protein attachment to the alveolar walls can form hyaline membranes.

Hemodynamic and Electrolyte Effects

Evaluations of near-drowning patients have not demonstrated severe electrolyte or hemoglobin abnormalities with either salt- or freshwater aspiration. This suggests that victims do not swallow or aspirate volumes sufficient to cause death through altered electrolyte or hemoglobin concentrations. Neither hemoglobin nor hematocrit measurements can be used to determine whether fresh or seawater has been aspirated.[53] Animal studies have found that the type of fluid aspirated (hypotonic, isotonic, or hypertonic) is not important in determining the hemodynamic response to near drowning. Pulmonary vascular resistance increases and cardiac output decreases with hypoxia, regardless of the tonicity of the fluid aspirated.[54] The heart becomes asystolic with persistent hypoxia.

> While the heart and the lungs are vital organ systems adversely affected by a drowning incident, it is the brain that sustains the long-term consequences.

DROWNING SEQUENCE AND INITIAL RESCUE (PREHOSPITAL CARE)

In 2004 the United States Lifeguard Association reported 48,514 rescues on the shores of U.S. beaches,[55] with estimates of eight cases of near drowning for each reported death.[56] The National Safe Kids Campaign reports that contrary to the notion of splashing and considerable noise of crying out for help, drowning generally occurs quickly and silently[31] and is a horrifying event. The sequence of events has been well documented[57] and consists of the following: (1) panic and immediate struggle, (2) suspension of movement—exhalation of a little air and frequent swallowing, (3) violent struggle, (4) convulsions—expiration of air and spasmodic inspiratory efforts with mouth wide open and disappearance of reflexes, and (5) death.[58]

The panicked and struggling victim can be dangerous, and it is for this reason that immediate intervention and rescue should entail adherence to the DRABC algorithm: danger (to rescuer, bystander, and casualty), response, airway, breathing, and circulation.[58] Pia[59] has described the *instinctive drowning response*, where contrary to the popularized depiction displayed in the movies, the victim does not wave and cry out for help. Pia goes on to say that breathing is instinctive and takes precedence, and the following occurs: the victim is typically in the upright position with arms extended laterally, thrashing and slapping the water; the victim will submerge and surface several times during this struggling time, and is unable to call for help. Pia has shown that children can struggle for only 10 to 20 seconds before final

> The body's instinctual desire for self-preservation exposes the well-intentioned and noble rescuer to increased risk. Be prepared to protect yourself when you assist in a drowning rescue.

submersion and that adults may be able to struggle up to 60 seconds.[59] This is why the would-be rescuer should take into account the need to protect him- or herself from this natural tendency for the victim to cling to life at all cost. Lifeguards are taught to approach the victim with caution and to use an intermediary object, such as a torpedo buoy, to assist in the rescue. Once this potential danger is overcome, the victim must be removed from the water, the ABCs followed as needed, and initial assessment begun. The primary aims of out-of-hospital treatment are relief of hypoxia, restoration of cardiovascular stability, prevention of further heat loss, and speedy evacuation to the hospital.[3] Achieving these desired aims requires skillful assessment of clinical features.

CLINICAL FEATURES

History

The initial assessment of drowning victims should be rapid and directed toward the victim's level of consciousness as well as the presence of pulse and respiration. Information from onlookers can also be very helpful in determining the extent of injury. If possible, the history should include information regarding the approximate length of time the patient was submerged, the type of fluid or water in which the victim was submerged, whether vital signs were present when the victim was removed from the water, the approximate length of time that transpired between submersion and the initiation of CPR, whether CPR was performed immediately after removal of the victim from the water, how long CPR was performed before vital signs returned, the approximate temperature of the water, the victim's age, and any other circumstances related to the near-drowning incident (e.g., diving or other accident, alcohol ingestion).

Physical Examination

Vital signs may be highly variable in near-drowning victims. Some victims may be in full cardiac arrest, while others may have a pulse and respirations within normal limits. The temperature of victims is variable depending on the temperature of the water in which they were submerged, their body surface area, and the duration of exposure. Hypothermia (less than 33°C [91.4°F]) can occur within a few minutes of exposure to frigid water, and although it may improve survival, careful rewarming of the patient is required. The cardiac effect of near drowning is usually bradycardia, which may be followed by asystole.[60] Hypothermia resulting from a near-drowning incident in more temperate regions (with warmer water temperatures) may indicate a longer submersion time and probably will not have a positive patient prognosis.

Neurological impairment from hypoxia results in (1) dilated pupils that respond slowly, or not at all, to light and (2) an impaired sensorium. The head and neck should be carefully inspected for possible trauma. Some near-drowning victims may have neck injuries from diving into shallow water. Suspected spinal cord injuries require immobilization before transport.

Auscultation over the chest may reveal one or both of the following: wheezing owing to bronchospasm or foreign-body aspiration and late-inspiratory crackles associated with atelectasis or pulmonary edema.[52] The presence of adventitious lung sounds (e.g., coarse crackles) suggests that the patient has aspirated and is at risk for pneumonia and ARDS.

The extremities of the near-drowning patient are often cool to the touch as a result of hypothermia and peripheral vasoconstriction in response to hypotension or sympathetic outflow stimulated by brain hypoxia. A slow capillary refill is present when peripheral circulation is reduced.

Arterial Blood Gases

Arterial blood gas (ABG) studies often reveal hypoxemia (especially when aspiration has occurred) and metabolic acidosis. The severity of the metabolic acidosis is usually related to the severity of the tissue hypoxia. Hemoglobin, hematocrit, and electrolyte concentrations may decrease when large volumes of fresh water are swallowed or aspirated. This is the result of the dilution effects of the water when it enters the circulating blood volume.

> The respiratory therapist's (RT's) assessment skills and knowledge of cardiorespiratory physiology become exceedingly valuable in the decision-making process and ultimate care of the drowning victim.

CLINICAL OUTCOMES

While no system can predict outcome with 100% accuracy, several scoring systems aid the initial assessment of near-drowning victims. Three commonly used systems are the Glasgow coma scale (GCS),[5,61-63] the Orlowski score,[5,61-63] and the postsubmersion neurological classification system published independently by Modell and associates[64] and Conn and colleagues.[65]

The GCS has three categories; the best response from each category is determined and given the numeric value assigned to that response (Box 10.3). Scores from each category are then added for a total score. A score of 3 is the lowest possible, a score of 7 or less indicates coma, and a score of 14 indicates full consciousness. Prognosis is then based on the initial GCS examination. Near-drowning patients with an initial GCS of 4 or less have an 80% chance of dying or having permanent neurological sequelae.[61] Patients with a GCS of 6 or higher have a very low risk for permanent neurological sequelae or mortality. Patients with a GCS of at least 13 can be safely discharged from the emergency department after 4 to 6 hours of observation if

Box 10.3 Glasgow Coma Scale*

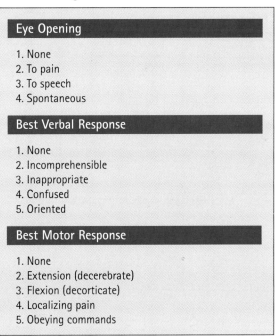

Eye Opening

1. None
2. To pain
3. To speech
4. Spontaneous

Best Verbal Response

1. None
2. Incomprehensible
3. Inappropriate
4. Confused
5. Oriented

Best Motor Response

1. None
2. Extension (decerebrate)
3. Flexion (decorticate)
4. Localizing pain
5. Obeying commands

*The Glasgow coma scale scores the patient's best response from each category. The numeric value to the left of each chosen response is then added together for all three categories for a total value. A total score less than 7 indicates presence of coma, whereas 14 signifies full consciousness.

SOURCE: From Orlowski, J: Drowning, near-drowning, and ice-water submersions. Pediatr Clin North Am 34(1):75, 1987, with permission.

Box 10.4 Orlowski Score*

Unfavorable Prognostic Factors
1. Age ≤ 3 years
2. Estimated submersion time longer than 5 minutes
3. No resuscitative measure attempted for at least 10 minutes
4. Patient comatose upon arrival at the emergency room
5. Arterial blood gas pH ≤ 7.10

*The Orlowski score is determined by the number of unfavorable factors listed that apply to the near-drowning victim. Lower scores are prognostic of a more favorable outcome.

SOURCE: From Orlowski, J: Drowning, near-drowning, and ice-water submersions. Pediatr Clin North Am 34(1):75, 1987, with permission.

they have a normal oxygen saturation on room air and a normal pulmonary examination.[66]

The Orlowski score[5,61-63] is based on evidence of unfavorable factors related to the patient's recovery (Box 10.4). It uses a scoring system that includes age less than three years, duration of submersion greater than 5 minutes, resuscitation attempts delayed for more than 10 minutes after incident, presence of coma on arrival to emergency department, and arterial pH less than or equal to 7.1.[2] Patients with two or fewer unfavorable prognostic factors have a 90% chance of a good recovery, compared to a 5% chance in patients with three or more unfavorable factors.

In 1980 Modell and associates[64] and Conn and colleagues[65] independently published a postsubmersion neurological classification system based on the near-drowning patient's initial level of consciousness with A = alert; B = blunted, and C = comatose (Box 10.5). Conn and colleagues subcategorized the coma group, whereas Modell did not. Cerebral damage may cause decorticate posturing upon (painful) stimulation, in which the arms, wrists, and fingers are bent upon themselves (flexed) and pulled inward toward the body (adducted). The legs are rigidly kept in a straight position (extension) and feet are rotated inward. Damage to the brain stem may result in decerebrate posturing upon stimulation, in which the arms are extended and rotated inward, while the spine, legs, and feet are rigid and hyperextended.

All patients in one retrospective study with an admission assessment of category A (Box 10.5) survived without complications.[64] Of the category B patients, 90% survived with complete recovery, but 10% died. Of category C patients, 55% completely recovered, but 34% died and 10% had permanent neurological sequelae.

Except for those recovered from frigid waters, near-drowning victims with submersion times greater than 10 minutes and an initial resuscitation lasting longer than

Box 10.5 Postsubmersion Neurological Classification System*

Category	Description
A Awake	Alert, fully conscious, and oriented
B Blunted	Blunted consciousness, lethargic but rousable; purposeful response to pain
C Comatose	Not arousable; abnormal response to pain
C_1	Decorticate flexion in response to pain
C_2	Decerebrate extension in response to pain
C_3	Flaccid or no pain response

*By Modell and Conn. Prognosis is determined by category, with those in categories A and B having an excellent prognosis. Prognosis worsens in category C according to the depth of coma.

SOURCE: From Conn A, et al: Cerebral salvage in near-drowning following neurological classification by triage. Can Anaesth Soc J 27(3):201, 1980, with permission.

25 minutes are predicted to have a poor prognosis (persistent vegetative state or death).[67] One group predicted a poor outcome in patients with nonreactive pupils in the emergency department and a GCS of 5 or less upon arrival to the intensive care unit (ICU).[68] Another group reported poor outcome in comatose patients with absent pupillary light reflex, patients with an increase in initial blood glucose, and male patients.[69] One report recommended that a neurologi-

> A dismal or gloomy neurological picture should not deter the RT from aggressively and persistently providing care. Many variables are at play in long-term disposition.

cal examination be performed 24 hours after the submersion to predict satisfactory versus unsatisfactory outcome. They found that all survivors who were awake and making purposeful movements 24 hours postimmersion had normal neurological function or mild deficits, whereas those who remained comatose died or had severe neurological deficits.[70] Another report suggested that prolonged in-hospital resuscitation and aggressive treatment of victims who lack vital signs and who are not hypothermic (less than 33°C [91.4°F]) is usually unsuccessful.[71]

TREATMENT

Basic life support[72] and activation of the emergency medical services (EMS) system should begin as soon as possible. The rescuer should carefully open the victim's airway and, if there is no breathing, perform rescue breathing, initially giving two slow breaths. If the apneic victim cannot be rapidly removed from the water, rescue breathing should be attempted in the water. Assessment for a heartbeat should be done when the victim is either brought to shore or placed on a flotation device large enough for both the rescuer and the victim. Chest compressions performed in the water will not restore brain perfusion and should not be attempted until the victim is ashore or placed on a flotation device. If the victim is recovered from cold water, the recommended pulse check should take up to 1 minute[5,73] to rule out bradycardia or a faint heartbeat. Chest compressions started in haste can result in ventricular fibrillation and can actually decrease cerebral perfusion. The victim should be transported to a medical center as soon as possible.

Do not perform the Heimlich maneuver unless an airway obstruction is present.[6] A drowning victim may swallow a large amount of water, and the Heimlich maneuver can result in vomiting and aspiration of the stomach contents. If breathing spontaneously, the drowning victim should be placed and transported in the right lateral decubitus position, with the head lower than the trunk to reduce the risk of aspiration. If rescue breathing is performed, cricoid pressure should be applied when possible to limit the risks of gastric aspiration.[3] Additionally, it is generally accepted that rewarming be commenced immediately with the use of blankets; warmed intravenous fluids; warmed gastric, bladder, or peritoneal lavage; and hemodialysis.

Health-care practitioners at the hospital should prepare appropriate equipment in anticipation of the near-drowning victim's arrival. Equipment for intubation needs to be present, including laryngoscope, an assortment of blades, various tube sizes, stylets, Magill forceps, syringe to check cuff patency and for cuff inflation, equipment for suctioning, tape to secure the endotracheal tube, and an appropriate bag-valve-mask device. An ABG kit should be available, as well as appropriate gowning provisions for universal precautions.

Treatment for near-drowning patients is based on initial assessment and categorization. The following summary is based on the postsubmersion neurological classification system.

Category A (Awake)

The neurological status of these patients is alert and awake with a GCS of 14, indicating minimal hypoxic injury. These patients should be hospitalized and placed under continuous observation for 12 to 24 hours to allow early intervention should pulmonary or neurological deterioration occur. Laboratory evaluation should include a complete blood count (CBC), serum electrolytes, chest radiograph, ABG, sputum cultures, blood glucose levels, and clotting times. A drug toxicological screen may also be necessary. A radiograph of the cervical spine should be obtained if there is a possibility of neck injury.

Treatment for this group is primarily symptomatic. Oxygen is delivered as needed via cannula or mask to maintain a PaO_2 above 60 mm Hg. An incentive spirometry device (volume type) may be helpful. Foreign-body aspiration can be evaluated by chest radiograph. Bronchospasm can be treated with aerosolized beta-agonist agents. IV access is important for fluid and electrolyte management and allows rapid intervention should deterioration occur.

Neurological deterioration may result from:

- Hypoxemia owing to worsening pulmonary condition
- An increase in intracranial pressure (ICP) caused by hypoxic injury
- Drug ingestion before the event

If the patient is stable and no neurological or pulmonary deterioration has occurred within 12 to 24 hours, the patient may be discharged. Physician follow-up within 2 to 3 days after discharge is strongly recommended to evaluate the patient for a potential pulmonary infection.

Category B (Blunted)

The neurological status of these patients is obtunded, or semiconscious but rousable. GCS is usually 10 to 13, indicating a more serious and prolonged episode of asphyxia. They have purposeful pain responses, normal respirations, and normal pupillary reactions. They may be irritable and combative. After resuscitation and initial evaluation in the emergency department, these patients should be placed in the ICU with close attention paid to any changes in neurological, pulmonary, or cardiovascular status. The hospital stay for category B patients is usually longer than that for category A patients. All testing and treatment mentioned earlier for category A patients should be implemented for category B patients. Blood, sputum, and possibly urine cultures should be performed initially and as indicated by signs and symptoms. Vitamin K administration may improve clotting times. Antibiotics should be implemented only when culture specimens show bacterial growth other than normal flora. Changes in the patient's neurological status can occur rapidly, and a normal routine for head injury should be followed. Pulmonary edema, intractable metabolic acidosis, and a prolonged resuscitation period generally indicate severe hypoxia (except in patients found in cold water). Hypoxemia may become refractory to increased inspired oxygen concentrations. Continuous positive airway pressure (CPAP) delivered via mask or mechanical ventilator may be necessary to maintain a PaO_2 of greater than 60 mm Hg or an SpO_2 of greater than 90%. Fluid restriction may be necessary, but serum osmolality should not exceed 320 mOsm/liter.

Category C (Comatose)

These severely ill patients are unarousable. The GCS is less than 7. Treatment should ultimately be directed toward maintaining normal oxygenation, ventilation, perfusion, blood pressure, blood sugar, and electrolyte levels.

Limited animal studies on brain resuscitation bring potential new hope for salvaging comatose patients with severe anoxic episodes.[74–87] The goals of brain resuscitation are to prevent increases in ICP and to preserve brain cells that are viable but nonfunctional. Treatment may include use of hypothermia, hyperventilation, calcium channel blockers, barbiturates, muscle relaxation or paralysis, etomidate, and fluorocarbon infusions. Unfortunately the results of brain resuscitation have been mixed, and the therapies remain controversial.[8] Some of these offer brain protection when applied before the hypoxic event, but not after, as in the near-drowning patient. A serious ethical issue is whether brain resuscitation improves postresuscitation quality of life or merely prolongs the dying process by creating a larger population of patients in a persistent vegetative state.

The following sections are based on Conn and colleagues' brain resuscitation recommendations.[65] They used the term *hyper* because seriously brain-injured patients are frequently *hyperhydrated*, *hyperventilating*, *hyperpyrexic*, *hyperexcitable*, and *hyperrigid*.

Hyperhydration

The hyperhydrated state may contribute to an increase in both ICP and pulmonary edema. In an attempt to control both, diuretics are usually implemented. Hemodynamic monitoring is used to avoid excessive fluid restriction that may lead to renal insufficiency and failure. Small doses of dopamine (less than 5 mg/kg/minute) act on dopaminergic receptors in the kidneys to increase renal perfusion and possibly urine output. Diuresis should not drive the serum osmolality above 320 mOsm/liter. Invasive hemodynamic monitoring requires use of a pulmonary artery catheter for monitoring central venous, pulmonary artery, and wedge pressures. Arterial lines may also be necessary if blood pressure is unstable or frequent ABG measurements are needed.

ICP monitoring was widely used during the 1980s to control or prevent increases in ICP. It is now most commonly used for patients in categories A or B who show signs of mental and neurological deterioration. It is hoped that hyperventilation, osmotic diuretics, and thiopental will reverse the cerebral edema resulting from ischemia. Unfortunately, successful control of ICP does not ensure survival with normal brain function.[88–91]

Hyperventilation

Patients requiring mechanical ventilation should be hyperventilated and $Paco_2$ kept between 25 and 30 mm Hg. Cerebral vascular resistance is controlled by the arterioles, which respond to changes in $Paco_2$. Hyperventilation causes cerebral vasoconstriction and can lower ICP. A patient's tidal volume (V_T) can be set in the range of 10 to 15 mL/kg at a rate necessary to achieve the appropriate reduction in $Paco_2$. ICP can also be somewhat relieved by elevating the head of the patient's bed by 30 degrees and keeping the patient's head midline.

Oxygen delivery to the tissues is an important goal in patients with more extensive lung involvement. Maintaining an arterial oxygen saturation (Sao_2) of greater than 96% (Pao_2 of 100 mm Hg) is ideal, but not always possible. Positive end-expiratory pressure (PEEP) is a valuable adjunct for achieving adequate oxygenation (Pao_2 greater than 60 mm Hg) when refractory hypoxemia is present. In adults and older pediatric patients, PEEP levels should be increased by increments of 5 cm H_2O until acceptable oxygenation is achieved. Smaller changes in PEEP should be made in younger patients.

Hyperpyrexia

Hypothermia (body temperature 29°C to 31°C [86°F to 88°F] or less) is known to protect the brain when induced before cerebral hypoxia. However, it has not improved neurological outcome in patients who have already sustained cerebral hypoxia and can induce other complications, such as suppression of normal immune response, a left shift in the oxyhemoglobin dissociation curve, and cardiac dysrrhythmias. Normothermia should be maintained via antipyretics and a cooling mattress when fever is present, since fever increases oxygen consumption.

Hyperexcitability

Barbiturates are thought to bring about reduction of ICP via cerebral vasoconstriction, suppression of seizure activity, and reduction of cerebral metabolic rate. Thiopental is probably the only barbiturate that may remove oxygen free radicals. Induction of a barbiturate coma has not been shown to improve survival or neurological outcome in near-drowning patients with severe deficit and may enhance cardiovascular instability. Barbiturate coma is no longer a part of the recommended treatment because of these problems.[90–92] Barbiturates are used, however, to control seizure activity. Steroid use was also advocated in near-drowning treatment in the hope of controlling ICP. Subsequent studies have shown steroids to be an ineffective treatment for postanoxic near-drowning patients. Steroid use may also inhibit normal immune responses to bacterial infection, resulting in a higher risk of sepsis.[8,92]

> It's not just the RTs' adeptness with basic cardiac life support (BCLS) and advanced cardiac life support (ACLS) that provides value in the care of the drowning victim but their unique knowledge and ability to institute mechanical ventilation and end expiratory pressure therapy that position them as key members of the health-care team.

Hyperrigidity

Decerebrate and decorticate rigid posturing are signs of raised ICP (cerebral or brain stem damage or both). ICP may be elevated as a result of brain swelling caused by hypoxia, mechanical ventilation, and PEEP; coughing; and the Trendelenburg position. Suctioning procedures may elevate ICP for as long as 30 minutes. ICP might be reduced in patients requiring mechanical ventilation with sedation and use of paralytic agents.

PROGNOSIS

Idris and associates determined that factors associated with prognosis and outcome of drowning can be categorized as either victim-related, incident-related, or identified at hospital admission. Victim-related factors include being male, being African American, the presence of a seizure disorder, and the use of alcohol or illicit drugs. Incident-related factors associated with death or bad outcome include failure to receive immediate resuscitative effort at the scene, prolonged duration of submersion, warm water conditions, and acute resuscitative efforts lasting longer than 25 minutes. Factors identified upon entry to the emergency department that are likely to produce poor or undesirable outcomes include prolonged unconsciousness, elevated serum glucose, hypothermia, and signs of brain stem dysfunction, such as absent pupillary reflex and absent spontaneous respiration.[13]

Moon and Long identified good prognostic signs and poor prognostic indicators for victims arriving in the emergency

Box 10.6 Good Prognostic Signs Upon Arrival in the ED

- Short submersion time
- Spontaneous respiration and heartbeat
- Glasgow coma scale >5

department. Their results are listed in Boxes 10.6 and 10.7.[58] While these indicators provide an approximate assessment of an individual's prognosis, some patients with numerous bad prognostic indicators have survived and all authors suggest that these indicators should not be used as criteria to withdraw or withhold treatment.[58]

Box 10.7 Poor Prognostic Indicators Upon Arrival in the ED

- Submersion duration >25 minutes
- Resuscitation time >25 minutes
- Ventricular tachycardia or fibrillation on initial ECG
- Fixed and dilated pupils on initial evaluation, GSC <5
- Severe acidosis (arterial ph <7)
- Apnea, absent heartbeat

PREVENTION

The literature is filled with commentary regarding the highly preventable nature of near drowning because some experts estimate that 80% of all drowning cases could have been prevented.[93] Salmonez and Vincent[2] suggested that preventive strategies for accidental drowning fall into one of two categories: human factors and site-specific factors. The human factors include inadequate supervision and/or less than complete surveillance, swimming ability and survival skills, use and abuse of alcohol, training in CPR, presence of lifeguards, and proper use of life jackets. Site factors include removing hazards and creating barriers or layers of safety. Specific site factors include draining unnecessary accumulations of water (such as tubs and buckets), implementing and enforcing mandatory isolation fencing (four-sided, at least 4 feet high, with no more than 4-inch gaps between slats), use of pool alarms, self-closing and self-latching gates, and installation of poolside phones to eliminate the need to leave the pool area as well as for use in emergency situations. Box 10–8 provides a list of common preventive strategies.

Like so many other cardiopulmonary conditions, drowning is a highly preventable event. It simply doesn't have to occur!

In a survey of members of the American Academy of Pediatrics by O'Flaherty and Pirie[11], the authors reported that most pediatricians do not routinely provide information (written materials) or anticipatory guidance to their patients or their patients' parents on drowning prevention. The Academy recognizes the power and influence it holds in the patient-physician relationship and also its strong history of child advocacy. It recognizes the criticality of incorporating education in pediatric practice and recommends drowning preventive strategies become a priority and be appropriately addressed in all routine visits.

Box 10.8 List of Common Preventive Strategies

Human factors:
- Supervision and/or complete surveillance
- Swimming ability and survival skills
- Alcohol
- Training in CPR
- Presence of lifeguards
- Proper use of life jackets

Site factors:
- Draining unnecessary accumulations of water
- Installation of isolation fencing
- Use of pool alarms
- Self-closing and self-latching gates
- Installation of poolside phones

Baby B

HISTORY

Baby B is a 13-month-old white male infant found upside down with face submerged and upper torso stuck in a bucket in his grandparents' washroom. The infant was missing for approximately 5 minutes. The infant's mother immediately began mouth-to-mouth resuscitation and he responded after four to five breaths. He began breathing spontaneously, cried, and vomited a large amount of water. He was taken to the local emergency medical services facility, where he was alert, active, and crying. His initial ABG analysis on room air was pH 7.34, $Paco_2$ 34 mm Hg, Pao_2 51 mm Hg, Sao_2 84%, HCO_3^- 19 mEq/liter, and base excess (BE) +2 mEq/liter. His temperature at that time was 38.8°C (101.8°F) (rectally), and chest auscultation revealed bilateral coarse crackles.

The patient was given oxygen by cannula and was warmed with blankets.

QUESTIONS	ANSWERS
1. What factor(s) contributed to this infants near drowning?	The primary factor was a lapse in adult supervision. Being inquisitive and adventuresome at this young age exposes a child to increased risk for a submersion incident.
2. Interpret the acid-base and oxygenation status of this patient's initial ABG. What accounts for the acid–base abnormality?	His acid-base status is consistent with a partially compensated metabolic acidemia. The metabolic acidosis is probably the result of lactic acidosis from anaerobic metabolism. He is moderately hypoxemic on room air.
3. What could be the cause of the coarse crackles?	The coarse crackles are most likely due to aspiration.

More on Baby B

PHYSICAL EXAMINATION

- **General.** Height 88 cm, weight 10.87 kg; patient alert, cooperative, oriented, and in no acute respiratory distress

- **Vital Signs.** Rectal temperature 35.8°C (96.4°F), pulse 156/min, respiratory rate 46/min, blood pressure 98/58 mm Hg, mean arterial pressure 72 mm Hg

- **HEENT.** Normocephalic; atraumatic; pupils equal, round, reactive to light and accommodation (PERRLA); sclera and conjunctiva nonicteric; nasopharynx showing nasal crusting, no nasal flaring; oropharynx clear; tympanic membranes showing erythema on left with a decreased light reflex on the right with some cerumen; head circumference 47.4 cm

- **Neck.** Supple, full range of motion without rigidity or tenderness

- **Lungs.** Coarse crackles anteriorly and posteriorly on auscultation of the lower lung fields

- **Heart.** Regular rhythm and normal S_1 and S_2; no murmurs, gallops, or rubs

- **Back.** Straight, without presacral edema or gross abnormalities

- **Extremities.** Full range of motion with + + pulses and normal reflexes

- **Skin.** Warm and pink

- **Neurological.** Patient is alert and oriented; cranial nerves II through XII fully intact; motor and sensory examination within normal limits.

QUESTIONS	ANSWERS
4. Based on the initial evaluation, what GCS would you give Baby B? What Orlowski score would you give him? Under what category would he be placed according to the Conn-Modell postsubmersion neurological classification system?	His GCS score is 14; his Orlowski score shows only one unfavorable prognostic factor (age ≤3 years); and his postsubmersion neurological classification is category A.
5. Based on these evaluation methods, what is Baby B's prognosis?	His prognosis is 100% full recovery without neurological deficit, although pneumonia and sepsis are possible and could be life threatening.

More on Baby B

Laboratory Evaluation

CBC	Value
White blood cell (WBC) count	14.9×10^3/mL
Red blood cell (RBC) count	4.41×10^6/mL
Hemoglobin (Hb)	12.0 g/dL
Hematocrit (Hct)	34.7%
Platelets	480×10^3/mL
Differential	
Segmented neutrophils	33%
Bands	47%
Lymphocytes	19%
Monocytes	1%
Electrolytes	**Value**
Na^+	133 mEq/liter
K^+	3.6 mEq/liter
Cl^-	106 mEq/liter
Total CO_2	18 mmol/liter
Blood urea nitrogen (BUN)	6 mg/dL
Creatinine	0.4 mg/dL

(box continued on page 240)

ABGs on 2 liters/minute	
ABG	Value
pH	7.37
Paco$_2$	33 mm Hg
Pao$_2$	73 mm Hg
Sao$_2$	94%
Cao$_2$	13.7 vol%
HCO$_3^-$	19 mEq/liter
BE	25 mEq/liter
Hb	10.7 g/dL

Chest Radiograph: Patchy opacifications in both lower lobes with the left clearer than the right, consistent with bibasalar subsegmental atelectasis. Mild central pulmonary congestion and interstitial edema consistent with noncardiogenic interstitial pulmonary edema (Figure 10.2).

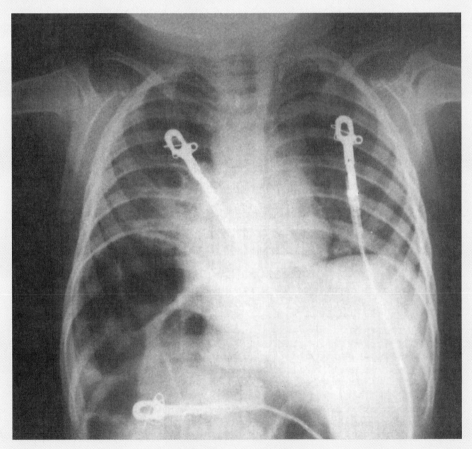

FIGURE 10.2 This radiograph is consistent with mild noncardiogenic interstitial pulmonary edema. Note the elevation of the left hemidiaphragm resulting from subsegmental atelectasis.

QUESTIONS	ANSWERS
6. Interpret the ABG analysis.	The acid-base status is consistent with a completely compensated metabolic acidosis. There is mild hypoxemia on 2 liters/min.
7. Electrolytes show a diminished Na^+. What might be the cause?	The drop in Na^+ is most likely due to dilutional hypervolemia resulting from swallowing large amounts of water. Dilution may also occur from aspiration and absorption of water through the lungs.
8. What pathophysiology might account for the hypoxemia?	The $Paco_2$ is low, ruling out hypoventilation as a source of hypoxemia. The Pao_2 response to supplemental oxygen would help determine whether the hypoxemia is due to $\dot{V}/\dot{Q}$ mismatching (which is associated with an improved Pao_2, as in this case) or shunt (which would not be associated with an improved Pao_2).
9. How soon could Baby B return home, and what follow-up is necessary?	The patient is stable and can be discharged after 12 to 24 hours of observation if he continues to improve and shows no signs of lung complications. He should be reevaluated after 2 to 3 days in the outpatient clinic.
10. What preventive measures could have been employed to decrease the likelihood of this event?	Complete surveillance and/or constant and immediate supervision. Education by the family pediatrician may also have proven helpful in warning family members of the possibility of this event.

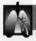

Child N

HISTORY

Child N is a 2-year-old African-American male who had been missing for 10 to 15 minutes and was found floating face down under the solar cover of a neighbor's above-ground swimming pool. He was unresponsive upon removal from the pool.

QUESTIONS	ANSWERS
1. What factors contributed to this child's near drowning?	The primary factor was a lapse in adult supervision. Black males in this age bracket are at greater risk for drowning, and toddlers in general tend to be more inquisitive and adventuresome, which can expose a child to increased risk for a submersion incident.

2. What treatment is indicated, and when should it be implemented?

The ABCs of CPR should be started immediately, as follows:

a. Determine unresponsiveness by shaking and shouting. Call for help! Open the airway.

b. Evaluate whether breathing is present by looking, listening, and feeling for breathing. Give two full breaths if the victim is apneic.

c. Assess whether circulation is present by monitoring pulse for 5 to 10 seconds; if there is no pulse during this interval, begin chest compressions. Continue CPR at a ratio of chest compressions to ventilations of 5:1. If this had been an adult victim, the ratio of chest compressions to ventilations would have been 15:2. Activate the EMS system as soon as possible!

3. Should the Heimlich maneuver be implemented? Why or why not?

The Heimlich maneuver should not be implemented at this time. It is used only when complete airway obstruction is present. Near-drowning patients frequently swallow large quantities of water, and the likelihood of vomiting and aspiration is increased when the Heimlich maneuver is performed.

 ## More on Child N

One family member starts CPR while another activates EMS. The paramedics arrive shortly thereafter and take over CPR. Child N is transported to the nearest facility, arriving there within 20 minutes from the time of initial discovery.

QUESTION	ANSWER
4. What airway preparations should you make before the patient arrives?	Make the following preparations:

a. Ensure that the appropriate intubation equipment is in good working condition: laryngoscope with various blade sizes (straight and curved), endotracheal tubes (cuffed and uncuffed), batteries, replacement bulbs for the blades, stylet, tape, Magill forceps, syringe for cuff inflation, nonpetroleum-base lubricating gel. Once the tube size is determined, if there is a cuff, determine cuff integrity by inflating and then removing the air. Insert stylet and lubricate the distal end of the tube.

b. Ensure that appropriate suctioning equipment is present (wall or portable suction device, reservoir, tubing, suction catheters, Yankauer's suctioning device) and is in good working condition.

c. Ensure that an appropriate bag-valve-mask device with a face mask assortment and an adequate 100% oxygen source is available and working.

d. Ensure that appropriate equipment is available for drawing arterial blood for ABG analysis.

e. Gown as appropriate for universal precautions.

More on Child N

Child N remains in full arrest upon arrival to the facility. The initial ABG with CPR in progress and the patient on 100% oxygen by bag-valve-mask device shows the following: pH 6.69, $Paco_2$ 55 mm Hg, Pao_2 70 mm Hg, BE–30 mEq/liter, and plasma HCO_3^- 7 mEq/liter. He is orally intubated with a 4.5-mm-diameter endotracheal tube and given one dose (0.2 mg IV) of epinephrine and 2 mEq of sodium bicarbonate ($NaHCO_3$). CPR continues, and after 10 minutes, a second round of drug therapy is administered.

QUESTIONS	ANSWERS
5. Interpret the initial ABG.	The acid–base status is consistent with a severe combined respiratory and metabolic acidemia. The oxygenation status is consistent with mild hypoxemia despite manual ventilation with 100% oxygen.
6. What treatment is indicated by the ABG results?	The extreme acidemia indicates the need for $NaHCO_3$ administration. The elevation of the $Paco_2$ indicates the need to increase alveolar ventilation.
7. After intubation, what should be done to determine endotracheal tube placement?	Assessment of endotracheal tube position can be done by auscultating the lungs for equal, bilateral breath sounds; by checking the linear measurement of the tube at the lip to determine how far it was inserted; and by reviewing the chest radiograph to assess proper tube placement. The right mainstem bronchus is shorter, wider, and straighter than the left mainstem bronchus, so the endotracheal tube will usually enter the right side if it is inserted too far. Intubation of the right mainstem bronchus usually leaves the left lung without ventilation and breath sounds.

More on Child N

Child N remains asystolic in the emergency department for about 1 hour. He requires several doses of epinephrine, $NaHCO_3$, and atropine. A nasogastric tube is inserted and 15 mL of clear fluid removed. The advanced cardiac life support measures restore Child N's heartbeat. An ABG is performed while he is receiving 100% oxygen via manual resuscitator. Results are as follows: pH 7.02, $Paco_2$ 11 mm Hg, Pao_2 464 mm Hg, BE–26 mEq/liter, and HCO_3^- 3 mEq/liter.

After resuscitation, Child N's initial temperature is 34.4°C (94.0°F) rectally; respirations are sporadic, requiring assistance; pulses range from 80 to 130/min; blood pressure varies from 99/25 to 134/69 mm Hg; and pupils are 4 mm and react sluggishly to light. Child N is unresponsive to stimuli (i.e., without eye opening, without verbal response) and exhibits decorticate posturing. His initial glucose level is 744 mg/dL. Initial electrolytes reveal the following: Na^+ 118 mEq/liter, K^+ 3.6 mEq/liter, Cl^- 92 mEq/liter, total CO_2 less than 5 mmol/liter, BUN 18 mg/dL, and creatinine 0.9 mg/dL. His initial CBC reveals the following: WBCs 7.2 $\times$ 10^3/mL, RBCs 4.5 $\times$ 10^6/mL, Hb 12.2 g/dL, Hct 35.6%, and a differential morphology showing segmented neutrophils 22% and lymphocytes 78%. Warming measures are started, and Child N is transported to a tertiary care facility. The initial chest radiograph shows proper endotracheal tube placement; bilateral fluffy infiltrates, more extensive on the left, consistent with noncardiogenic pulmonary edema; and a right-sided pleural effusion. The heart is normal in size, and the tip of the nasogastric tube is seen in the fundus of the stomach (Figure 10.3).

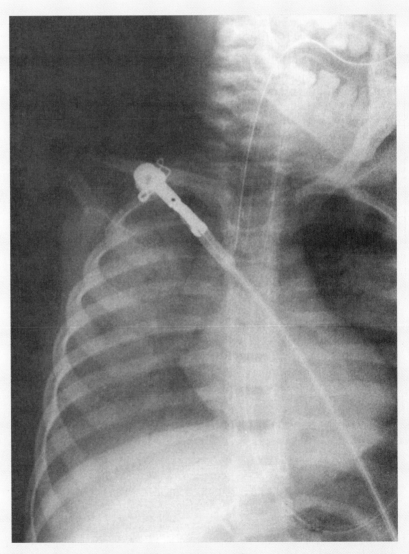

FIGURE 10.3 This radiograph is consistent with noncardiogenic pulmonary edema with probable right-sided pleural effusion.

QUESTIONS	ANSWERS
8. What GCS score would you give Child N? What Orlowski score would you give him? Under what category would you place him according to the Conn-Modell postsubmersion neurological classification system?	His GCS is 5. His Orlowski score shows four unfavorable prognostic factors (see Box 10.2). His postsubmersion neurological classification category is C_1.
9. What is Child N's prognosis?	According to the Conn-Modell system, there is approximately a 34% chance of mortality and a 55% chance of full recovery.
10. What do his initial electrolytes and CBC reveal, and what is the most likely cause of these results?	His electrolytes reveal hyponatremia and hypochloremia, which are likely caused by dilutional hypervolemia resulting from swallowing and aspirating water. The diminished total CO_2 is consistent with marked acidemia. His CBC reveals mild anemia, again consistent with dilutional hypervolemia.
11. What is indicated by the bilateral fluffy infiltrates and normal heart size on his chest radiograph?	The radiography results are consistent with aspiration or noncardiogenic pulmonary edema.
12. Should life support efforts be continued?	Yes, resuscitation should continue because there is a chance of full recovery.

More on Child N

PHYSICAL EXAMINATION

- **General.** Weight 35 pounds; patient responsive to deep pain only; difficult to assess secondary to decorticate movements involving all extremities, head, and trunk

- **Vital Signs.** Temperature 36.7°C (98.1°F), heart rate 169/min, respiratory rate 28/min by manual resuscitation, blood pressure 140/90 mm Hg

- **HEENT.** Head normocephalic, atraumatic; patient unable to focus; pupils sluggishly reactive, 4 mm, sclerae not icteric or injected; ears showing normally shaped pinna, auditory canals patent, tympanic membranes clear, without sign of infection; nose without nasal discharge; patient intubated

- **Neck.** No adenopathy or thyromegaly

- **Heart.** Regular rate and rhythm; normal S_1, S_2, without gallop

- **Lungs.** Coarse crackles heard throughout chest

- **Abdomen.** Soft, nondistended; no spleen tip or other masses palpated

- **Back.** Intact; no spina bifida, hair tuft, or sacral dimple

- **Extremities.** Pulses barely palpable in axillae, carotids, and femoral arteries; nail beds dusky

- **Skin.** Very poor perfusion, cool to the touch; no rashes noted on examination; no signs of trauma

- **Neurological.** Responds to deep pain only; hyper-reflexic deep tendon reflexes; decorticate posturing

QUESTIONS	ANSWERS
13. What is the significance of the sluggish pupils?	The sluggish pupils indicate an impaired neurological function that may be due to the hypoxic event.
14. What is the significance of dusky nail beds?	The dusky nail beds indicate poor cardiac output, poor peripheral perfusion, or hypothermia. In this case shock and poor cardiac output are the most likely causes.

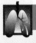

More on Child N

Ventilator settings are intermittent mandatory ventilation (IMV) at a rate of 20/min, FIO_2 0.70, V_T 170 mL, and PEEP 5 cm H_2O. An ABG taken on these parameters reveals pH 7.42, $Paco_2$ 30 mm Hg, Pao_2 75 mm Hg, BE−4 mEq/liter, HCO_3^- 19 mEq/liter.

During the first 8 hours, Child N's intake is 282 mL and output 497 mL. After 12 hours, his neurological status improves, showing some purposeful movements, pupils 4 mm bilaterally and reactive, purposeful response to pain, and occasional back arching. Breath sounds are improved. An electrocardiogram (ECG) shows a regular rate and rhythm. A foul-smelling, bloody discharge from his rectum is thought to be consistent with a compromised gastrointestinal tract caused by severe ischemia.

Laboratory Evaluation

Electrolyte Evaluation	
Measure	Value
Na^+	133 mEq/liter
K^+	3.3 mEq/liter
Cl^-	105 mEq/liter
Total CO_2	19 mol/liter
BUN	20 mg/dL
Creatinine	0.5 mg/dL
Glucose	181 mg/dL
Serum osmolality	273 mOsm/liter
CBC	**Value**
WBC	5.6×10^3/mL
RBC	Within normal limits
Hb	14.7 g/dL
Hct	42.8%
Platelet count	368×10^3/mL
Prothrombin time	13.3 seconds
Partial thromboplastin time	32 seconds

QUESTIONS	ANSWERS
15. Which data indicate persistent metabolic acidosis?	The parameters that indicate persistent metabolic acidosis include BE − 4 mEq/liter, HCO_3^- 19 mEq/liter, and total CO_2 19 mmol/liter.
16. How would you interpret the ABG?	The acid-base status is consistent with a completely compensated metabolic acidosis. There is mild hypoxemia on an F_{IO_2} of 0.70 and a PEEP of 5 cm H_2O. The calculated Ca_{O_2} is 18.5 vol%, which is within normal limits.
17. Why is the serum Na^+ rising?	The hyponatremia is resolving as diuresis occurs, ridding the body of the excess fluids.
18. What changes in ventilator parameters would you make, if any?	If tolerated, an increase in PEEP might improve his Pa_{O_2} and allow the F_{IO_2} to be decreased below 0.50. This would reduce the risk of oxygen toxicity.

 ## More on Child N

On the 14th hour of hospitalization, there is a sudden drop in the pulse oximeter saturation, accompanied by an increase in pulse and respiratory rate. The patient begins fighting the ventilator and is paralyzed. Auscultation reveals his breath sounds to be markedly diminished on the left side.

QUESTIONS	ANSWERS
19. What are possible causes of the sudden fall in the pulse oximeter saturation, increase in pulse and respiratory rate, and decreased breath sounds on the left side?	Causes of the sudden deterioration might include advancement of the endotracheal tube into the right mainstem bronchus, pneumothorax, or obstruction of the left mainstem bronchus by mucus and debris.
20. What should be done to confirm the cause and treat it?	Check the position of the endotracheal tube to determine if it has slipped. If so, reposition it and auscultate for equal bilateral breath sounds. Obtain a chest radiograph immediately to confirm endotracheal tube position and rule out pneumothorax and atelectasis. Pneumothorax may be corrected by chest tube placement. Mucus plugging can usually be corrected by chest physical therapy and postural drainage. Bronchoscopy may be used if these techniques fail to reverse the atelectasis.

Child N Conclusion

Child N's chest radiograph reveals a moderate-sized pneumothorax on the left side with pneumomediastinum. The bilateral diffuse pulmonary edema is essentially unchanged from the previous chest radiograph. Also, the endotracheal tube has retracted to the level of the thoracic inlet; a central venous line is present with the tip in the right atrium, and the naso-gastric tube tip remains in the fundus of the stomach (Figure 10.4). A chest tube is placed on the left side, and the follow-up radiograph shows marked decreases of the pneumomedi-astinum and left pneumothorax. The left hemidiaphragm is elevated, which is associated with atelectasis in the left lower lobe. The bilateral pulmonary edema appears to be worsening, as evidenced by the increased hazy opacification of the lungs (Figure 10.5). The ventilator parameters are changed to FIO_2 1.0 and PEEP 12 cm H_2O, which result in a PaO_2 of 77 mm Hg.

   Child N never regains consciousness, and after 6 weeks he dies of respiratory complications.

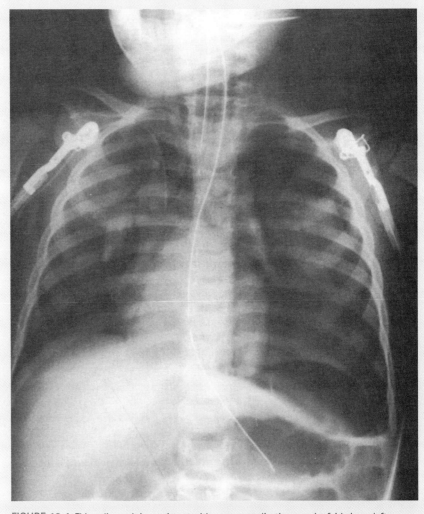

FIGURE 10.4 This radiograph is consistent with pneumomediastinum and a fairly large left pneu-mothorax. Also, there is persistent bilateral diffuse pulmonary edema, and subcutaneous emphysema extends into the soft tissue of the neck.

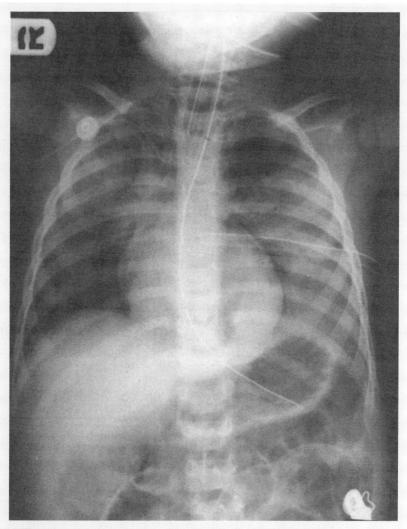

FIGURE 10.5 This radiograph is consistent with the presence of chest tube placement on the left, with reinflation of the left lung. Pneumomediastinum is present, and the bilateral pulmonary edema is worsening. Also, left lower lobe subsegmental atelectasis is present.

QUESTION	ANSWER
21. What preventive measures could have been employed to decrease the likelihood of this event?	A number of interventions could aid in the prevention of this drowning situation. First and foremost is complete surveillance and/or constant and immediate adult supervision in addition to creating barriers to entry into the neighbor's pool such as isolation fencing (four-sided, at least 4 feet high, and no more than 4-inch spaces between slats), a pool alarm, and a self-latching and self-closing gate. It should be noted that pool covers are no substitution for supervision and surveillance. Finally, education by the family pediatrician might have proved helpful in alerting family members of the potential for this problem ∎

KEY POINTS

- Respiratory therapists play a pivotal role in the assessment and management of the near-drowning patient.
- Drowning is the process of experiencing respiratory impairment from submersion or immersion in liquid.
- Near drowning is a critical predicament resolved by successful water rescue and entails successful resuscitation and survival for at least 24 hours.
- Globally, 500,000 people die annually, with the most in the Western Pacific Region and the least in the Americas.
- Drowning represents the seventh leading cause of unintentional death for all ages in the United States and the second leading cause of injury-related death for the 1 to 14 year old age group.
- Males account for 78% of drowning deaths in the United States.
- The two age groups with the highest incidence are toddlers age 1 to 4 and adolescents and young adults ages 15 to 24.
- Of children who drown, 55% of infants drown in bath tubs, 56% of children (1 to 4) drown in artificial pools, and 63% of older children drown in natural bodies of water.
- Drownings ranked fifth on the list of highest unintentional home injury deaths and were highest in Florida, Arizona, Nevada, and California.
- There has been a decline in the death rate for drowning for all age groups in the United States.
- Typical costs for near drowning range from $75,000 for initial care to $180,000 a year for long-term care.
- Drowning rates are inversely related to per capita income for all age groups.
- Drowning death rates for black and American Indian children are 50% to 70% higher than for white children.
- Drowning has the greatest seasonal variation of all causes of unintentional deaths and is highest during May through August.
- Inadequate supervision was the most common factor associated with submersion, and 88% of children were under some form of supervision when the incident occurred.
- A child can drown in as little as 2 inches of water and in less than 5 minutes.
- Alcohol is estimated to be involved in 30% to 50% of adolescent and adult drowning deaths, and a blood alcohol level of 0.10 or higher exposes an individual to a 16-fold increased risk of drowning.
- Swimming instruction along with water safety training and training in dealing with hazardous aquatic environments can better prepare an individual to deal with the risk of drowning.
- The American Academy of Pediatrics recommends children wait till they are at least 4 years of age before taking swimming lessons.
- Hypothermia provides beneficial and detrimental effects on near drowning—beneficial from delay of neurological consequences and detrimental from relentless drop of body temperature.
- Eighty-five to ninety percent of victims aspirate fluid into their lungs, while the remaining experience laryngospasm and dry lungs.
- Pulmonary consequences include ventilation-perfusion mismatch, intrapulmonary shunting, a decrease in residual capacity, and a decrease in lung compliance.

(key points continued on page 251)

KEY POINTS (CONTINUED)

- Evaluations of near-drowning patients have not shown severe electrolyte or hemoglobin abnormalities or renal dysfunction.
- The primary aims of out-of-hospital treatment are relief of hypoxia, restoration of cardiovascular stability, prevention of further heat loss, and speedy evacuation to the hospital.
- Initial assessment should be rapid and directed toward the victim's level of consciousness.
- Clinical assessment should include vital signs, neurological assessment, auscultation, and ABG analysis.
- Clinical outcomes can be determined through a variety of scoring systems (Galscow Coma Scale, Orlowski Score, and Postsubmersion Neurological Classification System).
- Treatment includes basic life support and activation of the emergency medical system.
- The Heimlich maneuver should not be routinely performed unless airway obstruction is present.
- The "hyper" brain resuscitation recommendations are controversial but still employed in the care of the drowning patient: hyperhydration, hyperventilation, hyperpyrexia, hyperexcitability, and hyperrigidity.
- Approximately 80% of drowning deaths can be prevented.
- Specific preventative measures include adequate supervision and complete surveillance, swimming ability and survival skills, refraining from alcohol, training in CPR, presence of lifeguards, use of personal flotation devices, isolation fencing, pool alarms, and self-closing and self-latching gates.
- Pediatricians can assist in lowering incidence by providing education related to prevention.

REFERENCES

1. Papa, L, Hoelle, R, Idris, A: Systematic review of definitions for drowning incidents. Resuscitation 65(3):255–264, 2005,
2. Salomez, F, Vincent, JL: Drowning: a review of epidemiology, pathophysiology, treatment and prevention. Resuscitation 63:261–268, 2004.
3. Orlowski, JP, Szpilman, D: Drowning: rescue, resuscitation, and reanimation. Pediatr Clin North Am 48(3):627–646, 2001.
4. Levin, D, et al: Drowning and near-drowning. Pediatr Clin North Am 40(2):321, 1993.
5. Orlowski, J: Drowning, near-drowning, and ice water submersions. Pediatr Clin North Am 34(1):75, 1987.
6. Ornato, J: The resuscitation of near-drowning victims. JAMA 256(1):75, 1986.
7. Neal, J: Near-drowning. J Emerg Med 3(1):41, 1985.
8. Gonzalez-Rothi, R: Near drowning: consensus and controversies in pulmonary and cerebral resuscitation. Heart Lung 16(5):474, 1987.
9. Martin, T: Near drowning and cold water immersion. Ann Emerg Med 13:263, 1984.
10. Spyker, D: Submersion injury: epidemiology, prevention, and management. Pediatr Clin North Am 32(1):113, 1985.
11. O'Flaherty, JE, Pirie, PL: Prevention of pediatric drowning and near drowning: a survey of members of the American Academy of Physicians, Pediatrics 99(2):169–174, 1997.
12. Brenner, RA, Committee on Injury, Violence, and Poison Prevention. Prevention of drowning in infants, children, and adolescents. Pediatrics 112(2):440–445, 2003
13. Idris, AH, Berg, RA, Bierens, J, et al: Recommended guidelines for uniform reporting of data from drowning. Circulation 108:2565–2574, 2003.
14. Modell, JH: Drowning: to treat or not to treat—an answerable question? Crit Care Med 21(3):313–315, 1993.

15. Model, JH: Drowning versus near-drowning: a discussion of definitions [Editorial]. Crit Care Med 9:351–352, 1981.

16. Subcommittee on Classification of Sports Injuries, Committee on the Medical Aspects of Sports, American Medical Association. Standard Nomenclature of Athletic Injuries. American Medical Association, Chicago, 1996.

17. Van Dorp, JCM, Knape, JTA, Bierens, JJLM: Recommendations: World Congress on Drowning, 2002, June 26–28, Amsterdam, The Netherlands. Available at: http://www.drowning.nl/.

18. Idris, AH, Berg, RA, Biernens, J, et al: Recommended guidelines for uniform reporting of data from drowning: the "Utstein Style." Resuscitation 59:45–57, 2003.

19. World Health Organization. Facts about injuries. In Drowning. See www.who.int/violence-injury-prevention.

20. CDC: 2002 National Vital Statistics Report. Leading Causes of Accidental Death in the United States. Available at: http://www.the-eggman.com/writings/death_stats.html.

21. CDC. Nonfatal and Fatal Drownings in Recreational Water Settings–United States, 2001–2002 MMWR 53(21):447–452, 2004.

22. Centers for Disease Control and Prevention. Web-based Injury Statistics Query and Reporting System (WISQARS). National Center for Injury Prevention and Control, Centers for Disease Control and Prevention (producer). Available at: www.cdc.gov/ncipc/wisqars.

23. Quan, L, Gore, EJ, Wentz, K, Allen, J, Novack, AH: Ten-Year Study of Pediatric Drownings and Near-Drownings in King County, Washington: Lessons in Injury Prevention. Pediatrics, 83:1035–1040, 1989.

24. Smith, GS, Brenner, RA: The changing risks of drowning for adolescents in the US and effective control strategies. Adolesc Med 6:153–170, 1995.

25. Ellis, AA, Trent, RB: Hospitalizations for near drowning in California: incidence and costs. Am J Public Health 85:1115–1118, 1995.

26. Pearn, J, Nixin, J, Wilkey, I: Freshwater drowning and near-drowning accidents involving children: a five-year total population study. Med J Aust 2:942–946, 1976.

27. Wintemute, GJ: Childhood drowning and near-drowning in the United States: prevention. Am J Dis Child 144:663–669, 1990.

28. CDC: Available at: www.cdc.gov/ncipc/factsheets/drown.htm.

29. Brenner, RA, Trumble, AC, Smith, GS, Kessler, EP, Overpeck, MD: Where children drown, United States, 1995. Pediatrics 108:85–89, 2001.

30. World Health Organization. Guidelines for Safe Recreational-Water Environments. Vol. 2. Swimming Pools, Spas, and Similar Recreational-Water Environments. Geneva, CH, 2000. Available at:

http://www.crid.or.cr/crid/CD_Agua/pdf/eng/doc14599/doc14599.htm.

31. Cody, BE, Quirashi, AY, Dastur, MC, Mickallide, AD: Clear danger: a national study of childhood drowning and related attitudes and behaviors. National SAFE KIDS Campaign, Washington, DC, 2004.

32. Baker, SP, O'Neil, B, Ginsburg, MJ, Li, G: The Injury Fact Book, ed. 2. Oxford University Press, New York, 1992.

33. Turner, J: Prevention of drowning in infants and children. Dimensions Crit Care Nurs 23(5):191–193, 2004.

34. Kane, BE, Mickalide, AD, Paul, HA: Trauma Season: A National Study of the Seasonality of Unintentional Childhood Injury. National SAFE KIDS Campaign, Washington, DC, 2001.

35. DeNicola, LK, Falk, JL, Swanson, ME, et al: Submersion injuries in children and adults. Crit Care Clin 13:477–502, 1997.

36. Howland, J, Mangione, T, Hingson, R, Smith, G, Bell, N: Alcohol as a risk factor for drowning and other aquatic injuries. In Watson, RR (ed): Alcohol, Cocaine, and Accidents. Drug and Alcohol Abuse Reviews. Vol. 7. Humana Press, Totowa, NH, 1995, pp. 85–104.

37. Driscoll, TR, Harrison, JA, Steenkamp, M: Review of the role of alcohol in drowning associated with recreational aquatic activity. Injury Prev 9:163–168, 2003.

38. U.S. Coast Guard, Department of Homeland Security. Boating Statistics. Available at: http://www.uscgboating.org/statistics/accidents_stats.htm.

39. Asher, KN, Rivara, FP, Felix, D, Vance, L, Dunne, R: Water safety training as a potential means of reducing risk of young children's drowning. Injury Prev 1(4):228–233, 1995.

40. Patetta, MJ, Biddinger, PW: Characteristics of drowning deaths in North Carolina. Public Health Rep 103(4):406–411, 1988.

41. Smith, GS: Drowning prevention in children: the need for new strategies. Injury Prev 1:216–217, 1995.

42. AAP Committee on Sports Medicine and Fitness, Committee on Injury and Poison Prevention. Swimming programs for infants and toddlers. Pediatrics 105:868–870, 2000.

43. Olshaker, J: Near drowning. Emerg Med Clin North Am 10:339, 1992.

44. Siebke, H, et al: Survival after 40 minutes' submersion without cerebral sequelae. Lancet 1:1275, 1975.

45. Stryer, L: Biochemistry, ed 3. WH Freeman, New York, 1988.

46. Darnell, J, et al: Molecular cell biology. Sci Am 15:617, 1986.

47. Modell, J, et al: Serum electrolyte concentrations after fresh-water aspiration. Anesthesiology 30(4):421, 1969.

48. Modell, J, et al: The effects of fluid volume in seawater drowning. Ann Intern Med 67(1):68, 1967.

49. Giammona, S, Modell, J: Drowning by total immersion: effects on pulmonary surfactant of distilled water, isotonic saline, and sea water. Am J Dis Child 114:612, 1967.

50. Halmagyi, D: Lung changes and incidence of respiratory arrest in rats after aspiration of sea and fresh water. J Appl Physiol 16:41, 1961.

51. Reidbord, H, Spitz, W: Ultrastructural alterations in rat lungs: changes after intratracheal perfusion with freshwater and seawater. Arch Pathol 81:103, 1966.

52. Nichols, D, Rogers, M: Adult respiratory distress syndrome. In Rogers, M (ed): Textbook of Pediatric Intensive Care. Williams & Wilkins, Baltimore, 1987.

53. Modell, J, et al: Clinical course of 91 consecutive near-drowning victims. Chest 70:231, 1976.

54. Orlowski, J, et al: The hemodynamic and cardiovascular effects of near-drowning in hypotonic, isotonic, or hypertonic solutions. Ann Emerg Med 18:1044, 1989.

55. U.S. Lifeguard Association. http://www.usla.org/ Statistics/current.asp?Statistics=Current.

56. Orlowski, JP. Ped Clin North America 48(3):630, 2001.

57. Karpovich, PV: Water in the lungs of drowned animals. Arch Pathol Lab Med 15: 828–833, 1933.

58. Moon, RE, Long, RJ: Drowning and near drowning. Emerg Med 14:377–386, 2002.

59. Pia, F: Reflections on lifeguard surveillance program. In Fletemeyer, JR, Freas, SJ (eds): Drowning: New Perspectives on Intervention and Prevention. CRC Press, Boca Raton, FL, 1999, pp. 231–243.

60. Gilbert, J, et al: Near drowning: current concepts of management. Respir Care 30(2):108, 1985.

61. Dean, J, Kaufman, N: Prognostic indicators in pediatric near-drowning: the Glasgow coma scale. Crit Care Med 9(7):536, 1981.

62. Frewen, T, et al: Cerebral resuscitation therapy in pediatric near-drowning. J Pediatr 106(4):615, 1985.

63. Allman, F, et al: Outcome following cardiopulmonary resuscitation in severe pediatric near-drowning. Am J Dis Child 140:571, 1986.

64. Modell, J, et al: Near-drowning: correlation of level of consciousness and survival. Can Anaesth Soc J 27(3):211, 1980.

65. Conn, A, et al: Cerebral salvage in near-drowning following neurological classification by triage. Can Anaesth Soc J 27(3):201, 1980.

66. Causey, AL, Tilelli, JA, Swanson, ME: Predicting discharge in uncomplicated near drowning. Am J Emerg Med 18:9–11, 2000.

67. Quan, L, Kinder, D: Pediatric submersions: prehospital predictors of outcome. Pediatrics 90:909, 1992.

68. Lavelle, J, Shaw, K: Near drowning: is emergency department cardiopulmonary resuscitation or intensive care unit cerebral resuscitation indicated? Crit Care Med 21(3):368, 1993.

69. Graf, W, et al: Predicting outcome in pediatric submersion victims. Ann Emerg Med 26:312, 1995.

70. Bratton, S, et al: Serial neurological examinations after near drowning and outcome. Arch Pediatr Adolesc Med 148:167, 1994.

71. Biggart, M, Bohn, D: Effect of hypothermia and cardiac arrest on outcome of near-drowning accidents in children. J Pediatr 117:179, 1990.

72. Textbook of Basic Life Support for Healthcare Providers. American Heart Association, Dallas, 1994.

73. Steinman, A: Cardiopulmonary resuscitation and hypothermia. Circulation 74(suppl IV):29, 1986.

74. Steen, P, Michenfelder, J: Barbiturate protection in tolerant and non-tolerant hypoxic mice: comparison with hypothermic protection. Anesthesiology 50:404, 1979.

75. Carlsson, C, et al: Protective effect of hypothermia in cerebral oxygen deficiency caused by arterial hypoxia. Anesthesiology 44:27, 1976.

76. Hagerdal, M, et al: Protective effects of combination of hypothermia and barbiturates in cerebral hypoxia in the rat. Anesthesiology 49:165, 1978.

77. Bleyaert, A, et al: Thiopental amelioration of brain damage after global ischemia in monkeys. Anesthesiology 49:390, 1978.

78. Lafferty, J, et al: Cerebral hypometabolism obtained with deep pentobarbital anesthesia and hypothermia (30 C). Anesthesiology 49:159, 1978.

79. Michenfelder, J, et al: Cerebral protection by barbiturate anesthesia: use after middle cerebral artery occlusion in Java monkeys. Arch Neurol 33:345, 1976.

80. Hoff, J, et al: Barbiturate protection from cerebral infarction in primates. Stroke 6:28, 1975.

81. Hankinson, J, et al: Effect of thiopental on focal cerebral ischemia in dogs. Surg Forum 25:445, 1974.

82. Bleyaert, A, et al: Amelioration of post ischemic brain damage in the monkey by immobilization and controlled ventilation. Crit Care Med 6:112, 1978.

83. Soloway, M, et al: The effect of hyperventilation on subsequent cerebral infarction. Anesthesiology 29:975, 1968.

84. Safar, P, et al: Resuscitation after global brain ischemia-anoxia. Crit Care Med 6:215, 1978.

85. Pappius, H, McCann, W: Effects of steroids on cerebral edema in cats. Arch Neurol 20:207, 1969.

86. Rovit, R, Hagan, R: Steroids and cerebral edema: the effect of glucocorticoids on abnormal capillary permeability following cerebral injury in cats. J Neuropathol Exp Neurol 27:277, 1968.

87. Wilkinson, H, et al: Diuretic synergy in the treatment of acute experimental cerebral edema. J Neurosurg 34:203, 1971.

88. Sarnaik, A, et al: Intracranial pressure and cerebral perfusion pressure in near-drowning. Crit Care Med 13(4):224, 1985.

89. Nussbaum, E, Galant, S: Intracranial pressure monitoring as a guide to prognosis in the nearly-drowned, severely comatose child. J Pediatr 102:215, 1983.

90. Dean, J, McComb, J: Intracranial pressure monitoring in severe pediatric near-drowning. Neurosurgery 9:627, 1981.

91. Bohn, D, et al: Influence of hypothermia, barbiturate therapy, and intracranial pressure monitoring on morbidity and mortality after near-drowning. Crit Care Med 14(6):529, 1986.

92. Conn, A, Barker, G: Fresh water drowning and near-drowning: an update. Can Anaesth Soc J 31(3):S38, 1984.

93. Mackie, IJ: Availability and quality of data to assess the global burden of drowning. In: Bierens, J (ed): Handbook on Drowning. Prevention, Rescue and Treatment. Netherlands, Springer, 2003.

11

Acute Respiratory Distress Syndrome

Robert L. Wilkins PhD, RRT, FAARC

James R. Dexter MD, FACP, FCCP

CHAPTER OBJECTIVES:

After reading this chapter you will be able to state or identify the following:

- The relationship between acute lung injury and acute respiratory distress syndrome (ARDS).
- The most common clinical problems associated with ARDS.
- The effect of ARDS on lung function.
- The clinical features, blood gas changes, and chest radiograph abnormalities associated with ARDS.
- The treatment of ARDS and how to apply mechanical ventilation to patients with this syndrome.
- The parameters used to monitor care of the ARDS patient.
- The parameters to use for determining when to wean the ARDS patient.

INTRODUCTION

In the 1960s during the Vietnam war a distinct form of respiratory failure was recognized as the result of acute, internal injury to both lungs. Soldiers who developed this disorder often had been resuscitated after trauma and/or shock but died days later from respiratory failure owing to oxygenation problems. The soldier would develop severe dyspnea and persistent hypoxemia despite oxygen therapy. In each case, the oxygenation failure was due to bilateral pulmonary edema and atelectasis. Some physicians initially described the syndrome as "shock lung," while others used the phrase "adult respiratory distress syndrome" because they perceived it as occurring only in adults. Subsequently, physicians recognized that this syndrome occurs in patients of all ages and the term **acute respiratory distress syndrome (ARDS)** is now preferred.

ARDS represents the clinical consequence of another syndrome known as **acute lung injury (ALI)**. ALI is characterized by persistent lung inflammation seen at the level of the alveolar capillary membrane with increased vascular permeability. ALI results in bilateral pulmonary edema and atelectasis despite no evidence of left heart failure (e.g., normal pulmonary capillary wedge pressure [PCWP]). The degree of ALI varies widely from patient to patient. In some, ALI is less severe, with minimal oxygenation problems. In others, the ALI is severe and oxygenation failure occurs despite aggressive treatment.

ARDS is present when the ALI results in such severe hypoxia that the Pao_2/Fio_2 ratio is 200 mm Hg or less. Approximately 10% to 15% of intensive care patients meet the criteria for ARDS in the typical ICU.[1–4]

ARDS is often accompanied by multiple organ system failure. Most commonly affected are the cardiovascular, renal, hepatic, and central nervous systems and bone marrow. When ARDS was first described, its mortality rate was approximately 90% and the majority of deaths were due to respiratory failure. Currently, the mortality rate is 35% to 40% and the cause of death is frequently due to nonrespiratory problems.[5–6]

ETIOLOGY

A large variety of clinical disorders can cause ARDS. Some cause it by direct insult on the lung (e.g., aspiration of gastric contents), while others indirectly cause acute lung injury by initiating an acute systemic inflammatory response (indirect insult).

The most common clinical problems associated with the onset of ALI and ARDS are sepsis, severe trauma, multiple transfusions, aspiration, severe pneumonia, and smoke inhalation. These factors along with at least 60 other medical conditions apparently have the ability to trigger a systemic inflammatory response as described later. Some of the other known causes of ALI and ARDS are listed in Box 11.1. The presence of multiple predisposing disorders substantially increases the risk of ARDS.

PATHOPHYSIOLOGY

ARDS affects lung mechanics, gas exchange, and the pulmonary vasculature of both lungs. Although both lungs are affected, the degree of lung involvement varies throughout each lung. In the most affected regions, intravascular fluid leaks from the pulmonary capillaries, overwhelms lymphatic drainage, and floods the bronchioles, thus diluting surfactant. Injury of type II pneumocytes decreases the production of surfactant. As a result, microatelectasis occurs and lung compliance decreases. These changes in lung mechanics increase the patient's work of breathing.

Box 11.1 Causes of ALI and ARDS

- Sepsis
- Pneumonia
- Major trauma
- Pulmonary aspiration and near drowning
- Burns
- Inhalation of noxious fumes
- Fat embolism
- Massive blood transfusion
- Amniotic fluid embolism
- Air embolism
- Eclampsia
- Poisoning
- Radiation

Alveolar flooding and atelectasis produce uneven pathological changes in the lung and areas of perfusion without ventilation (**shunt**). Ventilation-perfusion ($\dot{V}/\dot{Q}$) mismatch is present in both lungs. These abnormalities cause hypoxemia that responds poorly to supplemental oxygen administration (**refractory hypoxemia**).

Hypoxemia, microemboli, and capillary compression increase the pulmonary vascular resistance (PVR). This alters the distribution of blood flow through the lungs, contributes to the $\dot{V}/\dot{Q}$

mismatch, and produces pulmonary hypertension. Right ventricular pressure, size, and work increase to maintain cardiac output. Right ventricular failure may develop if the increased work placed on the heart exceeds its capabilities.

CLINICAL FEATURES

The clinical findings in the patient with ARDS vary according to the underlying cause and the severity of the lung damage. For example, fever and hypotension are the primary initial problems in the patient with sepsis as the cause. Despite the large variety of conditions that cause ARDS, the clinical course is very similar in each case once the lung injury phase begins. Respiratory deterioration is accompanied by dyspnea, an apparent increase in work of breathing, tachypnea, tachycardia, and possibly cough. Rapid and shallow breathing are present because of the significant drop in lung compliance. Auscultation reveals bilateral inspiratory crackles. Chest radiographs are initially normal but soon show bilateral fluffy infiltrates and air bronchograms. Arterial blood gases show an uncompensated respiratory alkalosis with moderate to severe hypoxemia and an increased $P(A-a)o_2$.

Over the next 12 hours the patient will continue to deteriorate, and intubation with mechanical ventilation is often needed. Arterial blood gases show hypoxemia that responds poorly to oxygen therapy alone but somewhat better to oxygen therapy with positive pressure ventilation. Leukocytosis is common when infection is the underlying cause. Pulmonary capillary wedge pressure readings are not elevated (<18 mm Hg), indicating that the pulmonary edema is due to leaky capillaries.

> The patient with bilateral pulmonary edema and severe dyspnea may have cardiogenic or noncardiogenic pulmonary edema. A normal or low PCWP is strong evidence that the pulmonary edema is due to ARDS.

TREATMENT

The treatment of ARDS is primarily supportive. Patient care includes treatment of the precipitating problem (e.g., antibiotics for sepsis and pneumonia), mechanical ventilation, and hemodynamic monitoring and support. Searching for and treating the precipitating cause is important and is the role of the attending physician. The emphasis below is placed on mechanical ventilation since this is where the respiratory therapist plays the largest role in caring for the patient with ARDS.

Mechanical Ventilation

Mechanical ventilation of the patient with ARDS is needed in most cases to maintain adequate oxygenation. Mechanical ventilators neither prevent nor directly treat ARDS, but keep the patient alive until the underlying problem resolves and the lungs heal enough to support the patient again. The most recent attempts at determining a better method of ventilation in ARDS involve strategies to limit airway pressures. The goal of these strategies is adequate oxygenation without the hemodynamic and pulmonary complications associated with high mean airway pressure that frequently occur with conventional volume-targeted ventilation.

Continuous mechanical ventilation (CMV) in ARDS is best administered using a tidal volume (V_T) range of 5 to 7 mL/kg and plateau pressures of <30 cm H_2O.[7]

Box 11.2 Guidelines for Provision of Mechanical Ventilation

- V_T appropriate to maintain PAP, frequently 5 to 7 mL/kg in ARDS
- PEEP 10 to 15 cm H_2O
- Eliminate inflection point on P-V curve
- Avoid air trapping and auto-PEEP
- Respiratory rate ≤20 to 25; limit set by development of auto-PEEP
- Inspiratory time limit set by development of auto-PEEP
- I:E generally ≤1:1; may be greater, but limited by the development of auto-PEEP

I:E = inhalation:exhalation ratio; PAP = peak alveolar pressure; PEEP = positive end-expiratory pressure.
SOURCE: From Kacmarek, RM, Hickling, KG: Permissive hypercapnia. Respir Care 38(4):390, 1993, with permission.

This strategy should be employed regardless of the precipitating event.[8] The patient should initially be sedated to minimize discomfort. Paralysis will rarely be needed.

> Mechanical ventilation in the ARDS patient has several benefits. It allows administration of a reliable FIO_2, it decreases the work of breathing, and it can recruit atelectatic lung units. Such benefits are only available when the ventilator is applied appropriately.

Both pressure- and volume-limited ventilation are acceptable modes for mechanical ventilation in ARDS patients. Pressure-limited ventilation reduces the chance of barotrauma but may result in low tidal volumes and reduced effective ventilation when lung compliance decreases. Small tidal volume ventilation with volumes limited to keep the plateau pressure <30 cm H_2O has been shown to improve survival of patients with ARDS.[8] This may result in hypercapnia. Hypercapnia that keeps the patient's pH above 7.20 is acceptable. This philosophy for mechanical ventilation is termed **permissive hypercapnia**.

Oxygenation is maintained by the adjustment of **positive end-expiratory pressure (PEEP)**. Atelectatic regions may be reopened by application of PEEP. PEEP converts areas of physiological shunt to functional gas exchange units, resulting in increased arterial oxygenation at a lower FIO_2. Recruitment of atelectatic alveoli also increases functional residual capacity (FRC) and pulmonary compliance. Generally, the goal of CMV with PEEP is to obtain a PaO_2 of greater than 60 mm Hg on an FIO_2 of less than 0.60.

Although PEEP is an important part of maintaining adequate gas exchange in the lungs of the ARDS patient, side effects are possible. Decreased pulmonary compliance from overdistended alveoli, decreased venous return and cardiac output, increased PVR, increased right ventricular afterload, and barotrauma may occur. For these reasons, the use of **optimal PEEP** is suggested, which is generally defined as the level of PEEP whereby the best O_{2del} is achieved at an FIO_2 of less than 0.60. PEEP levels that improve arterial oxygenation but significantly reduce cardiac output are not optimal because this causes O_{2del} to be reduced.

The **partial pressure of mixed venous oxygen** ($P\bar{v}O_2$) provides information related to tissue oxygenation. A $P\bar{v}O$ of less than 35 mm Hg indicates that tissue oxygenation is not optimal. Reductions in cardiac output (as may occur with the application of PEEP) typically result in a low $P\bar{v}O_2$. For this reason, $P\bar{v}O_2$ can also be used to monitor optimal PEEP. Saturation of central venous blood for oxygen ($ScvO_2$) is also used to monitor overall oxygenation. An $ScvO_2$ below 70% is abnormal.

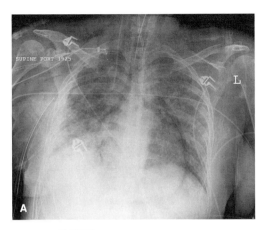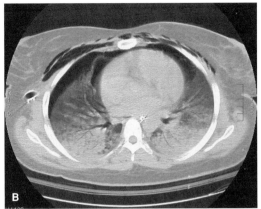

FIGURE 11.1 Redistribution of the lung densities due to gravity. This is not seen on the chest x-ray (A), but is clearly visible by CT (B).

Experimental Strategies

Numerous other ventilator strategies are available to manage the patient with ARDS. Such strategies include airway pressure release ventilation (APRV), high-frequency ventilation (HFV), tracheal gas sufflation (TGI), and extracorporeal membrane oxygenation (ECMO). None of these strategies have proven to be clearly beneficial in supporting the ARDS patient. They are employed as a last ditch effort in certain settings, however, when traditional modes have failed and the patient continues to deteriorate. Since they require significant resources and expertise, they are best reserved for those facilities that have extensive experience with them.

Prone positioning of the ARDS patient during mechanical ventilation has been done in an effort to improve $\dot{V}/\dot{Q}$ mismatching and thus oxygenation (Figure 11.1). Research has shown that proning the patient does improve oxygenation but does not improve mortality rates in ARDS patients.[9] Given the high degree of inconvenience associated with its use and the lack of data showing improved outcome, proning is not widely used. Some clinicians continue to use prone positioning however, since the risks are minimal when proning is done by experienced personnel. Some experts recommend its early use in patients failing to respond to high-pressure recruitment maneuvers who require PEEP >12 cm H_2O and an $FIO_2 >0.60$.[10]

Weaning from Mechanical Ventilation

Assurance of the patient's ability to survive without ventilator support is required prior to weaning the patient from the ventilator. The best criteria for weaning parameters are listed in Chapter 2. Mechanical indices such as maximum inspiratory pressure (MIP), vital capacity (VC), and spontaneous V_T measure respiratory muscle strength and the patient's ability to move air in and out of the chest. None of these measurements, however, reflects the endurance capabilities of the respiratory muscles. For this reason, the f/V_T ratio may be the best indicator of weaning readiness. Physiologic indices such as pH, dead space-V_T ratio ($VDS:V_T$), P(A-a)O_2, nutritional status, cardiovascular stability, and metabolic acid-base status reflect the patient's general reserve and ability to tolerate the stress of weaning.

Weaning from mechanical ventilation is done in a stepwise fashion to ensure that the patient has recovered to the point where weaning will be successful. Weaning is usually initiated when the patient is medically stable, FiO_2 requirement is less than 0.40, PEEP requirement is 5 cm H_2O or less, and the f/V_T ratio during spontaneous breathing is less than 100.

Weaning must be monitored to ensure its success. Significant (>20%) changes in blood pressure, heart rate, respiratory rate, a drop in SpO_2, or decreased mental function indicate *weaning failure*. Gradual lengthening of the weaning periods can help prevent weaning failure caused by fatigue while the patient regains independent pulmonary function. Taking each episode of weaning to the patient tolerance level provides an index of weaning progress from day to day. The different methods of weaning from mechanical ventilation and the benefits of each are described in more detail in Chapter 2.

Monitoring

Pulmonary artery pressure monitoring allows measurement of cardiac output, calculation of O_{2del}, and measurement of $P\bar{v}O_2$. These parameters are useful for the management of hemodynamic complications associated with mechanical ventilation or otherwise. Pulmonary artery monitoring also allows measurement of the filling pressures for the right (CVP) and left (PCWP) ventricles of the heart, which is useful in optimizing cardiac output (see Chapter 6) and for discriminating between cardiogenic and noncardiogenic pulmonary edema.

The use of a pulmonary artery catheter for hemodynamic monitoring in ARDS patients is controversial because there is risk in its use and there is no clear evidence that its use alters mortality rates. Some physicians use it only when the patient with ARDS is also having severe hemodynamic complications. Studies are underway to determine who is best served by use of the catheter.

Static compliance (C_{st}) gives valuable information regarding stiffness of the lungs and chest wall, whereas dynamic compliance (C_{dyn}) also provides information about airway resistance. C_{st} is calculated by dividing V_T by static (plateau) pressure (P_{stat}) less PEEP pressure:

$$C_{st} = V_T/(P_{stat} - PEEP)$$

P_{stat} is measured by obtaining a short inspiratory hold after a volume-limited breath. This hold can be achieved by using the pause control on the ventilator or by manual occlusion of the expiratory limb of the patient circuit. P_{stat} is monitored on the ventilator manometer during volume hold and should be less than the peak airway pressure (P_{pk}). C_{dyn} is similarly calculated, although P_{pk} is used instead of P_{stat}, as follows:

$$C_{dyn} = V_T/(P_{pk} - PEEP)$$

Normal C_{st} is from 60 to 100 mL/cm H_2O and may be decreased to around 15 or 20 mL/cm H_2O in severe cases of pneumonia, pulmonary edema, atelectasis, and ARDS. Because pressure is required to overcome airway resistance during ventilation, a portion of the peak airway pressure generated during the mechanical breath represents resistance to flow through the airways and ventilator circuit. C_{dyn} thus measures total impairment in airway flow caused by both compliance and resistance. Normal C_{dyn} is 35 to 55 mL/cm H_2O. All of the problems that decrease C_{st} can adversely affect C_{dyn}, as can factors that affect resistance (e.g., bronchoconstriction, airway edema, retained secretions, and airway compression by tumor).

> **V**entilator adjustments that keep the plateau pressure <30 cm H_2O improve survival for patients with ARDS.

Monitoring plateau pressure after a 0.50-second inspiratory hold (P 0.50) is useful. It is related to static compliance. Keeping this plateau pressure below 30 cm H_2O reduces the chance of barotrauma and increases the patient's chance of survival. The primary way in which the plateau pressure is kept below 30 cm H_2O is the use of small tidal volumes.

Ms. Y

HISTORY

Ms. Y is a 23-year-old woman who was feeling fine until the morning of admission, when she began having severe chills, vomiting, diarrhea, headache, and a fever of 40.3°C (104.5°F). The symptoms persisted throughout the day and caused her to seek medical attention at the local emergency department about 6 p.m. Ms. Y had an intrauterine device (IUD) inserted at a local family planning clinic 3 days prior to admission. At the time of admission she denied shortness of breath, wheezing, sputum production, cough, hemoptysis, orthopnea, chest pain, illicit drug use, and exposure to tuberculosis.

PHYSICAL EXAMINATION

- **General.** Patient well nourished, alert, and oriented to time, place, and person; appears anxious, but has no evidence of respiratory distress

- **Vital Signs.** Temperature 40.3°C (104.5°F), respiratory rate 24/min; heart rate 104/min; blood pressure 126/75 mm Hg lying and 90/40 mm Hg standing

- **HEENT.** Sinuses not tender, throat not inflamed

- **Neck.** Supple with full range of motion; trachea midline and mobile; carotid pulses ++ bilaterally with no bruits; no jugular venous distention; no cervical or supraclavicular lymphadenopathy

- **Chest.** Normal configuration and normal expansion with breathing; normal resonance to percussion bilaterally

- **Heart.** Regular rhythm with a rate of 104/min; no murmurs, heaves, or rubs noted

- **Lungs.** Clear breath sounds bilaterally

- **Abdomen.** Lower abdominal tenderness to palpation; no masses or organomegaly; bowel sounds present

- **Extremities.** No cyanosis, edema, or clubbing; pulses and reflexes ++ and symmetric

Laboratory Evaluation

Chest Radiograph (see Figure 11.2)

CBC	Value
White blood cells	15,500/mm^3
Bands	16%
Segmented neutrophils	65%
Hb	10.2 g/100 mL

Electrolytes	Value
Na$^+$	135 mEq/liter
K$^+$	4.5 mEq/liter
Cl$^-$	105 mEq/liter
HCO$_3$$^-$	15 mEq/liter

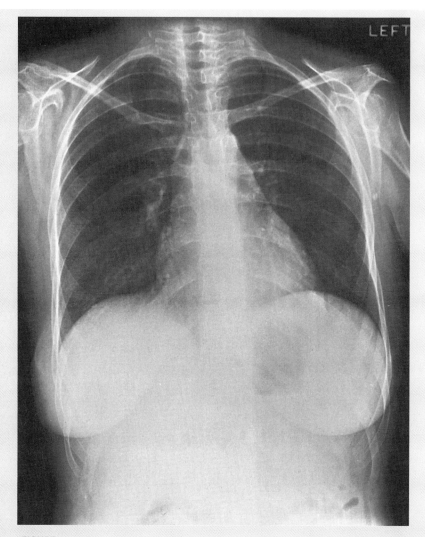

FIGURE 11.2 Chest radiograph showing normal appearance during the initial onset of ARDS.

QUESTIONS	ANSWERS
1. Does Ms. Y appear to have a pulmonary problem at this time?	No, the patient does not appear to have a pulmonary problem at this time, although the respiratory rate is slightly elevated.
2. Does Ms. Y's medical problem predispose her to developing ARDS?	Yes, the patient's problem may predispose her to developing ARDS. Severe chills and fever suggest that an infection may be present, and the most common cause of ARDS in medical intensive care units is infection.
3. What are the typical signs and symptoms of ARDS?	Typical signs of ARDS include dyspnea, tachypnea, tachycardia, increased work of breathing, use of accessory muscles of ventilation, and cyanosis. On laboratory evaluation, arterial blood gases (ABGs)

may reveal hypoxemia despite a normal chest film early in the course of the disorder.

QUESTIONS	ANSWERS
4. What is the significance of the lower abdominal tenderness?	Lower abdominal tenderness 2 to 4 days after placement of an IUD suggests infection in the lining of the uterus.
5. What is the significance of the CBC and electrolyte findings?	The elevated WBC suggests infection. The increase in bands and segmented neutrophils also suggests acute infection. Bands are immature forms of neutrophils used in defense against infection only under severe conditions. Electrolytes show a decreased serum HCO_3^-, which is consistent with metabolic acidosis or compensation for respiratory alkalosis.
6. Is fluid administration important?	Yes, fluid administration is important in this patient. There is evidence of orthostatic hypotension. Infection is often associated with relaxation of the arterioles causing relative hypovolemia. Studies evaluating early goal-directed therapy have shown improved patient outcomes with rapid and early fluid replacement in septic patients.[11]

More on Ms. Y

Ms. Y is started on IV antibiotic therapy. Results of a uterine swab show gram-negative diplococci, and a preliminary blood culture also shows gram-negative cocci. Twelve hours later, she begins complaining of increased shortness of breath. Respiratory rate is 34/min, heart rate 120/min, and temperature 39.6°C (103.3°F). Ms. Y is using her accessory muscles to breathe, and chest auscultation reveals fine, inspiratory crackles bilaterally.

A blood glucose is measured at 150 mg/dL.

An ABG is ordered immediately, with the following results: pH 7.25, $Paco_2$ 21 mm Hg, Pao_2 62 mm Hg, HCO_3 9 mEq/liter, base excess (BE)–7, and SaO_2 88% on room air. Based on these ABG results, the patient was placed on nasal cannula at 3 liters/min.

QUESTIONS	ANSWERS
7. What is the patient's acid–base and oxygenation status on the initial ABG?	The acid-base status of the patient is suggestive of metabolic acidosis, most likely as a result of lactic acidosis. Moderate hypoxemia is present with the patient on room air. The hypoxemia would probably be worse if the patient were not hyperventilating.
8. What is the most likely explanation for the sudden onset of dyspnea, tachypnea, and tachycardia?	The sudden onset of dyspnea, tachypnea, and tachycardia is most likely due to the acute onset of ARDS. The leakage of pulmonary edema into the lung causes surfactant dysfunction, atelectasis, hypoxemia, and a subsequent increase in the patient's work of breathing. These changes often occur suddenly and result in acute changes in the patient's clinical condition. Less likely causes of sudden onset of dyspnea would be pulmonary embolus and pneumothorax.

9. Why is the chest radiograph normal just 4 hours prior to the onset of the respiratory problems?

The chest radiograph is not sensitive to the early detection of damage to the alveolar capillary membrane. For this reason, it often lags behind the clinical findings in patients with ARDS.

10. What pathophysiology accounts for the adventitious lung sounds (fine, inspiratory crackles)?

Fine, inspiratory crackles are common in any disease that allows peripheral airways to shut during exhalation and pop open during subsequent inhalation. In ARDS patients, damage to the alveolar capillary membrane allows fluid to leak into the interstitial spaces and peripheral airways. The fluid sticks the small airways shut during exhalation and results in fine, inspiratory crackles over the entire chest.

11. What is the most likely cause of the accessory muscle usage?

The patient is using her accessory muscles to breathe because the lungs are much less compliant and more difficult to expand as a result of the pulmonary edema and atelectasis associated with ARDS.

12. What is indicated by the blood sugar of 150 mg/dL? Is this a sign of diabetes, and should it be treated?

An elevated blood sugar is common in sepsis since the severe infection often disrupts sugar metabolism. This patient is probably not diabetic. Studies have shown that careful management of blood sugar levels (80 to −120 mg/dL) in septic patients may improve survival.[12] The elevated blood sugar in this patient should be treated with insulin.

 ## More on Ms. Y

The patient continues to experience severe respiratory distress, and she is placed on an F_{IO_2} of 0.60 by entrainment device with the following ABG results: pH 7.26, Pa_{CO_2} 35 mm Hg, Pa_{O_2} 49 mm Hg, and HCO_3^- 16 mEq/liter. Her respiratory rate is now 38/min and heart rate is 134/min. A portable chest radiograph is obtained (Figure 11.3).

QUESTIONS

ANSWERS

13. Interpret the ABGs.

The ABGs show metabolic acidosis with moderate hypoxemia on 60% oxygen. Although the Pa_{CO_2} is not elevated, it is increased compared to the previous blood gas. This is suggestive of the relative hypoventilation that would accompany respiratory muscle fatigue.

14. What treatment is needed at this point?

Mechanical ventilation with PEEP is required because of the refractory nature of the hypoxemia. Refractory hypoxemia is most often caused by intrapulmonary shunting. PEEP holds the airways open and improves the distribution of ventilation, thereby reducing shunt and increasing Pa_{O_2}. PEEP allows adequate oxygenation at a lower F_{IO_2} and reduces the chance of oxygen toxicity. Mechanical ventilation may not be required initially, as the major problem is hypoxemia, but the patient with stiff lungs will soon tire and need ventilatory support.

15. What does the chest radiograph show, and are the findings typical of ARDS?

The chest radiograph now shows bilateral alveolar infiltrates, air bronchograms, and no cardiomegaly, which is typical of ARDS.

16. The attending physician writes orders for the administration of activated protein C. Why?

Numerous studies have shown that patients with sepsis have severe depletion of protein C.[13,14] Septic patients with low levels of protein C have higher mortality rates.[15] Treatment with activated protein C is considered for patients with sepsis syndrome and two organ system failures.[16]

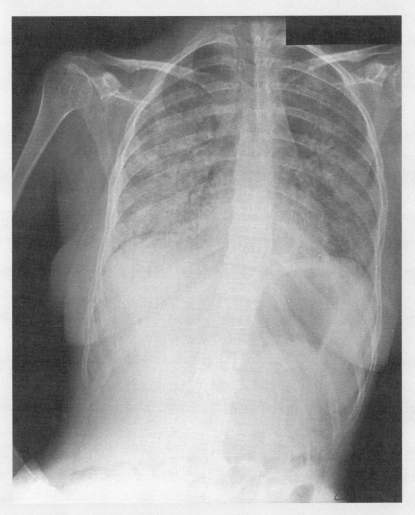

FIGURE 11.3 Portable chest radiograph taken approximately 12 hours after admission.

More on Ms. Y

The patient is sedated, intubated, and placed on a volume ventilator.

QUESTIONS	ANSWERS
17. What ventilator settings do you recommend? What are the targets of your ventilator adjustments?	The patient can be placed on a volume ventilator with a V_T of 5 to 7 mL/kg of ideal body weight. Since she weighs 55 kg, an ideal V_T would be about 300 to 400 mL. The ventilator should be set in the assist-control or intermittent mandatory ventilation (IMV) mode with a backup rate of 20 to 25/min. Initially, a PEEP of 5 cm H_2O and an FIO_2 of 0.60 is reasonable. The patient should be sedated for her comfort, as well as to control her ventilation. Paralysis could also be used if sedation does not allow adequate control of ventilation. Targets for mechanical ventilation: adjust PEEP for SpO_2 >90% with FIO_2 <0.65; adjust V_T for P_{plat} 0.5 sec of <30 ch H_2O and adjust respiratory rate to keep pH >7.20.
18. How should the position of the endotracheal tube be assessed?	The endotracheal tube position should be evaluated by listening to breath sounds bilaterally and by inspecting the chest x-ray. The tip of the tube should be 3 to 5 cm above the carina, as seen on the chest x-ray.

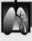

More on Ms. Y

After being placed on mechanical ventilation, Ms. Y has the following vital signs: pulse 120/min, respiratory rate 22/min, temperature 38.9°C (102°F), and blood pressure 90/60 mm Hg. A pulmonary artery catheter is inserted because of the hypotension, and an ABG shows the following results: pH 7.25, $PaCO_2$ 47 mm Hg, PaO_2 55 mm Hg, and HCO_3^- 20 mEq/liter. Chest auscultation reveals bilateral inspiratory crackles. A chest radiograph shows diffuse, bilateral, fluffy infiltrates and normal heart size consistent with noncardiogenic pulmonary edema. It also shows that the endotracheal tube is in a good position. During a mechanical breath, the P_{pk} was 60 cm H_2O and P_{stat} 45 cm H_2O with an exhaled V_T of 400 mL and a PEEP of 5 cm H_2O.

QUESTIONS	ANSWERS
19. What is Ms. Y's C_{st} and C_{dyn}, and how do you interpret the measurements?	C_{st} is calculated by dividing P_{stat} minus the PEEP level into the exhaled V_T. In this case, the C_{st} is calculated as follows: 400 mL/(45 − 5) cm H_2O = 10.0 mL/cm H_2O The C_{dyn} is calculated by dividing the peak pressure minus the PEEP level into the V_T. In this case, the C_{dyn} is calculated as follows: 400 mL/(60 − 5) cm H_2O = 7.2 mL/cm H_2O

Since normal C_{st} is 60 to 100 mL/cm H_2O and C_{dyn} is normally 35 to 55 mL/cm H_2O, the above values are well below normal. The measurements indicate that an increased pressure is required to inflate the lungs to a specific volume. This increases the work of breathing during spontaneous breathing and eventually will fatigue the respiratory muscles.

20. What pathophysiology accounts for the C_{st} measurement?

Pulmonary compliance is reduced when fluid moves from the injured pulmonary capillaries into the interstitial spaces, airways, and alveoli. Loss of surfactant, atelectasis, and fibrous tissue also reduce lung compliance.

21. To what hazards does the increased ventilating pressure predispose the patient?

Increased airway pressures predispose the patient to barotrauma (e.g., pneumothorax, cardiovascular compromise) and therefore further impairment in ventilation and oxygenation.

22. What changes in the mechanical ventilator mode of ventilation could be used to reduce the hazards of increased pressure?

Further reducing the V_T within the range of 5 to 7 mL/kg to limit peak airway pressures to 40 cm H_2O and P_{plat} <30 should allow adequate ventilation (although the $Paco_2$ will increase further) while minimizing the side effects of increased pressure. Because the PaO_2 is still less than 60 mm Hg on an FIO_2 greater than 0.60, an increase in PEEP is indicated. In addition, application of appropriate PEEP levels improves compliance by reducing alveolar opening pressures and increasing the distribution of ventilation.

 ## More on Ms. Y

Ms. Y is placed on a V_T of 330 mL and a respiratory rate of 20/min. A PEEP study is performed, yielding the following results:

PEEP (cm H_2O)	Pao_2 (mm Hg)	$P\bar{v}o_2$ (mm Hg)	PAP (mm Hg)	PCWP (mm Hg)	Cardiac Output (liters/min)	C_{st} (mL/cm H_2O)
5	55	32	28/14	18	4.2	13
10	71	36	27/16	22	4.1	25
15	82	33	32/20	29	3.1	18

QUESTIONS

ANSWERS

20. Based on the PEEP study, what is the optimal PEEP? Why?

The optimal PEEP level at present is 10 cm H_2O. At a PEEP level of 10 cm H_2O, the cardiac output and Pao_2 are both at an acceptable level. The cardiac output dropped significantly when the PEEP was increased to 15 cm H_2O, suggesting that tissue oxygenation is not as good as it was when the PEEP was 10 cm H_2O.

21. Are the PAP and PCWP readings believable at a PEEP level of 15 cm H_2O? Why or why not?

No, the pulmonary artery measurements are not believable at a PEEP level of 15 cm H_2O. A PCWP that is almost equivalent to the systolic PAP indicates that blood would be flowing backward through most of the cardiac cycle. This is probably impossible and certainly not consistent with life. Pressure from the airways is apparently being transmitted to the pulmonary artery catheter at higher PEEP levels. The catheter may be in a zone I position.

22. Why did the $P\bar{v}o_2$ drop when the PEEP was increased from 10 to 15 cm H_2O?

The $P\bar{v}o_2$ dropped when the PEEP was increased from 10 to 15 cm H_2O because of the drop in cardiac output and oxygen delivery to the tissues. A lack of adequate tissue oxygenation causes severe desaturation of the blood in the tissues, and venous blood returning to the heart thus has lower than normal oxygen levels.

23. Why did the C_{st} drop when the PEEP was increased from 10 to 15 cm H_2O?

Initially PEEP increases pulmonary compliance by increasing alveolar recruitment; however, as PEEP is increased beyond optimal levels, overdistention of alveoli can occur, reducing lung compliance.

24. How can the zone position of the pulmonary artery catheter be assessed?

Since patent blood vessels are present in true zone III conditions, a wedged catheter in zone III shows an undamped waveform with distinct A and V waves. Location of the wedged pulmonary artery catheter can also be assessed via chest radiograph. When positioned in zone III, the catheter tip will appear below the left atrium on a lateral chest radiograph.

25. If the $Paco_2$ on the next ABG was found to be 54 mm Hg, what would be the best course of action?

No changes are absolutely necessary at this point. A gradual rise in $Paco_2$ while allowing the kidneys to compensate is well tolerated and is the definition of permissive hypercapnia. In this mode, eucapnic ventilation is not the goal of therapy; rather, maintaining the patient's airway pressure at a reasonable level, while still achieving adequate oxygenation through changes in PEEP and Fio_2, is desired.

 More on Ms. Y

A few hours later Ms. Y has a sudden onset of labored breathing, a pulse rate of 140/min, and a blood pressure of 70/40 mm Hg. A check of the ventilator reveals a significant increase in the peak inspiratory pressure with each mechanical breath and frequent sounding of the pressure limit alarm. The patient's level of consciousness deteriorates, and peripheral cyanosis is present.

QUESTIONS	ANSWERS
26. What may be causing the sudden deterioration of Ms. Y?	The most likely causes of the sudden increases in peak pressure and clinical deterioration of the patient are pneumothorax, mucus plugging, or kinking of the endotracheal tube.
27. What assessment procedures should be done to identify the cause of the sudden clinical deterioration?	Auscultation should be done to see if bilateral breath sounds are present. A chest radiograph should be ordered immediately. Attempts to pass a suction catheter should help assess whether the endotracheal tube is blocked.
28. What therapeutic procedures should be done in response to each of the most likely causes of the patient's problem?	The patient's F_{IO_2} should be increased to 1.0. If breath sounds are present only on one side and increased resonance to percussion is present on the side with absent breath sounds, a pneumothorax is probably present. A chest radiograph would confirm the pneumothorax, but the patient may not survive the time needed to obtain and develop one. The attending physician should insert a large-bore needle between the ribs on the affected side if a pneumothorax is strongly suggested by the clinical findings and the patient is rapidly deteriorating. Once the patient is stable, a chest radiograph can be ordered and a chest tube inserted if the x-ray confirms the pneumothorax. If the endotracheal tube is blocked, it should be cleared or removed and replaced.

More on Ms. Y

A portable chest radiograph is taken immediately and confirms a right-sided pneumothorax. A chest tube is inserted, which results in immediate improvement in pulmonary and cardiovascular function. Ms. Y's condition stabilizes within a few hours.

Over the next 5 days, Ms. Y is maintained on mechanical ventilation with a PEEP of 10 to 12 cm H_2O and an F_{IO_2} of 0.40 to 0.45. Her vital signs remain stable, and body temperature gradually decreases to near normal. Her hemodynamic status stabilizes, and on day 6 her cardiac output is 5.2 liter/min with a PCWP of 14 mm Hg. Her C_{st} is calculated to be 35 mL/cm H_2O, and her chest radiograph shows minimal improvement in the alveolar infiltrates. Auscultation reveals bilateral inspiratory crackles, especially in the dependent regions. Spontaneous respiratory mechanics give a VC of 1100 mL, V_T of 420 mL, and MIP of -28 cm H_2O.

QUESTIONS	ANSWERS
29. Is Ms. Y ready to begin weaning from the mechanical ventilator? Why or why not?	The patient appears to be ready for weaning because the values for respiratory mechanics (VC, V_T, MIP) are acceptable, her C_{st} is much improved, her cardiovascular parameters and vitals (cardiac output, blood pressure, and PCWP) are stable, and the infection appears to be clearing.

| 30. What modes of ventilation can be used to wean Ms. Y? | Weaning can take place by using IMV and slowly decreasing the mechanical rate, by using pressure support, or by using continuous positive airway pressure for increasing periods of time, as tolerated. The ventilatory support should allow the patient to resume her own work of breathing gradually, without producing undue stress. The weaning can continue as long as the stress of weaning does not produce more than a 20% change in blood pressure, respiratory rate, or pulse rate. |
| 31. How should weaning proceed? | After the FIO_2 is less than 0.45, the PEEP can be decreased in increments of 3 to 5 cm H_2O, as tolerated, to approximately 5 cm H_2O. Waiting at least 3 to 4 hours to assess the patient's response to each decrease in the PEEP before proceeding is desirable. Mechanical support can then be decreased until the patient is breathing spontaneously. After 12 to 24 hours of stability, the endotracheal tube can be removed. |

 ## Ms. Y Conclusion

Over the next 24 hours Ms. Y is weaned from PEEP and mechanical ventilation. She is extubated and placed on a nasal cannula at 3 liters/min. Over the next several days, her chest radiograph continues to show improvement of the alveolar infiltrates with no residual fibrotic changes. Auscultation reveals improved breaths sounds, although scattered inspiratory crackles remain. Ms. Y is discharged on the 12th hospital day. ∎

 ### KEY POINTS

- ALI is characterized by persistent lung inflammation seen at the level of the alveolar capillary membrane with increased vascular permeability that results in bilateral pulmonary edema and atelectasis.
- ARDS is a severe form of ALI. ARDS is present when the ALI results in such severe hypoxia that the PaO_2/FIO_2 ratio is 200 mm Hg or less.
- ARDS is a common problem worldwide, and about 10% to 15% of ICU patients meet the criteria for it.
- The most common clinical problems associated with the onset of ALI and ARDS are sepsis, severe trauma, multiple transfusions, aspiration, severe pneumonia, and smoke inhalation.
- In ARDS patients, arterial blood gases show hypoxemia that responds poorly to oxygen therapy alone but somewhat better to oxygen therapy with positive pressure ventilation.
- The chest radiograph will show bilateral fluffy infiltrates and a normal heart shadow in most cases of ARDS.

KEY POINTS (CONTINUED)

- Mechanical ventilation of the patient with ARDS is needed in most cases to maintain adequate oxygenation.
- Mechanical ventilation in ARDS is best administered using a tidal volume (V_T) range of 5 to 7 mL/kg and plateau pressures of <30 cm H_2O.
- Adequate oxygenation with a modest increase in FIO_2 is obtained by the application of positive end-expiratory pressure (PEEP). Atelectatic regions may be reopened by the application of PEEP.
- PEEP levels should be kept at 15 cm H_2O or below to prevent lung injury in most cases.
- The use of a pulmonary artery catheter for hemodynamic monitoring in ARDS patients is controversial because there is no clear evidence that its use alters mortality rates.
- Measuring static compliance (C_{st}) gives valuable information regarding stiffness of the lungs and chest wall. Improvement in C_{st} with the addition of PEEP or new ventilator settings indicates recruitment of previously collapsed alveoli.

REFERENCES

1. Frutos-Vivar, F, Nin, N, Esteban, A: Epidemilogy of acute lung injury and acute respiratory distress syndrome. Curr Opin Crit Care 10:1, 2004.
2. Estenssoro, E, Dubin, A, Laffaire, E, et al: Incidence, clinical course, and outcome in 217 patients with acute respiratory distress syndrome. Crit Care Med 30:2450, 2002.
3. Esteban, A, Ansueto, A Frutos, F, et al: Characteristics and outcome in adult patients receiving mechanical ventilation: a 28 day international study. JAMA 287:345, 2002.
4. Zaccardelli, DS, Pattishall, EN: Clinical diagnostic criteria of of the adult respiratory distress syndrome in the intensive care unit. Crit Care Med 24:247, 1996.
5. Abel, SJC, Finney, SJ, Bret, SJ, et al: Reduced mortality in association with acute respiratory distress syndrome. Thorax 53:292, 1998.
6. Siegal, MD, Hyzy, RC: Mechanical ventilation in acute respiratory distress syndrome. Available at: uptodate.com (accessed December 31, 2004).
7. ARDS Network: Ventilation with lower tidal volumes as compared with traditional tidal volumes for acute lung injury and acute respiratory distress syndrome. N Engl J Med 342:1301, 2000.
8. Eisner, MD, Thompson, T, Hudson, LD, et al: Efficacy of low tidal volume ventilation in patients with different clinical risk factors for acute lung injury and acute respiratory distress syndrome. Am J Respir Crit Care Med 164:231, 2001.
9. Guerin, C, Gaillard, S, Lemasson, S, et al: Effects of systematic prone positioning in hypoxemic acute respiratory failure: a randomized controlled trial. JAMA 292:2379, 2004.
10. Schwartz, DR, Malhotra, A, Kacmarek, RA: Prone ventilation. Available at: www.uptodate.com (accessed March 30, 2005).
11. Rivers, E, Hguyen, B, Havstad, S, et al: Early goal directed therapy in the treatment of severe sepsis and septic shock. N Eng J Med 345:1368(1377, 2001.
12. Dellinger, RP, Carlet, JM, Masur, H, et al: Surviving sepsis campaign guidelines for management of severe sepsis and septic shock. Crit Care Med 32:858–673, 2004.
13. Yan, SB, Helterbrand, JD, Hartman, DL, et al: Low levels of protein C are associated with poor outcomes in severe sepsis. Chest 120:915–922, 2001.
14. Hesslevik JF, Malm, J, Dahlback, B, Blomback, M: Protein C, protein S, C4b-binding protein in severe infection and septic shock. Thomb Haemost 65:126–129, 1991.
15. Mesters, RM, Helterbrand, JD, Utterback, BG, et al: Prognostic value of protein C concentrations in neutropenic patients at high risk of severe septic complications. Crit Care Med 28:2209–2216, 2000.
16. Vincent, J, Abraham, E, Annane, D, Barnard, G, Rivers, E, Van den Berghe, G: Reducing mortality in sepsis: new directions. Crit Care 6(Suppl 3): S1–S18, 2002.

12

Chest Trauma

George H. Hicks, MS, RRT

Carl A. Eckrode, MPH, RRT

CHAPTER OBJECTIVES:

After reading this chapter you will be able to state or identify the following:

- The significance of trauma as a cause of death in the United States and the proportion of fatal trauma that is chest-related.
- The etiology of chest trauma, including the major subcategories and common causes for each.
- Injury patterns and pathophysiological changes associated with chest trauma, including fractures, parenchymal and pleural injuries, cardiac injuries, and the long-term outcomes of chest trauma and its treatment.
- The components of a chest trauma assessment, including application of a trauma scoring system.
- Immediate steps for treatment of a chest trauma patient, including airway, oxygen delivery, and mechanical ventilation strategies.

INTRODUCTION

Trauma is the leading cause of death in the United States in the first four decades of life,[1] with chest trauma second only to head trauma as the most common cause of traumatic death.[2] Motor vehicle crashes, falls, fire and burns, homicide, and suicide are the most common causes of death from traumatic injuries. In 2002, 161,269 people died of trauma-related injuries, resulting in an estimated 3,540,075 years of potential life lost.[3] However, many more victims of trauma survive their initial injuries. Seventy to eighty percent of chest injuries are the result of blunt trauma incurred during motor vehicle crashes; one-third of the patients hospitalized after motor vehicle crashes present with major chest trauma.[2] With the large number of trauma patients who present with thoracic injuries, and the high morbidity and mortality associated with these injuries, proper management of the pulmonary system and prompt treatment of associated chest trauma injuries is essential.

> Trauma is the leading cause of death in the United States in the first four decades of life. Chest trauma is second only to head trauma as a cause of traumatic death.

ETIOLOGY

Chest trauma can be classified as **penetrating, blunt**,[4] or a combination of the two (Table 12.1). Another type of chest trauma is **primary blast injury.** This is trauma to the chest caused directly by an explosive blast wave and is included in the category of blunt trauma. This form of chest injury is an important consequence of terrorist acts and industrial accidents. For example, in the 2004 Madrid training bombings, 63% of the critically ill victims sustained blast lung injury.[5]

Four general anatomical regions of the chest may be involved in chest trauma: the thoracic cage, the conducting airways, the lung parenchyma, and the pleura. The scope of traumatic chest injury includes damage to the chest wall, pleura, tracheobronchial tree, lungs, diaphragm, esophagus, heart, and great vessels (Figure 12.1).[2]

Acts of violence are an important cause of chest trauma; most penetrating injuries of the chest are the result of homicide, suicide, or their attempts. These penetrating wounds are most commonly produced by knives or high-speed and low-speed missiles, such as bullets and fragments from explosions. Low-speed penetrating stab wounds, such as those caused by knives or similar instruments, cause chest injuries that are largely localized to the tissues that have been pierced and the resulting hemorrhage. The injuries from high-velocity missiles are often less localized. The injuries produced by high-speed missiles are proportional to the kinetic energy they deliver to the body, with both the mass and design of the missile and its velocity determining the energy transfer and resultant damage. Velocity is

Table 12.1	Mechanisms of Injuries in Chest Trauma	
Mechanism	Example
Blunt Trauma:	
Acceleration/deceleration	Motor vehicle crashes and falls
Compression	Crushing and blasts
Penetration Trauma:	
High-speed impact/ penetration	Gunshot wound, bomb fragments
Low-speed penetration	Stab wound

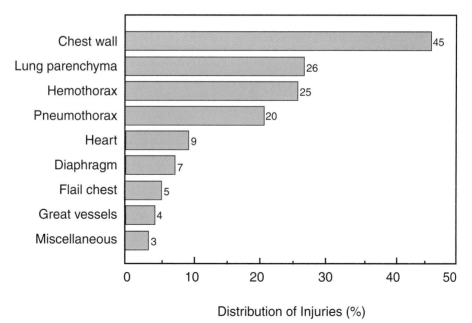

FIGURE 12.1 The distribution of specific types of injuries in 15,047 chest trauma patients from the North American Trauma Outcome Study. (Developed from data presented in LoCicero, J, Mattox, KL: Epidemiology of chest trauma. Surg Clin North Am 69:15–19, 1989.)

considered by most experts to be the most important factor in predicting the severity of injury from a penetrating wound.[6,7]

Missiles traveling at high speeds and possessing high kinetic energy can cause significant damage to both the organs they pierce and the surrounding tissues. The energy discharged to the tissues by high-speed projectiles can cause significant direct damage and destruction along their trajectory and can cause damage owing to cavitation effects. Cavitation often pulls external debris into the wound. In contrast, wounds from lower-velocity missiles are generally less severe.[7] However, the extent of damage from lower-velocity projectiles can be increased if the projectile is designed to inflict greater trauma. This occurs when the missile is made of softer materials, "wanders," expands, or breaks up on impact with bone or solid structures (e.g., unjacketed or partially jacketed lead and hollow-point bullets, multiple-part projectiles such as the Glaser Safety Slug, or flechettes). The resulting energy transfer increases the damage to surrounding tissue. Wounds from close-range shotgun blasts cause severe damage by producing a very large entrance wound, with extensive underlying tissue damage from pellet penetration. At point-blank ranges, this large wound damage is enhanced by the great volume of gas discharged at the muzzle. These wounds are further complicated by additional components of the shotgun round, such as paper or plastic barriers (wads) that separate and protect the projectiles and propellant prior to firing. These components can enter the tissue, contributing to further damage and increasing the risk of infection.[7] At greater distances, shotgun blast injuries are more typically numerous small-diameter pellet entrance wounds, with less deep tissue destruction.[7]

> **C**hest trauma can be classified as blunt or penetrating. Acts of violence account for the majority of penetrating chest trauma, and motor vehicle crashes are responsible for most blunt chest trauma.

Blunt force trauma to the chest causes severe damage by crushing tissue, fracturing bones, and shearing tissue after rapid acceleration or deceleration.[8–10] Sudden and severe deceleration causes violent motion of mobile structures, resulting in shearing forces that cause microscopic and macroscopic tears in the tissues. In the United States blunt chest trauma occurs most frequently as a result of motor vehicle crashes.[2]

PATHOPHYSIOLOGY

Chest Wall Injuries

Subcutaneous Emphysema

With the exception of major burn injuries, traumatic cutaneous injuries are rarely fatal, but they may be the source of considerable morbidity. Subcutaneous emphysema, a common manifestation of chest injuries, should lead the clinician to suspect airway injury, such as rupture. In this event, air migrates along the great vessels to the mediastinum and then into the soft tissues of the neck and chest. Subcutaneous emphysema is usually only a temporary cosmetic problem because of the skin's distensible characteristics; however, its presence may indicate underlying problems that could be life threatening.

Open Chest Wound

Open or "sucking" chest wounds can act as one-way valves that allow air to enter upon inspiration and to be trapped during exhalation. This can lead to a pneumothorax that can rapidly escalate to a life-threatening **tension pneumothorax**. The loss of lung volume, compromised alveolar ventilation, and ventilation-perfusion ($\dot{V}/\dot{Q}$) mismatching that result from an open chest wound and pneumothorax can lead to respiratory failure and shock.

Fractures

Clavicular fractures are rarely a clinical problem unless their sharp, bony ends lacerate the underlying blood vessels, brachial plexus, the lung, or a combination of these. Rib fractures, on the other hand, may present a wide range of morbidity and mortality. Rib fractures often cause pain, shallow breathing, guarded cough, atelectasis, or pneumonia. Rib fractures are more common in adults than children because children have highly elastic costochondral cartilage; the harder, less flexible ribs of adults are more likely to break on impact. Fractures to ribs 1 and 2 are rare because of the added protection and support provided by the bones and tissues of the shoulder girdle.[11] An impact great enough to fracture ribs 1 and 2 is often associated with severe injuries to the head, neck, lung, great vessels, and tracheobronchial tree; the mortality rate in these cases can approach 50%.[11] Ribs 4 through 10 are more likely to be broken by blunt trauma. Fracture of these ribs may lead to laceration of the lung, often resulting in hemothorax, pneumothorax, or a hemopneumothorax. These fractures often suggest the development of an underlying pulmonary tissue contusion.

Sternal fractures and costochondral separations are often the result of a high-speed deceleration impact to the anterior chest during a motor vehicle crash. These injuries are frequently associated with flail chest, cardiac contusion, great vessel rupture, or tracheobronchial rupture.[12] The most common site of sternal fractures is along the junction of the manubrium and sternal body or transversely through the sternal body.

Flail Chest

Flail chest is characterized by an unstable chest wall as a result of thoracic injury, which has an asymmetric or paradoxical motion during the breathing cycle.[11] This condition is rare but quite serious.[12] When multiple ribs are fractured in two or more places, the resulting instability can produce a paradoxical, or "flail," motion (Figure 12.2). During the inspiratory phase the unsupported region is pulled in while the rest of the chest expands; the reverse occurs during exhalation (Figure 12.3). Hypoxemia and CO_2 retention may occur as a result of both increased work of breathing and underlying pulmonary contusion and may become more apparent as the patient relaxes under sedation.[11–13] Often these patients require mechanical ventilation and have more respiratory complications and longer hospital stays.[14] Current practice is to stabilize the chest wall with positive pressure ventilation and to consider the need for surgical stabilization. Stabilization of the chest wall with the use of surgically placed rib plates or wiring has been successful in improving pulmonary function, reduced time on mechanical ventilation, reduced infection, improved quality of life, and achieving reductions in ventilator time.[15]

> Simple rib fractures often do not require any treatment. However, flail chest is a more severe problem and may require positive pressure ventilation or surgical intervention.

Lung Parenchymal Injuries

Pneumothorax, hemothorax, and **hemopneumothorax** are frequently associated with blunt force chest trauma and are characterized by the collection of air, blood, or a mixture of air and blood in the pleural cavity. These conditions are commonly caused by broken ribs that penetrate and lacerate the lungs, in the case of blunt chest trauma, or by other penetrating wounds. Bleeding from the low-pressure pulmonary circulation is relatively slow

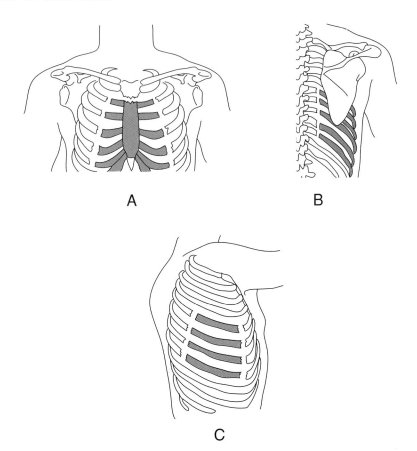

FIGURE 12.2 Areas of the thoracic cage involved in flail chests. (A) Anterior sternal flail. (B) Lateral flail. (C) Posterior flail. (From Pate, JW: Chest wall injuries. Surg Clin North Am 69:59–70, 1989, with permission.)

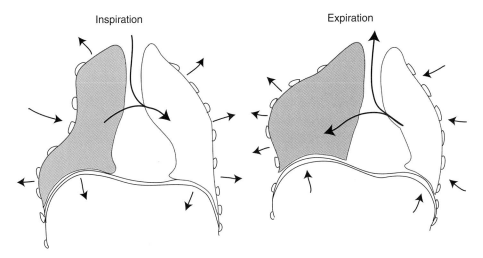

FIGURE 12.3 Paradoxical, or flail, motion of the chest following multiple rib fractures. The resulting motion produces a very inefficient movement of gas that can lead to respiratory muscle fatigue and respiratory failure. (From Wilkins, EW: Non-cardiovascular thoracic injuries: chest wall, bronchus, lung, esophagus, and diaphragm. In Burke, JF, Boyd, RJ, and McCabe, CJ (eds): Trauma Management. Year Book Medical, Chicago, 1988, with permission.)

and often self-limiting compared to that from higher-pressure intercostal arteries, which can produce more brisk bleeding. Air and blood in the pleural cavity decrease lung volume and cause increased ($\dot{V}/\dot{Q}$) mismatching.

Pneumothorax

Simple pneumothorax is usually not associated with significant physiologic impairment until more than 30% of the lung has collapsed. Open pneumothorax is more often associated with penetrating chest trauma; however, severe blunt trauma, such as from explosive blasts, may result in substantial tissue destruction, leading to an open pneumothorax. If the diameter of chest wall opening is greater than two-thirds the diameter of the trachea, air will flow through the chest wall rather than the airways, impairing oxygenation.[10,11] Tension pneumothorax is life-threatening because of the compression of the heart and great vessels. Tension pneumothorax will most likely be diagnosed as a result of hemodynamic instability, diminished or absent breath sounds on the affected side, and a tracheal shift to the unaffected side. Rapid decompression of the pneumothorax by emergent thoracotomy (either by needle or trocar) is required for patient survival. The diagnosis of simple pneumothorax is suggested by diminished breath sounds on the affected side and confirmed by chest radiographic or computed tomography (CT) findings of air or fluid, or both, in the pleural space. Placement of a chest tube is the treatment of choice to evacuate the air and blood and to reexpand the lung.

Bronchopleural Fistula

A **bronchopleural fistula** is characterized by persistent leakage of air into the pleural space despite proper chest tube placement and suction. Its occurrence is rare and is almost always associated with a severe lung laceration or tracheobronchial rupture and the use of positive pressure ventilation. In severe cases the leakage can exceed 50% of a delivered tidal breath during mechanical ventilation and can be further exacerbated by the application of positive end-expiratory pressure (PEEP). As the leakage increases, effective ventilation and oxygenation become more difficult. Rapid repair of the underlying injury is essential to prevent future formation of strictures and other negative sequelae.

Pulmonary Contusion

Pulmonary contusion is associated with interstitial edema and hemorrhage, generally localized to the area of lung underlying an impact site.[10] On occasion, contusions can occur on opposite sides of the chest or throughout both lungs as a result of high-impact shock waves from a blast. Regardless of etiology, the edema and bleeding in the contused region of the lung cause a progressive decline in local lung compliance and increased airway inflammation, leading to atelectasis or consolidation of the injured areas.[10] Additionally, the contusion may result in increased intrapulmonary shunting and impaired oxygenation. These changes can take between 8 and 24 hours to appear, though chest radiograph changes consistent with focal injury are normally apparent within 6 hours of the injury[10] and on CT immediately.[11,12] Pulmonary contusion injuries can progress to the development of acute lung injury (ALI; PaO_2/FIO_2 ratio < 300 to 200) or, the more severe form, acute respiratory distress syndrome (ARDS; PaO_2/FIO_2 ratio <200) (see Chapter 11), which increases mortality.[16]

The development of ALI or ARDS following blunt chest injury is strongly associated with the severity of injury (injury severity score >25), the presence of pulmonary contusion, age >65 years, hypotension on admission, and a 24-hour transfusion requirement >10 units.[17] Small contusions can be managed with supplemental oxygen, cough and deep breathing, and monitoring. Use of ventilatory support with lower tidal volumes (6 mL/kg) and PEEP coupled with careful use of fluid resuscitation, vasoactive drugs, and treatment for renal failure are needed in severe pulmonary contusions that lead to ALI or ARDS. These approaches have resulted in a decline in the length of ICU stay and mortality rate for trauma patients in general.[18]

Aspiration

Further injury to the lung parenchyma can result from aspiration. Aspiration of stomach contents is relatively common in the trauma patient, and should always be suspected in the unconscious patient with a reduced PaO_2/FIO_2 ratio. Airway obstruction and aspiration pneumonitis in the gravity-dependent portions of the lungs are the major complications of gastric aspiration. The signs of inflammatory changes in the lung are often delayed for 12 to 24 hours. The combination of chest trauma and aspiration increases a patient's risk of pneumonia and ARDS.[16]

> Lung parenchymal injuries can include pneumothorax, hemothorax, or hemopneumothorax. Tension pneumothorax is immediately life-threatening and requires emergent treatment by needle decompression. Other injuries, such as pulmonary contusion, can vary in their severity and need for treatment. Aspiration is common in the trauma patient and increases the risk of pneumonia and ARDS.

Infection

Chest trauma patients are at particular risk for infection because they frequently become immune compromised and have interventions that increase the risk of colonization. The most common infection in these patients is a bacterial pneumonia. Often the infectious organism(s) are those that are acquired after admission and colonization of their upper airway (e.g., *Staphylococcus* bacteria). These infections can progress from a ventilator-associated pneumonia to sepsis syndrome to ALI/ARDS and, in more severe cases, can develop into septic shock and multiple organ dysfunction syndrome (MODS). Care should always be exercised to reduce the chance of a ventilator- or hospital-associated infection in these and all acutely ill patients.

Airway Injuries

Blunt force injury to the larynx may produce sudden airway occlusion secondary to a crushed larynx or cricotracheal dislocation. A more common problem is progressive airway obstruction from edema. Most laryngeal injuries are caused by impacts to unrestrained drivers involved in motor vehicle crashes. Symptoms of laryngeal and tracheal injury include hoarseness, inability to lie supine, dysphasia, laryngeal tenderness, tracheal deviation, and subcutaneous emphysema.[19] These signs and symptoms provide important clues to tracheal injury. Lateral neck radiographs may be deceptively negative. A CT scan can provide a more accurate view of the laryngeal anatomy. Initial laryngoscopy should be done cautiously in the operating room in case sudden airway obstruction occurs and emergent tracheostomy is required. Placement of an endotracheal tube with the aid of a bronchoscope, or emergent tracheostomy if emergent bronchoscopy is impossible, is the treatment of choice for severe laryngeal trauma and airway obstruction.[20]

Sudden compression of the thorax can cause deceleration shearing of the trachea. Most of these injuries occur within five centimeters of the carina and result in pneumothorax and subcutaneous emphysema.[21] Victims of transection of the trachea frequently have two or more other major injuries.[20] Tracheal and bronchial laceration or rupture requires rapid evaluation and direct repair by thoracotomy. Emergent surgical repair of a lacerated trachea or bronchus is the treatment of choice, as massive bleeding can rapidly lead to asphyxiation. Therapeutic efforts are aimed at reducing the bleeding and maintaining airway clearance. Diagnostic and therapeutic bronchoscopy is an important tool in managing the patient with tracheobronchial injuries. If the exhaled

> In airway trauma, maintenance of a patent airway is the primary concern. This may require the use of difficult airway techniques, bronchoscopy, or surgery.

tidal volume (V_T) is significantly less than the delivered V_T, the presence of a bronchopulmonary fistula or tracheal rupture should be suspected and the cause explored.

Heart and Great Vessel Injuries

Chest trauma, whether blunt or penetrating, can lead to a variety of cardiac injuries, including penetration, rupture, cardiac tamponade, coronary artery lacerations and occlusion, myocardial contusion, pericardial effusion, septal defects,valvular injuries, air embolism, and great vessel rupture.[11] These injuries can be rapidly fatal. Cardiac penetrating injuries are most often caused by knife and gunshot wounds. Blunt trauma is more often associated with **cardiac contusion** or cardiac rupture injuries (the right atrium is the most common rupture site).[22,23] Single-chamber cardiac rupture has a survival rate of approximately 40%.[22] Blunt cardiac injury accounts for up to 20% of all motor vehicle deaths.[24]

Cardiac Tamponade

After rupture of a cardiac chamber or lacerations of the coronary or great vessels, blood rapidly fills the pericardial sac and results in **cardiac tamponade**. Collection of only 60 to 100 mL of blood in the pericardial cavity can produce cardiac tamponade, often resulting in cardiogenic shock secondary to reduced cardiac filling.[25] Puncture wounds through the pericardial sac and cardiac chamber result in brisk bleeding, which will dominate the clinical picture as a poorly responsive hypotension. Cardiac tamponade is often identified through recognition of the set of clinical signs known as **Beck's Triad**: distended neck veins, hypotension, and diminished heart tones.[12,25] However, Beck's Triad may not be observed in patients who are hypovolemic. A widened mediastinum on the chest radiograph or CT may suggest mediastinal bleeding or cardiac tamponade or both. In comparison to Beck's Triad or chest radiograph, echocardiography is often more helpful in establishing the diagnosis of cardiac tamponade. Emergency needle thoracotomy, surgical exploratory thoracotomy with heart-lung bypass circulatory support, surgical repair, and adequate transfusion are the corrective measures of choice for cardiac rupture and cardiac tamponade.[25]

> Cardiac rupture and tamponade are life-threatening injuries. They require rapid identification through physical assessment, chest radiograph, and echocardiography and emergent treatment.

Myocardial Contusion

Myocardial contusion after blunt chest trauma is not easily identified. In an autopsy study the incidence of cardiac contusion was 16% however, quantifying the incidence of myocardial contusion depends on the diagnostic criteria used, and reports of incidence thus vary from 8% to 71%.[23] Pathological changes in the contused heart can include intramyocardial hemorrhage, myocardial edema, coronary artery occlusion, myofibril degeneration, and myocardial cell necrosis.[23] These changes can lead to dysrhythmias and hemodynamic instability, very similar to changes found during and after a myocardial infarction.[23]

Electrocardiographic (ECG) findings often show tachycardia, ST-segment elevation, T-wave changes, and occasional premature ventricular contractions.[11,19] Cardiac enzyme levels in plasma (e.g., aspartate aminotransferase [AST], lactate dehydrogenase [LDH], and creatine kinase [CK]) are often elevated after blunt chest trauma and are therefore of little diagnostic value. CK-MB isoenzymes may be nondiagnostic.[22] However, in combination with a symptomatic ECG, serum cardiac Troponin I elevation is a reliable indication of myocardial contusion.[26,27] When cardiac contusion has been diagnosed, pulmonary artery catheterization is often useful in monitoring hemodynamic performance and for treating heart failure. Echocardiography, radionuclide angiography, serial ECG, hemodynamic monitoring, and serum cardiac Troponin I monitoring form the diagnostic array for detecting and monitoring myocardial contusion. Patients are treated as though they had a myocardial infarction, and long-term negative outcomes from blunt cardiac trauma are infrequent.[23,28]

> Myocardial contusion can be most accurately determined by serial symptomatic ECG and elevated serum Troponin I levels. Echocardiography, angiography, and hemodynamic monitoring play a part in the complete diagnostic array.

Aortic Rupture

Aortic rupture and exsanguination after blunt chest trauma in a motor vehicle crash leads to rapid death. Eighty to ninety percent of patients with thoracic aortic rupture die before arriving at the hospital.[22,29] The upper thoracic aorta, near the left subclavian artery, is the most common site of rupture.[22] If they survive to admission, patients frequently present with profound hypotension, often with chest radiographic findings showing a widened mediastinum.[22] If the patient presents in shock and with an obviously widened mediastinum, emergent thoracotomy, surgical repair, and transfusion are needed.

Diaphragmatic Injuries

Injuries to the diaphragm result from both blunt and penetrating trauma, though penetrating trauma is the most frequent cause of this injury.[11] Unless abdominal contents enter the thorax, this injury often goes undetected. Rupture of the left hemidiaphragm is more frequent and is often associated with splenic rupture; hemothorax; omentum, bowel, and spleen herniation into the thorax; impaired diaphragmatic motion; and ventilatory failure.[30] The diagnosis is usually made by evaluation of the chest and abdominal radiographs, by CT scans of the abdomen, or during exploratory laparotomy.[30] Diaphragmatic rupture requires surgical evaluation and closure.

Delayed and Long-Term Complications of Chest Wall Trauma

Chronic pain, recurring atelectasis, dyspnea, and pneumonia are among the most common long-term sequelae of chest trauma.[28,31,32] Chronic pain and dyspnea are usually managed with analgesics, oxygen therapy, and reassurance. Pleural infection can arise from a retained hemothorax or foreign body and can result in empyema, pleurisy, and fibrothorax.[28,32] Thoracotomy, pleural drainage, antibiotics, and pleural decortication are frequently used to treat poorly responding pleural infections and to avert the formation of a fibrothorax.

Penetrating and blunt chest injuries can lead to pulmonary dysfunction, chronic pain, ventricular aneurysm, cardiac insufficiency, and esophageal stricture or fistula.[32] Retained foreign bodies have been found to migrate or erode into other areas many years after the initial injury; migration of these foreign bodies can result in embolic events. These long-term complications often require acute, surgical, and rehabilitative care.[32]

> Chest trauma can involve a wide range of pathophysiologies. Chest wall injuries and fractures, injuries to the lung parenchyma, cardiac contusions, airway injuries, and diaphragm injury are among the many variants of chest trauma.

CLINICAL FEATURES AND LABORATORY FINDINGS

The clinical features of chest trauma vary widely by category and cause. A focused physical examination is the starting point for rapidly obtaining the clinical information needed to guide the resuscitation and treatment of a chest trauma patient. The primary survey is a rapid, focused, and careful physical examination that should include evaluation of the patient's airway, breathing rate and effort, oxygen saturation, heart rate, blood pressure, assessment of blood loss, level of consciousness and signs of other disability including the initiation of spinal cord injury precautions.[33,34] A trauma scoring system can aid in the rapid and systematic evaluation of the nervous, circulatory, and respiratory systems. This scoring system is a simple method for evaluating trauma patients and determining the severity of their injuries (Table 12.2). Assessment findings can then guide the care team in the selection of additional tests and the type of care to be provided.

The secondary survey of the trauma victim will determine more precisely the nature and extent of the injuries. It should include further evaluation of the relevant historical events, thorough physical evaluation, and imaging and laboratory examinations.[33] The patient is examined from head to toe for all signs of injury. During this examination, evaluating the thorax for signs of flail chest, the presence of subcutaneous emphysema, symmetry, and quality of breath sounds is also essential. Auscultation of the lungs is often definitive in diagnosing hemo- and pneumothoraces and can be life-saving in quick diagnosis of a tension pneumothorax. The portable anteroposterior chest radiograph is necessary and highly effective in the great majority of cases. The chest CT scan is highly sensitive in detecting thoracic injuries after blunt chest trauma and is superior to a routine chest radiograph in visualizing lung contusions, pneumothorax, and hemothorax.[35] The chest CT scan should be performed in the early management of the trauma patient who has chest injuries. However, definitive surgical treatment can be unnecessarily delayed by waiting for CT scans, and the clinician must weigh the value of information gathered against the time required for this procedure. Complete blood count (CBC), electrolytes, arterial blood gases (ABGs), and ECG are taken on admission and then serially. Toxicological studies may also be indicated,

> A systematic, focused assessment is required for successful resuscitation of the chest trauma patient. Attention to the basics of airway, breathing and circulation, combined with the effective use of a trauma scoring system, can guide the clinician toward a successful outcome. The use of chest radiograph, CT, and laboratory tests support the focused assessment.

Table 12.2 Trauma Score			
Glasgow Coma Scale	Systolic Blood Pressure	Respiratory Rate	Points
13–15	>89	10–29	4
9–12	76–89	>29	3
6–8	50–75	6–9	2
4–5	1–49	1–5	1
3	0	0	0
Example Case	POINTS		
Glasgow coma scale* = 15	4		
Blood pressure = 80	3		
Respiratory rate = 35	3		
Trauma score	10		

*Glasgow coma scale is a simple neurologic examination system that awards points according to the patient's best eye movement, verbal response, and motor response to various stimuli.

SOURCE: Adapted from Champion, HR, et al: A revision of the trauma score. J Trauma 29:623, 1989.

depending on the history obtained or other results of the assessment. More specialized studies such as bronchoscopy, magnetic resonance imaging, and angiography are done to gain a more precise determination of the extent of injuries.

TREATMENT

Survival of chest trauma is often contingent on rapid access to advanced life support and trauma center care. The phrase "the golden hour" is often used to refer to the time from identifying the need for care until definitive surgical or acute care is provided. An organized, preplanned approach to initial care of the trauma patient is essential for optimal outcomes.[33,34] A focused assessment and complete history of the events of the trauma are vital to determining the extent of injury and developing a care plan. Information about the nature of the motor vehicle crash (e.g., whether occupant restraints were used, whether the victim was ejected, the size and type of vehicle, degree of intrusion into the passenger compartment), the type of weapon used, the height of a fall, and how long the victim went untreated or was in shock are examples of useful information. It is important to gather any information regarding preexisting heart, lung, vascular, and renal disease, as well as a history of substance abuse, because these factors may complicate the response to, and treatment of, chest trauma.

Acute care for chest trauma includes maintenance of a patent airway, supplementary oxygen therapy with an F_{IO_2} of 1.0 via non-rebreathing mask, resuscitation bag with reservoir or other high-flow oxygen delivery system, placement of an artificial airway and initiation of mechanical ventilation, placement of arterial and IV catheters for monitoring blood pressure and for fluid or blood administration, chest tube placement, spinal fracture/injury precautions, and possibly direct admission to the operating room for emergency surgeries.[33,34] Placement of a pulmonary artery catheter is useful when managing a patient who is either hemodynamically unstable or requires large amounts of fluids to maintain fluid balance and blood pressure or both. However, this is typically not feasible in the emergency department.[34] Pain management is also important. Use of patient-controlled analgesia devices, epidural analgesia, and pleural infusions for the administration of pain medication (e.g., systemic infusion or thoracic epidural analgesia) improves the patient's pain tolerance, cooperation in deep breathing, and pulmonary function.[36,37]

Airway Management

Airway obstruction after trauma is a potential cause of preventable death. Airway obstruction is most commonly caused by the tongue obstructing the oropharynx. Aspiration of vomitus, blood, excessive saliva, or dentures and oral or laryngeal injuries with swelling are also causes of airway obstruction. Manual repositioning of the victim's head by an appropriate and safe maneuver and placement of an oropharyngeal airway facilitates a patent airway and bag-mask ventilation with 100% oxygen prior to intubation. Caution must be exercised in airway opening of the patient with suspected cervical spinal injury; the trauma jaw-thrust technique is recommended for these patients.[33,34]

A properly sized cuffed oral endotracheal tube is the airway of choice in most cases requiring emergency airway maintenance. It permits positive pressure ventilation, facilitates endotracheal suctioning, and helps protect the lungs from macro-aspiration. If the patient has a suspected cervical fracture, bronchoscopically assisted placement of a nasotracheal tube may be required; this method does not require extension of the head for endotracheal tube placement. Inadequate preoxygenation, mainstem intubation, esophageal intubation, respiratory alkalosis secondary to excessive ventilation, vasovagal reflex bradycardia, or a combination of these, may result in cardiac arrest during attempted endotracheal tube placement.

Careful examination of the endotracheal tube placement should be done to ensure proper tube placement and bilateral ventilation. Use of colorimetric or quantitative end-tidal capnometers or other placement confirmation devices can aid in preventing misplaced endotracheal tubes. A chest radiograph is indicated for every intubation, and fiberoptic bronchoscopy may be indicated to evaluate and treat excessive bleeding into the airway. Diagnostic and therapeutic fiberoptic bronchoscopy is also often very useful in patients with persistent or reoccurring atelectasis. The conversion to a tracheostomy tube may be necessary to facilitate secretion clearance and to avoid ventilator-associated pneumonia in patients requiring an artificial airway for more than 5 to 7 days. A double-lumen endotracheal tube may be required in cases of severe asymmetric lung contusion or tracheobronchial rupture necessitating independent lung ventilation.

When endotracheal intubation and tracheostomy tube placement are difficult or impossible, other airway adjuncts, such as the laryngeal mask airway (LMA) or CombiTube may be needed. In extreme situations, cricothyrotomy can be performed until it is possible to place a definitive airway. For emergent situations where no other airway access technique is available or successful, the insertion of one or several 12-gauge cricothyroid needles can provide short-term percutaneous transtracheal jet and ventilation until a tracheostomy tube can be placed.[38]

> Obtaining a patent airway is paramount to treating chest trauma. The endotracheal tube remains the airway of choice, but other techniques, such as the CombiTube, LMA, or percutaneous transtracheal jet ventilation must be considered for the difficult airway.

Ventilatory Support

The patient with chest injuries often adopts a rapid and shallow breathing pattern as a result of pain and declining respiratory system compliance.[36,37] This often begins a vicious cycle of lung volume decline, decreased oxygenation, and more rapid and shallow breathing. If this cyclic pattern is allowed to progress, the patient often declines into respiratory failure.

In patients who are alert and cooperative, the use of high-flow continuous positive airway pressure (CPAP) with a properly fitting mask has been found to be useful.[39–41] The fit of the mask and the patient's ability to cooperate is critical. The flow should be in excess of demand (e.g., 60 to 80 L/min), heated to 37°C, and humidified. The FIO_2 should be started at 1.0, and the initial CPAP should be set at 5 cm H_2O and adjusted in 2 cm H_2O increments to reach an arterial saturation of >92% and respiratory rate less than 30 to 35/min. If the patient fails to respond (saturation <92% and respiratory rate >35 /min) to 100% oxygen and 15 cm H_2O after 20 to 30 minutes, intubation and mechanical ventilation should be instituted.

A similar approach is the use of the noninvasive positive pressure ventilation (NPPV) modality also known as bilevel positive airway pressure (BiPAP). Several studies have demonstrated that some patients who develop hypoxemic respiratory failure can be effectively treated with NPPV, as it decreases the risks associated with intubation and reduces the length of stay in the ICU.[42,43] It should not be considered useful in all patients with significant trauma.[44] Those who have a higher injury severity score, an older age, ARDS or pneumonia, or fail to improve after a 30- to 60-minute trial, as with CPAP, are at much higher risk for respiratory failure and should be intubated and mechanically ventilated.[45]

Patients who present with apnea or frank respiratory failure (PaO_2 less than 60 mm Hg, $PaCO_2$ greater than 50 mm Hg, and pH less than 7.20) or who have impending respiratory failure (respiratory rate greater than 35/min and very shallow breathing) and are either unresponsive to or not candidates for CPAP or NPPV will require intubation and mechanical ventilation. Initial ventilator settings for a patient with an unknown degree of chest injury should be directed toward complete support with assist-control (AC) mode in either volume-controlled or pressure-controlled ventilation (PCV).[46] Pressure-regulated volume control (PRVC) or autoflow, forms of self-regulating PCV, may improve oxygenation, ventilation, and patient synchrony while lowering peak airway pressures when compared to volume-controlled ventilation. The V_T) setting should be 5 to 7 mL/kg, with a set rate of 12 to 20 min, an inspiratory:expiratory ratio of 1:3, and an FIO_2 of 1.0. Adjustments can then be made after further clinical examination and review of ABG results. A PEEP of 5 cm H_2O or greater is frequently necessary to improve lung volume and oxygenation. The use of *open lung* strategies have been shown, in some studies, to improve oxygenation in chest trauma patients.[47–49] Other ventilation strategies involving low tidal volumes, high rates, and PEEP titration based upon FIO_2 requirements have also been successful in managing the ventilation of the chest trauma patient.[18,50,51]

No matter what ventilation strategy is applied, caution is needed when using positive pressure ventilation and PEEP in chest trauma victims, because of an increased risk of hypotension and barotrauma. Thus, the clinician should attempt to maintain peak airway pressures of <35 cm H_2O and plateau pressures of <30 cm H_2O and utilize a *gentle ventilation* strategy whenever possible to avoid the development of ventilator-induced lung injury (VILI).[52]

A variety of techniques are available for management of more complicated cases that fail to respond to conventional mechanical ventilation. The use of recruitment maneuvers such as sustained breath holding with 30 to 40 cm H_2O pressure for 30 to 40 seconds to reexpand regions of lung that fail to respond to conventional levels of PEEP have been found to be useful in some patients. This and similar approaches have been found to improve lung volume and oxygenation.[53–55] However, a recent randomized cross-over study of patients with ALI and ARDS showed that the use of recruitment maneuvers resulted in variable response and short-term effect on oxygenation and may induce further VILI.[56] Use of recruitment maneuvers, therefore, is not recommended as part of routine care for these patients. Recruitment maneuvers may be considered for those who present with persistent atelectasis that does not respond to bronchoscopy and PEEP. Another approach to recruitment of collapsed lung is the placement of the patient in the prone position for long periods of time (8 to 20 hours). This effectively expands the atelectatic regions of the posterior lung segments and improves oxygenation in most patients.[57,58] While the use of prone position in ARDS does improve oxygenation, it does not improve survival unless there is improvement in alveolar ventilation and Pa_{CO_2}.[59] While the use of low-level inhaled nitric oxide has had mixed results in this patient population and is now generally not used, a recent report showed that it was useful in reducing right ventricular afterload and improving hemodynamics in myocardial contusion following blunt chest trauma.[60]

Several other techniques have been found to facilitate the use of the low tidal volume ventilation strategy in an attempt to help avoid or reduce VILI. Permissive hypercapnia, by reducing V_T to safer ranges, has allowed the reduction of peak inflation pressure to below 40 cm H_2O and improves survival in blast lung-injury victims.[61] The use of tracheal gas insufflation, addition of 5 to 10 L/min of 100% O_2 via a small bore catheter placed through the endotracheal tube down to the carina, enables the use of lower V_T and inflation pressures while maintaining the same Pa_{CO_2}.[62]

In severe cases of lung and vascular injuries, a variety of complex modes of support have been found to be successful in improving gas exchange. The use of inverse ratio ventilation in the form of pressure-controlled inverse-ratio ventilation (PCIRV) or airway pressure release ventilation (APRV) may improve lung volume, oxygenation, and ventilation and reduce high peak airway pressure when higher levels of airway pressure are needed.[63-65] Patients who present with severe asymmetric lung injury or significant air leak from one lung or who show signs of poor oxygenation despite the application of 100% oxygen and PEEP during conventional mechanical ventilation may improve with independent lung ventilation through a double-lumen endotracheal tube.[66-69]

High-frequency ventilation with jet and oscillating ventilators may also have utility in the chest trauma patient when the patient fails to respond to conventional ventilatory support.[70,71] In the most severe cases, extracorporeal membrane oxygenation (ECMO) may be required and should be available in level 1 trauma centers.[72] However, this modality may be contraindicated for patients with severe head trauma and may exacerbate cerebral hemorrhage. The use of heparin-bonded ECMO circuitry has been successful in support of the massively injured trauma victim and did not further their hemorrhaging.[73]

When the patient can effectively breathe spontaneously, a variety of support modes are available for matching the ventilator with the patient's breathing pattern, for example, pressure support (PS), volume support, and mandatory minute ventilation. Once patients are stabilized and improving (able to make breathing efforts, mean systemic blood pressure >90 mm Hg with minimal pressor support, FIO_2 <0.5, PEEP <8 cm H_2O), they should have a spontaneous breathing trial with FIO_2 of 0.5% and CPAP of 5 cm H_2O.[50] If the respiratory rate is less than 35/min and vital signs are stable, the patient should be advanced to pressure support of 20 cm H_2O (and titrated down to reduce the respiratory rate to less than 25/min) at the same FIO_2 and PEEP. If the patient has a spontaneous breathing trial that results in more than 35 breaths/min, the patient should be returned to AC or SIMV mode, and another breathing trial should be performed after the appropriate interventions are applied (e.g., suctioning, sedation, etc.).

Weaning from ventilatory support can be accomplished by switching from AC mode or by gradually decelerating the SIMV to pressure or volume support as the patient's respiratory muscles develop strength and stamina. If the patient tolerates PS at 5 cm H_2O and maintains a V_T of 4 to 5 mL/kg at a rate of

Mechanical ventilation of the chest trauma patient can be challenging. A wide variety of strategies and modes are available; the avoidance of high peak and plateau pressures and the careful use of PEEP are essential in any of these.

20 to 25/min with an F_{IO_2} of 0.4 at least 30 minutes, he or she can be placed on the same or slightly higher F_{IO_2} via a tracheostomy mask or Briggs T adapter and further assessed. In some trauma victims the use of NPPV has been found to be a successful weaning tool to facilitate the transition to effective spontaneous ventilation and reduce the length of ICU stay.[74]

Other Techniques of Respiratory Care

The patient with chest trauma often requires additional forms of respiratory care. Therapy using heated or cooled aerosol is frequently used for the management of secretions. Airway clearance is very important for those who have prosthetic airways or secretion retention. Chest physical therapy, whether by means of percussion or vibration, is often effective in mobilizing retained airway secretions and can be as effective as bronchoscopy in reexpanding atelectatic areas. Therapeutic bronchoscopy may be needed to remove mucus plugs and reoccurring atelectasis. Aerosolized bronchodilator therapy is frequently employed to reduce airway resistance, facilitate lung expansion, and reduce the work of breathing. These forms of respiratory care are important in the acute as well as long-term phases of treatment for chest trauma patients.

OUTCOME PREDICTION

A variety of measurements and scoring systems have been developed to help predict the outcome of trauma victims. The base deficit, routinely determined during arterial blood gas analysis, has been shown to be effective in predicting survival from trauma.[75,76] Patients who have a persistent base deficit below -6 mEq/liter in the first 24 hours generally had a poorer outcome, and these levels are associated with the development of ARDS and MODS.[77]

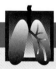

Mr. K

HISTORY

Mr. K is a 49-year old male, a daily user of alcohol, who was wearing his seat belt when he struck a logging truck on a rural two-lane road. He was unconscious when discovered a short while later. When paramedics assessed him in the field, he responded to a sternal rub by becoming combative. He underwent a prolonged extrication (more than 30 minutes). After his extrication, he was placed on a backboard, fitted with a cervical collar, and taken by helicopter to a level 1 trauma center, where he was assessed and trauma life support began.

QUESTIONS	ANSWERS
1. What signs and symptoms will need to be evaluated immediately upon Mr. K's arrival?	Signs of a patent airway, spontaneous breathing, quality of breath sounds and their symmetry, pulse rate, blood pressure, and level of consciousness should be evaluated.

2. What diagnostic techniques can be used to help determine the severity of Mr. K's injuries?	The nature and severity of his injuries can be better understood by determining the nature of the motor vehicle crash. A careful and rapid physical evaluation followed by radiographs of his spine, chest, abdomen, and extremities will be needed as indicated. Other important features include the degree and duration of shock, signs of gastric aspiration, signs of hypothermia, and any underlying medical conditions or history of substance abuse that may complicate his injuries.
3. What therapeutic support should be available upon Mr. K's arrival?	Oxygen therapy (cannula or non-rebreathing mask), intubation equipment, manual resuscitation bag with proper mask, oxygen reservoir and a PEEP capability, venous and arterial line placement equipment, fluids for vascular support, resuscitation drugs, chest tube placement equipment, and medications for pain and agitation should be available. Patients in shock as a result of internal bleeding must have direct access to the operating room upon arrival at the hospital.

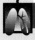 **More on Mr. K**

PHYSICAL EXAMINATION

- **General.** The patient has an approximate weight of 100 kg; is awake and frequently combative. The patient is supine on a backboard with a cervical collar on, and is spontaneously moving all extremities. The patient has an SpO_2 of 92% while breathing room air; his Glasgow coma scale score is 13.

- **Vital Signs.** Temperature 37.9°C; respiratory rate 17/min; blood pressure 120/90 mm Hg; heart rate 120/min; capillary refill 5 seconds.

- **HEENT.** Pupils equal and reactive to light; no obvious nasal flaring, left mandibular fracture, left ear laceration.

- **Neck.** Trachea midline; no signs of inspiratory stridor or contusion to the larynx; carotid pulses ++ bilaterally without bruit; no signs of lymphadenopathy or thyroidomegaly.

- **Chest.** Abrasions over the left chest; obvious flail motion of the left lateral and anterior chest with 1 to 2 cm depression on inspiration; subcutaneous air felt over the anterior and lateral left chest; breath sounds diminished in the left lung compared to the right lung with coarse crackles on the left.

- **Heart.** Regular rhythm at a rate of 110 to 120/min without murmurs, gallops, or rubs.

- **Abdomen.** Within normal limits.

- **Extremities.** Moving right extremities and left arm; signs of left femur fracture or hip dislocation with posterior displacement; no clubbing and no obvious cyanosis.

QUESTIONS	ANSWERS
4. What signs and symptoms indicate chest injuries?	Chest injuries are indicated by the presence of chest wall abrasions, flail motion, tachypnea, accessory muscle tensing, subcutaneous emphysema, and diminished breath sounds in the left lung.
5. How will the chest injuries influence respiratory function?	Flail chest will result in increased work of breathing and decreased efficiency of gas exchange. ABGs are almost always abnormal as a result of this type of injury.
6. What are the possible causes of Mr. K's respiratory distress?	His respiratory distress is probably due in part to the flail chest and pain from broken ribs. Other possible causes include pneumothorax or hemopneumothorax, lung contusion, tracheobronchial rupture, cardiac contusion, great vessel fracture, diaphragmatic herniation, and intraabdominal injuries. These changes may be inducing increased airway resistance, decreased pulmonary compliance, $\dot{V}/\dot{Q}$ mismatching, hypoxemia, and ventilatory failure.
7. In addition to the physical examination, how should Mr. K's cardiorespiratory status be further evaluated?	To evaluate his cardiorespiratory distress further, ABGs, ECG monitoring, and a chest radiograph are needed. Placement of peripheral venous, central venous, and arterial lines will be needed to guide and maintain hemodynamic stability. Because his mandibular fracture may point to more severe head injury, a CT of the head and a cross-table and C-spine radiograph are also indicated.
8. What other laboratory tests would be helpful?	Laboratory assessment of CBC, electrolytes, and standard blood chemistry and screening for alcohol and other substances are indicated. Alcohol consumption prior to the crash may be contributing to altered mental status and will require care and continued monitoring, but care must be used to avoid missing potential head injuries that may be masked by the presence of alcohol. Abdominal injuries should be evaluated by peritoneal lavage for the presence of blood.

 More on Mr. K

BEDSIDE AND LABORATORY EVALUATIONS

ECG: Sinus tachycardia of 117/min without any other abnormalities

Chest Radiograph: Subcutaneous air over the left hemothorax. Ribs 1 through 6 fractured on the left. Hemopneumothorax in the left pleural space. Signs of hazy infiltrate in the left, which is consistent with pulmonary contusion. Normal mediastinal width and no sign of pneumomediastinum. No foreign bodies visible.

ABGs: pH 7.35, $Paco_2$ 53 mm Hg, Pao_2 83 mm Hg, HCO_3^- 30 mEq/liter while breathing approximately 0.35 Fio_2 by nasal cannula

Hematology: Hematocrit (Hct) 19.2%; no other values available at this time

Chemistry and Toxicology: Results pending

CT: Reveals a left subarachnoid hemorrhage

QUESTIONS	ANSWERS
9. How would you interpret the ECG and blood pressure?	The ECG findings indicate a compensatory tachycardia in response to blood loss and stress.
10. What does the chest radiograph indicate, and what should be done based on these findings?	The chest radiographic findings reveal the magnitude of injuries after a severe blunt-impact injury to the left chest. The hemopneumothorax indicates the need for chest tube placement to drain blood and air. A chest CT should be considered.
11. How would you interpret the ABG data?	The ABG shows a fully compensated respiratory acidosis, hypoventilation, and hypoxemia. After severe blunt chest injuries, these findings are consistent with one or more of the following: shock, $\dot{V}/\dot{Q}$ abnormality, diffusion defect, and venous–arterial intrapulmonary shunting.
12. What do the hematologic data indicate?	The hematologic data may indicate anemia secondary to severe blood loss and require prompt location and ending of the bleeding.
13. What hemodynamic support is indicated at this time, and how should it be evaluated?	Fluid resuscitation with crystalloid IV infusion should be started. Blood should be given as soon as available. Evaluation of central venous pressure, systemic blood pressure, and renal output should be monitored to avoid hypotension or fluid overload. If hemodynamic instability develops, placement of a pulmonary artery balloon catheter for monitoring preload pressures, cardiac output, and afterload may be needed.
14. What complications may occur in the next 24 to 48 hours?	The severity of his blunt-impact injuries and shock provide multiple risk factors for the development of ARDS and multiple organ failure. He will require intensive care for continued ventilatory support, IV fluid administration, and monitoring of neurologic, cardiovascular, pulmonary, and renal function. Additionally, the subarachnoid hemorrhage may worsen, with negative sequelae.

More on Mr. K

On admission and evaluation at the trauma center, Mr. K's problem list now includes the following:

1. Shock from blunt trauma to the chest and head

2. Multiple rib fractures, flail chest, lung contusion, and subcutaneous emphysema on the left side

3. Midline abdominal incision after repair of multiple abdominal injuries

4. Closed head injury with potential hypoxic brain injury

5. Rule out spinal injuries and hip fracture

The goals of his initial treatment at the trauma center concentrate on improving cardio-vascular stability, respiratory function, and neurologic status. In the trauma unit, Mr. K is prepared for the insertion of a chest tube. While preparing for the procedure, he again becomes combative and tachypneic, with shallow breaths. An ABG drawn at this time and analyzed with a handheld device reveals: pH 7.31, $Paco_2$ 53 mm Hg, Pao_2 104 mm Hg while breathing approximately 100% oxygen by non-rebreather mask.

QUESTIONS	ANSWERS
15. What respiratory care is indicated at this time, and how should it be evaluated?	The patient will need to be fully supported. After intubation, visual inspection of chest motion and breath sounds will be needed for initial determination of proper tube placement. To help correct the hypoxemia and acidosis, his initial ventilator support could include the following parameters: PRVC mode, set V_T at 700 mL, set rate at 18/min, an I:E ratio of 1:3, set PEEP at 0 cm H_2O, and set Fio_2 at 1.0. Place chest tubes in the left hemothorax. A repeat physical examination, vital signs, ABG, and chest radiograph should be done to determine the patient's initial response to therapy.

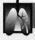

More on Mr. K

In the trauma unit, Mr. K is orally intubated using a rapid sequence technique, with an 8.5-mm cuffed tube, and placed on mechanical ventilation with 100% oxygen. Peripheral venous and arterial lines are in place. A 36-French chest tube is placed in the left pleural space, and 25 cm H_2O of suction is applied by underwater seal drainage systems. Air and 600 mL of blood are immediately removed.

Shortly after intubation and placement of the chest tube and central catheter, Mr. K's bedside findings, vital signs, chest radiograph, ventilator settings, and laboratory data are as follows:

Mr. K is lying in a semi-Fowler's position and is orally intubated, with a chest tube exiting his left thorax. A small amount of blood (less than 20 mL/hour) is continuously draining from the chest tubes, and no air leaks are crossing the water seal. He periodically becomes combative, requiring reassurance, anxiolytic/amnesics for agitation (Versed), analgesics for pain (Morphine), and anesthetic agents (Fentanyl) for sedation. He is following the set rate of the Servo 300A ventilator through an endotracheal tube (8.5-mm internal diameter). The endotracheal tube has 25 cm H_2O pressure in the cuff, and no gas leakage is heard over the cuff site. The airway is secured to the upper lip with waterproof tape and is showing the 24-cm mark at the lip. The left hemithorax is noted to have a flail motion if he becomes agitated and makes spontaneous efforts to breathe. His breath sounds are generally diminished over the left lung, with better aeration noted in the right lung, with coarse rhonchi heard on the left. On suctioning his airway, small amounts of mucoid sputum are removed. In-line ventilator circuit delivery of 4 to 6 puffs of albuterol via metered-dose inhaler (MDI) and spacer is being given every 4 hours and as needed (prn).

Bedside Findings

Vital Signs and Hemodynamics	
Measure	Value
Rectal temperature	37.9°C
Respiratory rate	18/min
Heart rate	110/min
Systemic arterial blood pressure	170/90 mm Hg
Central venous pressure	9 mm Hg
Urine output	approximately 100 mL/hour since admission
Chest Radiograph: See Figure 12.4	

Ventilator Settings and Findings	
Measure	Value
PRVC ventilation	rate set 18/min
V_T	set 0.7 liter
V_T	exh 0.72 liter
F_{IO_2}	1.0
Total respiratory rate	18/min
V_E	12.8 liters/min
Peak pressure	33 cm H_2O
Set PEEP	5 cm H_2O

Laboratory Evaluation

ABG	Value
pH	7.35
Pa_{CO_2}	44 mm Hg
Pa_{O_2}	350 mm Hg
HCO_3^-	23 mEq/liter
$P(A-a)O_2$	308 mm Hg
Pa_{O_2}/F_{IO_2}	350
Sa_{O_2}	100% (calculated)
Sp_{O_2}	99% (pulse oximeter)

Toxicology: Alcohol and marijuana found
Microbiology: Blood, sputum, and wound smear and cultures pending

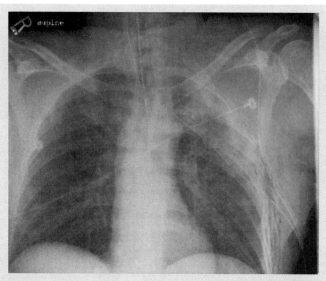

FIGURE 12.4 Chest radiograph shortly after intubation in the trauma center.

QUESTIONS	ANSWERS
16. What do Mr. K's airway care and breath sounds indicate? What would be recommended at this time?	The airway is appropriate and its position appears acceptable. Cuff pressure is effectively sealing the trachea at a safe pressure and is high enough to help avoid silent aspiration of saliva around the cuff. Placement of a tracheostomy tube is not indicated at this time. Breath sounds indicate reduced ventilation of the right lung and retained secretions. The in-line aerosolization of albuterol is appropriate. The sputum removed from the airway does not suggest pulmonary hemorrhage or infection at this time. Special attention to the airway, its maintenance, and sterile technique are necessary to help avoid complications.
17. How would you describe Mr. K's hemodynamics?	The hemodynamic values are acceptable after fluid replacement. The right heart filling pressure (central venous pressure) indicates that he has an adequate blood volume at this time.
18. How would you describe the radiographic findings?	The portable anteroposterior chest radiograph taken shortly after admission to the trauma center shows subcutaneous emphysema in the lateral left hemothorax with generalized loss of lung volume. Ribs 1 through 6 are fractured, and a left lung pulmonary contusion with air bronchograms is present. A chest tube is seen in the left thorax, the endotracheal tube is 4 cm above carina, and a nasogastric tube has been placed.

19. How would you describe the ventilator settings, breathing pattern, and pulmonary mechanics? Are the ventilator settings appropriate for Mr. K's condition? What should be recommended at this time?

The ventilator settings indicate that he is receiving substantial ventilatory support while in a state of mild tachypnea with a potentially toxic FIO_2. The V_T setting of 0.7 liter (7 mL/kg) is at the upper limit of acceptable for his frame size. The PEEP is necessary to improve $\dot{V}/\dot{Q}$ matching, prevent further development of atelectasis, and allow FIO_2 reduction, though caution is indicated in the presence of his head injury. His respiratory pattern is not resulting in any additional auto-PEEP, although he may start gas trapping if his rate increases.

His PaO_2 is excessive, and his FIO_2 should be titrated with continuous pulse oximetry to maintain a targeted SpO_2 of greater than 90%. The $P(A-a)O_2$ is significantly increased and indicates a diffusion defect, shunting, $\dot{V}/\dot{Q}$ mismatching, or a combination of these. His oxygen content is acceptable at 18 mL/dL. The $PaCO_2$ is normal but is requiring elevated minute ventilation as a result of an increased metabolic rate, dead space ventilation, or both. The acid–base balance is acceptable.

 ## More on Mr. K

After assessment of Mr. K's condition, his oxygen is gradually decreased to 50% over the next two hours. He undergoes a successful surgery for open reduction of a left acetabular fracture. However, over the next three days, his breath sounds become progressively coarser sounding, with bilateral inspiratory and expiratory rhonchi and wheezes, and are diminished on the left. His secretion output increases to the degree that he requires tracheobronchial suctioning every half an hour to maintain a patent airway. Aerosolized bronchodilation continues, and he undergoes fiberoptic bronchoscopy for therapeutic and diagnostic reasons. Secretion samples are sent to the lab for culture and sensitivity.

For the next week his ventilatory requirements continue at the same level, and he cannot tolerate weaning attempts in SIMV without becoming excessively tachypneic, desaturated (by pulse oximetry), tachycardic, and hypertensive. Cyclic fever spikes and episodic atelectasis with infiltrates occur during this period. These pulmonary changes require rigorous pulmonary hygiene and a second therapeutic bronchoscopy for removal of mucus plugs. His chest tube remains in place, and a second chest tube is placed after the first tube is obstructed by a blood clot. His nutritional status is maintained through regular central line alimentation until nasogastric tube feedings are tolerated.

Seven days after his injury his temperature increases to 38.3°C. The cultures from the repeat bronchoscopies reveal significant (4+) levels of *H. influenzae* and *S. aureus*. A chest radiograph taken at this time (Figure 12.5) shows increasing infiltrates with a loss of lung volume. The endotracheal tube and other invasive catheters all appear to be in their proper positions. Treatment is started with Vancomycin, and aggressive airway care and aerosolized bronchodilator therapy is continued. Over the next 48 hours Mr. K's breath sounds, sputum production, and chest radiograph improve. Ventilatory support is gradually reduced to PS of 18 cm H_2O and 40% oxygen. Over the next week, this pattern of fever spike, breath-sound changes, purulent sputum with heavy bacterial counts, chest radi-

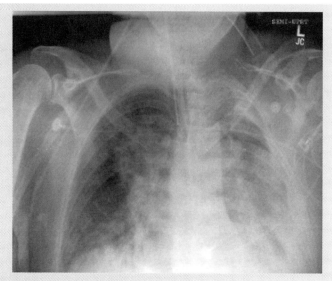

FIGURE 12.5 Chest radiograph 7 days after admission to the trauma center.

ographic findings consistent with pneumonia, increasing ventilatory support requirements, antibiotic treatment with Clindamycin and Ciprofloxin in addition to the Vancomycin, and intensive airway care is repeated. His ventilatory support is adjusted between pressure support and volume support modes, as indicated by clinical impression. His chest tube remains in place. Though the subarachnoid hemorrhage has not continued or expanded, his level of consciousness has not improved; he is in alcohol withdrawal, combative and not responsive to instruction or verbal stimuli. It is believed that he will require prolonged ventilatory support because of his unchanged mental status and pneumonia. He is percutaneously tracheostomized with an 8.0 tracheostomy tube in place, and ventilatory support continues. His bedside findings, vital signs, chest radiograph, ventilator settings, and laboratory data are as follows:

Mr. K is sitting up in bed, tracheostomized. He is spontaneously initiating every breath from the Servo 300A. The left hemothorax is still noted to have some flail motion when he makes vigorous efforts to breathe. His breath sounds are generally diminished over the left lung, with better aeration noted in the right lung; inspiratory and expiratory rhonchi are heard bilaterally. Moderate amounts of mucoid sputum are periodically removed during airway care. In-line ventilator circuit delivery of eight puffs of albuterol by MDI continues every 4 hours and prn.

Bedside Findings

Vital Signs, Hemodynamics, and Urine Output	
Measure	Value
Temperature	38.5°C
Respiratory rate	21/min (total rate observed while on ventilator)
Heart rate	100/min
Systemic arterial blood pressure	105/50 mm Hg
Urine output continuing at about	70 mL/hour

Chest Radiograph

Multiple rib fractures on the left and patchy infiltrates bilaterally, which are in the process of clearing. Tracheostomy tube and other invasive devices apparently in their proper positions.

Ventilator Settings and Findings

mode	PS + PEEP
PS	10 cm H_2O
PS exhaled V_T	0.425 to 0.635 liter
FIO_2	0.30
Set PEEP	5 cm H_2O
Gas temperature	34°C (93.2°F)
Total respiratory rate	21/min
V_E	11.6 liters/min
Peak pressure	15 cm H_2O

Laboratory Evaluation

ABG	Value
pH	7.42
$PaCO_2$	38 mm Hg
PaO_2	96 mm Hg
HCO_3^-	24 mEq/liter
$P(A-a)O_2$	68 mm Hg
PaO_2/FIO_2	320
Hb	14 g/dL
SaO_2	98% (calculated)
SpO_2	97%
CaO_2	18.6 mL/dL

QUESTIONS	ANSWERS
20. How would you interpret Mr. K's vital signs?	His vital signs indicate a mild stress response with the presence of mild tachypnea and tachycardia. Urine output and temperature are within normal limits.
21. What do the current ventilator settings and breathing pattern indicate about Mr. K's ventilator support?	He is currently in a spontaneous mode of pressure support ventilation with a low level of PEEP. His respiratory pattern shows mild tachypnea, acceptable tidal ventilation (5 to 7 mL/kg), and moderately elevated minute ventilation. Approximately 75% or more of his pressure support is overcoming the airway resistance imposed by the endotracheal tube. The FIO_2 is modestly elevated but well below a toxic level.
22. What do the ABGs indicate?	His most recent ABG data indicate acceptable oxygenation with slight elevation of the $P(A-a)O_2$ consistent with persistent but improving $\dot{V}/\dot{Q}$ mismatching. The $PaCO_2$ indicates normal alveolar ventilation despite the elevated minute ventilation. The relatively high minute ventilation may be due to elevated metabolism or dead space, or both. The acid-base data indicate a normal balance.

23. What course of action would you recommend at this time? Why?

He should remain in PS ventilation to stabilize his respiratory, cardiovascular, and psychological status. A gradual approach to his weaning from ventilatory support will be necessary. The placement of a tracheostomy tube should facilitate his weaning and secretion management and should prevent further laryngeal injury from the endotracheal tube.

A number of weaning strategies can be used. Short trials of low-level PS (e.g., 5 cm H_2O) for 5 to 30 minutes three to four times per day could be tried. These trials can then be lengthened as he develops more respiratory muscle endurance and less dyspnea. Continued assessment of his head injury; respiratory tract secretions; pain; and nutritional, psychological, and fluid and electrolyte status should be made.

Mr. K Conclusion

Mr. K is continued in PS ventilation, and it is decided to attempt T-tube trials with adequate oxygen three times per day for 30 minutes, as tolerated. T-tube trials continue over the next week until he is able to remain off the ventilator throughout the day and most of the night without excessive dyspnea. Thirty days after his injury, he tolerates removal from the ventilator. He does well on 30% oxygen via cool aerosol to a tracheostomy collar. Over time, his pulmonary condition improves enough for him to be decannulated, and his fractures, hemopneumothorax, and infiltrates resolved (Figure 12.6). Unfortunately, his mental status does not improve, and the patient requires either sedation or constant interaction with caregivers to prevent him from injuring himself. Mr. K requires transfer to a rehabilitation program for long-term care. ■

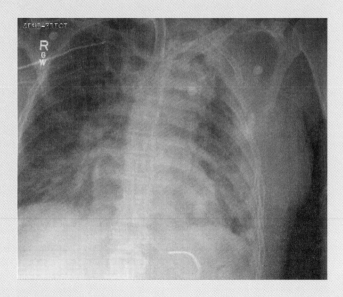

FIGURE 12.6 Chest radiograph 30 days after admission to the trauma center.

KEY POINTS

- Chest trauma is second only to head trauma as a cause of death in the United States, with trauma overall as the leading cause of death in the first four decades of life.
- Chest trauma can be classified as penetrating, blunt, or a combination of the two.
- Homicide, suicide, and other acts of violence are the causes of most penetrating chest trauma.
- Motor vehicle crashes are the most common cause of blunt chest trauma.
- Four general anatomic regions of the chest may be involved in chest trauma: the thoracic cage, the conducting airways, the lung parenchyma, and the pleura.
- The scope of traumatic chest injury includes damage to the chest wall, pleura, tracheobronchial tree, lungs, diaphragm, esophagus, heart, and great vessels.
- Penetrating wounds are most commonly produced by knives or high-speed and low-speed missiles, such as bullets or fragments from explosions.
- The pathophysiology of chest trauma includes chest wall injury, lung parenchymal injury, cardiac injury, airway injury, and diaphragm injury. Each injury type has a wide range of severity.
- Flail chest, tension pneumothorax, tracheal injury, and cardiac rupture or tamponade are severe, often life-threatening injuries that require emergent treatment.
- In limited cases, the use of NPPV techniques such as CPAP and BiPAP may have some utility in treating respiratory distress in the trauma patient.
- Positive pressure ventilation must be performed using the lowest peak and plateau pressures possible.
- Low tidal volumes and careful use of PEEP help to attain the goal of low pressures in these patients.
- The use of permissive hypercapnea and tracheal gas insufflation permits the use of lower tidal volumes.
- Consider adjunctive therapies, such as proning, to attain acceptable levels of oxygenation.
- Special modes of ventilation (such as high-frequency ventilation, ECMO, and inhaled nitric oxide) may be of utility in limited patient populations.
- The chest trauma patient can benefit from a variety of respiratory therapies in addition to mechanical ventilation. Appropriate bronchodilator therapy, postural drainage, percussion and vibration, and, in some cases, therapeutic bronchoscopy, may be required.
- Poor outcome from chest trauma is associated with a persistent base deficit of less than -6 mEq/L in the first 24 hours post-injury.

REFERENCES

1. 20 Leading Causes of Death, United States 2002, All Races, Both Sexes. Centers for Disease Control and Prevention, 2004.
2. Kulshrestha, P, et al: Profile of chest trauma in a level I trauma center. J Trauma 57:576, 2004.
3. 2002 United States Unintentional Injuries, All Ages, All Races, Both Sexes. Centers for Disease Control and Prevention, 2004.
4. Peters, R: Biomechanics of chest injury. In Nahum, AM, Melvin, J (eds): The Biomechanics of Trauma. Appleton-Century-Crofts, Norwalk, CT, 1985.
5. de Ceballos, JP, et al: 11 March 2004: The terrorist bomb explosions in Madrid, Spain: an analysis of the logistics, injuries sustained and clinical management of casualties treated at the closest hospital. Crit Care 9:104, 2005.

6. Bartlett, C: Clinical update: gunshot wound ballistics. Clin Orthop 1:28, 2003.

7. Fackler, M: Gunshot wound review. Ann Emerg Med 28:194, 1996.

8. Kirsh, MM: Acute thoracic injuries. In Siegel, JH (ed): Trauma: Emergency Surgery and Critical Care. Churchill Livingstone, New York, 1987.

9. Perchinsky, M, et al: Trauma-associated dissection of the thoracic aorta. J Trauma 45:626, 1998.

10. Keough, V, Pudelek, B: Blunt chest trauma: review of selected pulmonary injuries focusing on pulmonary contusion. AACN Clin Issues 12:270, 2001.

11. Wilson, RF: Trauma. In Shoemaker WC, et al (eds): Textbook of Critical Care, ed. 2. WB Saunders, Philadelphia, 1989.

12. Wanek, S, Mayberry, JC: Blunt thoracic trauma: flail chest, pulmonary contusion, and blast injury. Crit Care Clin 20:71, 2004.

13. Mizushima, Y, et al: Changes in contused lung volume and oxygenation in patients with pulmonary parenchymal injury after blunt chest trauma. Am J Emerg Med 18:385, 2000.

14. Velmahos, GC, et al: Influence of flail chest on outcome among patients with severe thoracic cage trauma. Int Surg. 87:240, 2002.

15. Tanaka, H, et al: Surgical stabilization of internal pneumatic stabilization? A prospective randomized study of management of severe flail chest patients. J Trauma. 52:727, 2002.

16. Hudson, LD, et al: Clinical risks for development of the acute respiratory distress syndrome. Am J Respir Crit Care Med 151:293, 1995.

17. Miller, PR, et al: Acute respiratory distress syndrome in blunt trauma: identification of independent risk factors. Am Surg. 68:845, 2002.

18. Navarrete-Navarro, P, et al: Acute respiratory distress syndrome among trauma patients: trends in ICU mortality, risk factors, complications and resource utilization. Intensive Care Med 27:1133, 2001.

19. Ecker, RR, et al: Injuries of the trachea and bronchi. Ann Thorac Surg 11:289, 1971.

20. Fuhrman, GM, et al: Blunt laryngeal trauma: classification and management protocol. J Trauma 30:87, 1990.

21. Pate, JW: Tracheobronchial and esophageal injuries. Surg Clin North Am 69:111, 1989.

22. Neal, D: Blunt Thoracic Trauma. Available at www. trauma.org.

23. Feghali, NT, Prisant LM: Blunt myocardial injury. Chest 108:1673, 1995.

24. Schultz, JM, Trunkey DD: Blunt cardiac injury. Crit Care Clin 20:57, 2004.

25. Spodick, DH: Current concepts: acute cardiac tamponade. N Engl J Med 349:684, 2003.

26. Salim, A, et al: Clinically significant blunt cardiac trauma: role of serum troponin levels combined with electrocardiograph findings. J Trauma 50:237, 2001.

27. Velmahos, GC, et al: Normal electrocardiography and serum troponin I levels preclude the presence of clinically significant blunt cardiac injury. J Trauma 54:45, 2003.

28. Symbas, PN, Gott, JP: Delayed sequela of thoracic trauma. Surg Clin North Am 69:135, 1989.

29. Ott, MC, et al: management of blunt thoracic aortic injuries: endovascular stents versus open repair. J Trauma 56:565, 2004.

30. Haciibrahimoglu, G, et al: Management of traumatic diaphragmatic rupture. Surg Today 34:111, 2004.

31. Kishikawa, M, et al: Pulmonary contusion causes long-term respiratory dysfunction with decreased functional residual capacity. J Trauma 31:1203, 1991.

32. Yeo, TP: Long-term sequelae associated with blunt thorax trauma. Orthop Nurs 20:35, 2001.

33. Advanced Trauma Life Support Course, American College of Surgeons, Chicago, 1997.

34. Richards, CF, Mayberry, JC: Initial management of the trauma patient. Crit Care Clin 20:1, 2004.

35. Trupka, A, et al: Value of thoracic computed tomography in the first assessment of severely injured patients with blunt chest trauma: results of a prospective study. J Trauma 43:405, 1997.

36. Karmakar, MK, Ho, AM: Acute pain management of patients with multiple fractured ribs. J Trauma 54:615, 2003.

37. Haenel, JB, et al: Extrapleural bupivacaine for amelioration of multiple rib fracture pain. J Trauma 38:22, 1995.

38. Divatia J, et al: Failed intubation managed with subcricoid transtracheal jet ventilation followed by percutaneous rracheostomy. Anesthesiology 96:1519, 2002.

39. Trinkle, JK, et al: Management of flail chest without mechanical ventilation. Ann Thorac Surg 19:355, 1975.

40. Hurst, JM, et al: Use of CPAP mask as the sole mode of ventilatory support in trauma patients with mild to moderate respiratory insufficiency. J Trauma 25:1065, 1985.

41. Branson, RD: PEEP without endotracheal intubation. Respir Care 33:598, 1988.

42. Antonelli, M, et al: A comparison of noninvasive positive-pressure ventilation and conventional mechanical ventilation in patients with acute respiratory failure. N Engl J Med 339:429, 1998.

43. Ferrer M, et al: Noninvasive ventilation in severe hypoxemic respiratory failure: a randomized clinical trial. Am J Respir Crit Care Med 168:1438, 2003.

44. Keenan, SP, et al: Does noninvasive positive pressure ventilation improve outcome in acute hypoxemic respiratory failure? A systematic review. Crit Care Med 32:2516, 2004.

45. Antonelli, M, et al: Predictors of failure of noninvasive positive pressure ventilation in patients with acute hypoxemic respiratory failure: a multi-center study. Intensive Care Med 27:1718, 2001.

46. Sharma, S, et al: Ventilatory management of pulmonary contusion patients. Am J Surg 171:529, 1996.

47. Schreiter, D, et al: Alveolar recruitment in combination with sufficient positive end expiratory pressure increases oxygenation and lung aeration in patients with severe chest trauma. Crit Care Med 32:968, 2004.

48. Böhm, S, et al: The open lung concept. In Vincent, JL (ed): Yearbook of Intensive Care and Emergency Medicine.. Berlin, Springer Verlag, 1998.

49. Lachmann, B: Open up the lung and keep the lung open. Intensive Care Med 18:319, 1992.

50. The Acute Respiratory Distress Syndrome Network: Ventilation with lower tidal volumes as compared with traditional tidal volumes for acute lung injury and the acute respiratory distress syndrome. N Engl J Med 342:1301, 2000.

51. Levy, MM: Optimal PEEP in ARDS: changing concepts and current controversies. Crit Care Clin 18:15, 2002.

52. Michaels, AJ: Management of post traumatic respiratory failure. Crit Care Clin 20:83, 2004.

53. Gattinoni, L, et al: How to ventilate patients with acute lung injury and acute respiratory distress syndrome. Curr Opin Crit Care. 11:69, 2005.

54. Tugrul, S, et al: Effects of sustained inflation and postinflation positive end-expiratory pressure in acute respiratory distress syndrome: focusing on pulmonary and extrapulmonary forms. Crit Care Med 31:738, 2003.

55. Johannigman, JA, et al: Influence of low tidal volumes on gas exchange in acute respiratory distress syndrome and the role of recruitment maneuvers. J Trauma 54:320, 2003.

56. Brower, RG, et al: Effects of recruitment maneuvers in patients with acute lung injury and acute respiratory distress syndrome ventilated with high positive end-expiratory pressure. Crit Care Med 31:2592, 2003.

57. Voggenreiter, G, et al: Intermittent prone positioning in the treatment of severe and moderate post-traumatic lung injury. Crit Care Med 27:2375, 1999.

58. Ward, NS: Effects of prone position ventilation in ARDS. An evidence-based review of the literature. Crit Care Clin 18:35, 2002.

59. Gattinoni, L, et al: Decrease in $PaCO_2$ with prone position is predictive of improved outcome in acute respiratory distress syndrome. Crit Care Med 31:2727, 2003.

60. Meaudre, E, et al: Nitric oxide inhalation is useful in the management of right ventricular failure caused by myocardial contusion. Acta Anaesthesiol Scand 49:415, 2005.

61. Sorkine, P, et al: Permissive hypercapnea ventilation in patients with severe pulmonary blast injury. J Trauma 45:35–38, 1998.

62. Nakos, G, et al: Tracheal gas insufflation reduces the tidal volume while $PaCO_2$ is maintained constant. Intensive Care Med 20:407, 1994.

63. Wang, SH, Wei, TS: The outcome of early pressure-controlled inverse ratio ventilation on patients with severe acute respiratory distress syndrome in surgical intensive care unit. Am J Surg 183:151, 2002.

64. Rasanen, J, et al: Airway pressure release ventilation during acute lung injury: a prospective multicenter trial. Crit Care Med 19:1234, 1991.

65. Frawley, PM, Habashi, NM: Airway pressure release ventilation: theory and practice. AACN Clin Issues 12:234, 2001.

66. Kanarek, DJ, Shannon, DC: Adverse effect of positive end expiratory pressure on pulmonary perfusion and arterial oxygenation. Am Rev Respir Dis 112:457, 1976.

67. Glass, DD, et al: Therapy of unilateral pulmonary insufficiency with double lumen endotracheal tube. Crit Care Med 4:323, 1976.

68. Branson, RD, et al: Synchronous independent lung ventilation in the treatment of unilateral pulmonary contusion: a report of two cases. Respir Care 29: 361, 1984.

69. Katsaragakis, S, et al: Independent lung ventilation for asymmetrical chest trauma: effect on ventilatory and haemodynamic parameters. Injury 36:501, 2005.

70. Derdak, S: High-frequency oscillatory ventilation for acute respiratory distress syndrome in adult patients. Crit Care Med 31 (Suppl.):S317, 2003.

71. Riou, B, et al: High-frequency jet ventilation in life-threatening bilateral pulmonary contusion. Anesthesiology 94:927, 2001.

72. Dauphine, C, et al: Selective use of cardiopulmonary bypass in trauma patients. Am Surg 71:46, 2005.

73. Perchinsky, MJ, et al: Extracorporeal cardiopulmonary life support with heparin-bonded circuitry in the resuscitation of massively injured trauma patients. Am J Surg 169:488, 1995.

74. deBoisblanc, MW, et al: Weaning injured patients with prolonged pulmonary failure from mechanical ventilation in a non-intensive care unit setting. J Trauma 49:224, 2000.

75. Rutherford, EJ, et al: Base deficit stratifies mortality and determines therapy. J Trauma 33:417, 1992.

76. Rixen, D, et al: Base deficit development and its prognostic significance in posttrauma critical illness: an analysis by the trauma registry of the Deutsche Gesellschaft fur unfallchirurgie. Shock 15:83, 2001.

77. Rixen, D, Siegel, JH: Metabolic correlates of oxygen debt predict posttrauma early acute respiratory distress syndrome and the related cytokine response. J Trauma 49:392, 2000.

13

Postoperative Atelectasis

Thomas P. Malinowski, BS, RRT, FAARC

CHAPTER OBJECTIVES:

After reading this chapter you will be able to identify the following:

- The definition of atelectasis.
- Factors predisposing patients to develop atelectasis.
- Clinical features associated with atelectasis.
- Treatment options for patients with atelectasis.

INTRODUCTION

Atelectasis is a clinical condition characterized by regions of the lung that are collapsed or airless. Atelectasis commonly occurs during and after surgery, and unless properly managed can lead to pneumonia, respiratory failure, and an increase in hospital stay.[1] Weight, age, anesthetics, surgical site, and intra-operative management all influence a patient's risk for postoperative atelectasis.[2]

Adults are not the only patients susceptible to postoperative atelectasis. Atelectasis has been reported to occur in about 10% to 30% of postoperative surgical cases involving infants and children.[3]

ETIOLOGY

Three factors may combine or independently contribute to the development of atelectasis: inadequate lung distending forces, obstruction of the airways leading to absorption of alveolar air, and insufficient surfactant levels.[4] All three of these factors may occur in surgical patients, especially during the postoperative period.

Inadequate Lung Distention

Lung expansion depends on (1) the ability of the respiratory muscles to generate negative intrapleural pressures and (2) an intact chest cage. Factors that weaken or alter respiratory muscle function reduce the ability to generate normal negative inspiratory pressures. This reduction in transpulmonary pressure leads to alveolar collapse or atelectasis.

The risk for atelectasis can begin prior to surgery. Any condition that reduces a patient's inspiratory capacity decreases the ability to recruit collapsed alveoli. For example, patients who have limited diaphragm movement because of their larger abdomen (morbid obesity, pregnancy) have lower functional residual capacity (FRC) and a propensity to airway closure. These patients show radiographic evidence of atelectasis prior to anesthesia induction and have more severe and prolonged atelectasis postoperatively.[5]

Elderly patients who are malnourished may be unable to generate the inspiratory force necessary for deep breathing and coughing. Patients with chest wall abnormalities (e.g., kyphosis, scoliosis) have limited lung expansion because of their thoracic cage malformation. Diaphragmatic movement may be limited in those with neuromuscular disease. Pulmonary fibrosis causes the lung to expand poorly in response to normal negative intrapleural pressure changes.

Although numerous intraoperative factors affect lung distention, the most significant may be the type of anesthesia. General anesthesia causes a reduction in FRC within minutes of induction. Atelectasis and induced airway collapse have been implicated in 75% of the patients experiencing hypoxia during general anesthesia.[6] Atelectasis occurs in both spontaneously breathing and mechanically ventilated anesthetized patients.[7] Both inhaled and intravenous agents produce this result. Ketamine is the only anesthetic agent that does not produce this effect, unless used in combination with a paralytic agent.[8] When patients are supine and given anesthetics and paralytics, the diaphragm relaxes and the posterior section displaces cephalad.[9] In addition, prolonged use of paralytic agents may be associated with diaphragmatic muscle atrophy and may result in a reduction in diaphragmatic strength. In some patients use of steroidal preparations in combination with paralytic agents results in a neuromyopathy and weaning failure.[10]

Newborns and infants are prone to alveolar collapse under anesthesia. FRC constitutes 40% to 50% of total lung capacity (TLC) in awake infants. The FRC is strongly influenced by diaphragmatic and intercostal tone, and to a lesser extent by active cessation of exhalation. In sedated patients upper airway tone is depressed, chest wall and diaphragm excursion reduced, and FRC falls to 10% to 15% of TLC, resulting in ventilation-perfusion ($\dot{V}/\dot{Q}$) mismatch and hypoxemia.[11]

Body positioning also impacts atelectasis development. Adults reclining from an upright to supine position experience a reduction in FRC even when awake. Anesthesia results in a further reduction. Proning patients from a supine position slightly increases FRC. Lateral decubitus positioning results in a reduction in FRC in the dependent lung, with a comparable increase in FRC in the nondependent lung.[7]

The type, location, and duration of the surgical procedure also affect lung distention.[2,12–14] Upper abdominal procedures present the greatest risk for atelectasis, followed by thoracic, lower abdominal, and peripheral procedures. Diaphragmatic function may be compromised by fluid accumulation in the abdominal space (ascites, peritoneal fluid) and pleural space (pleural effusion). Following upper abdominal surgery, postoperative pain may lead to decreased respiratory effort and a reduction in pleural and intra-abdominal pressures, resulting in atelectasis.[2] Patients who have thoracic surgery are also at risk for postoperative atelectasis. Topical cooling of the left phrenic nerve during cardiac surgery can cause inadequate diaphragmatic movement postoperatively and can contribute to left lower lobe atelectasis.[15] In the postoperative period the inadequate lung distention may persist for 2 to 10 days, especially in the presence of complications such as excessive pain or pleural effusion.[16]

Newborns and infants also are susceptible to atelectasis in the postoperative period. Lung expansion is limited by poor ventilatory reserve (i.e., less diaphragmatic muscle mass and strength) and a less effective cough secondary to muscle weakness. In addition, diaphragmatic enervation may be immature and insufficient to respond to an increased ventilatory need (Box 13.1).

Box 13.1 Factors that Decrease Ability to Generate Adequate Lung Distention

> Anesthesia
> Pain
> Reduction in lung volume
> Diaphragmatic apraxia: phrenic neuropathy, myopathy
> Chest wall disorders
> Obesity, ascites, pregnancy
> Malnutrition

Obstruction and Absorption of Alveolar Air

The development of postoperative atelectasis can also occur as a result of retained secretions in the bronchi.[4,17] Secretion retention occurs when mucociliary transport is diminished, cough is weak or absent, secretion volume is excessive, or hydration is inadequate. Anesthetic agents impair mucociliary activity and depress tidal volume and cough. Humidity is rarely added during anesthesia, and the anesthesiologist frequently administers pharmacological agents that dry respiratory secretions.[9] Pathological conditions associated with excessive secretions and impaired mucus transport such as smoking and chronic bronchitis increase the risk of secretion retention.[14] Mucus plugs lead to atelectasis with absorption of gases distal to the obstruction. This condition is enhanced during breathing of anesthetic gases and/or high inspired oxygen concentrations because these gases are more readily absorbed into the pulmonary blood flow.[18,19]

Intubated infants and children are particularly susceptible to secretion retention and partial obstruction of both the endotracheal tube and the airways. Limited collateral ventilation and reduced airway diameter make neonatal and pediatric patients susceptible to lobar atelectasis from secretion retention (Box 13.2).

Box 13.2 Factors Predisposing to Obstruction and Absorption of Alveolar Air

> Anesthetics
> Dry, inspired gases
> Intubated children, infants
> Diseases associated with excessive secretions, impaired
>   mucus transport
> Bronchiectasis, COPD, cystic fibrosis, asthma
> Elevated inspired oxygen concentration (>0.80 FIO_2)

Surfactant Depletion

An adequate quantity and quality of **surfactant** is necessary to maintain alveolar stability and prevent collapse. Pulmonary edema, smoke inhalation, inhaled anesthetics, lung contusion, pulmonary embolus, acute respiratory distress syndrome (ARDS), high FIO_2 concentrations, and prolonged breathing at low tidal volumes reduce the quantity and quality of surfactant.[4,7] Cardiopulmonary bypass may result in an inadequate perfusion of the lung and alveolar epithelium leading to insufficient release of surfactant.[20]

> Atelectasis develops when lung volume is reduced, leading to a fall in FRC. Atelectasis can be present before surgery but often develops in the operating room during anesthesia. Anesthesia depresses respiratory muscle tone and function. Patients requiring abdominal surgery with major incisions are at most risk for atelectasis.

PATHOPHYSIOLOGY

Atelectasis results in a decrease in FRC and lung compliance. This, in turn, results in alterations in the distribution of the inhaled gas without corresponding changes in perfusion. As a result, ventilation-perfusion ($\dot{V}/\dot{Q}$) mismatching occurs and leads to hypoxemia. General anesthesia also inhibits hypoxic pulmonary vasoconstriction reflexes in the lung, which further contributes to $\dot{V}/\dot{Q}$ mismatching and hypoxemia.[7,20]

Increased surface tension holds collapsed alveoli shut and requires higher distending pressures to reinflate the affected regions of the lung. Unaffected lung regions are more compliant and easier to inflate. The more compliant regions receive a greater proportion of the tidal volume than atelectatic areas and may be easily overinflated when large tidal volumes are used with mechanical ventilation.

Patients with moderate to severe atelectasis exhibit significant increases in work of breathing. Increased work of breathing adds a significant work load to the muscles of breathing and contributes to the onset of respiratory failure, especially in those with preexisting lung disease.

CLINICAL FEATURES

History

Signs and symptoms of atelectasis vary with the amount of lung involved, the patient's previous health status, and the duration of the problem. Dyspnea is the most common symptom but may not be present if the patient has minimal lung involvement and is otherwise healthy. When atelectasis involves larger portions of the lung or when the patient has a chronic lung disease, dyspnea can become severe. Atelectasis is a likely diagnosis in patients with a recent history of abdominal or thoracic surgery.

Physical Examination

Tachypnea commonly occurs with atelectasis. Respiratory rates usually increase in proportion to the amount of lung involved. Decreased lung compliance associated with atelectasis results in the patient breathing smaller tidal volumes with minimal variations in the depth of the breath.[17,21] To maintain adequate gas exchange, the patient must breathe at a more rapid rate to compensate for the smaller tidal volume. Tachycardia and fever may indicate infection associated with retention of secretions.

Auscultation is often helpful in detecting the onset of atelectasis. Late-inspiratory crackles are heard with deep inspiratory efforts and represent the sudden opening of atelectatic regions. Initially, these inspiratory crackles are usually heard in the dependent regions of the lung and may clear after the patient takes several deep breaths. Bronchial breath sounds and bronchophony over the affected region indicate airway patency in the atelectatic area. Diminished or absent breath sounds indicate that the airways are plugged or collapsed in the affected region. Accessory muscle usage suggests a significant increase in the work of breathing and is typically the result of a decreased lung compliance.

Abnormal or adventitious breath sounds rarely assist in establishing the diagnosis of atelectasis in the intubated infant. An alternate technique is observation of chest expansion. Mechanically ventilated infants with severe atelectasis often demonstrate unequal or reduced chest expansion.

Chest Radiograph

The chest radiograph often suggests the diagnosis of chest atelectasis before it is clinically apparent.[4,17] Obliteration of typical radiographic shadows may indicate the location of atelectasis. For example, the right heart border is often obscured with right middle lobe atelectasis but is visible with right lower lobe atelectasis. Other signs of lung volume loss include elevation of the hemidiaphragm and mediastinal shifts toward the affected side. Collapse of the lung tissue around inflated airways results in air bronchograms. When present, air bronchograms indicate that the atelectasis is not due to mucus obstruction of the airways. Computerized tomography (CT) scans provide greater resolution and may reveal reduction in lung volume and opacification not apparent with standard chest radiographs.[22] This type of radiographic testing is used only in cases where the diagnosis is in question following the routine chest film.

Arterial Blood Gases

Arterial blood gases (ABGs) often reveal hypoxemia in patients with atelectasis. The severity of hypoxemia does not necessarily correlate with the extent of atelectasis on the chest radiograph. Profound hypoxemia may exist as a result of microatelectasis that is not apparent radiographically. Hypoxemia frequently causes mild respiratory alkalosis.

Pulmonary Function Studies

Because patients with pulmonary disease are at greater risk for postoperative complications, bedside spirometry is useful to identify high-risk patients before surgery. Spirometry is especially useful to assess patients with a significant smoking history or those scheduled for upper abdominal or thoracic surgery.[23] Postoperative bedside spirometry indicates the severity of the decrease in lung volumes (vital capacity [VC] and inspiratory capacity [IC]) associated with atelectasis. Severe decreases in VC indicate that the simple techniques used to correct atelectasis may not be sufficient (see later discussion).

> Tachypnea, dyspnea, and mild to moderate hypoxemia are hallmarks of the severity of atelectasis. Chest x-rays help make the diagnosis, but CT scans provide more detailed information.

TREATMENT

Preoperative evaluation by the respiratory therapist (RT) should identify factors that might contribute to postoperative complications. Patients with a long history of smoking or pulmonary symptoms should undergo spirometry to identify obstructive or restrictive lung disease. Patients with moderate to severe chronic obstructive pulmonary disease (COPD) have a greater risk for postoperative respiratory complications. Preoperative bronchial hygiene techniques focusing on secretion clearance are applied. Avoid high inspired oxygen concentrations (>80%) whenever possible, as this favors the development and recurrence of atelectasis.[24] Patients on mechanical ventilation should be placed on F_{IO_2} <0.4 for at least 10 minutes prior to extubation to reduce the incidence of atelectasis.[25]

Following the diagnosis of postoperative atelectasis, the severity of respiratory compromise determines the therapy. Asymptomatic patients require only incentive spirometry.

Symptomatic or nonambulatory patients with atelectasis need more intensive postoperative respiratory care.

Lung Inflation Techniques

Lung inflation techniques either recruit the lung by increasing IC or prevent alveolar collapse by maintaining or increasing FRC. Deep breathing and coughing maneuvers aid recruitment and secretion clearance. They are as effective as any of the more costly techniques for the treatment and prevention of atelectasis in the cooperative patient.[26] Incentive spirometry may benefit patients who require additional coaching, and it can serve as an indicator of improvement in pulmonary function.

Intermittent application of 10 to 15 cm H_2O continuous positive airway pressure (CPAP) or positive expiratory pressure (PEP) help prevent alveolar collapse and are often effective in the treatment of atelectasis when simple IC maneuvers are ineffective. Lower values of CPAP have not been as effective.[27–30] The American Association for Respiratory Care (AARC) clinical practice guidelines on positive airway pressure adjuncts to bronchial hygiene therapy provides concise guidelines for the application of CPAP and PEP.[31] In adults most complications associated with CPAP occur in the greater than 20 to 25 cm H_2O range. In infants and children complications may develop at lower pressures. Periodic application of CPAP (every 1 to 3 hours) often assists the resolution of atelectasis and may support patients who are unable to cooperate or who have recurrent or persistent forms of atelectasis. PEP is effective in improving postoperative pulmonary function when applied on an hourly basis.[29] Some PEP devices provide inspiratory flow assistance, augmenting IC maneuvers.

Patients who are unable to perform more simple maneuvers for lung inflation and whose VC is less than 10 to 15 mL/kg may benefit from intermittent positive-pressure breathing (IPPB). Volume-oriented IPPB can improve lung volumes and promote a more effective cough.[32]

Even though the complication rate is low, patients treated with positive-pressure ventilation (e.g., CPAP, IPPB) should be closely monitored for the adverse effects of raised intrathoracic pressure (i.e., hyperinflation, reduced perfusion, barotrauma, and gastric inflation). The application of positive pressure must be used in conjunction with bronchial hygiene techniques when secretion retention is the cause of the atelectasis.

Some patients require mechanical ventilation after major surgery. Significant lung recruitment postanesthesia occurs when inflation pressures of up to 40 cm H_2O for brief durations of 15 to 20 seconds are followed by the application of 8 to 12 cm H_2O of PEEP. The higher sustained inflation pressures recruit lung units, and the PEEP maintains alveolar recruitment after the inspiratory maneuver is completed.[24]

> Resolving atelectasis requires lung volume to be recruited and then for the lung volume to be maintained. Airways and alveoli must maintain sufficient volume and patency to prevent the reoccurrence of atelectasis.

Secretion Removal

When retained mucus results in atelectasis, treatment should emphasize removal of airway secretions in addition to lung inflation. Encouraging the patient to generate an effective cough is often all that is necessary. If this therapy is not effective and radiographic evidence suggests the characteristic lobar atelectasis pattern (i.e., radiographic density, absent air bronchograms, fissure displacement, mediastinal shift, diaphragmatic elevation, compensatory hyperinflation), bronchial hygiene maneuvers are indicated. Oscillatory PEEP devices (e.g., Acapella™, Flutter™) assist in secretion clearance. The use of manual or mechanically aided chest physiotherapy techniques should be limited to patients with large amounts of secretions.

Lobar atelectasis often responds to a short, vigorous course of chest physical therapy (CPT), usually within 6 hours, and compares favorably with bronchoscopy in removing retained secretions.[33,34] If secretions persist, their removal with the use of endotracheal suctioning or bronchoscopy is indicated.[35] Postoperative management of patients with COPD should also include bronchodilators and humidity therapy to facilitate a better cough and secretion expectoration. CPT has not proven to be effective in preventing postoperative atelectasis in infants and newborns, and on the contrary, may be associated with an increased risk of atelectasis.[36]

The simulated cough maneuver may prove effective as a treatment regimen in intubated children with various degrees of lung collapse unresponsive to conventional CPT.[37] The therapy consists of endotracheal instillation of saline, followed by manual lung inflation with a momentary inflation hold, release of the hold, and simultaneous forced exhalation and vibration to simulate cough. Endotracheal suctioning completes the procedure. The maneuver is usually repeated three to five times. The maneuver has been most successful in infants with airway occlusion secondary to mucus (without air bronchograms on x-ray).

> Secretion clearance techniques should be considered when lung recruitment maneuvers are not effective or a patient is prone to mucus plugging.

Intrapulmonary percussive ventilation (IPV) is a positive-pressure maneuver that delivers a high-velocity gas into the airways at rates of 100 to 300 cycles/minute. The IPV device (Percussionaire, Sand Point, Idaho) is a pneumatic high-frequency positive-pressure ventilator. Treatments are administered on an intermittent basis (e.g., every 2 hours, every 4 hours) for a duration of 15 to 20 minutes. Peak airway pressures may vary from 5 to 25 cm H_2O. Theoretically, IPV loosens secretions and maintains positive airway pressures, allowing secretions to migrate to larger airways for clearance. Published case reports identify IPV as a safe and effective therapy in enhancing secretion removal and reversing lung consolidation in children and adults unresponsive to conventional therapy.[38]

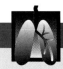

Mrs. M

HISTORY

Mrs. M is a 47-year-old morbidly obese Caucasian female who was admitted to the ICU postoperatively following gastric bypass surgery. She was maintained on continuous mechanical ventilation for 1 day. She was extubated on day 2 and placed on a 40% high-flow oxygen aerosol mask. Two days after extubation, she began complaining of "not being able to catch her breath." Her present chief complaint is dyspnea.

Her past medical history includes systemic hypertension and diabetes (both being managed medically) and obstructive sleep apnea. She is moderately compliant with her nasal CPAP (8 cm H_2O) at night. She denies any history of smoking, alcohol abuse, or drug abuse.

QUESTIONS	ANSWERS
1. What clinical conditions could cause Mrs. M's acute dyspnea?	Dyspnea may be due to an increased work of breathing associated with decreased lung compliance from atelectasis, diaphragmatic compression from the abdomen, or pulmonary edema. Other potential causes of dyspnea in this case would include pulmonary embolus and pneumonia.
2. What factors would limit diaphragmatic excursion and predispose Mrs. M to developing atelectasis?	Obesity, surgical site, anesthesia, body habitus, pain. All factors could reduce diaphragmatic motion, limit inspiratory capacity, and reduce FRC. There is a direct relationship between postoperative complications and the proximity of the surgical incision to the diaphragm. Atelectasis is much more likely with upper abdominal than peripheral surgery and less likely with endoscopy procedures.
3. What physical examination procedures would you suggest be done at this point?	Assessment of the respiratory rate, pulse rate, body temperature, breathing pattern, and breath sounds would help evaluate Mrs. M's pulmonary status. Cardiac examination for a third or fourth heart sound, jugular venous distention, and hepatojugular reflex would help rule out pulmonary edema. Evaluation for a pleural friction rub and palpation of the calf for tenderness would suggest pulmonary embolism, if present.

More on Mrs. M

PHYSICAL EXAMINATION

- **General.** Patient fatigued and in moderate respiratory distress; mildly diaphoretic, lying in a semi-Fowler's position in bed
- **Vital Signs.** Temperature 38.5°C (101.3°F), respiratory rate 38/min, blood pressure 148/57 mm Hg, pulse 124/min
- **HEENT.** Pupils equal, round, and reactive to light and accommodation (PERRLA); tympanic membranes clear; no nasopharyngeal lesions, masses, or exudates; nasal flaring with inspiration
- **Neck.** Trachea midline and mobile to palpation; no stridor; no carotid bruits, lymphadenopathy, thyromegaly, or jugular venous distention; tension of sternocleidomastoid muscles noted during inspiration
- **Chest.** Symmetrical chest expansion with rapid, shallow breathing pattern; decreased resonance to percussion of lower lung fields
- **Heart.** Regular rhythm with a rate of 124/min; no murmurs, gallops, or rubs
- **Lungs.** Diminished breath sounds in all lung fields, with late-inspiratory crackles heard in the posterior bases
- **Abdomen.** Markedly obese, distended, tender; no bowel sounds
- **Extremities.** No clubbing, cyanosis, or edema; capillary refill less than 3 seconds; pulses and reflexes +1 and symmetrical

QUESTIONS	ANSWERS
4. What pathophysiology is suggested by the rapid, shallow breathing pattern?	Rapid, shallow breathing suggests that the patient is experiencing a significant drop in her lung compliance. This leads to breathing with smaller tidal volumes and a more rapid rate. Common causes of decreased lung compliance include pulmonary edema, atelectasis, and pneumonia.
5. What is the cause of the late-inspiratory crackles in the bases? What characteristic of these crackles should the RT identify?	Late-inspiratory crackles are caused by the sudden opening of many collapsed peripheral airways. This occurs when the patient with atelectasis inhales deeply enough to re-expand atelectatic regions. Determine whether the crackles diminish as the patient repeatedly inhales deeply. This would suggest that the crackles are due to atelectasis.
6. What could be causing Mrs. M's tachycardia?	A number of factors might result in tachycardia: abdominal compression of the diaphragm, hypoxemia, inadequate pain management, fever, and anxiety. The patient has systemic hypertension that might predispose her to heart disease.
7. Why is Mrs. M using her accessory muscles to breathe?	The diaphragm, the primary inspiratory muscle, is much less effective for several weeks or months after abdominal surgery. Lungs are also less compliant and more difficult to expand after major surgery. Atelectasis may worsen the problem, and assistance may be needed from the accessory breathing muscles to maintain ventilation. The patient's total work of breathing is increased.
8. What laboratory tests would you recommend at this point?	Laboratory tests that would be helpful are aimed at narrowing the list of problems that could cause the patient's current distress. Such tests include a CT scan, chest radiograph, ABG analysis, bedside spirometry, complete blood count (CBC) and electrolyte evaluation, and an electrocardiogram (ECG).

More on Mrs. M

Laboratory Evaluation

Chest Radiograph (see Figure 13.1)

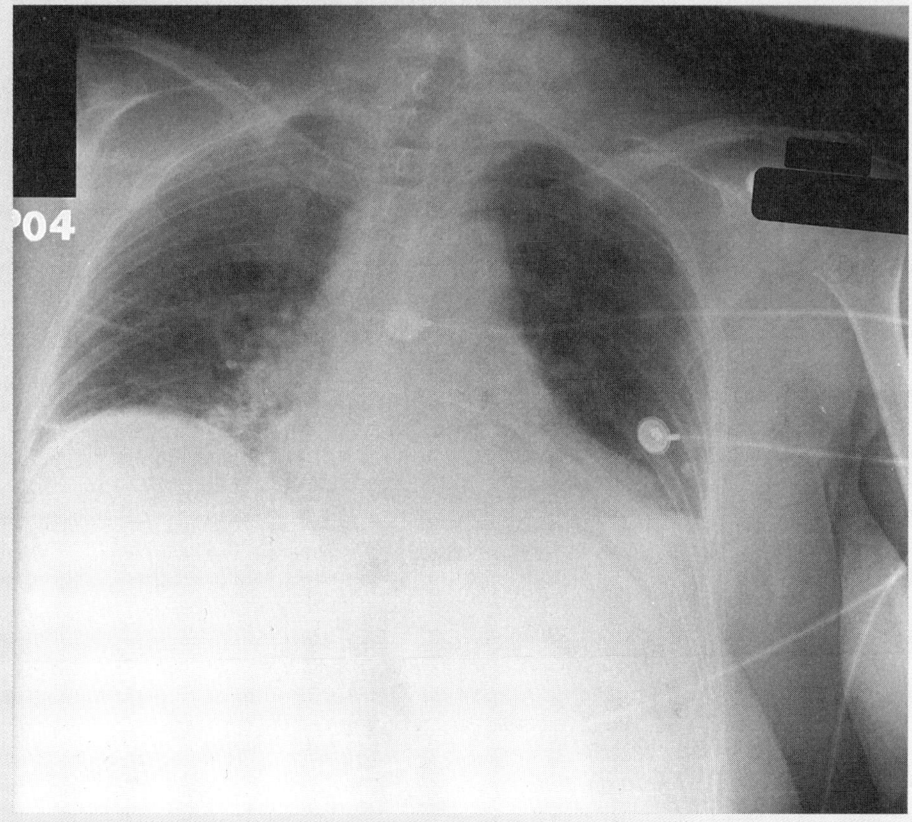

FIGURE 13.1 Portable chest radiograph of Mrs. M 48 hours after surgery.

ABG	Value
pH	7.46
Pa_{CO_2}	33 mm Hg
Pa_{O_2}	54 mm Hg on F_{IO_2} 0.40
HCO_3^-	24 mEq/liter

(box continued on page 310)

Laboratory Evaluation (CONTINUED)

Spirometry: Slow inspiratory capacity 1.0 liter; patient unable to perform a VC maneuver

CBC	
Measure	Value
WBCs	16,500/mm^3, with 65% segmented neutrophils and 11% bands
RBCs	3.9 million/mm^3
Hb	9.9 g/dL
Hct	37%
Platelets	155,000/mm^3

Chemistry	
Measure	Value
Na$^+$	139 mEq/liter
K$^+$	3.2 mEq/liter
Cl$^-$	102 mEq/liter
Blood urea nitrogen	17 mg/dL
Total proteins	6.7 g/dL (albumin 3.2 g/dL)
Glucose	78 mg/dL

QUESTIONS	ANSWERS
9. How would you interpret the ABG and spirometry results?	The ABGs reflect moderate hypoxemia with mild uncompensated respiratory alkalosis, indicating that the patient is hyperventilating. The Pao$_2$ of 54 mm Hg on 0.40 Fio$_2$ suggests that the hypoxemia is somewhat refractory to oxygen therapy. The spirometry results are consistent with a poor effort or a severely restrictive condition. The patient's inability to perform a VC maneuver indicates significant fatigue.
10. How would you interpret the chest radiograph?	The chest radiograph suggests poor inspiratory effort or reduced lung volumes. Obliteration of the right heart border is consistent with right middle lobe atelectasis. Presence of air bronchograms suggests a lack of mucus plugs in the affected regions.
11. How would you interpret the CBC and electrolyte values?	The WBCs are elevated, consistent with infection. The increase in bands indicates that young WBCs have been recruited to fight an acute infection. Hb, Hct, and RBCs are reduced, indicating hemodilution or blood loss. This reduces oxygen-carrying capacity, requiring an increased cardiac output to maintain adequate

oxygen delivery. The potassium is slightly reduced and should be replenished, especially if heart rhythm abnormalities develop. Circulating total proteins and albumin are reduced, which is a common finding after major surgery. This slightly reduces oncotic pressure, making the patient susceptible to fluid accumulation in the lungs.

12. What are your therapeutic objectives for respiratory care?

The therapeutic goals are to re-expand collapsed areas of the lung using lung inflation techniques and to treat the hypoxemia.

13. What would be your treatment plan?

Initial recommendations for treatment should focus on lung recruitment maneuvers, correction of hypoxemia, and continued obstructive sleep apnea management:

a. Incentive spirometry (IS) with multiple, maximal inspiratory capacity maneuvers should be performed hourly.

b. Lung volume improvement should be monitored.

c. Poor response to IS would warrant PEP mask therapy or intermittent CPAP, usually with initial pressures of 8 to 10 cm H_2O. Pressures may need to be increased if the initial settings do not prove effective.

d. Supplemental oxygen therapy should continue, using a high-flow oxygen system at a specific FIO_2. A high-flow system helps ensure that FIO_2 concentrations will not vary with changes in the tidal volume, pattern, or rate. Because the patient's ventilation ($PaCO_2$) is adequate, monitoring improvement in oxygenation can be done with intermittent pulse oximetry. A repeat ABG analysis is indicated if the clinical condition fails to improve or deteriorates.

e. Continuation of nasal CPAP for nighttime use.

f. Hb and Hct should be monitored; transfusion may be indicated if values continue to drop.

14. How would you evaluate Mrs. M's response to therapy?	Patient compliance and proper coaching are extremely important for successful lung inflation therapy. Excessive secretions do not appear to be the cause of this patient's atelectasis, so CPT or bronchoscopy are not indicated.
	Evaluate the patient's response to oxygen therapy by monitoring heart rate, respiratory rate, perceived dyspnea, pulse oximetry, and ABGs.

More on Mrs. M

Initial treatment included IS along with encouraging deep breathing and coughing. Six hours after IS is initiated by the respiratory care practitioner (RCP), the patient remains alert and oriented but continues to complain of dyspnea. Her inspiratory capacity is 1.3 liters, respiratory rate 26/min, and pulse 116/min. She remains febrile, continues to use her accessory muscles for breathing, and continues to have diminished breath sounds in the bases along with some inspiratory crackles. Pulse oximetry reveals an oxygen saturation of 92% on an F_{IO_2} of 0.45. Results of a repeat chest radiograph are pending.

QUESTIONS	ANSWERS
15. Are the therapeutic objectives being met?	The therapeutic objectives were to improve oxygenation and lung expansion. It appears that oxygenation has improved, although it remains less than optimal. Lung expansion has not improved significantly.
16. What is your assessment of Mrs. M's condition after IS therapy for 6 hours?	Assessment of the patient after 6 hours of IS reveals persistent atelectasis. This assessment is based on the continued tachypnea, diminished breath sounds and crackles, and reduced inspiratory capacity.
17. Would you suggest any changes in the treatment plan?	Treatment at this point should include the application of intermittent CPAP or PEP. This is needed because of the slow resolution of the atelectasis with IS.
18. What is Mrs. M at risk for with regard to her pulmonary status?	The patient is at high risk for respiratory failure, which could occur when the excessive work of breathing tires the respiratory muscles and results in fatigue. This would be recognized by deterioration of the ABGs, vital signs, and sensorium.

Mrs. M Conclusion

PEP-mask therapy is started every hour for 15 breaths at 8 cm H_2O and increased to 12 cm H_2O. Four hours after initiating PEP, dyspnea improves, respiratory rate is 18/min, and pulse oximetry is 97% on an FIO_2 of 0.40. A repeat chest radiograph shows improvement (Figure 13.2). The patient's nasal CPAP system is checked for safe operation and applied at nighttime at 8 cm H_2O. PEP frequency is reduced to every 3 hours, and IS is maintained every hour while awake. The patient is switched to nasal cannula at 4 liters/min, and 24 hours later is transferred to a step-down unit. IS and oxygen orders continue for 2 days after her transfer. ■

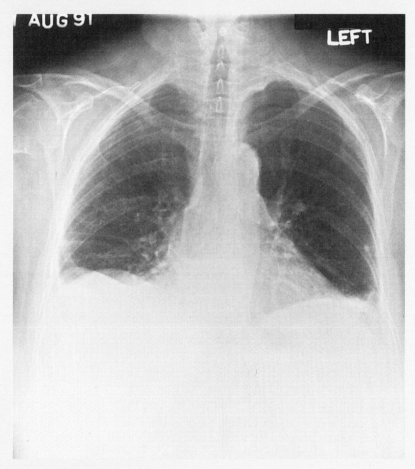

FIGURE 13.2 Portable chest radiograph showing improvement with better lung expansion.

KEY POINTS

- Atelectasis is a clinical condition characterized by regions of the lung that are collapsed or airless.
- Three factors may combine or independently contribute to the development of atelectasis: inadequate lung distending forces, obstruction of the airways leading to absorption of alveolar air, and insufficient surfactant levels.
- Upper abdominal procedures present the greatest risk for atelectasis, followed by thoracic, lower abdominal, and peripheral procedures.
- Atelectasis results in a decrease in FRC and lung compliance, which results in alterations in the distribution of the inhaled gas without corresponding changes in perfusion.
- Dyspnea is the most common symptom associated with atelectasis but may not be present if the patient has minimal lung involvement and is otherwise healthy.
- Tachypnea commonly occurs with atelectasis. Respiratory rates usually increase in proportion to the amount of lung involved.
- Auscultation is often helpful in detecting the onset of atelectasis. Late-inspiratory crackles are heard with deep inspiratory efforts and represent the sudden opening of atelectatic regions.
- The chest radiograph often suggests the diagnosis of chest atelectasis before it is clinically apparent.
- Following the diagnosis of postoperative atelectasis, the severity of respiratory compromise determines the therapy. Asymptomatic patients require only incentive spirometry. Symptomatic or nonambulatory patients with atelectasis need more intensive postoperative respiratory care.
- Deep breathing and coughing maneuvers aid recruitment and secretion clearance. They are as effective as any of the more costly techniques for the treatment and prevention of atelectasis in the cooperative patient.
- Intermittent application of 10 to 15 cm H_2O continuous positive airway pressure (CPAP) or positive expiratory pressure (PEP) help prevent alveolar collapse and are often effective in the treatment of atelectasis when simple IC maneuvers are ineffective.
- When retained mucus results in atelectasis, treatment should emphasize removal of airway secretions in addition to lung inflation.
- Lobar atelectasis often responds to a short, vigorous course of CPT, usually within 6 hours, and compares favorably with bronchoscopy in removing retained secretions.
- If secretions persist, their removal with the use of endotracheal suctioning or bronchoscopy is indicated.

REFERENCES

1. McAllister, FA, Bertsch, K, et al: Incidence of and risk factors for pulmonary complications after nonthoracic surgery. Am J Respir Crit Care Med 171: 514, 2005.
2. Luce, JM: Clinical risk factors for postoperative pulmonary complications. Respir Care 29:484, 1984.
3. Rivera, R, Tibballis, J: Complications of endotracheal intubation and mechanical ventilation in infants and children. Crit Care Med 20:193, 1992.
4. Johnson, NT, Pierson, DJ: The spectrum of pulmonary atelectasis: pathophysiology, diagnosis, and therapy. Respir Care 31:1107, 1986.
5. Eichenberger, AS, Projetti, S, et al: Morbid obesity and postoperative pulmonary atelectasis: an underestimated problem. Anesth Analg 95:1788, 2002.
6. Magnusson, L, Spahn, DR: New concepts of atelectasis during general anaesthesia. Br J Anaesth 91:61, 2003.
7. Duggan, M, Kavanagh, BP: Pulmonary atelectasis: a pathogenic perioperative entity. Anesthesiology 102:838, 2005.
8. Tokics, L, Hedenstierna, G: Lung collapse and gas exchange during general anesthesia: effects of spontaneous breathing, muscle paralysis, and posi-

tive end-expiratory pressure. Anesthesiology 66:157, 1987.

9. Didier, EP: Some effects of anesthetics and the anesthetized state on the respiratory system. Respir Care 29:463, 1984.

10. Deem, S, Lee, CM, Curtis, JR: Acquired neuromuscular disorders in the intensive care unit. Am J Respir Crit Care Med 168:735, 2003.

11. Lam, WW, Chen, PP, et al: Sedation versus general anaesthesia in paediatric patients undergoing chest CT. Acta Radiol 39:298, 1998.

12. Stein, M, Cassara, EL: Preoperative pulmonary evaluation and therapy for surgery patients. JAMA 211:787, 1970.

13. Wightman, JAK: A prospective survey of the incidence of postoperative pulmonary complications. Br J Surg 55:85, 1968.

14. Hodgkin, JE: Preoperative assessment of respiratory function. Respir Care 29:496, 1984.

15. Benjamin, JJ, et al: Left lower lobe atelectasis and consolidation following cardiac surgery: the effect of topical cooling on the phrenic nerve. Radiology 142:11, 1982.

16. Craig, DG: Postoperative recovery of pulmonary function. Anesth Analg 60:46, 1981.

17. Marini, JJ: Postoperative atelectasis: pathophysiology, clinical importance, and principles of management. Respir Care 29:516, 1984.

18. Dale, WA, Rahn, H: Rate of gas absorption during atelectasis. Am J Physiol 170:606, 1952.

19. Webb, SJS, Nunn, JF: A comparison between the effect of nitrous oxide and nitrogen on arterial PO_2. Anaesthesia 22:69, 1967.

20. Matthay, MA, Wiener-Kronish, JP: Respiratory management after surgery. Chest 95:424, 1989.

21. Askanazi, J, et al: Patterns of ventilation in postoperative and acutely ill patients. Crit Care Med 7:41, 1979.

22. Lundquist, H, Hedenstierna, G, et al: CT assessment of dependent lung densities in man during general anesthesia. Acta Radiol 36:626, 1995.

23. Stoller, JK: Pulmonary function testing as a screening technique. Respir Care 34:611, 1989.

24. Rothen, HU, Sporre, B, et al: Airway closure, atelectasis, and gas exchange during general anesthesia. Br J Anaesth 81:681, 1998.

25. Benoit, Z, Wicky, S, et al: The effect of increased FIO_2 before tracheal extubation on postoperative atelectasis. Anesth Analg 95:1777, 2002.

26. Celli, BR, et al: A controlled trial of intermittent positive pressure breathing, incentive spirometry, and deep breathing exercises in preventing pulmonary complications after surgery. Am Rev Respir Dis 130:12, 1984.

27. Pasquina, P, Merlani, P et al: Continuous positive airway pressure versus noninvasive pressure support ventilation to treat atelectasis after cardiac surgery. Anesth Analg 99:1001, 2004.

28. Branson, RD: PEEP without endotracheal intubation. Respir Care 33:598, 1988.

29. Ricksten, SE, et al: Effects of periodic positive pressure breathing by mask on postoperative pulmonary function. Chest 89:774, 1986.

30. Ford, TG, Guenter, CA: Toward prevention of postoperative complications. Am Rev Respir Dis 130: 4, 1984.

31. American Association for Respiratory Care: AARC clinical practice guideline: use of positive airway pressure adjuncts to bronchial hygiene therapy. Respir Care 38:516–521, 1993.

32. O'Donohue, WJ Jr: Maximum volume IPPB for the management of pulmonary atelectasis. Chest 76:683, 1979.

33. Marini, JJ, et al: Acute lobar atelectasis: a prospective comparison of fiberoptic bronchoscopy and respiratory therapy. Am Rev Respir Dis 119:971, 1979.

34. Stiller, KB, et al: Acute lobar atelectasis: a comparison of two chest physiotherapy regimens. Chest 98:1336, 1990.

35. Mahajan, VK, et al: The value of fiberoptic bronchoscopy in the management of pulmonary collapse. Chest 73:817, 1978.

36. Al-Alaiyan, S, et al: Chest physiotherapy and postextubation atelectasis in infants. Pediatr Pulmonol 21:227–230, 1996.

37. Galvis, A, et al: Bedside management of lung collapse in children on mechanical ventilation. Pediatr Pulmonol 17:326–330, 1994.

38. Birnkrant, D, et al: Persistent pulmonary consolidation treated with intrapulmonary percussive ventilation: a preliminary report. Pediatr Pulmonol 21:246–249, 1996.

14

Interstitial Lung Disease

N. Lennard Specht, MD, FACP

CHAPTER OBJECTIVES:

After reading this chapter you will be able to identify:

- Key definitions related to interstitial lung disease (ILD) including pulmonary fibrosis, asbestosis, silicosis, and pneumoconiosis.
- The etiology for ILD including the proportion of patients with ILD who have an identifiable cause.
- The inflammatory response believed to be responsible for the pathological changes associated with ILD.
- The clinical features often seen in patients with ILD including pulmonary function and radiographic studies.
- The treatment for patients with various types of ILD.

INTRODUCTION

Interstitial lung disease (ILD) is made up of a large group of diverse diseases that cause lung damage that results in fibrosis of the lung and reduced lung volumes and lung surface area. The term pulmonary fibrosis is also applied to these diseases because fibrosis of the lung is the ultimate result of ILD. As many as 81 of every 100,000 people in the United States have some form of ILD.[1] The many types of ILD can be categorized based on identifying the cause, or etiology, of the disease. ILDs with no known cause include: sarcoidosis, rheumatoid arthritis, and idiopathic pulmonary fibrosis. In contrast, some forms of ILD may be caused by identifiable factors. For example, inhalation of harmful dusts will cause asbestosis, silicosis, or hypersensitivity pneumonitis. Exposure to toxic chemicals or drugs such as chemotherapy used for cancer or amiodarone can cause ILD. Even exposing the lung to radiation like that used for cancer treatments may cause ILD.

The consequences of ILD have been seen for centuries, but most forms of ILD have been described within the past 50 years. The earliest descriptions of ILD involved workers exposed to inorganic dusts. Hypocrites told stories of miners who had difficulty breathing. Nineteenth century Dutch pathologists noted a sandy texture to the lungs in patients who had worked in mines. Nineteenth century English medical literature contains many good descriptions of dust-related lung disease (pneumoconiosis).[2,3] Coalminer's pneumoconiosis generated a tremendous amount of publicity in the early twentieth century. Worker safety concerns generated intense political debate and resulted in the "Black Lung

Laws," which allow employees with coalminer's pneumoconiosis to be compensated financially for their lung disease. While cutaneous sarcoidosis was first described in 1869 by two dermatologists, sarcoid lung involvement was not noted for several more decades.[4] Idiopathic pulmonary fibrosis was first described in 1944—a recent discovery in comparison to other forms of ILD.[5] Many forms of ILD, particularly the group of diseases called idiopathic interstitial pneumonias, are still being described and reclassified.

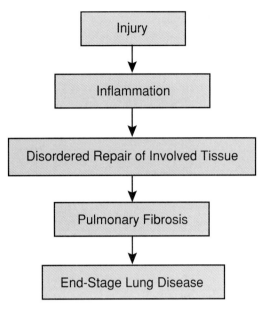

FIGURE 14.1 Cascade of events thought to represent the steps leading from the initiation of interstitial lung disease and culminating with pulmonary fibrosis and end-stage lung disease. Each of these stages may be present simultaneously in a given patient.

Most forms of ILD follow a common chain of events (Figure 14.1). In this scheme the disease is initiated by an injury. The injury promotes a vigorous immune reaction and inflammation. Inflammation leads to destruction of lung tissue. The destroyed lung tissue cannot regenerate, so healing leads to a disorganized repair process and scarring (fibrosis). The disordered repair and fibrosis lead eventually to end-stage lung disease.

Of all the ILDs perhaps the most puzzling are the group of diseases known as idiopathic interstitial pneumonias (IIP). The most common disease within the IIP group is idiopathic pulmonary fibrosis (IPF).[6] IPF has no known cause and is usually relentlessly progressive. It typically affects patients between the ages of 40 to 70 years of age. Recent research suggests IPF is caused when pulmonary epithelial cells release cytokines that promote fibrosis following certain types of injury.[7] This mechanism does not depend on inflammation for the disease to progress and would explain why the lungs of patients with IPF have so little inflammation when biopsied. The lack of inflammation also would explain why patients with IPF rarely respond to medications that suppress inflammation.[8]

ETIOLOGY

A large number of diseases can initiate the process of ILD. These diseases are usually classified according to the type of agent that causes the lung injury (Table 14.1). Only about one third of patients with ILD have an identifiable agent responsible for inducing lung injury. Typical inorganic dusts that may induce ILD include asbestos, silica (sand), coal, and talc. These agents injure the epithelium or endothelium of the lung directly via a toxic effect[9] or indirectly by leading to the production of toxic metabolites or activating immune responses.[10] Perhaps the most infamous disease caused by the inhalation of inorganic dusts is coalminer's pneumoconiosis, which occurs in about 0.4% of people who are regularly exposed to coal dust.[11] More recently, asbestos-related lung disease has been the source of much legislation and litigation.

Table 14.1 Classification of Interstitial Lung Disease	
Known Etiology	Unknown Etiology
Inorganic dusts	Sarcoidosis
Hypersensitivity	Collagen vascular disease
Pneumonitis	Idiopathic pulmonary fibrosis
Drugs	Other
Toxins	
Oxygen	
Radiation	
Infection	

Organic Dust

Inhalation of organic dusts may create a form of ILD known as hypersensitivity pneumonitis. Hypersensitivity pneumonitis is associated with repeated exposure to organic antigens. In susceptible patients, repeated exposure to the antigen leads to an abnormal allergic response that is destructive to the lung. Many different antigens can cause hypersensitivity pneumonitis. One of the more notorious antigens is from a group of bacteria called thermophilic *Actinomyces*. Thermophilic *Actinomyces* break down leaves and other vegetative matter, and they thrive at temperatures between 45°C (113°F) and 60°C (140°F). Repeated exposure to dusts from decomposing vegetation containing thermophilic *Actinomyces* will precipitates the disease in susceptible individuals. A number of forms of hypersensitivity pneumonitis are named for organic materials that contain thermophilic *Actinomyces* as they decompose. These forms include humidifier lung (air conditioning or humidifier ducts), bagassosis (sugar cane), mushroom worker's lung (mushroom compost), farmer's lung (hay), and grain handler's lung (grain). Thermophilic *Antinomyces* is only one group in a wide array of organisms that provide antigens that cause hypersensitivity pneumonitis. Other organisms include various fungi, *actinomycetes*, bacteria, parasites, insects, and birds as well as the hair and dander of mammals.

Box 14.1 Partial List of Drugs Associated with Development of Interstitial Lung Disease

Antibiotics

- Nitrofurantoin

Anti-Inflammatory Agents

- Aspirin
- Gold
- Penicillamine

Cancer Chemotherapy

- Bleomycin
- Busulfan
- Cyclophosphamide
- Methotrexate
- Cytosine arabinoside

Cardiovascular Drugs

- Amiodarone
- Tocanide

Illicit Drugs

- Heroin
- Methadone
- Propoxyphene
- Talc

Drugs

Drug-induced ILD is an important medical problem because healthcare providers caring for patients who require these drugs should be alert to the possible development of ILD. Early recognition of drug-induced injury will allow discontinuation of the offending drug, will usually stop further injury, and may reverse the disease process. A large number of drugs are known to induce lung injury (Box 14.1).

Many of drugs that are well known for causing ILD are used in the treatment of cancer.

Drug-induced lung disease is a major cause of morbidity and mortality in patients undergoing chemotherapy for cancer.[12] Of patients undergoing chemotherapy who are found to have diffuse infiltrative changes in their lungs, up to 20% are diagnosed with ILD.[13] Many patients die as a result of chemotherapy-induced ILD.[14] Most chemotherapy agents induce a pulmonary reaction within weeks of exposure, but some may result in lung disease many months after the last dose.

Amiodarone is a potent antidysrhythmic drug used for patients with serious cardiac dysrhythmias that do not improve with other treatments. Amiodarone can cause two forms of lung disease: chronic lung damage and acute amiodarone-mediated lung injury.[15] The chronic lung damage associated with amiodarone use is related to the dose the patient receives.[16] Patients receiving high doses of amiodarone have a greater incidence of toxicity than those who receive a lower dose.[16] The incidence of pulmonary complications caused by amiodarone is between 1% and 18%. Acute amiodarone lung toxicity is often seen following cardiac surgery.[17] Amiodarone lung disease improves as the drug is cleared from the body. The clearance of amiodarone is extremely slow, with a half life of at least 30 days.

Nitrofurantoin is a particularly effective antibiotic for treating urinary tract infections, but on rare occasions, its use can give rise to ILD.[18] The pulmonary toxicity from nitrofurantoin is either an acute reaction that begins hours to a few days following the first dose or a chronic reaction that develops after months to years of drug use.

Illicit drugs, particularly narcotics such as heroin, may produce an acute form of noncardiogenic pulmonary edema. Talc is occasionally mixed into illicit drugs either to dilute ("cut") the drug or because the drug was prepared for injection from talc-containing tablets. The IV injection of talc creates a granulomatous reaction in small blood vessels and the interstitium of the lung.

Oxygen at high concentrations over several hours or days may induce acute lung injury. Pathological pulmonary changes develop in animals after as little as 12 hours of exposure to 100% oxygen. The pathological changes progress with continued exposure to 100% oxygen, and by 48 hours pulmonary edema develops. Pathological changes similar in appearance to acute respiratory distress syndrome (ARDS) follow the development of pulmonary edema.

> Most patients diagnosed with interstitial pulmonary fibrosis do not have a known cause.

PATHOPHYSIOLOGY

The architecture of the lung can be viewed as a very delicate collection of small bubbles (alveoli). The bubbles connect to the trachea through a complex network of airways. The walls of the alveoli consist of an extremely thin layer of tissue and blood vessels that provide little resistance to the diffusion of gas between the capillary and alveolar air. The epithelial cells responsible for most of the alveolar lining are type I alveolar cells (pneumocytes). These cells are very flat with a large surface area that conforms to the shape of the underlying capillary bed. Scattered among the type I cells are a few type II cells that are much rounder and thicker; these are responsible for the secretion of surfactant. This fragile structure becomes the principal focus of the events associated with ILD.

The pathological appearance of the lungs in most patients with early ILD is characterized by inflammation. Sometimes the pattern of inflammation is characteristic enough that a skilled pathologist can determine the form of ILD by reviewing a biopsy. As the ILD progresses, the inflammation is replaced with fibrosis and cysts. Biopsies of fibrotic lung with cystic changes is usually unhelpful in establishing a diagnosis because the ILDs are virtually indistinguishable by the time they reach the end stage. If the ILD is due to an identifiable crystal such as talk or silica a pathologist can see the crystals within the lung.

In most patients with ILD, pulmonary inflammation develops after lung injury. The alveoli are the most frequent sites of inflammation, but the vasculature and smaller airways may be involved as well. The inflammatory response is characterized by migration into the alveolus and alveolar wall of one or more of the following: neutrophils, eosinophils, lymphocytes, macrophages, and plasma cells. The influx of immune cells is accompanied by fluid accumulation in the alevolar walls and alveolar airspace. This immune reaction damages the alveoli. The flat type I pneumocytes are destroyed and replaced with secretory type II cells. The alveolar walls become thickened and distorted by the inflammation. The alveoli are eventually destroyed as the disease progresses and are ultimately replaced with fibrotic connective tissue and cystic airspaces. The cystic airspaces that result from this process are lined with cuboidal or columnar epithelium and do not participate in gas exchange.[19]

In contrast with the inflammatory forms of ILD, IPF is characterized by areas of progressive fibrosis intermixed with areas of normal-appearing lung and areas of honeycomb cysts. It is rare to find dense inflammation in this form of ILD.[6]

CLINICAL FEATURES

History

The symptoms of lung involvement are similar regardless of the underlying cause. In addition, the symptoms of lung involvement are nonspecific and could suggest many other causes, including obstructive lung disease, heart disease, or pulmonary vascular disease. The first symptom of ILD is usually progressive dyspnea on exertion or a nonproductive cough. Patients initially notice dyspnea only during heavy exertion. Minimal exertion induces breathlessness as the process advances. In advanced stages of the disease, dyspnea occurs at rest.

ILD may lead to pulmonary hypertension and then right heart failure (cor pulmonale). Cor pulmonale causes edema to accumulate primarily in the lower extremities, elevated jugular venous pressure, and a hepatojugular reflex. Patients primarily complain of swollen ankles.

If exposure to a dust or a drug caused a patient to develop ILD, the exposure must be identified and stopped. Some treatment decisions may also depend on the identification of the exposure that caused the ILD. To determine whether the patient was exposed to agents known to cause ILD a careful history must include an employment record and a review of the patient's environment. A thorough review of the patient's medical history and current and previous medications is also important.

Physical Examination

Results of the physical examination in patients with ILD are often very nonspecific. There may be no abnormal findings early in the course of the disease. As the process progresses, tachypnea and fine, late-inspiratory crackles are present. These crackles are often called Velcro crackles, as they sound similar to Velcro being slowly pulled apart. A prominent pulmonic component of the second heart sound (loud P_2) will occur if pulmonary hypertension is present from prolonged hypoxemia. Distention of the jugular veins and edema of the lower extremities are signs of cor pulmonale and suggest more severe disease. Clubbing of the digits is a frequent finding, particularly with asbestosis and idiopathic pulmonary fibrosis.

If the cause of ILD is a systemic disease, then additional abnormalities specific to the disease can often be found on examination. For example, rheumatoid lung is almost always accompanied by arthritis. Patients with sarcoidosis may have a rash, swollen lymph nodes or cardiac rhythm irregularities. A complete physical examination is vital because it may guide the clinician to the etiology of ILD and it provides an indication of the severity of the disease.

> The first symptom seen in patients with IPF is usually dyspnea on exertion. The dyspnea is progressive, occurring with less and less exertion over time.

Arterial Blood Gases

Arterial blood gas (ABG) levels are normal early in ILD. As the process develops, the alveolar-arterial difference in partial pressure of oxygen (P[A-a]O_2) increases.[20,21] Hypoxemia during exercise is a frequent finding that may progress to hypoxemia at rest as the disease advances. Hypercapnia may occur during the terminal stages of ILD.

Pulmonary Function Studies

Lung volumes and flow rates are initially normal, but both decrease throughout the course of the disease.[22] Pulmonary function testing usually shows a purely restrictive defect in most patients with ILD. This is characterized by a decrease in forced vital capacity (FVC) and forced expiratory volume in 1 second (FEV_1). The loss of FEV_1 is proportional to FVC loss, so that the ratio of FEV_1 to FVC remains normal. Other measurements of lung volume, such as total lung capacity (TLC) and residual volume (RV), are also usually reduced.

The compliance of the lungs decreases as lung involvement progresses. This is due in part to fibrosis of the pulmonary parenchyma and the formation of cystic airspace.[23] Diffusion capacity of the lung (DLCO) is a good reflection of alveolar capillary surface area. Destruction of lung parenchyma results in a reduction in DLCO as ILD progresses. An abnormal DLCO may be the earliest evidence of ILD found on standard pulmonary function tests.[21,24]

Oxygen desaturation during exercise is a frequent finding in patients with ILD and is usually the earliest detectable pulmonary abnormality.[20,21] Exercise desaturation is caused by an alveolar capillary diffusion limitation and a worsening of ventilation-perfusion ($\dot{V}/\dot{Q}$) matching.[25]

> The first abnormality seen during pulmonary function studies of a patient with IPF is usually a reduced DLCO.

Chest Radiograph

The chest radiograph is occasionally normal early in the course of ILD. ILD creates several different chest appearances. All the chest radiograph appearances have one thing in common: they diffusely affect both lungs. The diffuse inflammation often seen early in ILD causes a ground-glass appearance of the lungs on chest films. The ground-glass appearance is seen as a diffuse increase in the density of the lungs, as though you were looking at the lungs through a ground-glass filter. If there is consolidation of the inflammation, the chest film will develop small ill-defined nodules. The walls of cysts cause short 0.5- to 1.0-cm linear (line like) densities to develop over the film. The pattern of numerous linear densities is called reticular. When both reticular and nodular findings are seen on the same film, the

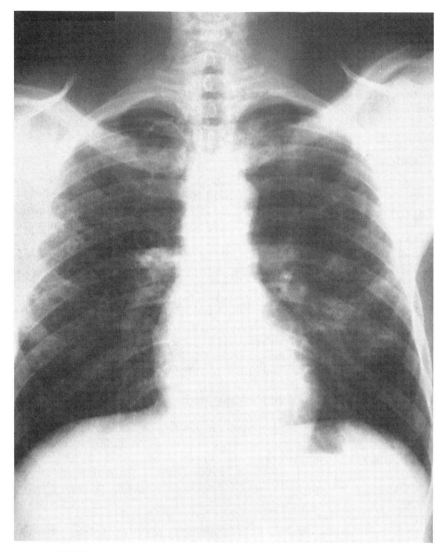

FIGURE 14.2 A diffuse reticular nodular pattern is visible throughout both lungs.

pattern is called reticulonodular (Figure 14.2). Most ILDs cause a progressive increase in the opacities on the radiograph and culminate with the development of honeycomb lung. The honeycomb-like appearance is created by numerous cysts superimposed one on top of the other (Figure 14.3).

Some chest radiographs contain specific findings that are suggestive of a particular disease process. For example, sarcoidosis is often associated with swelling of the lymph nodes in the hilum of the lung (hilar lymphadenopathy; Figure 14.4). Wegener's granulomatosis is associated with lower lobe cavities and nodules. Asbestosis may be associated with calcified pleural plaques (Figure 14.5).

ILD causes characteristic changes to the lung parenchyma that can be seen using computed tomography (CT). A normal CT scan examines a 10-mm-thick slice of tissue for each image. The densities in the 10-mm slice of lung are then averaged to create each image. Averaging the densities within a 10-mm slice of tissue eliminates much of the fine structural

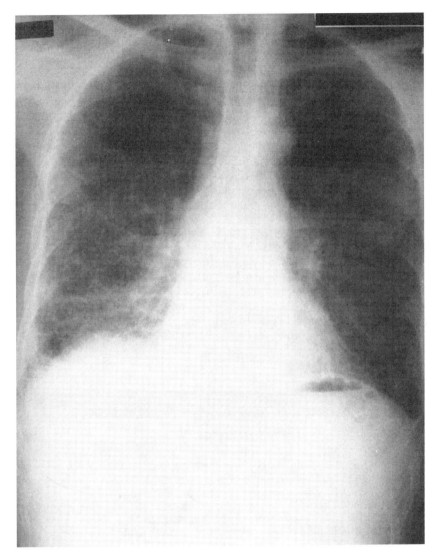

FIGURE 14.3 Dense reticular changes and cystic air spaces can be seen on this film—a pattern often called "honeycomb lung." This film is typical of end-stage ILD.

detail of the delicate lung parenchyma (Figure 14.6). The best way of viewing the lung parenchyma is to use a high-resolution CT scan, which examines only 1 mm of lung at each level, thus revealing some of the lung parenchyma's delicate architecture (Figure 14.7).

A high-resolution CT scan provides a wealth of information on the structural changes of the lung caused by the disease processes.[26,27] This information can be used to assist in the diagnosis of ILD and evaluate the severity of the disease (Figure 14.8). While high resolution CT scans provide marked improvement in imaging the lung parenchyma, the patient is exposed to as much as 2.8 times the radiation of a normal CT scan.[26]

Lung Biopsy

Confirmation of ILD frequently requires a lung biopsy in addition to a meticulous history and physical examination, as well as laboratory and radiographic evaluations.

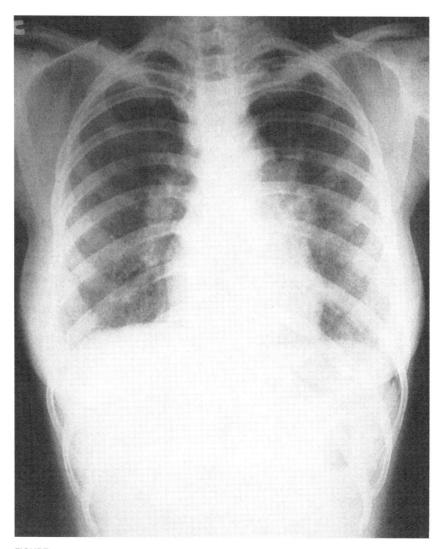

FIGURE 14.4 This chest radiograph shows a reticular pattern throughout both lungs. In addition, lymphadenopathy is visible in both hilar regions.

ILD typically involves all lobes of both lungs. When the lung is examined micro-scopically, however, the stage of involvement is extremely variable from one area of the specimen to another. Portions of lung that reveal characteristic pathological find-ings are often scattered among areas of normal lung with areas of end-stage fibrosis. To be certain that areas with characteristic changes are sampled, an open lung or tho-racoscopic[28,29] biopsy is often required. Sarcoidosis has such diffuse and characteristic pathologic changes that only very small pieces of lung are required to establish the diagnosis. These smaller specimens can be obtained with a bronchoscope using a tech-nique called transbronchial biopsy. To perform transbronchial biopsy, the broncho-scope is positioned in a smaller airway and a forceps is passed beyond the view of the operator into the periphery of the lung. The forceps can then be used to take small biopsies of lung tissue.

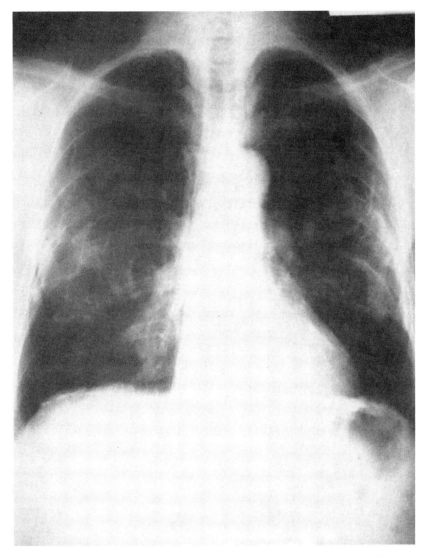

FIGURE 14.5 This chest radiograph discloses asbestos-related calcified pleural plaques. The plaques are easiest to see on the diaphragmatic surface as dense raised areas on both hemi-diaphragms. Pleural plaques are also visible, superimposed over the middle of both lungs. The plaques overlying the lung are more difficult to see than the diaphragmatic plaques because visualization is through the flat surface rather than the end of the plaque.

Bronchoalveolar Lavage

Bronchoalveolar lavage is another diagnostic technique performed by passing a broncho-scope into a segmental or smaller bronchus. The area beyond the bronchoscope is washed with saline. The saline that is then aspirated back through the bronchoscope contains a small number of cells. The cells that are recovered include many from the alveoli and are representative of the cells associated with the inflammatory process. The pathological evaluation of these cells may provide data on the cause of the ILD and may also be useful in following the inflammatory activity of the lung during therapy.[30,31]

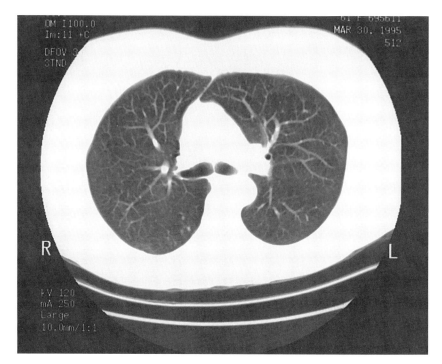

FIGURE 14.6 Normal CT scan of the chest with a 10-mm-thick slice, averaged for image.

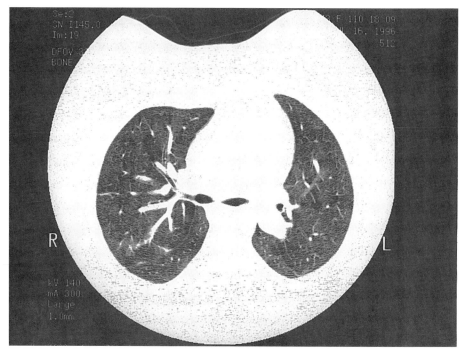

FIGURE 14.7 Normal high-resolution CT scan of chest, using a 1-mm-thick slice, averaged for image.

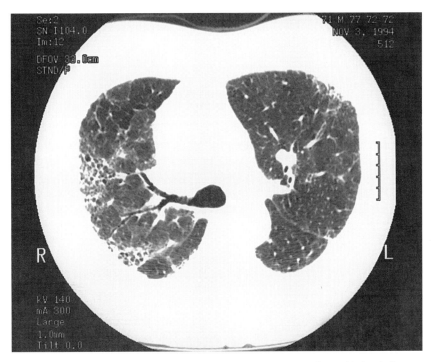

FIGURE 14.8 High-resolution CT scan of a patient with interstitial lung disease. Notice the large number of cystic air spaces typical of honeycomb lung.

TREATMENT

Specific Therapy

For most forms of ILD, the events that cause ILD begin with lung injury, which leads to lung inflammation, which results in irreversible ILD and end-stage lung disease. The goal of therapy is to prevent further irreversible damage to the lung. This is achieved by prevention of further injury and suppression of the inflammatory response. The most obvious treatment for lung injury induced by a known agent is preventing the patient from being exposed to more of the injurious substance. Although such avoidance of exposure is often adequate treatment and arrests the disease, an offending agent is identified in only about one third of patients with ILD. If the source of injury cannot be removed, or if removal of the source of injury is insufficient to avoid disease progression, treatment is aimed at suppressing inflammation. The drug most commonly used to suppress the inflammatory process initially is prednisone. In addition to prednisone, other immunosuppressive drugs such as cyclophosphamide[32] and azathioprine[33] are also used.

Sarcoidosis is the most common form of interstitial lung disease. In the vast majority of cases it is well controlled with corticosteroid therapy. Treatment with corticosteroids is recommended for sarcoid patients if they have symptoms or are at an advanced stage. It also appears that treatment is helpful for asymptomatic patients who have both lung involvement and enlarged lymph nodes in their chest radiograph.[34]

Patients with IPF are not likely to benefit from strategies to isolate them from environmental factors or from immunosuppression. New strategies designed to inhibit the growth of fibroblasts and thereby inhibit the development of fibrosis are being pursued. Among the more promising new drugs are interferon gamma 1b[35,36] and pirfenidone.[37]

Supportive Therapy

Exertional dyspnea associated with exercise hypoxemia is frequently improved by the addition of supplemental oxygen.[38] Oxygen at rest is required in the latter stages of the disease when resting hypoxemia develops.

Transplantation

Patients with progressive interstitial lung disease that continues to progress despite immuno-suppressive therapy may require lung transplantation. Transplanting only one of the patient's diseased lungs is usually adequate.[39] Lung transplantation is appropriate for interstitial lung disease only when the patients are in the end stages of the disease. Although this therapy is successful at improving lung function and quality of life, as many as 40% of patients who undergo lung transplantation die within the first 2 years following the surgery.[40]

PROGNOSIS

The prognosis for patients with interstitial lung disease is extremely variable. Early therapy can be helpful but does not alter the prognosis for a large number of interstitial lung diseases. Some diseases, for example sarcoidosis, do extremely well with treatment, with complete resolution of the findings in most cases. Other diseases are progressive and difficult to control even with aggressive therapy. These diseases include IPF, many forms of drug-induced lung disease, and some of the lung diseases associated with collagen vascular disease.

Mr. J

HISTORY

Mr. J is a 28-year-old African American man currently employed as a savings-and-loan computer analyst. He noticed increasing fatigue over the past several months, which progressed to the point where he stopped jogging and he felt listless and tired most of the time. This began as a flu-like illness and left him with a nonproductive cough. He denied having fever, chills, sore throat, coryza, headaches, or wheezing. He noted no sputum production, hemoptysis, or abnormalities in his hands or feet. After further questioning he agreed that the fatigue he experienced was probably dyspnea. He could walk indefinitely on level ground, but if he were to climb more than one flight of stairs, he would have to stop to catch his breath. He did not awaken with breathlessness, nor did he notice having dyspnea at rest.

As a child he had chickenpox, but not measles or mumps. He has had no surgeries but had broken his leg in a skiing accident at age 22. Mr. J never smoked and drank alcoholic beverages only socially. The only prescription medication he took was ampicillin once or twice for upper respiratory infections. He took aspirin for minor pain control, usually once a month. His mother has hypertension, but his father is healthy; his maternal grandfather has lung carcinoma, but his maternal grandmother is well. Both of his paternal grandparents died in a motor vehicle crash. He has two children, and both are well. Two healthy birds are kept as pets in the house.

Mr. J works as a manager of a small group of computer technicians. He has not been exposed to any dusts or fumes while performing his duties. He has worked as a computer manager since graduating from college. While in college he worked in a gas station pumping gas; in high school he worked at a local drive-through restaurant.

He is an avid sports fan and spends his leisure time watching professional sports. None of his hobbies places him at risk for lung disease.

QUESTIONS	ANSWERS
1. What is Mr. J's principal problem? Is there anything in the history that would help you characterize the problem?	Mr. J's principal complaint is dyspnea. The dyspnea is present only on exertion and has been progressive. The four major types of illness that can cause exertional dyspnea include (1) obstructive lung diseases such as asthma, emphysema, and chronic bronchitis; (2) interstitial lung disease; (3) pulmonary vascular disease such as primary pulmonary hypertension and chronic thrombotic obstruction of the pulmonary artery; and (4) heart diseases such as ischemic and valvular heart disease. This patient lacks the typical symptoms of bronchospastic lung disease such as wheezing and experiencing episodic dyspnea that occurs at rest or awakens him from sleep. He also lacks a history of previous cardiac problems that are typical of many patients with exertional dyspnea caused by heart problems. There is no history of previous deep vein thrombosis to suggest chronic thrombotic obstruction of the pulmonary artery.
2. What possible diagnosis could explain Mr. J's dyspnea on exertion?	Despite a careful history, none of these diagnoses can be excluded from consideration. The history does, however, clarify the problem we are dealing with and allows one to formulate a preliminary differential diagnosis.
3. Do the jobs Mr. J has performed place him at risk for lung disease? What jobs are typically related to exposure to inhaled inorganic dusts?	Mr. J is young and has worked primarily as a manager. None of the jobs he describes are likely to have caused lung disease. A careful exposure history should also include a history of exposure to pets and hobbies. The birds that are kept in his home as pets are a possible source of hypersensitivity pneumonitis or infection. The most common forms of inorganic pneumoconiosis are coalminer's pneumoconiosis, asbestosis, and silicosis. Coalminer's pneumoconiosis is caused by repeated exposure to coal dust. This occurs in miners and people who load coal for shipment. Asbestosis occurs in workers who are exposed to dust from asbestos. These people have usually

worked directly with asbestos as it is machined or installed. Asbestos is hazardous only when it is in the form of a dust that can be inhaled. Asbestos-containing products that do not shed dust are not dangerous as long as they remain undisturbed. Silicosis occurs in miners, sand blasters, foundry workers, and anyone who deals with sand dust on a regular basis.

4. Although Mr. J denies using illicit drugs, what form of lung disease do these drugs cause?

Illicit drugs can cause lung disease in two ways: (1) by inducing noncardiogenic pulmonary edema or (2) by vasculitis induced by the IV injection of talc. Talc is sometimes used to dilute (cut) the active drug or may have contaminated the drug as it was extracted from talc-containing tablets.

5. What are your goals for the physical examination?

The major goal of the physical examination is to help clarify the cause of Mr. J's dyspnea. Obstructive lung disease may be associated with an increase in the anteroposterior (AP) diameter of the chest and wheezes over the lung. Interstitial lung disease is usually associated with pulmonary crackles. Pulmonary vascular disease is characterized by the signs of pulmonary hypertension. The physical examination findings in pulmonary hypertension are a loud pulmonic component to the second heart sound (P_2) and possibly right ventricular heave or lift. Patients with chronic heart disease may have an abnormal heart rhythm, resulting in an abnormal extra heart sound such as a cardiac murmur, which suggests valvular heart disease, or an S_3 or S_4 heart sound, which suggests heart failure.

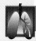

More on Mr. J

PHYSICAL EXAMINATION

- General. An athletic-appearing man in no respiratory distress

- Vital Signs. Temperature 36.3°C (97.3°F), pulse 62/min, respiratory rate 14/min, blood pressure 156/96 mm Hg

- HEENT. Head normal; nose patent without discharge; pupils equal, round, and reactive to light; mucous membranes moist without cyanosis

- Neck. Carotid arteries normal in contour and intensity; jugular neck veins not distended; trachea in midline of neck; swelling of submandibular salivary glands and several 1 to 2 cm lymph nodes in anterior cervical region

- Chest. Configuration and expansion of the chest normal; diffuse, fine, inspiratory crackles throughout both lungs without wheezing found upon auscultation; normal resonance noted over all portions of the chest with percussion

- **Heart.** Regular rate with no murmur or gallop; S_1 and S_2 have normal intensity and splitting; cardiac impulse in the fourth interspace 1 cm medial to the midclavicular line

- **Abdomen.** Soft, nontender; bowel sounds active; no masses or organ enlargement noted; abdominal wall rising with each inspiration

- **Extremities.** No edema noted; no clubbing or cyanosis seen; extremities warm with good capillary refill

QUESTIONS	ANSWERS
6. What is your interpretation of the vital signs?	With the exception of the blood pressure, the vital signs are normal. The elevation of blood pressure may be due to hypertension or it may be a response to stress in a healthy person. Treatment of hypertension of this magnitude is not necessary unless multiple measurements have shown chronic elevation of blood pressure.
7. How would you interpret the pulmonary findings? How might they affect your assessment of Mr. J?	It was noted that Mr. J had diffuse, fine, inspiratory crackles over both lungs, which is consistent with the diagnosis of interstitial lung disease or pulmonary edema owing to heart failure. Wheezing and increased AP diameter of the chest, signs of obstructive lung disease are absent. The lung examination indicates that heart failure and ILD are the most likely explanations for Mr. J's exertional breathlessness. It is still possible, though much less likely, that this represents an atypical presentation of obstructive lung disease or pulmonary vascular disease.
8. How would you interpret the cardiac findings? How might they affect your assessment?	Results of the heart examination were normal. There were no extra heart sounds and no increase in P_2. The location of the cardiac impulse was normal. The lack of abnormal findings on cardiac examination makes it less likely, but not impossible, that Mr. J's dyspnea is related to pulmonary hypertension or heart failure.
9. Does Mr. J have evidence of cor pulmonale?	Cor pulmonale is right heart failure that is the result of lung disease. Right heart failure causes systemic venous congestion, which is characterized by distention of the jugular veins, pedal edema, and hepatojugular reflux. In addition to systemic congestion, the heart examination is also abnormal when cor pulmonale is present. Right ventricular strain causes an abnormal pulsation (heave) over the lower left sternal border and an S_3 or S_4 that can be heard over this same area. Mr. J has none of these findings and therefore does not have cor pulmonale.

10. What is the significance of the swelling of multiple structures in Mr. J's neck?

Swelling of lymph nodes (lymphadenopathy) can result from an infection or inflammatory process occurring either in the area drained by the lymph node or in the lymph node itself. Sarcoidosis is associated with cervical lymphadenopathy and enlargement of salivary glands.

11. Describe the normal relationship between the respiratory cycle and movement of the abdominal wall.

The diaphragm is the major muscle of respiration. Contraction of the diaphragm causes it to descend, drawing air into the lungs. Diaphragmatic descent also causes the abdominal wall to rise during inspiration, as is seen in this patient. If a patient has a very high inspiratory muscle load or diaphragmatic fatigue, the diaphragm rises on inspiration. This paradoxical movement of the diaphragm causes the abdominal wall to fall on inspiration. This would be a sign of respiratory failure.

12. What pathology typically accounts for the fine, inspiratory crackles heard in Mr. J? Are crackles commonly heard in patients with restrictive lung disease or obstructive lung disease?

Inspiratory crackles are caused by sudden opening of peripheral lung units with inspiration. This finding is typical of patients with ILD, atelectasis, or pulmonary edema. Fine, late-inspiratory crackles are consistent with restrictive lung disease.

13. Does the lack of cyanosis indicate that hypoxemia is not present?

A lack of cyanosis does not indicate that hypoxemia is not present. The disease process that is causing Mr. J to experience dyspnea is probably an ILD, but this has not been proved.

14. What laboratory work would be most useful to determine the etiology of Mr. J's dyspnea?

Pulmonary function testing including spirometry and D$_{LCO}$ would help determine whether restrictive or obstructive lung disease is present and would also determine the severity of the disease. A chest radiograph should be ordered to help classify the pulmonary disease. An ABG analysis should be ordered to determine Mr. J's ability to ventilate and oxygenate.

More on Mr. J

Laboratory Evaluation

Chest Radiograph: (see Figure 14.9)

ABG (on room air)	Value	
pH	7.45	
Pa_{O_2}	65 mm Hg	
Pa_{CO_2}	32 mm Hg	
HCO_3^-	21 mEq/liter	
$P(A-a)_{O_2}$	44 mm Hg	
O_2 content	17.5 mL/dL	

CBC	Observed	Normal
White blood cells/mm^3	9100	4000–11,000
Red blood cells (million/mm^3)	4.3	4.1–5.5
Hemoglobin (g/dL)	14.2	14–16.5
Hematocrit (%)	41	40–54

Differential		
Segmented neutrophils (%)	69	40–75
Band neutrophils (%)	9	0–6
Lymphocytes (%)	17	20–45
Monocytes (%)	3	2–10
Eosinophils (%)	1	0–6
Basophils (%)	1	0–1

Chemistry		
Na^+ (mEq/liter)	142	137–147
K^+ (mEq/liter)	4.1	3.5–4.8
Cl^- (mmol/dL)	108	98–105
HCO_3^- (mEq/liter)	22	22–29
Blood urea nitrogen (mg/dL)	19	7–20
Creatinine (mg/dL)	1.1	0.7–1.3
Calcium (mmol/liter)	2.5	2.1–2.55
Phosphate (mg/dL)	2.9	2.7–4.5
Uric acid (mg/dL)	6.9	4.5–8.2
Albumen (g/dL)	4.8	3.5–5.0
Protein (g/dL)	8.2	6.4–8.3

Pulmonary Function Testing		
	Value	(%) of Predicted
Spirometry		
FVC (liters)	2.79	63
SVC (liters)	2.61	59
FEV$_1$ (liters)	2.12	67
FEV$_1$/FVC (%)		76
FEF$_{25-75\%}$ (liters/minute)	4.11	98
Body plethysmography		
RV (liters)	1.20	118
TLC (liters)	3.99	74
D$_{LCO}$ (mL/min per mm Hg)	11.35	38

FEF = forced expiratory flow; SVC = slow vital capacity.

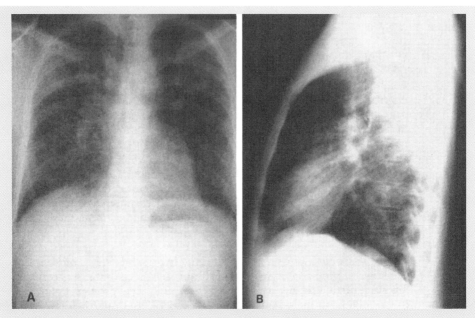

FIGURE 14.9 Chest radiograph of Mr. J at presentation. (A) Posteroanterior (PA) view; (B) lateral view.

QUESTIONS	ANSWERS
15. How do you interpret the chest radiograph?	The chest radiograph shows diffuse reticulonodular opacification of both lungs. There is bilateral hilar enlargement as well. The heart is of normal size and configuration. This chest radiograph is consistent with interstitial lung disease. The presence of hilar lymphadenopathy suggests the diagnosis of sarcoidosis.
16. How would you evaluate and interpret Mr. J's ABG values?	Chronic respiratory alkalosis is demonstrated in these ABG values. The patient has mild hypoxemia with an increase in the $P(A-a)o_2$.
17. Interpret the results of the pulmonary function test. How do these tests affect possible diagnosis of interstitial lung disease or obstructive lung disease?	The reduction of lung volumes on spirometry suggests restrictive lung disease. The loss of FEV_1 is proportional to the loss of vital capacity (FEV_1/FVC is normal), suggesting restrictive lung disease. Measurements obtained from body plethysmography suggest restrictive lung disease. TLC is decreased. The normal RV indicates that some obstructive lung disease may also be present. The abnormal D_{LCO} indicates a loss of alevolar capillary surface area and strongly suggests that lung destruction is occurring. These findings are consistent with ILD.

18. What testing may be helpful in determining whether the patient will be helped by supplemental oxygen?	The initial ABG analysis does not indicate that supplemental oxygen is required. Patients with ILD become desaturated upon exercise and may benefit from supplemental oxygen during exercise. Treadmill exercise testing with ABG samples and exhaled gas collection would determine whether Mr. J requires oxygen with exertion.
19. What additional testing will be needed to determine the cause of this patient's disease?	At this point there is strong evidence that Mr. J has a form of ILD. It is important to determine the type of ILD in order to devise an appropriate therapeutic plan. Lung biopsy is the most effective way to determine with accuracy what disease is responsible for Mr. J's symptoms. There are several reasons to suspect that Mr. J has sarcoidosis. Because sarcoidosis is the most likely diagnosis, transbronchial biopsy is the diagnostic test of choice.

More on Mr. J

Mr. J undergoes pulmonary stress testing. He exercises for 8 minutes and 32 seconds using a modified Bruce protocol exercise test. He stops because of extreme dyspnea. No cardiac abnormalities are noted on the electrocardiogram.

Stress Test	Value	% of Predicted
$\dot{V}O_2$ max (mL/min)	1201	37
$\dot{V}CO_2$ max (mL/min)	1528	
RQ	1.27	
Lowest O_2 saturation (%)	81	

RQ = respiratory quotient; $\dot{V}CO_2$ max = maximum CO_2 consumption; $\dot{V}O_2$ max = maximum O_2 consumption

ABGS (on room air at rest and during peak exercise)	
At Rest	
pH	7.43
PaO_2	65 mm Hg
$PaCO_2$	33 mm Hg
HCO_3^-	22 mEq/liter
$P(A-a)O_2$	44 mm Hg
O_2 content	17.5 mL/dL
Peak Exercise Value	
pH	7.31
PaO_2	47 mm Hg
$PaCO_2$	28 mm Hg
HCO_3^-	14 mEq/liter
$P(A-a)O_2$	67 mm Hg
O_2 content	15.6 mL/dL

A bronchoscopy with transbronchial biopsy and a bronchoalveolar lavage is performed. The airways appear normal on examination. A modest amount of bleeding was encountered following transbronchial biopsy. The transbronchial biopsy contains numerous noncaseating granulomas without infectious organisms. The pathological diagnosis is sarcoidosis. The bronchoalveolar lavage shows numerous lymphocytes with alveolar macrophages and occasional neutrophils.

QUESTIONS	ANSWERS
20. What is a plausible explanation of Mr. J's dyspnea on exertion?	There are many reasons for persons with ILD to experience dyspnea. In Mr. J, hypoxemia develops with exercise. This exertional desaturation may in part explain the breathlessness he develops when jogging.
21. Interpret the ABG analysis taken at peak exercise. What physiologic changes are responsible for each of the changes you see?	There is profound hypoxemia with exercise. There is also a mixed acid-base disorder with a respiratory alkalosis and a metabolic acidosis. The hypoxemia in this case is caused by worsening of $\dot{V}/\dot{Q}$ matching and reduction in the red blood cell transit time through the alveolar capillaries. The drop in Pa_{CO_2} may be driven by hypoxia and acidosis. The drop in HCO_3^- is caused by lactic acidosis owing to anaerobic metabolism of exercising muscle.
22. What is a respiratory quotient? What does Mr. J's RQ indicate?	The RQ is the ratio of carbon dioxide produced to oxygen consumed. At rest, the RQ of a healthy person is about 0.8. With anaerobic metabolism, such as occurs during vigorous exercise, the amount of carbon dioxide produced exceeds the amount of oxygen consumed. When an individual makes a transition from aerobic to anaerobic metabolism, he or she is said to have crossed the "anaerobic threshold." Mr. J had an RQ of 1.27, which indicates that he crossed his anaerobic threshold.
23. How is a transbronchial biopsy obtained? What type of tissue will it provide for examination?	Transbronchial biopsy is a technique for sampling alveoli and small airways without performing major surgery. A bronchoscope is used to locate the airway that leads to the portion of the lung that is to be sampled. Biopsy forceps are then passed several inches beyond the bronchoscope, and the biopsy is taken from the small airways. The samples of tissue that are obtained are very small and therefore inadequate for diagnosing many forms of ILD. This technique is popular, however, because it can easily diagnose diseases such as sarcoidosis, tumors, and infections and does not require a general anesthetic or skin incision.

24. How is bronchoalveolar lavage obtained? What types of samples will it provide for examination?

Like transbronchial biopsy, bronchoalveolar lavage is a bronchoscopic technique. The purpose of the lavage is to wash a small number of cells from the alveoli for pathologic examination. The bronchoscope is passed into the smallest airway it can enter. Saline (50 to 200 mL) is injected into the bronchial lumen. The saline washes out to the small airways and is then aspirated back out through the bronchoscope. Unlike biopsy, bronchoalevolar lavage obtains cells with no surrounding structure. This technique is useful for diagnosing and staging ILD, diagnosing certain lung infections (particularly *Pneumocystis carinii* pneumonia), and diagnosing some forms of lung cancer.

25. Will oxygen therapy help relieve Mr. J's breathlessness? If oxygen is given to this patient, how should he use it?

Yes, Mr. J has a marked tendency toward desaturation with moderate exercise levels. The use of supplemental oxygen with exertion may help his exertional dyspnea. There is no need at this time to have him use oxygen 24 hours a day.

26. What therapy should Mr. J receive for his sarcoidosis? What is the goal of that therapy?

Sarcoidosis is one of the forms of ILD that has no known cause. As a consequence, therapy cannot be directed at preventing further exposure to an injuring agent. Instead, therapy is aimed at suppressing inflammation, which is usually accomplished with corticosteroids, cyclophosphamide, or azathioprine, or a combination of these drugs. In sarcoidosis, therapy with corticosteroids such as prednisone is usually very effective at stopping progression of the disease.

Mr. J Conclusion

One year after the initial diagnosis of sarcoidosis, Mr. J feels much better. He has taken prednisone for 1 year, after which his chest radiograph shows improvement. He has less dyspnea on exertion and no longer requires oxygen therapy. He continues to have a restrictive defect on spirometry and a reduction in his D_{LCO}, but both of these parameters are improved.

QUESTIONS

ANSWERS

28. If the sarcoidosis had progressed to its end stage, what would Mr. J's lungs have been like radiographically and pathologically?

End-stage ILD is characterized by replacement of normal lung tissue by cystic airspaces and fibrotic tissue. On radiograph, the cystic airspaces can be seen surrounded by fibrous connective tissue in a pattern called honeycomb lung.

29. If ILD were to progress to its end stage despite anti-inflammatory medication, what treatment options would be available?

End-stage ILD may require single lung transplantation to control the symptoms of interstitial lung disease. Single lung transplantation improves a patient's symptoms, exercise tolerance, and quality of life if the patient survives the surgery and tolerates the immunosuppression necessary to prevent rejection of the transplanted lung. ∎

KEY POINTS

- Interstitial lung disease (ILD) includes a large group of diverse diseases that cause lung damage that results in fibrosis of the lung, reduced lung volumes and lung surface area.
- The term **pneumoconiosis** refers a form of ILD related to the inhalation of inorganic dust.
- Only about one third of patients with ILD have an identifiable agent responsible for inducing lung injury. Typical inorganic dusts that may induce ILD include asbestos, silica (sand), coal, and talc.
- Many of drugs that are well known for causing ILD are used in the treatment of cancer. Drug-induced lung disease is a major cause of morbidity and mortality in patients undergoing chemotherapy for cancer.
- The pathological appearance of the lungs in most patients with early ILD is characterized by inflammation. As the ILD progresses, the inflammation is replaced with fibrosis and cysts.
- The first symptom of ILD is usually progressive dyspnea on exertion or a nonproductive cough.
- There may be no abnormal physical examination findings early in the course of the disease. As the process progresses, tachypnea and fine, late-inspiratory crackles are present.
- Pulmonary function studies usually show a purely restrictive defect in most patients with ILD. This is characterized by a decrease in forced vital capacity (FVC) and forced expiratory volume in 1 second (FEV_1).
- An abnormal D_{LCO} may be the earliest evidence of ILD found on standard pulmonary function tests.
- Oxygen desaturation during exercise is a frequent finding in patients with ILD.
- The diffuse inflammation often seen early in ILD causes a ground-glass appearance of the lungs on chest films.
- Most ILDs cause a progressive increase in the opacities on the radiograph and culminate with the development of honeycomb lung. The honeycomb-like appearance is created by numerous cysts superimposed one on top of the other.
- The most obvious treatment for lung injury induced by a known agent is preventing the patient from being exposed to more of the injurious substance.
- If the source of injury cannot be removed, or if removal of the source of injury is insufficient to avoid disease progression, treatment is aimed at suppressing inflammation. The drug most commonly used to suppress the inflammatory process initially is prednisone.
- Patients with progressive ILD that continues to progress despite immunosuppressive therapy may require lung transplantation.

REFERENCES

1. Coultas, DB, et al: The epidemiology of interstitial lung diseases. Am J Respir Crit Care Med 150:967, 1994.
2. Morgan, WKC, Seaton, A: Occupational Lung Diseases, ed 2. WB Saunders, Philadelphia, 1984.
3. Becklake, MR: Pneumoconiosis. In Murray, JF, Nadel, JA (eds): Textbook of Respiratory Medicine. WB Saunders, Philadelphia, 1988, pp. 1556–1592.
4. Johns, CJ: Sarcoidosis. In Fishman, AP (ed): Pulmonary Disease and Disorders. McGraw-Hill, New York, 1988, pp. 619–641.
5. Hammon, L, Rich, AR: Acute interstitial fibrosis of the lung. Bull Johns Hopkins 74:177, 1944.

6. American Thoracic Society/European Respiratory Society: International multidisciplinary consensus classification of the idiopathic interstitial pneumonias. Am J Respir Crit Care Bed 165:277, 2001.

7. Khalil, N, O'Connor, R: Idiopathic pulmonary fibrosis: current understanding of the pathogenesis and the status of treatment. CMAJ 171:153, 2004.

8. King, T, et al: Idiopathic pulmonary fibrosis: relationship between histopathologic features and mortality. Am J Respir Crit Care Med 164:1025, 2001.

9. Stachura, I, et al: Mechanisms of tissue injury in desquamative interstitial pneumonitis. Am J Med 68:733, 1980.

10. Fox, RB, et al: Pulmonary inflammation due to oxygen toxicity: involvement of chemotactic factors and polymorphonuclear leukocytes. Am Rev Respir Dis 123:521, 1981.

11. Guidotti, TL: Coal workers' pneumoconiosis and medical aspects of coal mining. South Med J 72:456, 1979.

12. Batist, G, Andrews, JL: Pulmonary toxicity of antineoplastic drugs. JAMA 246:1449, 1981.

13. Cockerill, FJ, et al: Open lung biopsy in immunocompromised patients. Arch Intern Med 145:1398, 1985.

14. Rosenow, EC, Martin, WJ: Drug induced interstitial lung disease. In Schwarz, MI, King, TE (eds): Interstitial Lung Disease, BC Decker, Toronto, 1988, pp. 123–137.

15. Donaldson, L, Grant, IS, Naysmith, MR, et al: Acute amiodarone-induced lung toxicity. Intensive Care Med 24:626, 1998.

16. Kndenchyk, PJ, et al: Prospective evaluation of amiodarone pulmonary toxicity. Chest 86:541, 1984.

17. Ashrafian, H, Davey, P: Is amiodarone an under-recognized cause of acute respiratory failure in the ICU?. Chest 120(1):275–282, 2001.

18. Suntres, ZE, Shek, PN: Nitrofurantoin-induced pulmonary toxicity: in vivo evidence for oxidative stress-mediated mechanisms. Biochem Pharmacol 43:1127, 1992.

19. Flint, A: Pathologic features of interstitial lung disease. In Schwarz, MI, King, TE (eds): Interstitial Lung Disease. BC Decker, Toronto, 1988, pp. 45–62.

20. Crystal, RG, et al: Idiopathic pulmonary fibrosis: clinical, histologic, radiographic, physiologic, scintigraphic, cytologic and biochemical aspects. Ann Intern Med 85:769, 1976.

21. Fulmer, JD: The interstitial lung diseases. Chest 82:172, 1982.

22. Carrington, CB, et al: Natural history and treated course of usual and desquamative interstitial pneumonia. N Engl J Med 298:801, 1978.

23. Fulmer, JD: An introduction to the interstitial lung diseases. Clin Chest Med 3:457, 1982.

24. Crystal, RG, et al: Interstitial lung disease: current concepts of pathogenesis staging and therapy. Am J Med 70:542, 1981.

25. Wagner, PD: Ventilation-perfusion matching during exercise. Chest 101:192S, 1992.

26. Engeler, CE, et al: Volumetric high resolution CT scan in the diagnosis of interstitial lung disease and bronchiectasis: diagnostic accuracy and radiation dose. AJR 163:31, 1994.

27. Nishimura, K, et al: The diagnostic accuracy of computed tomography in diffuse infiltrative lung diseases. Chest 104:1149, 1993.

28. Nasim, A, et al: Video-thoracoscopic lung biopsy in diagnosis of interstitial lung disease. J R Coll Surg Edin 40:22, 1995.

29. Krasna, MJ, et al: The role of thoracoscopy in the diagnosis of interstitial lung disease. Ann Thorac Surg 59:348, 1995.

30. American Thoracic Society: Clinical role of bronchoalveolar lavage in adults with pulmonary disease. Am Rev Respir Dis 142:481, 1990.

31. Costabel, U, Guzman, J: Bronchoalveolar lavage in interstitial lung disease. Curr Opin Pulmonary Med 7:255, 2001.

32. Johnson, MA, et al: Randomized controlled trial comparing prednisolone alone with cyclophosphamide and low dose prednisolone in combination in cryptogenic fibrosing alveolitis. Thorax 44:280, 1989.

33. Raghu, G, et al: Azathioprine combined with prednisone in the treatment of idiopathic pulmonary fibrosis: a prospective double-blind randomized placebo-controlled clinical trial. Ann Rev Respir Dis 144:291, 1991.

34. Pietinalho, A, et al: Early treatment of stage II sarcoidosis improves 5-year pulmonary function. Chest 121:24, 2002.

35. Ziexche, R, et al: A preliminary study of long-term treatment with interferon gamma-1b and low dose prednisolone in patients with idiopathic pulmonary fibrosis. N Engl J Med 341:1264; 1999.

36. Raghu G, et al: A placebo-controlled trial of interferon gamma-1b in patients with idiopathic pulmonary fibrosis. N Engl J Med 350:125, 2004.

37. Raghu G, et al: Treatment of idiopathic pulmonary fibrosis with a new antifibrotic agent, pirfenidone. Am J Respir Crit Care Med 159:1061, 1999.

38. Harris-Eze, AO, et al: Oxygen improves maximal exercise performance in interstitial lung disease. Am J Respir Crit Care Med 150:1616, 1994.

39. Egan, TM, et al: Isolated lung transplantation for end-stage lung disease: a viable therapy. Ann Thorac Surg 53:590, 1992.

40. Cooper, JD, et al: Current status of lung transplantation: report of the St. Louis International Lung Transplant Registry. Clin Transpl 77:81, 1992.

15

Neuromuscular Diseases

N. Lennard Specht, MD, FACP

Rebekah Bartos Specht, MSN, FNP

CHAPTER OBJECTIVES:

After reading this chapter you will be able to:

- Describe the role of the respiratory therapist (RT) in evaluating and treating the patient with neuromuscular disease.
- Identify the function of the neuromuscular system and its components with regard to breathing.
- Identify the defects in the neuromuscular system that can cause respiratory failure.
- Identify the names of neuromuscular disorders that often cause respiratory failure.
- List the common clinical features associated with the different types of neuromuscular disease.
- State the general and specific treatment needed for patients with various neuromuscular diseases.

INTRODUCTION

Neuromuscular diseases are a large group of syndromes that affect the central nervous system, the peripheral nervous system, or the muscles. Neuromuscular disorders can threaten every activity from walking to breathing. They may be temporary and completely resolve, or they may be permanent, resulting in paralysis or even death. Regardless of the specific type of neuromuscular disorder present, the patient needs to be accurately diagnosed so he or she receives the best treatment and achieves the best possible outcome.

Respiratory therapists (RTs) often play a key role in the evaluation and care of the patient with neuromuscular disease, especially when the disorder threatens the muscles of breathing or reflexes that protect the lungs from aspiration. Dyspnea is a frequent problem associated with neuromuscular disease, but early in the disease process it may be inappropriately attributed to other problems, such as asthma or chronic obstructive pulmonary disease (COPD). RTs are often in a good position to recognize impending respiratory failure or respiratory muscle weakness inaccurately diagnosed as asthma or COPD. For this reason, it is vital that RTs be familiar with this group of medical problems. A review of the anatomy and physiology associated with the neuromuscular system controlling breathing is helpful as an introduction to the subject of specific neuromuscular diseases.

NORMAL NEUROMUSCULAR FUNCTION IN BREATHING

Normal breathing during rest, exercise, and sleep requires a healthy respiratory pump for effective movement of air in and out of the chest. The respiratory pump consists of four major components:

1. Chemoreceptors, which respond to oxygen and carbon dioxide levels and signal the respiratory centers in the brain stem
2. The respiratory centers in the brain stem, which control the rate and depth of breathing.
3. The peripheral nerves that conduct impulses from the respiratory centers to the respiratory muscles
4. The respiratory muscles.

Chemoreceptors

Chemoreceptors are located in the great vessels (peripheral) and in the brain stem (central). Both create neural impulses based on the concentration of oxygen or carbon dioxide and transmit these impulses to the respiratory centers.

The peripheral chemoreceptors are located in the carotid bodies and the aortic bodies. The carotid bodies are located in the back of the bifurcation of the common carotid arteries, and the aortic bodies are located in the arch of the aorta. The location of the peripheral chemoreceptors allows monitoring of gasses in arterial blood. The peripheral chemoreceptors sense oxygen and carbon dioxide. The output of oxygen receptors increases as the Pa_{O_2} drops. The carbon dioxide receptors increase their output as Pa_{CO_2} levels rise.

The central chemoreceptors are located in the ventral surface of the medulla. These receptors are responsive to the concentration of hydrogen ions in the surrounding cerebrospinal fluid (CSF). The extracellular fluid is largely controlled by the blood-brain barrier. This barrier strictly regulates the flow of ions and water into the brain. Three molecules are the major determinants of central chemoreceptor activity: bicarbonate ions (HCO_3^-), hydrogen ions (H^+[pH]), and carbon dioxide (CO_2). The brain is protected from sudden shifts in ion concentrations in the blood by an impermeable layer of cells separating the blood from the brain. This layer of cells is called the blood-brain barrier. The blood-brain barrier regulates the movement of virtually all substances into and out of the brain. Bicarbonate and H^+ movement is carefully regulated by the blood-brain barrier, but CO_2 can freely cross it. The enhanced mobility of CO_2 makes the central chemoreceptors much more responsive to changes in blood CO_2 than to changes in blood pH.

Respiratory Centers

The respiratory centers are located in multiple areas within the medulla and pons in the brain stem. Three major components form the respiratory centers. The medullary center is responsible for maintaining a regular rhythmic respiratory pattern. The apneustic and pneumotaxic centers work together to regulate respiratory frequency and volume.

The respiratory centers receive input from oxygen sensors in the carotid and aortic bodies, carbon dioxide receptors in the aortic bodies, hydrogen ion sensors in the brain stem, mechanoreceptors in the lung, and the cerebral cortex. The respiratory centers interpret this information and produce a signal that is sent through peripheral nerves to the respiratory muscles. As the impulse leaves the brain stem, it travels down

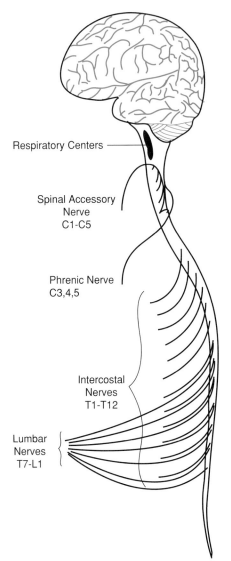

Respiratory Centers

Spinal Accessory
Nerve
C1-C5

Phrenic Nerve
C3,4,5

Intercostal
Nerves
T1-T12

Lumbar
Nerves
T7-L1

FIGURE 15.1 The neural pathways necessary for the respiratory pump.

the spinal cord, exits to the peripheral nerves, and travels to the neuromuscular junction. Here the impulse connects to the respiratory muscles, which respond to the stimulus by contraction.

Peripheral Nerves

The three nerve groups that are most important to respiration are the phrenic, the intercostal, and the abdominal wall muscle nerves (Figure 15.1). The phrenic nerves arise from the cervical spinal cord at the C3 to C5 level. These nerves leave the spinal canal, travel through the neck and into the mediastinum and then over the pericardium, and insert into the diaphragm on either side of the heart. The intercostal nerves arise from the thoracic spinal cord at levels T1 to T12. These nerves lie under each rib and supply the intercostal muscles. The abdominal muscle nerves arise from the thoracic and lumbar spine (T7 to L1).

Each nerve ending is connected to a muscle fiber by a neuromuscular junction. An impulse transmitted along a nerve reaches a nerve ending at the neuromuscular junction. The nerve ending releases acetylcholine when stimulated by a nerve impulse. The presence of acetylcholine at the neuromuscular junction causes the muscle to contract. The acetylcholine that is released into the neuromuscular junction is rapidly degraded by acetylcholinesterase to prevent excessive muscle stimulation.

Respiratory Muscles

There are several muscles of respiration (Figure 15.2). The diaphragm is the largest and most important inspiratory muscle. Contraction of the diaphragm pushes down on the abdominal contents, which are held in place by the abdominal wall, and uses them as a fulcrum to raise the anterior portion of the ribs. This causes the pressure in the chest to drop, and air rushes in through the trachea, inflating the lungs. Other inspiratory muscles include the external intercostal, scalene, and sternocleidomastoid muscles. These muscles become active during heavy exercise in healthy persons or at rest in patients with compromised diaphragmatic function.

The expiratory muscles are the internal intercostal and abdominal wall muscles, including the rectus abdominus, internal and external oblique, and transverse abdominus muscles. They are called on only during forceful exhalation, as with a cough. They are not needed during passive exhalation to the point of functional residual capacity in healthy persons.

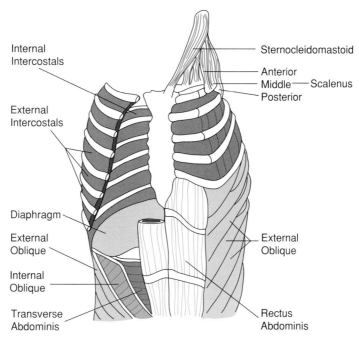

FIGURE 15.2 The major respiratory muscles.

PATHOPHYSIOLOGY

In healthy people the respiratory pump is an efficient servomechanism, sensing respiratory gasses, determining from the gas information the necessary depth and rate of ventilation, and transmitting ventilatory depth and rate impulses through the nerves to the muscles to obtain the required ventilation. This servomechanism allows for rapid changes in ventilation when blood gas concentrations change. Changes in blood gas concentrations are rapidly sensed by the chemoreceptors, and the output of the respiratory pump will be altered rapidly. The respiratory pump is vulnerable to injury; damage to any portion of the pump may lead to respiratory failure.

Respiratory Centers

Because the respiratory centers are located in several parts of the brain stem, they are relatively invulnerable to direct injury. In fact, the respiratory centers are frequently one of the last neurologic functions still evident in patients with severe head injury or strokes. While protected from injury, the respiratory centers are affected by a number of disease processes and drugs.

Sedative drugs, particularly narcotics, can suppress respiration by depressing the respiratory centers. An overdose of narcotics, barbiturates, or even benzodiazepines can lead to hypoventilation or apnea in severe cases.

Central sleep apnea is an example of a disease caused by an abnormality in the respiratory center. It is characterized by lapses of breathing effort during sleep. This disorder most often affects adults with cerebrovascular disease, but it may also play a role in sudden infant death syndrome (SIDS).

Primary alveolar hypoventilation is another example of a disease caused by insufficient respiratory drive in the absence of an obvious defect of the respiratory pump or lungs. These patients hypoventilate while awake and during sleep, but when asked to, they can voluntarily lower their $Paco_2$ to normal levels.

Nerve Interruption

If signals from the respiratory centers to the respiratory muscles are interrupted, the respiratory pump will be unable to provide ventilation. There are many sites along the pathway where nerve damage can result in compromise of the respiratory system.

Trauma is the most frequent cause of nerve damage that affects the respiratory pump. Spinal cord injury (SCI) blocks transmission of nerve impulses below the level of injury. Nerves that arise from the spinal cord below the level of injury, as well as muscles supplied by those nerves, are therefore nonfunctional. Injuries to the cervical spinal cord create much more difficulty than injuries to the thoracic and lumbar spine (Table 15.1). Damage to the midthoracic spine leads to loss of function of the abdominal and some of the intercostal muscles. Cervical spine injuries in the C6 to C7 area lead to loss of function of all intercostal and abdominal muscles. A cervical spinal cord transection to the C1 to C3 area will lead to apnea because almost all respiratory muscles are affected. Approximately 200,000 people in the United States live with significant SCI, many of whom need some form of respiratory care.[1]

> The location of the SCI is important in predicting the degree of respiratory compromise. The higher up the spinal cord the injury is located, the greater the chance of pulmonary complications.

The phrenic nerve arises from C3 to C5. Within the respiratory pump, the phrenic nerve is the peripheral nerve that is most vulnerable to injury. Temporary interruption of a phrenic nerve may occur during coronary artery bypass surgery. Cooling measures used to protect the heart from ischemia while the bypass grafts are being completed may cool the phrenic nerves excessively. Excessive cooling of the phrenic nerve causes interruption of the nerve and resultant diaphragmatic paralysis. This paralysis is frequently temporary but may take months to resolve.

Nontraumatic processes can also interrupt nerves. Polio is a viral illness that destroys the motor neurons in the anterior horn of the spinal cord. The destruction of motor neurons may involve nerves that innervate respiratory muscles. Paralysis of the respiratory muscles from polio may become so pronounced that respiratory failure and apnea develop. Respiratory failure from polio was a common occurrence until the development of the polio vaccine in the 1950s. Modern mechanical ventilation was developed in part as a treatment for polio patients with respiratory failure. Negative pressure ventilators known as iron lungs were frequently used to ventilate patients with polio (Figure 15.3). Widespread use of mechanical ventilation began with polio wards in the 1950s.

Amyotrophic lateral sclerosis (ALS) is a progressive fatal neurological disease also known as Lou Gehrig's disease. Despite extensive research, no etiology for ALS has been discovered. As in polio, patients with ALS lose muscle function because of loss

Table 15.1 **Respiratory Muscle Innervation**	
Spinal Cord Level	Peripheral Nerve(s)/Muscle(s)
C1–2	Spinal accessory/sternocleidomastoid
C3–5	Phrenic/diaphragm
C4–8	Cervical/scalene
T1–12	Intercostal/intercostal
T7–L1	Abdominal/abdominal wall

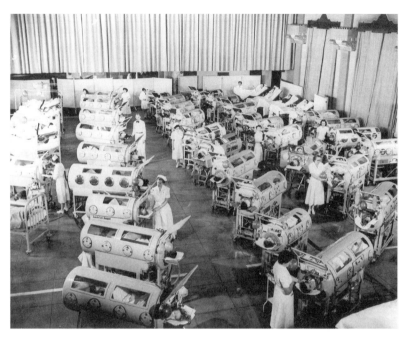

FIGURE 15.3 Polio ward with iron lungs. Photograph provided by Rancho Los Amigos National Rehabilitation Center.

of motor neurons in the anterior horn of the spinal cord. Respiratory failure invariably develops in ALS patients (Table 15.2). About 7,000 new cases of ALS are diagnosed in the United States each year.[2]

Patients with Guillain-Barré syndrome (GBS) have a progressive, ascending paralysis caused by an inflammatory destruction of the myelin sheath around peripheral nerves. Acute postinfectious polyneuropathy, another name for GBS, is frequently preceded by a viral-type illness. The viral syndrome is followed by inflammation of spinal roots and peripheral nerves. The inflammation of the spinal roots causes destruction of the myelin sheaths. The loss of myelin sheaths causes the associated nerve to malfunction. Most often, the inflammation resolves and the myelin sheaths regenerate.

Neuromuscular Junction

The nerve impulse can be interrupted at the synapse of the neuromuscular junction. This interruption can be caused by failure of a nerve to release acetylcholine, as in botulism poisoning. Destruction of acetylcholine receptors on the muscle, as in myasthenia gravis, will also lead to muscle weakness and potentially to respiratory pump failure (see Table 15.2). Myasthenia gravis

Table 15.2 Neuromuscular Disorders

Location of Defect	Disorder
Central nervous system	Ondine's curse
	Central sleep apnea
	Primary alveolar hypoventilation
	Sedative hypnotic overdose
Neuronal pathway	Spinal cord injury
	Multiple sclerosis
	Amyotrophic lateral sclerosis
Neuromuscular junction	Myasthenia gravis
	Botulism poisoning
	Organophosphate poisoning
Muscular function	Muscular dystrophy
	Myotonic dystrophy

is a classic example of a neuromuscular disease that affects the neuromuscular junction. It is probably a immunologic disease resulting from circulating antibodies directed against acetylcholine receptors in the junction. As a result, nerve impulses do not result in forceful muscle contraction when stimulated. Some toxins, such as organophosphate insecticides and chemical-warfare nerve gases, block the breakdown of acetylcholine in the neuromuscular junction. Blocking the breakdown of acetylcholine keeps the muscles from relaxing appropriately, causing muscle spasms, tetany, and respiratory failure.

Muscle Diseases

Myopathy is a disorder of the muscle. Several congenital myopathies lead to progressive muscular weakness. Muscular dystrophies are one of the most common examples of this type of disease. Muscular dystrophy leads to progressive muscle weakness and loss of function. Loss of muscle function eventually becomes so profound that a poor cough develops, lung volumes become reduced, and eventually respiratory failure develops. Patients with muscular dystrophy frequently die of respiratory failure or pneumonia.

CLINICAL FEATURES

> Spontaneous respiratory rate and vital capacity are good predictors of impending respiratory failure in the patient with neuromuscular disease. Respiratory rates above 35/min at rest and a vital capacity below 1.0 liter indicate that the patient is in trouble.

A patient with neuromuscular disease may not initially develop respiratory complications. Signs and symptoms of respiratory failure will occur, however, as the muscular weakness progresses to the point where the muscles of breathing are compromised. As the inspiratory muscles weaken, the patient's lung volumes decrease, and a rapid and shallow breathing pattern develops. The patient often complains of dyspnea, especially on exertion. Weakness of expiratory muscles leads to a poor cough and inability to clear excessive secretions from the airways. Retention of sputum in the lung may lead to mucus plugging, atelectasis, and pneumonia, which are common complications of neuromuscular disease.

Initial arterial blood gas (ABG) findings may be normal in the patient with mild neuromuscular disease; however, with severe weakness of the respiratory muscles, the ABG values demonstrate hypoxemia, an increased Pa_{CO_2}, and decreased pH. Hypoxemia is common because of ventilation-perfusion ($\dot{V}/\dot{Q}$) mismatching and the increase in alveolar P_{CO_2} (Pa_{CO_2}). The hypoxemia typically responds rapidly to supplemental oxygen therapy. If a patient also has a complicating pneumonia, more severe hypoxemia may be present. In general, ABG abnormalities are a late sign of acute respiratory failure in patients with neuromuscular disease and should not be relied on to determine the severity of the disease or when to start ventilatory support for the patient.

Bedside assessment of pulmonary function will reveal a reduced vital capacity (VC). Severe disease is marked by a reduction in the VC below 1.0 to 1.5 liters in the adult. The maximum inspiratory pressure (MIP) decreases as the inspiratory muscles weaken. MIP is a useful tool for quantifying the degree of muscle weakness and identifying trends in the course of the disease. An MIP measurement of less than -20 to -30 cm H_2O usually indicates severe weakness of the inspiratory muscles. RTs should measure MIP against a closed mouthpiece after the patient has exhaled to residual volume. Exhaling to residual volume provides the inspiratory muscles with the best mechanical advantage for performing the MIP maneuver.

GBS may occur at any age and has no discernible geographic or seasonal distribution. A preceding viral infection is commonly seen in patients diagnosed with GBS. Initial symptoms often include weakness of the lower extremities and paresthesia (sensations of numbness or tingling) in the fingers and toes. The lower extremity weakness is usually symmetrical, and the weakness progresses to the muscles of the abdomen, diaphragm, arms, and face. The patient with GBS may experience difficulty swallowing and a poor gag reflex as the muscles of the throat become involved. This may lead to aspiration. Hypertension or cardiac dysrhythmias develop in some GBS patients owing to involvement of the autonomic nervous system. Cardiac dysrhythmias may be serious enough to cause death if appropriate treatment is not implemented. Measurement of CSF protein level may be useful in making the diagnosis of GBS. CSF protein levels above 100 mg/100 mL are consistent with GBS.

Myasthenia gravis can occur at any age, but the incidence increases in early adulthood and in the elderly. In young adults, women outnumber men 2 to 1 in the incidence of the disease. The patient with myasthenia gravis usually presents with weakness of certain muscles when used repeatedly. The extraocular muscles are often affected initially and cause the patient to experience blurred vision (diplopia) and droopy eyelids (ptosis). The symptoms increase with repeated use of the involved muscles and may improve with rest. Some patients with myasthenia gravis experience gradual progression of the disease to other muscle groups, including the pharyngeal, laryngeal, arm, trunk, and leg muscles. Respiratory symptoms usually do not develop in individuals with milder cases of myasthenia gravis; however, respiratory failure is likely to occur when the diaphragm is affected by the disease. A number of factors (e.g., infection, surgery, menstruation, immunizations, certain drugs, emotional distress) can precipitate a myasthenia gravis crisis in a patient with a previously stable case.

The Tensilon test helps establish the diagnosis of myasthenia gravis. This test involves IV injection of 10 mg of Tensilon (edrophonium) while the areas of major muscle weakness are carefully observed. Muscle weakness will resolve within 20 to 30 seconds and remains nearly normal for a few minutes if myasthenia gravis is the cause of the patient's weakness.

Patients with ALS most often initially experience progressive weakness of distal muscle groups, such as the hands. Occasionally, the initial symptom is difficulty with swallowing. The disease may cause asymmetric weakness, atrophy, and tremors. A characteristic feature of ALS is the development of muscle fiber twitching called fasciculations. ALS usually advances over a period of 3 to 4 years and eventually causes weakness of all four extremities as well as the breathing muscles. Dyspnea occurs at rest, and the patient begins having difficulty coughing, swallowing, and talking as the disease progresses. Respiratory failure and death most often occur 3 to 4 years after the onset of symptoms. Some patients with ALS have brain stem involvement early in the course of their disease. These patients are said to have a bulbar form of ALS. Patients with the bulbar form of ALS develop respiratory failure early in the course of the disease and are less likely to respond to noninvasive ventilation.[3,4]

Respiratory symptoms of the patient with an SCI will vary with the location of the lesion. High cervical injuries above the C3 level produce nearly complete respiratory muscle paralysis. In these cases the patient is unable to breathe effectively, talk, or cough. The lack of effective breathing causes the rapid onset of respiratory acidosis and hypoxemia. Breath sounds are very diminished or absent. The diaphragm is elevated and immobile. Bedside VC is at best 20% of predicted.

The patient with a spinal lesion at the level of C4 to C8 is quadriplegic but usually retains some use of the respiratory muscles. VC is markedly reduced immediately after the injury but improves somewhat over the initial 12 months. Pneumonia or atelectasis commonly complicate the care of patients with spinal cord injury because of their inability to breathe deeply and cough effectively. ABG results usually demonstrate mild hypoxemia and a normal $PaCO_2$ during the daytime.

Disruption of the spinal cord below C8 does not usually cause a significant reduction in lung volumes. A mid to low spinal-cord lesion often attenuates expiratory muscle function to the point where the patient's cough may be weak and ineffective. As a result, secretion retention and atelectasis is a potential complication.

TREATMENT

Neuromuscular disease may weaken the respiratory muscles and cause the patient to have difficulty clearing airway secretions. Bronchial hygiene techniques, including postural drainage, cough assistance, and humidity therapy, are often beneficial. Intermittent positive-pressure breathing may be useful to prevent or treat atelectasis and dyspnea. Intubation may be needed when aspiration is likely to occur as a result of loss of the gag reflex or when respiratory failure is imminent.

Ventilatory Failure

Careful monitoring of the vital signs, breathing pattern, ability to cough, VC, and MIP is essential to identify the need for ventilatory assistance. A decline in the ABG measurements is often a late clinical manifestation and should not be relied on exclusively to determine the need for mechanical ventilation. Ventilatory assistance is indicated if VC drops below 15 mL/kg ideal body weight, if respiratory rate is greater than 35 per minute at rest, or progressive dyspnea is present. Once it is clear that ventilatory support is needed, it can be initiated using invasive or noninvasive ventilation. Noninvasive positive pressure ventilation (NIPPV) is usually delivered by a nasal or face mask connected to a form of pressure cycled ventilation. Among the most common forms of pressure cycled ventilation is Bilevel positive airway pressure ventilation (BiPAP). NIPPV only works with patients who are alert and cooperative. Obtunded or combative patients should be intubated and given routine mechanical ventilation. NIPPV has been successfully used to manage respiratory failure from neuromuscular disease and has been shown to improve the quality of life in ALS patients.[5–8] NIPPV may be initially successful but fail later as the disease worsens.[9] It is most likely to be successful when applied by experienced clinicians, and it's use lowers the risk of ventilator-associated pneumonia as compared to patients who are intubated and given PPV.[10]

> Intubation of the patient with neuromuscular disease provides protection of the airway, easier removal of retained secretions, and application of mechanical ventilation.

Invasive ventilation requires endotracheal intubation and mechanical ventilation. Invasive ventilation is initiated for patients who cannot ventilate adequately using noninvasive ventilation and cannot protect their airways or clear their airway of excessive pulmonary secretions. Once the patient is intubated, the RT should keep the airway clear with suctioning. Pressure support, assist-control pressure support, and assist-control ventilation have been shown to be effective ventilatory strategies in patients with neuromuscular disease.[11] Tracheostomy is useful when long-term mechanical ventilation is needed, as in the case of a high cervical spine fracture. Tracheostomy is usually not used during the first 2 weeks of mechanical ventilation for reversible conditions such as GBS or myasthenia gravis. After 10 to 14 days of intubation, however, if the patient has not shown any signs of improvement, tracheostomy is considered.

Clinicians caring for the patient with neuromuscular disease should anticipate complications such as pneumonia and pulmonary emboli. Antibiotics should be given if fever and pulmonary infiltrates develop. Prophylactic use of various forms of heparin or pneumatic compression socks are useful techniques to reduce the likelihood of deep venous thrombosis and pulmonary embolism.

Weaning from mechanical ventilation is reasonable when the patient is free of infection, is hemodynamically stable, and has significantly improved respiratory muscle function. Signs of improvement include a VC greater than 1.5 liters, an MIP greater than -30 cm H_2O, and a spontaneous tidal volume (V_T) greater than 300 mL. Improvement in lung mechanics is not likely to occur in patients with high neck fractures or ALS.

Specific Treatments

Treatment of the GBS patient is primarily supportive. Plasmapheresis has been used with some success and is reserved for severe cases. It involves removal of a portion of the circulating blood, which is then centrifuged to separate the red blood cells (RBCs) from the plasma. The plasma is discarded, and the RBCs are mixed with fresh plasma and reinfused into the patient. This process is continued until a major portion of the plasma is replaced, causing dilution of the offending antibody. Corticosteroids are controversial and are not commonly used to treat the GBS patient. Careful monitoring of the patient is crucial because respiratory failure represents the most immediate threat to life. Mechanical ventilation is needed in about 25% of cases.[12] After a period of stability the patient will usually begin to recover, but it often takes several weeks or months for complete recovery. The prognosis is usually very good unless serious complications occur.

Specific treatment of myasthenia gravis includes anticholinesterase medications such as neostigmine. The patient with myasthenia gravis should be admitted to the hospital any time he or she has difficulty breathing or swallowing. Careful monitoring of respiratory function is essential, as previously mentioned. Plasmapheresis and thymectomy (surgical removal of the thymus gland) have been used with some success to treat severe cases.[13,14]

Treatment for the patient with ALS is nonspecific and supportive. Careful monitoring of respiratory function is important, as respiratory failure can occur with little warning. Intermittent mechanical ventilatory support using a negative-pressure body respirator may prove useful for the patient with a severe case of chronic neuromuscular disease, as occurs with ALS. Nocturnal ventilation with a body respirator has a distinct advantage in that an artificial airway does not need to be placed in order to achieve ventilation. This type of mechanical ventilation may allow the fatigued diaphragm to rest at night, resulting in better gas exchange and sleep during the night.[15,16] Nocturnal intermittent positive-pressure ventilation (NIPPV) via nasal mask is an alternative to negative-pressure ventilation for patients with severe, chronic neuromuscular disease. NIPPV appears to be safe and effective and is less cumbersome to implement than negative-pressure ventilation.[17]

Care of patients with spinal cord injury must be tailored according to the location of the lesion. Those with a high neck fracture (above the level of C3) require intubation and mechanical ventilation to survive. Once stabilized, tracheostomy is needed for long-term ventilatory assistance. Patients with fractures below C3 require careful assessment to determine the extent of respiratory muscle paralysis. Most patients with neck fracture below the C3 level do not need continuous mechanical ventilation but may need nocturnal ventilatory support and assistance with secretion removal. In general, the lower the site of the neck fracture, the less respiratory care the patient will need. Chest physical therapy is applied to patients with cervical or thoracic SCI. This should include deep breathing, frequent turning, postural drainage, nasotracheal suctioning, and cough assistance as needed.[1]

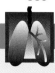

Mrs. E

HISTORY

Mrs. E is a 25-year-old white woman who came to the emergency department complaining of extremity weakness and difficulty swallowing. Mrs. E stated that 10 days earlier she had an episode of fever, headache, and general malaise. Her physician diagnosed her condition as influenza. She was given acetaminophen for the headache and told to drink plenty of fluids and rest until the symptoms resolved. The next day she noticed dizziness, extremity weakness, and numbness. The extremity weakness had progressed to the point where she could not stand without assistance. During the past 24 hours, she had difficulty swallowing and frequently choked. She stated that she became short of breath during moderate exertion. She denied having dyspnea at rest, chest pain, cough, sputum, fever, or nausea.

QUESTIONS	ANSWERS
1. What conditions are suggested by this medical history?	The symptoms suggest either a neuromuscular disease (e.g., myasthenia gravis, GBS, ALS) or flu with dehydration.
2. What is the significance of Mrs. E having difficulty swallowing?	The difficulty swallowing is significant because it suggests that neuromuscular control of the gag reflex may be in jeopardy, which could result in aspiration.
3. What is the significance of the recent history of flu symptoms?	A recent history of flu symptoms is common in patients with GBS. Approximately 65% of patients diagnosed with GBS have had a recent episode of respiratory or gastrointestinal flu within the previous 8 weeks.
4. Should Mrs. E be admitted? If so, why?	Mrs. E should be admitted because of her difficulty swallowing and because the respiratory muscles may weaken, resulting in a rapid onset of respiratory failure.

More on Mrs. E

PHYSICAL EXAMINATION

- **General.** The patient is alert, well oriented, and in no apparent distress. She is moderately obese for her height (height 5 feet 4 inches, weight 155 lb)

- **Vital Signs.** Temperature 36.6°C (97.9°F), heart rate 88/min, respiratory rate 20/min, blood pressure 150/110 mm Hg

- **HEENT.** Normocephalic with no signs of trauma; pupils equal, round, and reactive to light and accommodation (PERRLA); tympanic membranes intact; carotid pulses ++ bilaterally; trachea midline and without stridor; no ptosis noted, even upon repeated blinking

- **Lungs.** Clear breath sounds bilaterally; normal chest configuration; no evidence of trauma

- **Heart.** Irregular rate and rhythm without murmurs; normal S_1 and S_2, with no S_3 or S_4; point of maximal intensity not palpable

- **Abdomen.** Obese, soft, nontender; positive bowel sounds; no hepatomegaly

- **Extremities.** Deep tendon reflexes of the extremities absent; noticeable weakness of legs and feet; grip weak in both hands; no evidence of cyanosis, edema, or clubbing; extremities warm to touch

QUESTIONS	ANSWERS
5. What are the key findings of the physical examination and what problems do they suggest?	The key findings on the physical examination are the muscular weakness and loss of deep tendon reflexes of the extremities and the irregular heartbeat and hypertension. The extremity weakness and loss of reflexes suggests that the neuromuscular system is not functioning properly.
6. What may explain the hypertension and irregular heartbeat?	The hypertension and irregular heartbeat may indicate that the neuromuscular disease involves the autonomic nervous system. It is also possible, however, that the irregular heartbeat is the result of an unrelated heart condition.
7. Why did the examining physician ask Mrs. E to blink her eyelids repeatedly?	Asking Mrs. E to blink repeatedly is useful to check for myasthenia gravis. The eyelids will rapidly tire and begin to droop if myasthenia gravis is present. In Mrs. E's case, myasthenia gravis is not the likely diagnosis, as the eyelids remained functional.
8. What neuromuscular disease usually causes an ascending paralysis, as seen in this case?	GBS typically causes an ascending paralysis, as is seen in this case.
9. What laboratory and bedside tests would be useful in this case to identify the cause of the problem?	Laboratory tests that would be useful include a CSF protein count, a bedside analysis of VC and MIP, a complete blood count (CBC), and an electrolyte measurement. A chest radiograph may be useful to assess the condition of the lungs. An ABG assessment is not needed at this point, as there is no evidence of respiratory complications.
10. Should the attending physician administer the Tensilon test? What is the purpose of this test?	The Tensilon test is useful to confirm the diagnosis of myasthenia gravis. Because the evidence suggests that myasthenia gravis is not the cause of Mrs. E's weakness, the Tensilon test would not be useful.

More on Mrs. E

Laboratory Evaluation

CBC

Measure	Value
WBCs	9.5 thousand/mm^3
Segmented neutrophils	71%
Bands	6%
Lymphocytes	14%
Monocytes	8%
Basophils	1%
RBCs	4.2 million/mm^3
Hemoglobin (Hb)	13 g/100 mL
Hematocrit (Hct)	38%
Electrolytes	Normal, except for reduced total CO_2 (21 mEq/liter)

Other Tests

MIP	-35 cm H_2O
Bedside VC	2.4 liters (predicted normal 3.6 liters)
Chest Radiograph	Low lung volumes bilaterally with no evidence of infiltrates

QUESTIONS	ANSWERS
11. How would you interpret the CBC results?	The CBC is normal.
12. What could explain the reduced CO_2 on the electrolyte panel?	The reduced total CO_2 on the electrolyte panel represents reduced plasma HCO_3^-. This is commonly seen in patients who have been hyperventilating long enough for the kidneys to compensate for the resultant respiratory alkalosis by excreting plasma HCO_3^-. A reduced plasma HCO_3^- concentration also indicates metabolic acidosis.
13. How would you interpret the bedside MIP and VC?	The MIP and VC are reduced, which suggests that the respiratory muscles are probably affected by the disease and that the patient needs careful monitoring.
14. Is the chest radiograph consistent with the tentative diagnosis of neuromuscular disease? If so, why?	The chest radiograph finding of reduced lung volume is consistent with neuromuscular disease. As the diaphragm weakens, the lung recoil is less opposed and the lung volumes tend to diminish.

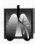

More on Mrs. E

The diagnosis at this point is neuromuscular disease, probably owing to GBS. Mrs. E is admitted to the intensive care unit (ICU) for careful monitoring. A spinal tap is done to measure the CSF protein level, which is found to be elevated. This provides more evidence to support the diagnosis of GBS. Plasmapheresis is started. Four hours after admission, Mrs. E begins complaining of shortness of breath after minimal exertion. Bedside assessment reveals a VC of 1.6 liters and an MIP of -20 cm H_2O. Mrs. E's respiratory rate has increased to 36/min, and her heart rate is 128/min. Her blood pressure remains moderately elevated. ABG results at this point are as follows: pH 7.45, $Paco_2$ 30 mm Hg, Pao_2 89 mm Hg, Sao_2 95%, HCO_3^- 19 mEq/liter on room air.

QUESTIONS	ANSWERS
15. What is plasmapheresis, and why is it used to treat GBS?	Plasmapheresis is the process of removing a portion of the patient's blood and centrifuging it to separate the blood cells from the plasma. The plasma is discarded, and the remaining blood cells are mixed with fresh plasma and reinfused into the patient. The purpose of plasmapheresis is to dilute the offending antibody present in the plasma.
16. How would you interpret the changes in the VC and MIP measurements?	The VC and MIP are reduced significantly from the previous measurement. This suggests that the respiratory muscles are weaker and that the patient is at high risk for respiratory failure.
17. How would you interpret the ABG results?	The ABG results demonstrate compensated respiratory alkalosis with adequate oxygenation on room air. The ABG results reflect adequate lung function. Respiratory failure, however, may occur in the very near future despite the relatively normal ABG results.
18. What therapy is indicated at this point?	Based on the trend of decreasing respiratory muscle strength, increasing respiratory rate, and increasing dyspnea, intubation and mechanical ventilation are indicated. It is usually better to perform the intubation while the patient with neuromuscular disease remains somewhat stable. Once respiratory failure is present, attempts to intubate are often rushed and the patient is at greater risk for complications.

More on Mrs. E

After being given an explanation regarding the procedure, Mrs. E is intubated nasally and placed on mechanical ventilation. Initial settings are assist-control mode with a backup rate of 12/min and a tidal volume (V_T) of 600 mL, a fraction of inspired oxygen (Fio_2) of 0.35, and no positive end-expiratory pressure (PEEP). A chest film confirms appropriate placement of the endotracheal tube. The ABG results 20 minutes after the initiation of mechanical ventilation with a mechanical rate of 16/min are as follows: pH 7.45, $Paco_2$ 31 mm Hg, Pao_2 105 mm Hg, HCO_3^- 20 mEq/liter, and Sao_2 98%. The patient continues to complain of weakness and extremity numbness.

QUESTIONS	ANSWERS
19. What changes in the ventilator settings would you suggest based on the ABG findings.	Because the oxygenation is more than adequate, a slight reduction in the Fio_2 from 0.35 to 0.30 is reasonable. A reduction in the mechanical minute ventilation would help increase the $Paco_2$ to normal range. This could be accomplished by reducing the V_T; however, a smaller V_T may promote atelectasis. Lowering the backup rate may decrease the minute volume, but only if the patient does not trigger the ventilator. Sedation may help reduce the patient's anxiety and reduce the hyperventilation. An alternative would be to switch the ventilator to the intermittent mandatory ventilation (IMV) mode (see Chapter 2). This would allow the patient to take spontaneous breaths between the mechanical breaths and should lower the overall minute volume. The IMV rate should be set high enough, however, to maintain adequate ventilation and allow the muscles to rest (e.g., 10 to 12/min).
20. What complications should be anticipated in this case?	Complications in this case could include pulmonary embolus, atelectasis, pneumonia, cardiovascular compromise from the mechanical ventilation, and pneumothorax.
21. What should Mrs. E be told about her prognosis?	The patient should be told that a full recovery is expected. A majority of GBS patients recover fully within a few weeks or months.
22. Should a tracheostomy be performed to avoid permanent damage to the larynx by the endotracheal tube?	At this point a tracheostomy is not needed. It is possible that the patient will recover enough to breathe on her own within 1 to 2 weeks. A tracheostomy should be considered if after 7 to 10 days the patient has not made any progress toward recovery.

More on Mrs. E

During the next week Mrs. E is maintained on mechanical ventilation with an IMV rate of 10/min and a mechanical V_T of 600 mL. Plasmapheresis is repeated daily. Mrs. E's spontaneous V_T varies but usually is in the range of 200 to 300 mL. On day 7 her MIP is -25 cm H_2O and she states that she feels stronger. The bilateral extremity numbness is greatly reduced and her grip is noticeably stronger. Her vital signs remain stable except for an elevation in body temperature to 38.3°C (100.9°F). Secretions suctioned from the endotracheal tube are white. The chest radiograph shows bibasilar atelectasis. The ABG findings on day 7 are as follows: pH 7.43, $Paco_2$ 36 mm Hg, Pao_2 84 mm Hg, and Fio_2 0.30.

QUESTIONS	ANSWERS
23. What treatment should be given for the bibasilar atelectasis?	The bibasilar atelectasis should be treated with chest physical therapy and postural drainage. Frequent changes in position may also be helpful. The sputum sample should be sent to the laboratory for a Gram stain and culture. If the sputum demonstrates numerous pus cells and bacterial growth, antibiotics should be started.
24. Should weaning from mechanical ventilation be started? Why or why not?	It appears that Mrs. E is improving, but weaning from mechanical ventilation should not begin until the fever and atelectasis have cleared.

Mrs. E Conclusion

On day 14 Mrs. E has a normal body temperature, and the chest radiograph shows significant clearing of the infiltrates. The weaning parameters at this point are VC 2.1 liters, MIP -35 cm H_2O, and spontaneous V_T 350 mL. Mrs. E tolerates an IMV rate of 4/min, which yields normal ABG results. On the evening of day 14 Mrs. E is extubated, and she tolerates the procedure well. She states that she still feels weak but much improved. Her cough is weak but improves daily. Her breath sounds remain clear, and vital signs stable. Neurologic examination reveals improved deep tendon reflexes and nearly normal responses to stimuli. Mrs. E is transferred from the ICU to the rehabilitation unit on day 18 and is sent home on day 21 without further complications.

Mr. R

HISTORY

Mr. R is a 62-year-old man with a 6-month history of ALS. Approximately 8 months earlier, he noticed weakness in his hands and legs. His initial problem involved gripping objects such as a cup or doorknob. He then had difficulty getting out of a chair. The disease had progressed rapidly over the past 6 months until he was unable to walk, grip anything, or lift anything more 1 to 2 lb with his arms. Speaking had become more difficult, but his mind was clear and he still communicated well with his family. His neurologist had referred him for an evaluation of his respiratory status.

Mr. R was experiencing mild dyspnea, most notably when he talked or assisted in transferring himself to a wheelchair. His family noted that he could not complete a sentence without stopping to catch his breath. When he was at rest and not talking, he appeared in no distress. One month before his visit, he acquired pneumonia of the right lower lobe, which was treated with ampicillin and resolved. No other significant problems in Mr. R's history were identified. He was a dentist who had been in practice until 8 months ago, when the ALS was first discovered.

Mr. R understood that this disease would lead to respiratory failure and was terminal. He felt that his quality of life was good enough at present and that he would like to have ventilatory support, if needed, to prolong his life. In addition, Mr. R expressed that if his ALS progressed to the point where his quality of life did not warrant continued ventilatory support, he would like to have mechanical ventilation discontinued at that time.

QUESTIONS	ANSWERS
1. What part of the nervous system does ALS affect, and what is the etiology of the disease?	ALS is a degenerative disease of motor neurons that has no known cause. The disease specifically destroys the Betz neurons in the cerebral cortex and the motor neurons in the anterior horns of the spinal cord.
2. The initial sign of Mr. R's muscle weakness was a weak grip. Is this pattern of weakness typical of proximal or distal muscle weakness?	Weakness of the hands and feet are signs of distal muscle weakness. The fact that distal muscle weakness was the initial symptom suggests that the disease is a neuromuscular disorder such as ALS or GBS. Proximal muscle weakness is characteristically seen in the arm and thigh, most notably when a patient gets up from a chair. Proximal muscle weakness is characteristic of muscle diseases such as muscular dystrophy.
3. Is it reasonable to provide mechanical ventilation for Mr. R considering that his disease is progressive and terminal?	Patients do have the right to decide which therapies they are willing to undergo. Because Mr. R is approaching respiratory failure, mechanical ventilation is a treatment option. Ideally, one of the roles of health care providers is to educate patients regarding the benefits and costs of such therapy. It is important that Mr. R's caregivers inform him of the discomfort associated with such therapy, as well as the intrusion into his life associated with mechanical ventilation. In addition, he needs to understand the nature and prognosis of the disease process that led to the requirement for this therapy. Only after patients (or close family members) have been fully educated in all aspects of their disease and the proposed therapy can they make an educated decision.
4. If you were to initiate mechanical ventilation for Mr. R and he later decided he wanted to stop ventilatory support and die, should you assist his death by discontinuing mechanical ventilation?	As discussed in the previous answer, Mr. R has the right to decide whether to initiate therapy and when to terminate therapy. If Mr. R were to decide to discontinue life support, it would probably be wise to make certain that he arrived at his decision after careful consideration and that the family understands and respects the decision before discontinuing mechanical support.
5. What characteristic muscle movements would you expect to see during your examination of the patient?	Muscle fasciculations, which are characterized by a visible twitching of muscle fibers from the affected muscles, develop in ALS patients.

More on Mr. R

PHYSICAL EXAMINATION

- **General.** Patient sitting in wheelchair and in no respiratory distress; vital signs stable; respiratory rate 24/min

- **HEENT.** No significant abnormalities

- **Heart.** Regular, with a normal rate; both S_1 and S_2 normal; no murmurs

- **Lungs.** A few fine, inspiratory crackles heard over the bases of both lungs; weak cough

- **Abdomen.** Soft, nontender; normal, active bowel sounds; no masses palpated

- **Extremities.** Equal pulses in all extremities; no peripheral edema noted

- **Neurological.** Alert, articulate; short sentences spoken, with pauses to take a breath every three to five words; cranial nerve function normal except for weakness of sternocleidomastoid, trapezius, and facial muscles; sensory examination normal; extreme weakness of extremities revealed upon motor examination; legs move and gestures weak; fasciculations noted over forearm and thigh muscles

QUESTIONS	ANSWERS
6. In this setting, what is the most likely reason for Mr. R's pulmonary crackles? Why do the crackles remain after coughing?	The principal pulmonary problem that patients with neuromuscular disease have is weakness of the respiratory pump. Weakness of respiratory muscles predisposes patients to difficulty expanding lung units, resulting in atelectasis. In addition, these patients may have difficulty clearing secretions, so atelectasis may develop as a result of mucus plugging. In patients with neuromuscular disease the airway may not be protected, which is why aspiration and subsequent pneumonia can develop.
7. What tests are most important in determining when mechanical ventilation should be instituted?	The profound respiratory muscle weakness that is common among patients with neuromuscular disease makes it difficult for these patients to breathe deeply and cough well enough to reverse atelectasis completely.
8. Should Mr. R be admitted to the hospital at this time?	The test that is most commonly used to determine whether patients with neuromuscular disease require mechanical ventilation is the measurement of VC. If the VC is less than 1 liter, then mechanical ventilation is usually indicated.
	If mechanical ventilation becomes necessary, the patient will then be admitted, and both the patient and family will be trained in the use of the ventilator. The physician may need to perform a tracheostomy if long-term mechanical ventilation is required.

More on Mr. R

Laboratory Evaluation

CBC		
Measure	Observed	Normal
WBCs/mm^3	5100	4000–11,000
RBCs (million/mm^3)	4.5	4.1–5.5
Hb (g/dL)	14	14–16.5
Hct (%)	42	37–50

Differential		
Segmented neutrophils (%)	61	38–79
Bands (%)	4	0–7
Lymphocytes (%)	29	12–51
Monocytes (%)	5	0–10
Eosinophils (%)	1	0–8
Basophils(%)	0	0–2

Chemistry		
Measure	Observed	Normal
Na$^+$ (mEq/liter)	141	136–146
K$^+$ (mEq/liter)	4.2	3.5–5.1
Cl$^-$ (mEq/liter)	93	98–106
HCO$_3^-$ (mEq/liter)	37	22–29
Blood urea nitrogen (mg/dL)	8	7–18
Creatinine (mg/dL)	0.5	0.5–1.1
Calcium (mmol/liter)	2.2	2.1–2.55
Phosphate (mg/dL)	2.9	2.7–4.5
Uric acid (mg/dL)	2.1	4.5–8.2
Albumin (g/dL)	3.9	3.5–5.0
Protein (g/dL)	7.2	6.4–8.3

Chest Radiograph: See Figure 15.4

ABG (on room air)	
Measure	Value
pH	7.38
Pao$_2$	67 mm Hg
Paco$_2$	58 mm Hg
HCO$_3^-$	33 mEq/liter
Alveolar-arterial oxygen gradient P(A-a)o$_2$	10 mm Hg
O$_2$ content	16.8 mL/dL

Spirometry	
Forced vital capacity (FVC)	0.92 liters
Negative inspiratory pressure	−12 cm H$_2$O

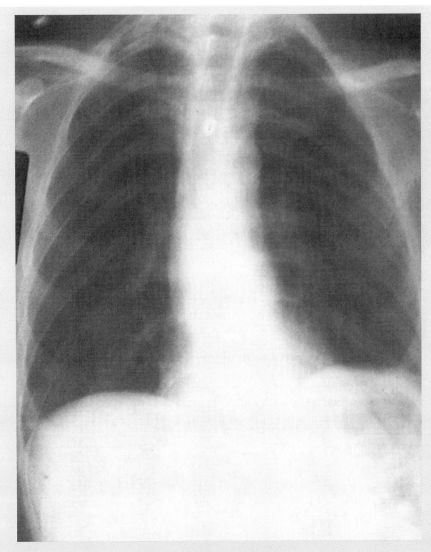

FIGURE 15.4 Portable chest radiograph.

QUESTIONS	ANSWERS
9. How would you interpret the chest radiograph?	The lungs are hyperinflated as a result of preexisting COPD. A slight degree of scoliosis is visible.
10. How would you interpret the results of the ABG?	The ABG indicates chronic respiratory acidosis, indicating that the hypoxemia is primarily due to the hypoventilation. The $P(A-a)o_2$ is normal.
11. How would you interpret the spirometry results?	The spirometry is consistent with profound respiratory muscle weakness.
12. What treatment options would you recommend to the physician at this point?	Having chronic respiratory acidosis and profound respiratory muscle weakness, Mr. R is at risk for acute respiratory failure due to ALS. Mr. R wanted

to begin mechanical ventilation when necessary, and this is an appropriate time to do so. The patient should be admitted and educated, along with the family members, regarding the procedure.

There are two different mechanical-ventilation options for patients in neuromuscular respiratory failure. One option is to perform a tracheostomy and initiate volume-cycled mechanical ventilation; the other option is to begin mechanical ventilation with nasal mask intermittent positive-pressure ventilation (NIPPV). The advantage of the second option is that no tracheostomy is required. At home, NIPPV or a negative-pressure body respirator may prove useful.

Mr. R Conclusion

Mr. R is admitted to the hospital. NIPPV is instituted for nocturnal use. The patient and family are instructed in the use of the ventilator, and after a few days of stabilization on the new regimen, the patient is discharged home.

For several weeks after the institution of NIPPV, Mr. R feels more energetic and finds breathing and talking easier. His ABGs improve, showing a normal $Paco_2$ during NIPPV use and during the daytime.

Over the next several months Mr. R's functioning deteriorates as the ALS progresses. His ventilatory requirements increase, and his breathlessness worsens. He finds that he requires NIPPV 24 hours a day and cannot easily talk or communicate with his family. He is now unable to perform even the simplest task without assistance. At this point Mr. R decides that the burden of the NIPPV is greater than the benefits he is deriving. He does not want a tracheostomy or other, more invasive forms of mechanical ventilation. He decides he will stop using the NIPPV. He and his family fully understand the consequences of this step. After talking with his family and caregivers, he stops the ventilator on his own. He dies a few minutes later. ■

KEY POINTS

- Respiratory therapists (RTs) often play a key role in the evaluation and care of the patient with neuromuscular disease, especially when the disorder threatens the muscles of breathing or reflexes that protect the lungs from aspiration.
- The respiratory pump consists of four major components: (1) Chemoreceptors, which respond to oxygen and carbon dioxide levels, (2) the respiratory centers in the brain stem, which control the rate and depth of breathing, (3) the peripheral nerves that conduct impulses from the respiratory centers to the respiratory muscles, and (4) the respiratory muscles. Disease may affect any part of this system.
- Sedative drugs, particularly narcotics, can suppress respiration by depressing the respiratory centers. An overdose of narcotics, barbiturates or even benzodiazepines, can lead to hypoventilation or apnea in severe cases.
- Trauma is the most frequent cause of nerve damage that affects the respiratory pump. Spinal cord injury (SCI) blocks transmission of nerve impulses below the level of injury.
- A cervical spinal cord transection to the C1 to C3 area will lead to apnea because almost all respiratory muscles are affected.
- Nontraumatic processes can also interrupt nerves. Polio is a viral illness that destroys the motor neurons in the anterior horn of the spinal cord. The destruction of motor neurons may involve nerves that innervate respiratory muscles.
- Amyotrophic lateral sclerosis (ALS) is a progressive fatal neurological disease also known as Lou Gehrig's disease. Despite extensive research, no etiology for ALS has been discovered. As in polio, patients with ALS lose muscle function because of loss of motor neurons in the anterior horn of the spinal cord.
- Myasthenia gravis is a classic example of a neuromuscular disease that affects the neuromuscular junction. It is probably an immunologic disease resulting from circulating antibodies directed against acetylcholine receptors in the junction. As a result, nerve impulses do not result in forceful muscle contraction when stimulated.
- As the inspiratory muscles weaken with neuromuscular disease, the patient's lung volumes decrease, and a rapid and shallow breathing pattern develops. The patient often complains of dyspnea, especially on exertion.
- Initial arterial blood gas (ABG) findings may be normal in the patient with mild neuromuscular disease; however, with severe weakness of the respiratory muscles, the ABG values demonstrate hypoxemia, an increased Pa_{CO_2}, and decreased pH.
- Severe NM disease is marked by a reduction in the VC below 1.0 to 1.5 liters in the adult.
- The maximum inspiratory pressure (MIP) decreases as the inspiratory muscles weaken. MIP is a useful tool for quantifying the degree of muscle weakness and identifying trends in the course of the disease. An MIP measurement of less than -20 to -30 cm H_2O usually indicates severe weakness of the inspiratory muscles.
- Guillain-Barré may occur at any age and has no discernible geographic or seasonal distribution. A preceding viral infection is commonly seen in patients diagnosed with GBS.
- Initial symptoms of GBS often include weakness of the lower extremities and paresthesia (sensations of numbness or tingling) in the fingers and toes.
- Myasthenia gravis can occur at any age, but the incidence increases in early adulthood and in the elderly. In young adults, women outnumber men 2 to 1 in the incidence of the disease.

(key points continued on page 362)

KEY POINTS (CONTINUED)

- The patient with myasthenia gravis usually presents with weakness of certain muscles when used repeatedly. The extraocular muscles are often affected initially and cause the patient to experience blurred vision (diplopia) and droopy eyelids (ptosis).
- The Tensilon test helps establish the diagnosis of myasthenia gravis. This test involves IV injection of 10 mg of Tensilon (edrophonium) while the areas of major muscle weakness are carefully observed. Muscle weakness will resolve within 20 to 30 seconds and remains nearly normal for a few minutes if myasthenia gravis is the cause of the patient's weakness.
- Patients with ALS most often initially experience progressive weakness of distal muscle groups such as the hands. Occasionally, the initial symptom is difficulty with swallowing.
- Bronchial hygiene techniques, including postural drainage, cough assistance, and humidity therapy, are often beneficial. Intermittent positive-pressure breathing may be useful to prevent or treat atelectasis and dyspnea. Intubation may be needed when aspiration is likely to occur as a result of loss of the gag reflex or when respiratory failure is imminent.
- Ventilatory assistance is indicated if VC drops below 15 mL/kg ideal body weight, respiratory rate is greater than 30 per minute, or progressive dyspnea is present. Once it is clear that ventilatory support is needed, this support can be initiated using invasive or noninvasive ventilation.
- Invasive ventilation is initiated for patients who cannot ventilate adequately using noninvasive ventilation and cannot protect their airways or clear their airway of excessive pulmonary secretions.
- Treatment of the GBS patient is primarily supportive. Plasmapheresis has been used with some success and is reserved for severe cases.
- Specific treatment of myasthenia gravis includes anticholinesterase medications such as neostigmine. The patient with myasthenia gravis should be admitted to the hospital any time he or she has difficulty breathing or swallowing.
- Treatment for the patient with ALS is nonspecific and supportive. Careful monitoring of respiratory function is important, as respiratory failure can occur with little warning.
- Those with a high neck fracture (above the level of C3) require intubation and mechanical ventilation to survive. Once stabilized, tracheostomy is needed for long-term ventilatory assistance.

REFERENCES

1. Lieberman, SL, Brown, R: Respiratory complications of spinal cord injury. Available at: up-to-date.com.
2. Maragakis, NJ, Galvez-Jimenez, N: Epidemiology and pathogenesis of amyotrophic lateral sclerosis. Available at: up-to-date.com.
3. Severa, E, Sancho, J, Zafra, MJ, Catala, A, Vergara, P, Marin, J. Alternatives to endotracheal intubation for patients with neuromuscular disease. Am J Phys Med Rehabil 84(11):851–857, 2005.
4. Farrero, E, et al: Survival in amyotrophic lateral sclerosis with home mechanical ventilation: the impact of systematic respiratory assessment and bulbar involvement. Chest 127:2132, 2005.
5. Haegerstrand, C, et al: Bi-level positive airway pressure ventilation maintains adequate ventilation in post-polio patients requiring home mechanical ventilation. Chest 128:1955(s), 2005.
6. Rabinstein, A, Wijducks, E: Bipap in acute respiratory failure due to myasthenic crisis may prevent intubation. Neurology 59:1647, 2002.
7. Martin, TJ, Hovis, JD, Costantino, JP, et al: A randomized prospective evaluation of noninvasive

ventilation for acute respiratory failure. Am J Respir Crit Care Med 161:807–813, 2000.

8. Bourke, SC, Bullock, RE, Williams, TL, Shaw, PJ, Gibson, GJ: Noninvasive ventilation in ALS: indications and effect on quality of life. Neurology 22:171–177, 2003.

9. Ferrero, E, et al: Survival in amyotrophic lateral sclerosis with home mechanical ventilation: the impact of systematic respiratory assessment and bulbar involvement. Chest 127:2132, 2005.

10. Hess, DR: Noninvasive positive-pressure ventilation and ventilator associated pneumonia. Respir Care 50(7):924–929, 2005.

11. Chadda, K, Clair, B, Orlikowski, D, Macadoux, G, et al: Pressure support ventilation versus assisted controlled noninvasive ventilation in neuromuscular disease. Neurocrit Care 1(4):429–434, 2004.

12. Ropper, AH: Severe acute Guillian-Barré syndrome. Neurology 36:429, 1986.

13. Gracey, DR, et al: Plasmapheresis in the treatment of ventilator-dependent myasthenia gravis patients. Chest 85:739, 1984.

14. Dau, PC: Respiratory failure in myasthenia gravis. Chest 85:721, 1985.

15. Holtackers, TR, et al: The use of the chest cuirass in respiratory failure of neurologic origin. Respir Care 27:271, 1982.

16. Curran, FJ: Night ventilation by body respirators for patients in chronic respiratory failure due to late stage Duchenne muscular dystrophy. Arch Phys Med Rehabil 62:270, 1981.

17. Leger, P, et al: Home positive pressure ventilation via nasal mask for patients with neuromuscular weakness or restrictive lung or chest-wall disease. Respir Care 34:73, 1989.

16

Bacterial Pneumonia

Robert L. Wilkins, PhD, RRT, FAARC

James R. Dexter, MD, FACP, FCCP

CHAPTER OBJECTIVES:

After reading this chapter you will be able to list or identify the following:

- The epidemiology for pneumonia.
- The common causes of pneumonia.
- The pathological changes in the lung typical for pneumonia.
- The clinical features of pneumonia.
- The treatment and prognosis for pneumonia.

INTRODUCTION

The term pneumonia refers to inflammation of the lung parenchyma and is most often used to describe inflammation caused by infection. Pneumonia is caused by a variety of infectious agents, including bacteria, viruses, and fungi. This chapter, however, focuses on bacterial pneumonia. Bacterial pneumonia continues to be a common medical problem despite the advent of antibiotics, and it is now is returning as a serious public health problem because of the emergence of antibiotic-resistant organisms.

Each year approximately five to six million people contract pneumonia in the United States, about one-fifth of whom need to be hospitalized.[1,2] Pneumonia is the sixth leading cause of death and the most common cause of death from infection. Most cases of pneumonia are contracted outside the hospital and are referred to as community-acquired pneumonia. This type of pneumonia is often easily treated on an outpatient basis. Pneumonia that occurs in the hospitalized patient is referred to as nosocomial pneumonia. Although other types of nosocomial infections (e.g., urinary tract infection) occur more often in hospitalized patients, pneumonia is the most common fatal nosocomial infection. Pneumonia represents a more serious medical problem among hospitalized and elderly patients whose immune systems are often inadequate.

ETIOLOGY

The distal airways are usually sterile because of the wide variety of mechanical and chemical systems that protect the lungs from infectious agents (Box 16.1). These protective systems may be sabotaged by factors such as cigarette smoking, alcohol abuse, chronic lung disease, neuromuscular disease, intubation, or acute viral upper respiratory tract infection. Pneumonia is increasingly common in the elderly and those with coexisting illness. Neuromuscular disorders are particularly troublesome because they may reduce the effectiveness of the patient's cough and interfere with the protective reflexes of the upper airway that prevent aspiration.

The distal airways can become contaminated with pathogenic organisms once the protective upper airway mechanisms are damaged. Infection is much more likely if the defense mechanisms of the lower airways are also compromised or if the organism is particularly virulent. Systemic disorders such as diabetes, cirrhosis, renal failure, malnutrition, acquired immune deficiency syndrome (AIDS), and cancer may render the patient's immune system compromised and contribute to the onset of pneumonia (Box 16.2). AIDS patients frequently acquire *Pneumocystis carinii* pneumonia. The use of steroids can suppress a patient's immune system and may contribute to the onset of pneumonia. For example, steroids used to treat obstructive lung disease may contribute to the onset of atypical infections in the lung, such as fungal pneumonia.

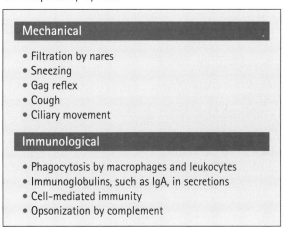

Box 16.1 Summary of the Protective Mechanisms of the Respiratory System

Mechanical

- Filtration by nares
- Sneezing
- Gag reflex
- Cough
- Ciliary movement

Immunological

- Phagocytosis by macrophages and leukocytes
- Immunoglobulins, such as IgA, in secretions
- Cell-mediated immunity
- Opsonization by complement

In addition to aspiration, potentially pathogenic organisms can enter the lung by inhalation and through the blood. Inhalation of small pathogen-carrying droplets is not common when the upper airway is healthy and capable of filtering the inspired gas. If the upper airway is diseased or bypassed, as with tracheotomy or intubation, organisms are more likely to be deposited in the lower airways. Systemic infections may result in the offending organism's traveling to the lung via blood flow. Once the organism reaches the lung from the blood or airways and begins to grow, pneumonia is likely to result.

Pneumonia remains a common medical problem treated around the world. Community-acquired pneumonia is usually treated on an outpatient basis with few problems; nosocomial pneumonia however, is often difficult to treat and more life-threatening.

PATHOPHYSIOLOGY

Infections of the lung parenchyma incite a reaction that causes an outpouring of fluid, inflammatory proteins, and white blood cells (WBCs). Interstitial and alveolar spaces become flooded with edema and exudative material. The inflammatory exudate makes the distal lung spaces dense and consolidated. Some cases of bacterial pneumonia are limited to small areas of lung parenchyma, but others quickly spread to surrounding tissue and to the pleura and pericardium.

Some bacterial organisms such as *Staphylococcus* and *Pseudomonas* can become severe enough to cause abscesses and permanently damage lung tissue. Pneumonia causing permanent damage to the lung tissue is called **necrotizing** pneumonia.

Box 16.2 Factors that Predispose Patients to Pneumonia

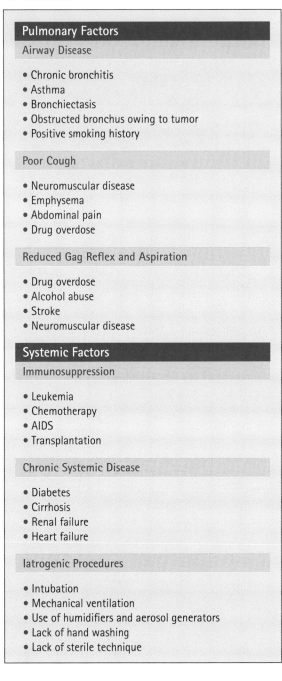

Pulmonary Factors

Airway Disease

- Chronic bronchitis
- Asthma
- Bronchiectasis
- Obstructed bronchus owing to tumor
- Positive smoking history

Poor Cough

- Neuromuscular disease
- Emphysema
- Abdominal pain
- Drug overdose

Reduced Gag Reflex and Aspiration

- Drug overdose
- Alcohol abuse
- Stroke
- Neuromuscular disease

Systemic Factors

Immunosuppression

- Leukemia
- Chemotherapy
- AIDS
- Transplantation

Chronic Systemic Disease

- Diabetes
- Cirrhosis
- Renal failure
- Heart failure

Iatrogenic Procedures

- Intubation
- Mechanical ventilation
- Use of humidifiers and aerosol generators
- Lack of hand washing
- Lack of sterile technique

Acute inflammation and consolidation of the lung leads to a reduction in ventilation and gas exchange in the affected region. Perfusion of the affected lung segments in areas that have poor ventilation results in severe ventilation-perfusion ($\dot{V}/\dot{Q}$) mismatching, or shunt.

Lung consolidation associated with pneumonia reduces lung compliance in the affected region. This increases the patient's work of breathing and causes a sensation of breathlessness. Lung volumes are typically reduced during the acute stages of pneumonia but will usually return to normal once the infection resolves.

CLINICAL FEATURES

History

The patient with typical bacterial pneumonia usually complains of an abrupt onset of fever, cough, and sputum production and may complain of shortness of breath and chest pain. Dyspnea is more common when the pneumonia involves multiple regions of the lung or when it is superimposed on chronic pulmonary disease. When chest pain is present, it is usually pleuritic. Symptoms such as headache, skin rash, and diarrhea may be present with some types of pneumonia. The past medical history is often positive for a chronic systemic or pulmonary disorder in the patient with acute pneumonia. The patient with a past history of chronic obstructive pulmonary disease (COPD) is prone to pneumonia.

Physical Examination

The patient often appears acutely ill at the onset of common bacterial pneumonia. Assessment of the vital signs often reveals a rapid heart and respiratory rate. Rapid breathing occurs with the drop in lung compliance and when fever or hypoxemia is present. Fever increases the patient's metabolic rate, which increases demand on the heart and lungs to provide additional oxygen to the tissues.

In the presence of severe pneumonia, inspection may reveal cyanosis and use of accessory muscles to breathe. A unilateral reduction in chest expansion may be seen with lobar pneumonia. This finding results from the poor expansion of the involved lobe caused by consolidation. Increased tactile fremitus and bronchial breath sounds are commonly found over the consolidated lung if the lobar bronchus associated with the affected region is patent. Sound travels more readily through consolidated lung tissue, so the turbulent flow sounds of the larger airways are more easily heard over areas of consolidation. The breath sounds will be markedly diminished or absent if the bronchus is obstructed. Reduced resonance to percussion is present over areas of consolidated lung. Inspiratory crackles are often present. Coarse crackles imply excessive airway mucus and are a common finding late in the course of bacterial pneumonia. A pleural friction rub may be present when pleural inflammation is complicating the pneumonia.

Laboratory Findings

Examination of the peripheral blood sample will reveal leukocytosis in most cases of bacterial pneumonia. Acute bacterial infection stimulates the bone marrow to increase the neutrophils in the circulating blood. As the infection worsens, the number of immature WBCs (bands) also increases. Leukopenia is seen in cases of severe bacterial pneumonia that overwhelm the immune system. A normal WBC count is commonly encountered with atypical pneumonias such as Mycoplasma or nonbacterial pneumonias.

Chest Radiograph

The chest radiograph is considered the gold standard for confirming the diagnosis of pneumonia. It is often needed because the signs and symptoms associated with pneumonia often occur in other disorders such as upper respiratory tract infection and pulmonary embolism. To avoid over utilization of the chest x-ray in children suspected of having pneumonia, x-ray should be obtained only in those with significant tachypnea and fever.[3] In adults the clinical signs of pneumonia are less predictive for disease, and the clinical judgment of the physician is most important.[4] The presence of multiple signs (e.g., fever, tachypnea, abnormal breath sounds, etc.) at the same time suggests that the chest film is needed and will be positive.[5] Clear breath sounds and normal breath rate indicate that the chest film is not needed in most cases.[6]

The chest radiograph also provides information about the extent of lung involvement and the onset of complications such as pleural effusion. Radiographic changes associated with pneumonia include areas of increased density with air bronchograms. In some cases the pneumonia may involve an entire lobe (lobar pneumonia), whereas in other cases the infiltrates occur along the airways and have a patchy segmental distribution (bronchopneumonia) (Figures 16.1, 16.2, and 16.3). Necrotizing pneumonia produces areas of radiolucency (caused by lung destruction) seen in the areas of increased density. Viral pneumonia most often causes interstitial infiltrates throughout both lungs (Figure 16.4). The chest film may take as long as 3 months to clear completely after bacterial pneumonia. There is no need to document complete resolution of the infiltrate if the patient improves clinically unless he or she is at risk for bronchogenic carcinoma (e.g., a cigarette smoker more than 40 years of age).

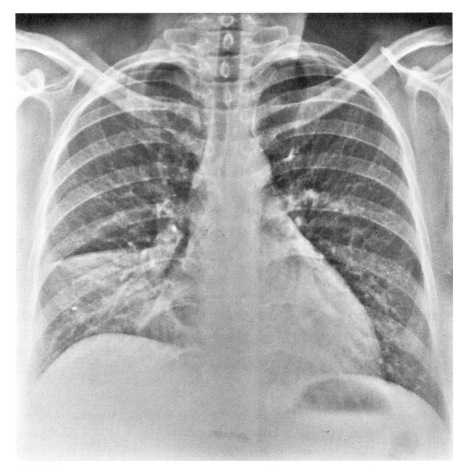

FIGURE 16.1 Lobar pneumonia as seen on posteroanterior (PA) chest radiograph. In this case the pneumonia is located in the right middle lobe.

Arterial Blood Gases

Arterial blood gases (ABGs) are usually not needed in routine cases of pneumonia. When obtained they often reveal hypoxemia and respiratory alkalosis. In severe cases severe hypoxemia and metabolic acidosis may be present. Respiratory acidosis is uncommon unless the patient also has COPD or neuromuscular disease.

Sputum Analysis

Microbiological evaluation of sputum is done to identify the pathogen responsible for the respiratory infection and is best performed before antibiotics are administered. In many cases a representative sample of lung pathogens is difficult to obtain because many patients do not have a productive cough and when sputum is produced most sputum specimens are contaminated with oral secretions as they pass through the mouth. Screening of the sputum sample is useful to identify significant contamination with oral secretions. Sputum samples should be discarded when 10 or more squamous epithelial cells per low-power field (lpf) are present because this signifies that the sample is heavily contaminated by oral secretions. A good sample is recognized by identifying many

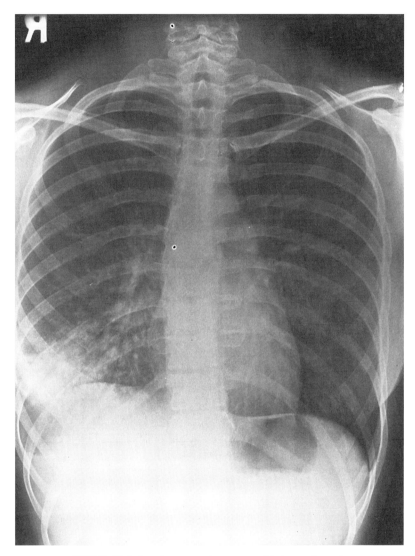

FIGURE 16.2 Bronchopneumonia as seen on PA chest radiograph.

(greater than 25/lpf) polymorphonuclear WBCs in the presence of few epithelial cells. A Gram stain and culture are more likely to be helpful when a good specimen has been obtained. The Gram stain does not take long and often (40% to 60% of the time) identifies the general category of bacteria causing the infection. If positive, the Gram stain allows the physician to start more specific antibiotic therapy before culture results are available. Cultures may identify the specific pathogen responsible for a pneumonia, and the sensitivity testing identifies effective antibiotics for the organism.

The classic clinical findings seen in typical bacterial pneumonia include abrupt fever, chills, cough, and shortness of breath. Abnormal breath sounds and tachypnea are also common. The chest film is most likely to be positive when more than one of these findings are present.

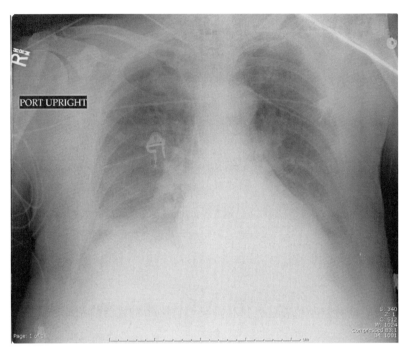

FIGURE 16.3 Bilateral pneumonia with pleural effusions.

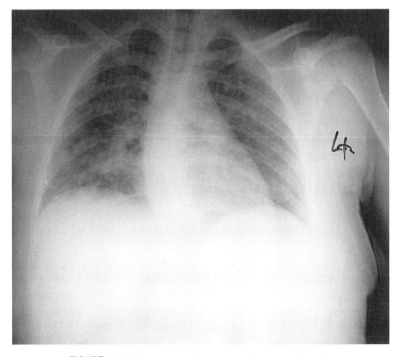

FIGURE 16.4 Viral pneumonia as seen on PA chest radiograph.

Many severely ill patients with pneumonia have trouble expectorating a sputum sample. In these cases invasive procedures may be considered such as transtracheal and transthoracic aspiration, bronchoscopy, and open lung biopsy. Most often these patients are treated with empiric antibiotics based on the clinical history.

TREATMENT

Some patients may be treated for pneumonia as outpatients, but severe cases should be managed in the hospital. Severe pneumonia is more common in the elderly and those with a coexisting illness. The criteria for severe pneumonia are listed in Box 16.3. Several algorithms have been developed to predict severity of pneumonia and need for hospitalization and whether placement in the hospital should be in the intensive care unit (ICU). Severe cases generally require supportive care in addition to antibiotic therapy. Supportive care includes fluid and nutritional therapy, oxygen, aerosol therapy, cooling measures if fever is high, and deep venous thrombi (DVT) prophylaxis if the patient is bedbound. Oxygen therapy is important in the presence of hypoxemia; 3 to 5 liters/min by nasal cannula is most often adequate unless the pneumonia is widespread. Aerosol or humidity therapy can be useful when thick secretions are difficult to expectorate. Chest physical therapy is not useful in treating the typical case of bacterial pneumonia unless it is complicated by bronchiectasis. Respiratory failure requiring mechanical ventilation is uncommon unless the pneumonia is unusually severe or is superimposed on a chronic lung disease.

Antibiotics

The attending physician can predict the most likely offending organism causing the pneumonia in most cases simply by careful bedside examination or radiographic analysis. Therefore, the choice and dosage of initial antibiotic therapy is necessarily determined empirically (i.e., on the basis of experience) in most cases. The initial empirical antibiotic therapy is based on the severity of the pneumonia and the presence of either coexisting illness or advanced age (more than 65 years). Patients with severe pneumonia, coexisting illness, or advanced age often have different pathogens causing the infection compared to other patient groups, and therefore they need a different antibiotic therapy.

An appropriate antibiotic should be started as soon as possible, although several days of the drug are needed to reach full effectiveness. In the patient who is not severely ill, a short delay in the onset of antibiotic therapy is reasonable while appropriate sputum and blood samples are obtained. Most quality criteria state that time of presentation for medical assistance for pneumonia to initial antibiotic administration should be less than 4 hours. The preliminary diagnostic results, such as the Gram stain and chest x-ray, may provide important clues regarding the offending organism. If gram-positive, elongated diplococci typical of pneumococci are seen, oral ampicillin or penicillin were the drugs of choice until penicillin-resistant pneumococci became common. Now higher doses of amoxicillin or cephalosporins are most commonly used for treatment of pneumococcal pneumonias. The

Box 16.3 Criteria for Diagnosis of Severe Pneumonia*

Respiratory rate >30/min at rest
Pao_2 <60 mm Hg on Fio_2 >0.30
Chest radiograph showing multiple lobe involvement
Evidence of shock (systolic BP <90 mm Hg or diastolic BP <60 mm Hg)
Low urine output (<20 mL/hour)

*Severe pneumonia is diagnosed when a patient presents with one or more of these clinical signs.

presence of gram-negative coccobacilli on the sputum sample is most likely *H. influenza* and suggests that ampicillin or a second-generation cephalosporin would be preferred. Once the culture results are available, the most specific agent that is effective against the offending organism should be given. In many cases, however, the responsible pathogen is not identified, even with extensive testing. Antibiotics are given for 5 to 7 days to patients with uncomplicated pneumonia and for 10 days (at least several days after the fever is gone) in severe cases.

Hospital Admission

The decision to admit the patient with pneumonia is based not only on the severity of the infection, but also on the presence of certain risk factors.[7] Patients with advanced age, coexisting illness, high fever, or leukopenia are at greater risk for severe, life-threatening pneumonia and should be more strongly considered for admission. Admission to the ICU is needed when predicted risk is high or if shock or respiratory failure are present.[8]

> The presence of hypotension, severe hypoxemia, and high fever or a high risk score on the severity prediction algorithm suggest the patient should be admitted to the ICU for close observation until therapy is started and begins to improve the patient's clinical condition.

The patient admitted for pneumonia is at risk for acquiring a nosocomial infection (superinfection), especially if the patient requires ventilator therapy. Careful hand washing between visits with each patient and use of sterile technique during airway care is crucial for preventing the spread of organisms from one patient to the next in the ICU. This point is emphasized by the fact that many nosocomial pneumonias are caused by gram-negative organisms, which may be easily spread by fluid carried on the health-care worker's hands. Gram-negative organisms are often relatively resistant to therapy, which makes treatment difficult and increases the risk of infection-related death.

PROGNOSIS

The prognosis for patients with community-acquired pneumonia treated on an outpatient basis is excellent. Mortality rates for such cases are about 1% to 3%. The mortality rate climbs to about 12% for those admitted to the hospital and to as high as 40% for patients admitted to the ICU.[9]

Mr. C

HISTORY

Mr. C is a 60-year-old African-American man who lives in his 1958 Nash Rambler. He earns money by collecting aluminum cans along the roadside and from trash dumpsters. He states that he has been coughing up about 1/4 cup of white sputum each morning for the past 20 years. About 1 week ago, he noticed a sudden onset of shaking, chills, fever, sweating, malaise, chest pain, and shortness of breath at rest. He also began coughing up rust-colored sputum that was thicker than his normal sputum production. Mr. C admits to current consumption of two packs per day of cigarettes (i.e., a 70 pack-year smoking history). He admits to occasional alcohol use but denies having orthopnea, ankle edema, nausea, vomiting, diarrhea, weight loss, dysuria, wheezing, or hemoptysis.

QUESTIONS	ANSWERS
1. What are the key symptoms in this case, and what disease do they suggest?	The key symptoms in this case are fever, sputum production, shortness of breath, and chest pain. These symptoms strongly suggest pneumonia.
2. What is the significance of the place of residence and source of income?	The fact that Mr. C lives in his car and earns money from collecting aluminum cans suggests that he may not have adequate nutritional intake. This decreases immune response and makes him more prone to pneumonia. It also makes him more likely to develop a severe or overwhelming pneumonia.
3. What is the significance of the smoking history?	Mr. C's smoking history is very significant and suggests that he is a candidate for lung cancer, COPD, and heart disease. COPD would increase his susceptibility to infections. His current use of cigarettes adds to his susceptibility to pneumonia, since they reduce the defensive mechanisms of the lung.
4. What is the significance of Mr. C's chronic sputum production?	Chronic sputum production is typical of patients with chronic bronchitis. Poor clearance of secretions in the lung makes infection, including pneumonia, more common.
5. What physical examination techniques are useful in this case, and what purpose do they serve?	The physical examination should begin with a general assessment and evaluation of the patient's vital signs. This will help assess the severity of Mr. C's illness and provides a baseline for later comparison. The chest should be inspected for chest wall configuration and breathing pattern, percussed for resonance, palpated for tactile fremitus, and auscultated for the presence of bronchial breath sounds, adventitious lung sounds, and pleural friction rubs. This will help identify the presence of lung consolidation and help determine whether the pleura is involved. The heart should be auscultated for evidence of failure (gallops) and murmurs. The extremities are examined for the presence of cyanosis, edema, or clubbing. The examiner should look for evidence of COPD.

More on Mr. C

PHYSICAL EXAMINATION

- **General.** Chronically ill–appearing elderly male in mild to moderate respiratory distress at rest; alert, oriented to person and place, and of nearly normal intellect, with long-term memory better than short-term memory

- **Vital Signs.** Temperature 39°C (102.2°F), heart rate 122/min, respiratory rate 32/min, blood pressure 110/60 mm Hg, height 150 cm, weight 65 kg

- **HEENT.** Cyanosis of the lips and mouth

- **Neck.** Supple with full active range of motion; trachea midline and mobile and without stridor or wheezing; carotid pulsation ++ and symmetrical with no bruits; mild supra-clavicular and cervical lymphadenopathy bilaterally; no jugular venous distention

- **Chest.** Anteroposterior diameter abnormally large, with diminished excursion noted on right side with each inspiratory effort; diminished resonance to percussion and increased tactile fremitus noted over right lower lobe posteriorly

- **Lungs.** Bronchial breath sounds over right lower lobe posteriorly; clear but diminished breath sounds over entire left lung and right middle and upper lobes; pleural friction rub heard over right lateral chest wall

- **Heart.** Regular rate and rhythm; no murmurs, gallops, or rubs noted; point of maximal impulse felt in epigastric area

- **Abdomen.** Normal in appearance, without tenderness to palpation; bowel sounds present; no masses, and no organomegaly

- **Extremities.** Cool, moist, and slightly dusky; cyanosis noted in fingertips; no clubbing or edema; pulses slightly diminished and symmetrical

QUESTIONS	ANSWERS
6. What is the significance of Mr. C's poor short-term memory?	Poor memory is an indication of reduced mental acuity and may be related to a number of adverse events, including hypoxia, alcohol abuse, sepsis, and chronic disease. Short-term memory is usually affected more severely by any cerebral insult compared to long-term memory.
7. How would you interpret the vital signs?	The vital signs demonstrate fever, hypotension, tachycardia, and tachypnea. These findings are consistent with a more severe case of acute pneumonia.
8. What is the significance of an increase in anteroposterior diameter?	The increase in anteroposterior diameter is consistent with COPD. Since COPD is a common predisposing factor for pneumonia, and since it may influence treatment, clinicians should be careful to note such findings.
9. What explains the unilateral chest expansion?	A unilateral reduction in chest expansion is commonly seen in lobar pneumonia. The affected lobe does not expand as well as the unaffected side with inspiration and lags behind the normal contralateral side.
10. What explains the decrease in resonance and increase in tactile fremitus?	The decrease in resonance with percussion suggests that the tissue underlying the chest wall in the affected region is dense, which is common with pneumonia. Other conditions, such as pleural effusion and lung tumors, may cause the same finding. An increase in tactile fremitus is also

11. What is the cause and significance of the bronchial breath sounds?	consistent with lung consolidation. The vibrations generated at the larynx travel much better through dense lung tissue compared to air-filled tissue.
	The bronchial breath sounds are consistent with lung consolidation. The turbulent flow sounds of the larger airways travel through consolidated lung more directly as compared to normal air-filled lung. The bronchus leading into the affected lung region must be patent to hear bronchial breath sounds over the affected region.
12. What is the significance of the pleural friction rub?	The pleural friction rub suggests that pleural inflammation is present. This finding indicates that the pneumonia is adjacent to the pleura.
13. Why are the extremities cool, moist, and dusky?	The extremities are cool, moist, and cyanotic because of the release of catecholamines in response to stress. The catecholamines cause sweating and peripheral vasoconstriction, which reduces blood flow to the extremities. As a result, the hands and feet become sweaty, cool, and cyanotic.
14. What laboratory tests are useful in this case?	Useful laboratory tests in this case would include a complete blood count (CBC), blood culture, chemistry profile, sputum Gram stain with culture and sensitivity, ABG, and chest x-ray.

More on Mr. C

Laboratory Evaluation

CBC	
Measure	Value
WBCs	4000/mm^3
Segmented neutrophils	60%
Bands	30%
Lymphocytes	10%
Hemoglobin	10.4 g

ABG on room air	
Measure	Value
pH	7.47
Paco$_2$	32 mm Hg
Pao$_2$	44 mm Hg
HCO$_3^-$	23 mEq/liter

Chest X-Ray: Right middle lobe consolidation; right heart border not visible (Figure 16.5) Sputum: Numerous gram-positive cocci with many WBCs and no epithelial cells

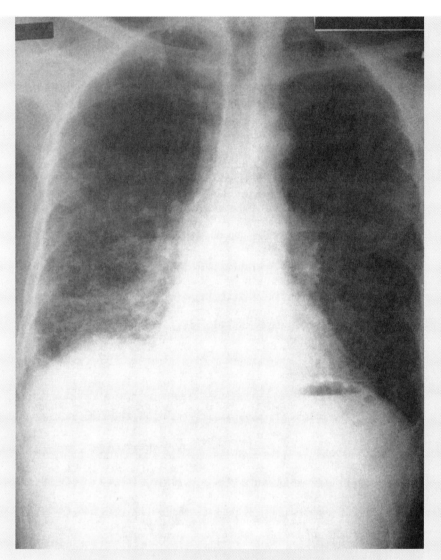

FIGURE 16.5 Right middle lobe pneumonia as seen on PA chest radiograph.

QUESTIONS	ANSWERS
15. How would you interpret the CBC?	The reduced WBC count in the presence of infection is consistent with an overwhelming infection. The WBC differential shows a large number of immature neutrophils (bands) that are not usually called into action unless the infection is severe. The hemoglobin is consistent with mild anemia.
16. How would you interpret the ABG results? Why are the Pa_{CO_2} and Pa_{O_2} reduced?	The ABG measurements are consistent with acute respiratory alkalosis and moderate hypoxemia. The Pa_{O_2} would be lower if the patient were not hyperventilating. The patient may be hyperventilating in response to both hypoxemia and sepsis. The Pa_{O_2} is reduced because of $\dot{V}/\dot{Q}$ mismatching in the lung.

17. What is the significance of the lack of visibility of the right heart border on the chest x-ray?

The inability to see the right heart border is evidence that the pneumonia is located in the right middle lobe. If the density were located in the right lower lobe, the right heart border would probably be visible.

18. What is the significance of gram-positive cocci found on the sputum Gram stain? What is the significance of the numerous WBCs and no epithelial cells?

The gram-positive cocci found on the Gram stain indicate that beta lactam–resistant antibiotics such as amoxicillin or a cephasporin should be used. The numerous leukocytes and lack of epithelial cells indicate a valid sputum sample representative of lower airway secretions.

19. Should Mr. C be treated as an outpatient, on the ward, or in the ICU?

The patient should be admitted to the ICU, where he can be closely monitored. This is needed because of the presence of shock and because he is at risk for respiratory failure. Also, there is evidence (via the low WBC count) that the pneumonia is overwhelming the patient's immune system.

20. What treatment should be provided?

The patient should be started on IV antibiotics—either a first-generation cephalosporin or a penicillin derivative. Respiratory care should start the patient on oxygen with an F_{IO_2} of 0.40 to 0.50 and titrate his F_{IO_2} to an arterial oxygen saturation (Sa_{O_2}) of approximately 90%. After his Sa_{O_2} is stable, a follow-up ABG would confirm his ventilatory, acid-base, and oxygenation status. IV fluids are needed to maintain hydration, as sepsis often decreases vascular tone and causes a relative hypovolemia. Sepsis-related vascular relaxation can result in profound hypotension requiring large amounts of fluid. Central venous pressure monitoring would be important if hypotension were to develop.

More on Mr. C

Mr. C is admitted to the ICU, where IV fluids and penicillin are started. Oxygen is given by mask at an F_{IO_2} of 0.40 with a heated aerosol. A cardiac monitor is attached to his chest to allow continuous assessment of heart rate and rhythm. Repeat ABGs 30 minutes after the start of oxygen therapy reveal the following: pH 7.47, Pa_{CO_2} 33 mm Hg, and Pa_{O_2} 53 mm Hg. Vital signs at this time are as follows: pulse 134/min, respiratory rate 36/min, body temperature 38.2°C (100.8°F), and blood pressure 105/65 mm Hg. Mr. C complains of increased dyspnea and cough. No change is noted in his right pleuritic chest pain. A blood sample is sent to the laboratory for culture.

QUESTIONS	ANSWERS
21. How would you interpret the repeat ABG results?	The acid-base status of the repeat ABG has not changed significantly from the initial ABG. Respiratory alkalosis with moderate hypoxemia continues.
22. What probably explains why the Pa_{O_2} did not increase very much with the increase in F_{IO_2} to 0.40?	Simple $\dot{V}/\dot{Q}$ mismatching causes hypoxemia that usually improves with supplemental oxygen therapy. Shunt is the likely explanation when the Pa_{O_2} increases little or not at all in response to an increase in F_{IO_2}. Pneumonia can lead to lung consolidation, which prevents air from entering the alveoli and coming in contact with blood in the pulmonary capillaries. An increase in F_{IO_2} will not increase the Pa_{O_2} significantly unless the affected region is participating in gas exchange.
23. Why is the Pa_{CO_2} not lower in response to the severity of the hypoxemia?	The Pa_{CO_2} is not lower in this case because of the presence of COPD. A high work of breathing and a large physiologic dead space associated with COPD make it difficult for the patient to increase ventilation enough to reduce his Pa_{CO_2} more than the ABG now shows.
24. What is your assessment of the patient's condition in the ICU as compared to previously?	The patient's condition appears to be deteriorating. The fever will increase his metabolic rate, which will require increased ventilation and blood flow, putting additional stress on his heart and lungs. Most patients do not tolerate respiratory rates greater than 30/min for a prolonged time, and an increasing respiratory rate is evidence of respiratory distress. The patient is experiencing increased dyspnea, which also suggests that he may be tiring and on the brink of respiratory failure.
25. What treatment is indicated based on your updated assessment? Should you be concerned about oxygen-induced hypoventilation?	The F_{IO_2} should be increased in an effort to obtain a Pa_{O_2} of 60 to 80 mm Hg. Given this patient's poor response to initial increases in the F_{IO_2} and the deteriorating vital signs, he will probably need intubation and mechanical ventilation to ensure adequate gas exchange. Oxygen-induced hypoventilation is not a concern in this case because the patient's previous ABGs reveal a reduced Pa_{CO_2}. Adequate oxygenation should never be sacrificed to avoid an increase in Pa_{CO_2}, even when Pa_{CO_2} is already elevated.

More on Mr. C

Mr. C's dyspnea and vital signs deteriorate further during the next hour. The cardiac monitor shows frequent premature ventricular contractions and tachycardia with a rate of 144/min. An endotracheal tube is placed, and mechanical positive pressure ventilation is started when Mr. C becomes confused and disoriented.

QUESTIONS	ANSWERS
26. What is the significance of Mr. C's sudden confusion and frequent premature ventricular contractions seen on the ECG monitor?	The sudden confusion and premature ventricular contractions suggest that Mr. C has become more hypoxic or septic, or both, and that he has inadequate cerebral perfusion. This is a sign that the patient's cardiopulmonary system is failing.
27. What mode of ventilation, tidal volume (V_T), respiratory rate, and FIO_2 would you recommend?	Mr. C can be ventilated with assist/control or intermittent mandatory ventilation. A mechanical respiratory rate of 10 to 14/min with a V_T of 390 to 520 mL (6 to 8 mL $\times$ 65 kg = 390 to 520 mL). An FIO_2 of 1.0 should be used initially, since he is showing signs of hypoxia.
28. How should the intubation and mechanical ventilation be assessed?	Placement of the endotracheal tube can be assessed by the following: a. Listening for airflow at the tube orifice as the patient makes respiratory efforts b. Auscultating for bilateral breath sounds on the lateral chest wall c. Listening for air entering the stomach with ventilator (or bag-valve-mask) driven breaths d. Examining a chest x-ray The mechanical ventilation can be assessed by ABG, breathing pattern, and vital signs.

More on Mr. C

Mr. C is placed on a volume ventilator in the assist/control mode with a backup rate of 12/min, a V_T of 500 mL, and an FIO_2 of 1.0. Initial auscultation reveals bilateral breath sounds with bronchial breath sounds over the right lower lobe. ABGs 20 minutes later reveal the following: pH 7.46, PaO_2 125 mm Hg, $PaCO_2$ 35 mm Hg, and HCO_3^- 27 mEq/liter. Mr. C has the following initial vital signs while on the ventilator: heart rate 128/min, respiratory rate 16/min, blood pressure 110/68 mm Hg, and temperature 38.5° C (101.3° F). A repeat chest x-ray reveals appropriate placement of the endotracheal tube and no change in the right lower lobe infiltrate. A Foley catheter is placed, and initial urine output is 25 mL for the first hour.

QUESTIONS	ANSWERS
29. What changes in the ventilatory settings would you recommend based on the most recent assessment data?	The initial ABG shows a relatively high Pa_{O_2} on an F_{IO_2} of 1.0. The oxyhemoglobin dissociation curve demonstrates that nearly as much O_2 is carried by blood with a Pa_{O_2} of 60 mm Hg as by blood with a Pa_{O_2} greater than 100 mm Hg. An F_{IO_2} of 1.0 puts the patient at risk for oxygen toxicity, and it should be titrated down to achieve an Sa_{O_2} of approximately 90% (Pa_{O_2} of about 60 to 65 mm Hg). Since the Pa_{CO_2} is within normal range, no change in the V_T or rate is needed.
30. What is the significance of the urine output of 25 mL for the first hour?	The initial urine output of 25 mL/hour suggests that the patient has poor renal perfusion, which may be caused by low relative blood volume. A normal urine output is approximately 60 mL/hour. IV fluid therapy is usually provided as initial therapy for patients with low urine output or low blood pressure associated with sepsis. Evidence that fluids might not be appropriate would include elevated jugular venous pressure, gallops in heart rhythm (third or fourth heart sound), hepatojugular reflex, and peripheral edema.
31. Is Mr. C at risk for nosocomial infection? If so, why? How can bedside clinicians reduce the risk?	Mr. C is at high risk for nosocomial infection because of his compromised immune system, intubation, and mechanical ventilation. Careful hand washing by all bedside clinicians before caring for each ICU patient is very important to prevent spread of bacteria from one patient to the next. The use of sterile technique for suctioning the airway is also important.

Mr. C Conclusion

Over the next 24 hours, Mr. C steadily improves. His temperature drops to 37.5°C (99.5°F), and his heart rate drops to 95/min. A repeat CBC reveals a WBC of 6000/mm^3 with 65% segmented neutrophils and 20% bands. IV penicillin and fluids are continued. ABGs at this time are as follows: pH 7.44, Pa_{CO_2} 39 mm Hg, Pa_{O_2} 72 mm Hg, and F_{IO_2} 0.50.

On day 3, Mr. C's weaning parameters are good and he is weaned from mechanical ventilation without difficulty. His vital signs are normal except for a respiratory rate of 28/min. The endotracheal tube is removed, and he tolerates spontaneous breathing well. He is given heated aerosol by mask with an F_{IO_2} of 0.50 after extubation. A repeat chest x-ray on day 3 shows that the right middle lobe infiltrate is less dense. The patient is switched to a nasal cannula at 3 liters/min, which he tolerates well. After his temperature is normal for 24 hours, the IV antibiotics are discontinued and oral antibiotics started. The patient is sent home on day 5 on oral penicillin. A follow-up visit with his physician is scheduled for 1 week later.

QUESTIONS	ANSWERS
32. What risk factors placed Mr. C at risk for pneumonia?	Mr. C's risk factors included a positive smoking history, COPD, possible alcohol abuse, and malnutrition.
33. How long might it take for the infiltrate to completely clear on the chest film? Should Mr. C have follow-up chest films to document complete resolution of the pneumonia? If so, why?	The infiltrate of bacterial pneumonia seen on the chest radiograph generally clears in 2 weeks in young, healthy patients but may take as long as 3 months to clear in older patients with lung disease. Yes, this patient should have follow-up chest films taken to document complete resolution of the pneumonia. He is also at high risk for bronchogenic carcinoma (see Chapter 20). The chest radiograph is needed because the infiltrate may be caused by airway obstruction from bronchogenic carcinoma; in such cases, the infiltrate will not clear completely with antibiotics. A nonresolving pneumonia requires further evaluation, most likely with bronchoscopy. ■

KEY POINTS

- Each year approximately five million persons contract pneumonia in the United States, about one fifth of whom need to be hospitalized.[1] Pneumonia is the sixth leading cause of death and the most common cause of death from infection.
- Infections of the lung parenchyma incite a reaction that causes an outpouring of fluid, inflammatory proteins, and white blood cells (WBCs). Interstitial and alveolar spaces become flooded with edema and exudative material.
- The patient with bacterial pneumonia usually complains of an abrupt onset of fever, cough, and sputum production and may complain of shortness of breath and chest pain. Dyspnea is more common when the pneumonia involves multiple regions of the lung or when it is superimposed on chronic pulmonary disease.
- The chest radiograph is considered the gold standard for confirming the diagnosis of pneumonia. It is often needed because the signs and symptoms associated with pneumonia often occur in other disorders such as upper respiratory tract infection and pulmonary embolism. It usually reveals a dense area of consolidation when pneumonia is present.
- Microbiological evaluation of sputum is done to identify the pathogen responsible for the respiratory infection and is best performed before antibiotics are administered. In many cases a representative sample of lung pathogens is difficult to obtain because many patients do not have a productive cough and when sputum is produced, most sputum specimens are contaminated with oral secretions as they pass through the mouth.
- An appropriate antibiotic should be started as soon as possible, although several days of the drug are needed to reach full effectiveness. In the patient who is not severely ill, a short delay in the onset of antibiotic therapy is reasonable while appropriate sputum and blood samples are obtained. If gram-positive, elongated diplococci typical of pneumococci are seen, oral ampicillin or penicillin is the drug of choice. Intravenous penicillin G is given if the patient appears ill.

(key points continued on page 382)

KEY POINTS (CONTINUED)

- The decision to admit the patient with pneumonia is based not only on the severity of the infection, but also on the presence of certain risk factors. Patients with advanced age, coexisting illness, high fever, or leukopenia are at greater risk for severe, life-threatening pneumonia and should be more strongly considered for admission. Admission to the ICU is needed when shock is present.

REFERENCES

1. Mandell, LA, Bartlett, JG, Dowell, JG: Update of practice guidelines for the management of community-acquired pneumonia in immunocompetent adults. Clin Infect Dis 37:1405, 2003.
2. Niederman, MS, Mandell, LA, Anzueto, A: Guidelines for the management of adults with community-acquired pneumonia. Diagnosis, assessment of severity, antimicrobial therapy, and prevention. Am J Respir Crit Care Med 163:1730, 2001.
3. Palafox, M, Guiscafre, HR, Munoz, O, Martinez, H: Diagnostic value of tachypnea in pneumonia defined radiologically. Arch Dis Child 82:41–45, 2000.
4. Basi, SK, Marrie, TJ, Huang, JQ, et al: Patients admitted to hospital with suspected pneumonia and normal chest radiographs: epidemiology, microbiology, and outcomes. Am J Med 117:305–311, 2004.
5. Lynch, T, Platt, R, Gouin, S, Larson, C, Patenaude, Y: Can we predict which children with clinically suspected pneumonia will have the presence of focal infiltrates on chest radiographs? Pediatrics 113:186–189, 2004.
6. Heckerling, PS: The need for chest roentgenograms in adults with acute respiratory illness. Clinical predictors. Arch Intern Med 146:1321–1324, 1986.
7. American Thoracic Society: Guidelines for the management of adults with community acquired pneumonia. Am Rev Respir Dis 163:1730, 2001.
8. Tuomanen, E: Pneumococcal pneumonia in adults. Available at up-to-date.com accessed: 11-5-05.
9. Fine, MJ, Smith, MA, Carson, CA, et al: Prognosis and outcomes of patients with community acquired pneumonia. A meta-analysis. JAMA 275:134, 1996.

17

Pneumonia in the Immunocompromised Patient

Philip M. Gold, MD, MACP, FCCP
N. Lennard Specht, MD, FACP

> ## CHAPTER OBJECTIVES:
>
> After reading the chapter you will be able to identify:
>
> - The definition of opportunistic infections.
> - The structure and function of the immune system.
> - The common causes of immunosuppression.
> - The typical signs and symptoms consistent with opportunistic pulmonary infections.
> - The treatment of pneumonia in the immunosuppressed patient.
> - The prophylactic treatment of patients with immunodeficiencies.

INTRODUCTION

The respiratory system has an extremely large surface area exposed to inhaled gases. At times, inhaled gases contain microorganisms that can result in serious lung infections. In healthy individuals the immune system is one of several factors that defend against the development of pulmonary infections. Highly infectious microorganisms such as *Streptococcus pneumoniae*, however, can cause pulmonary infections despite a strong immune system. Less infectious organisms that are easily controlled and eradicated by a normal immune system can cause serious pulmonary infections if the immune system is damaged. Infections caused by organisms that do not usually affect people with a healthy immune system are called **opportunistic infections**.

Defects in the immune system can be mild, causing only a slight increase in the frequency of infections, or severe, causing life-threatening infections. The source of the defect can be congenital (primary) or acquired (secondary). Primary immune deficiency diseases are not common and can be difficult to diagnose and treat.[1,2] One example of primary immunodeficiency is selective IgA deficiency. Chemotherapy, infections, radiation, and malnutrition are examples of factors that can cause acquired immunodeficiencies.

Respiratory therapists encounter patients with immunodeficiencies with increasing frequency. The emergence of **acquired immunodeficiency syndrome (AIDS)**, the increasing use of transplantation, and aggressive chemotherapy regimens all contribute to this trend.

ETIOLOGY

Basic Function of the Immune System

The immune system is a complex group of defense mechanisms designed to eliminate foreign organisms. Immunity has three principal characteristics that govern its behavior: ability to differentiate self from nonself, specificity, and memory. The vast majority of immune system attacks are directed at invading microorganisms, not the host. This selectivity is critical to prevent indiscriminate immune responses from damaging the host. In diseases such as rheumatoid arthritis, systemic lupus erythematosis, and scleroderma, the immune system attacks the host. These diseases are called **autoimmune diseases**.

The immune response detects molecules with specific molecular configurations unique to the organism it is attacking. These uniquely configured molecules are called antigens. The recognition and targeting of specific antigens enables the immune system to attack invading microorganisms and differentiate host from nonhost. The immune system remembers when it has been invaded by an organism and provides a more rapid, larger response when it is invaded by the same organism a second time. This principle, called immune memory, is the basis of vaccinations. A vaccination consists of a collection of antigens that resemble an organism, which when given to a patient, provides protection against that organism.

> The immune system aids in resisting and fighting infection. It is responsible for an organism's ability to distinguish between self and nonself and is characterized by specificity and memory.

The Immune System

The immune system is not confined to one area of the body. There are collections of immune cells scattered throughout the body that mobilize and circulate to specific areas as they are needed. Polymorphonuclear cells, such as neutrophils, basophils, and eosinophils, originate in the bone marrow. Lymphocytes congregate in the spleen, thymus, and lymph nodes.

The immune system is made up of many different types of cells (Figure 17.1). Lymphocytes and monocytes comprise the majority of the immune cells. The populations of lymphocytes are broadly divided into T and B lymphocytes. B lymphocytes can develop into antibody-secreting cells called plasma cells. Antibodies, also called immunoglobulins (Ig), are molecules that identify and bind to specific foreign antigens to assist the immune system in recognizing and destroying foreign invaders.

The five classes of immunoglobulins are IgG, IgM, IgE, IgA, and IgD. IgM antibodies are usually the first antibody produced at the onset of an infection. The level of IgM quickly rises to a peak and then declines as IgM is replaced by IgG as the primary antibody fighting the infection. IgA antibodies are produced in tissue adjacent to mucous membranes. These antibodies are then secreted onto the surface of the mucosa. On the mucosal surface, IgA inhibits binding of organisms to the membrane's surface and forms the initial barrier to entry of organisms across the mucosa. IgE antibodies mediate allergic reactions.

As they mature, T lymphocytes differentiate into three types that serve distinct functions. One subpopulation called natural killer cells has a direct cytotoxic effect on targeted cells. Another subgroup, called helper T lymphocytes, promotes the development of antibodies by B lymphocytes and assists in the development of natural killer cells. Helper T lymphocytes have the CD4+ antigen on their surface. The CD4+ antigen is used to recognize helper T cells in the clinical laboratory. Suppressor T cells inhibit the immune

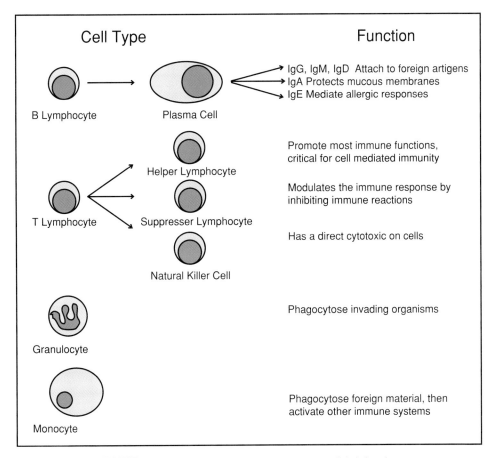

Cell Type

Function

B Lymphocyte

Plasma Cell

IgG, IgM, IgD Attach to foreign artigens
IgA Protects mucous membranes
IgE Mediate allergic responses

Helper Lymphocyte

Promote most immune functions, critical for cell mediated immunity

T Lymphocyte

Suppresser Lymphocyte

Modulates the immune response by inhibiting immune reactions

Natural Killer Cell

Has a direct cytotoxic on cells

Granulocyte

Phagocytose invading organisms

Monocyte

Phagocytose foreign material, then activate other immune systems

FIGURE 17.1 The major cells of the immune system and their function.

responses. This effect is important for inhibiting attacks on the host and regulating the immune response following antigen exposure. Suppressor T cells have the CD8+ antigen on their surfaces.

Helper T lymphocytes are significant in cell-mediated immunity. They are responsible for defense against specific types of organisms, including *Mycobacterium tuberculosis*. The reaction of the cell-mediated immunity to an antigen is called delayed hypersensitivity. The strength of the delayed hypersensitivity reaction can be assessed with a skin test.

Monocytes and macrophages are larger than lymphocytes. These mononuclear cells play a critical role in the immune response. Monocytes circulate in the blood and may migrate into tissue to become macrophages. Macrophages engulf foreign material and degrade it (**phagocytosis**). Important antigens in the degraded foreign material are then used by macrophages to activate the immune response by other cells, such as helper T lymphocytes.

Because of their phagocytic function, granulocytes provide another important defense against infection. Granulocytes are formed in the bone marrow and circulate in the blood as neutrophils, eosinophils, or basophils. As granulocytes develop, their nuclei become segmented with multiple lobules, giving these cells the appearance of multiple nuclei. For this reason they are often called polymorphonuclear cells. Neutrophils are the most common granulocytes. They are responsible for detecting invading microorganisms,

> The immune system has both cellular and humoral components.

phagocytosing them, killing them, and degrading their remains. Neutrophils often die in the process of destroying invading organisms. Neutrophils—both living and dead—are the major constituent of pus, which is found in infected tissue (e.g., boils).

PATHOPHYSIOLOGY

Immunosuppression and Disease

Depressed immunity has numerous causes. Each form of immunosuppression leads to decreased function of a distinct portion of the immune system (Table 17.1). When a portion of a patient's immune system is not functioning properly, the patient is prone to infection. Infections are frequently caused by organisms that are normally best controlled by the portion of the immune system that is damaged. To understand an opportunistic infection, you must also understand the immune system of the patient who has acquired the infection. An understanding of a patient's immune defect allows one to predict the organisms most likely to cause an infection. Some of the more commonly encountered forms of immune diseases are discussed here to illustrate the interaction among immune disease, the resulting infection, and optimal therapy.

> Impaired immunity may be congenital or acquired. Knowing the type of immune deficiency present helps predict the type of infection the patient may develop or has developed.

Antibody Deficiency

An inadequate level of antibodies increases a patient's susceptibility to infection. In patients with this form of immunosuppression, infections are usually caused by organisms that can also affect individuals with normal immunity. In patients with an antibody deficiency, however, these infections are more frequent and severe than they would be if the patient's immune systems were normal. Infections in these patients are therefore not typically classified as opportunistic because they also occur in patients with normal immunity.

A complete or partial absence of antibodies leads to repeated infections with bacteria such as *S. pneumoniae* or *Haemophilus influenzae* and other encapsulated bacteria. The

Table 17.1 Types of Immune System Deficiencies

Type of Immunity	Cause of Deficiency	Example
Antibodies	Congenital	IgA deficiency
Cell-mediated immunity	Infection	AIDS
	Congenital	MHC* class II deficiency
	Medications	Transplantation immunosuppression
Phagocytic immunity	Chemotherapy	Neutropenia
	Congenital	Chronic granulomatous disease

*MHC = major histocompatibility complex

respiratory tract is the usual target for these infections, but meningitis or septicemia can also develop. The most severe form of antibody deficiency is X-linked agammaglobulinemia. Starting 6 to 9 months after birth, infants affected with this disorder begin to acquire recurrent infections if they are not treated. Without treatment, patients with this disorder die at a very young age. Immunoglobulin replacement therapy is effective, but these patients may still be susceptible to respiratory infections because transfused IgA is not secreted onto the surface of mucous membranes.

Selective IgA deficiency is the most common form of immunoglobulin deficiency. IgA deficiency can lead to chronic, recurrent pulmonary infections. Not every patient with IgA deficiency acquires an unusual number of infections. Many of these patients are asymptomatic throughout life. Patients with IgA deficiency do not benefit from IgA transfusions and must rely on antimicrobial treatment of infections as they develop.

Defects in Cellular Immunity

Cell-mediated immunity is the portion of the immune system provided by T lymphocytes. A good example of this immunity is the body's defense against intracellular pathogens, such as *M. tuberculosis*. Cell-mediated immunity is regulated by helper T lymphocytes and suppressor T lymphocytes. Helper T lymphocytes have an important part in determining which antigens will be reacted to. Helper T cells also determine which immune cells are most effective for a given situation. They then mobilize that immune cell type into the area of infection.

Another cell-mediated response is cytotoxicity. Cytotoxic cells, like natural killer lymphocytes, bind to target cells and lyse them. Cytotoxic reactions are triggered when the host's natural killer lymphocytes recognize antigens or antibodies bound to the cell surface. A good example of antigens that are recognized and attacked as foreign are the major histocompatibility complex (MHC) antigens, which are expressed on the surface of the host's cells in a pattern unique to each individual. Cytotoxic cells recognize the unique MHC pattern as self and will attack any cells that do not express that pattern. The MHC antigens are an important factor in transplantation. Ideally the MHC pattern of a donor graft should be as close as possible to the recipient's pattern.

Deficiencies of cell-mediated immunity include rare, inherited forms and the more common acquired deficiencies (Box 17.1). AIDS is by far the most common acquired defect of cell-mediated immunity.

Defects in Phagocyte Function

Phagocytic cells are important in fighting infections caused by pyogenic bacteria. A significant decrease in the number of circulating phagocytes, or their ability to function, may result in overwhelming bacterial infections. Most of the circulating phagocytes are neutrophils.

Box 17.1 Types of Cell-Mediated Immunodeficiencies

Inherited

- MHC* class II deficiency
- DiGeorge's syndrome
- Hereditary ataxia-telangiectasia
- Wiskott-Aldrich syndrome

Acquired

- Acquired immunodeficiency syndrome

*MHC = major histocompatibility complex

Neutropenia (an abnormally low number of circulating neutrophils, usually less than 500/dL) can be congenital or acquired. Hereditary defects in phagocyte function include chronic granulomatous disease and leukocyte adhesion deficiency. Acquired neutropenia is frequently caused by cancer chemotherapy. Chemotherapy drugs can reduce the number of circulating granulocytes for several days or weeks. If an infection develops during the period of granulocytopenia, the infection can rapidly become overwhelming. Because infections in patients with neutropenia are so serious, patients are treated with intravenous antibiotics at the first sign of fever.

CLINICAL FEATURES

History

Opportunistic pulmonary infections occur when the effectiveness of the immune system has been reduced. Frequently, the cause of immunocompromise is clear when a patient presents for care. On occasion, however, immunosuppression may not be obvious on initial evaluation. A careful history and review of the laboratory data will usually uncover evidence suggesting that immunosuppression is present. Opportunistic pneumonia should be considered in any patient with recurrent bouts of pneumonia or a case of pneumonia that does not resolve with treatment. The interview should document whether the patient has a personal or family history of an acquired or inherited immunodeficiency or is at risk of an acquired immunodeficiency (Box 17.2).

Physical Examination

In most cases, the signs and symptoms of opportunistic pneumonias are similar to more common pneumonias. Symptoms of cough, dyspnea, and fever are common but not universal. Fever, in a neutropenic patient following chemotherapy, usually represents a serious infection. Patients with pyogenic pneumonias may also experience pleuritic chest pain, the production of purulent sputum, occasional hemoptysis, malaise, and recent weight loss.

The physical examination of an immunocompromised patient with pneumonia will often reveal features of both the acute pulmonary infection and the immunosuppression. Localized crackles or consolidation usually indicate

Box 17.2   Risk Factors for Acquired Immunodeficiency
            Syndromes

AIDS

- Multiple sexual partners
- Intravenous drug abuse

Neutropenia

- Leukemia
- Lymphoma
- Recent chemotherapy

Miscellaneous

- Immunosuppression for prevention of a transplant rejection
- Corticosteroid use
- Transfusions

Immune deficiency leads to "opportunistic" infections—infections that would not usually occur in a healthy individual. Systematic evaluation involves obtaining a history, physical examination, and obtaining a variety of tests and imaging studies.

localized pneumonia, whereas diffuse crackles or consolidation indicate widespread infection. In an immunocompetent patient an opportunistic pneumonia is more likely to be widespread than a bacterial pneumonia.

Laboratory Findings

Several laboratory tests may indicate immunosuppression. An abnormally low number of lymphocytes, particularly CD4+ cells, indicates a defect in cell-mediated immunity (e.g., AIDS). Neutropenia is characterized by a neutrophil count less than 500/mL on a blood count. Patients with pneumonia, either diffuse or localized, have some deterioration in gas exchange. This may be seen either as hypoxemia in severe cases or as an increase in the alveolar-arterial difference in partial pressure of oxygen (P[A-a]O$_2$) in milder cases.

Chest Radiograph

The chest radiograph of a patient with a healthy immune system who acquires pyogenic pneumonia usually reveals a localized area of increased density (frequently called an infiltrate) in the infected portion of the lung. In patients with an immunodeficiency, pneumonia is frequently diffuse, often affecting all portions of the lung. The chest radiograph of an immunocompromised patient with pneumocystis pneumonia usually reveals a diffusely increased density that often includes multiple portions of the lung.[3] The diffuse chest radiograph markings from pneumocystis pneumonia are occasionally subtle, having a ground-glass appearance; however, as the disease progresses, the markings become obvious, diffuse, interstitial infiltrates. If symptoms suggest pneumocystis pneumonia but the chest radiograph is normal, a gallium scan or an evaluation of lung diffusion capacity (DLCO) may be useful[4,5] in determining whether such an infection is present. Chest radiographs of patients with mild immunocompromise and tuberculosis reveal unilateral or bilateral upper lobe cavitating densities. These findings are similar to those of patients with tuberculosis without evidence of immune compromise.[6] Chest radiographs of patients with severe immunocompromise and tuberculosis may show diffuse pulmonary infiltrates and lymph node enlargement without cavitation.[7]

Microbiology

A wide variety of organisms can infect the immunocompromised patient, including bacteria, fungi, parasites, and viruses. Empiric treatment for all of these possibilities may be necessary but can be very toxic and expensive. For this reason it is important to identify the organism causing pneumonia in an immunocompromised patient as rapidly as possible. Unfortunately it is not always possible to identify the infecting organism, even with invasive testing procedures. These procedures should be used as soon as possible after opportunistic pneumonia is suspected. Empiric treatment is started until the results of diagnostic testing are available. The type of immunosuppression dictates which empiric treatment is best (see Treatment section).

Culture and microscopic examination of the sputum are the least invasive and most readily available techniques for identifying infectious agents. Initially, a Gram stain and acid-fast stain are used to stain the sputum. Cultures are performed for bacteria, acid-fast bacilli, and fungi. A stain should also be performed for *Pneumocystis jaroveci* if the patient has a defect in cell-mediated immunity. To obtain optimal sputum samples, many centers are meticulous in their sputum collection. Specimens are collected in the early morning, just after the patient has awakened. The patient brushes his or her teeth and oral cavity extensively and then gargles with water. Next a 3% saline solution is nebulized to induce the specimen. Using these techniques patients with pneumocystis pneumonia can be identified without an invasive test in as many as 75% of cases.[8] Specimens to be cultured are collected in a sterile container and sent immediately to the microbiology laboratory. For *P. jaroveci* evaluation, specimens are sent to a cytopathology laboratory for staining and review for the organism. A number of stains are used to identify the pneumocystis organisms, including monoclonal antibodies, Papanicolaou, Giemsa, and Grocott.[9]

If an induced sputum fails to determine which organism is responsible for the infection, a bronchoscopy with bronchoalveolar lavage[10,11] or transbronchial biopsy[12] may help establish the diagnosis. An open lung biopsy may be required to establish the etiology if bronchoscopy fails to reveal the infectious organism and the patient is not improving.[13]

SPECIFIC IMMUNE SYNDROMES

Some diseases that cause immunodeficiency are very uncommon. A few immunodeficiencies have become progressively more frequent. It is useful to focus our discussion on the more common immunodeficiency syndromes that respiratory care practitioners may encounter in their practice.

Acquired Immunodeficiency Syndrome

An infection by the human immunodeficiency virus (HIV) causes AIDS. HIV infection usually causes an unrelenting, slowly progressive loss of cell-mediated immunity. A patient infected with HIV is said to have developed AIDS when the immunocompromise becomes so severe that it causes an opportunistic infection or another complication, such as a tumor. HIV preferentially infects cells that have the CD4+ antigen. As the infection progresses, the helper T lymphocytes that express the CD4+ antigen are destroyed. The immune system becomes compromised when the number of helper T cells decreases from a normal concentration of 800 to 1200/μL to less than 600/μL. The risk of both opportunistic and nonopportunistic infections progressively increases as the CD4+ count drops. The number of circulating CD4+ cells is a rough indication of AIDS severity and the infections that are most likely to occur (Table 17.2).

Table 17.2 Frequent Infections in Patients with Acquired Immunodeficiency Syndrome[26,27]

Number of Circulating CD4+ Cells	Likely Infections/disorders
CD4+ >200/μL	*Mycobacterium tuberculosis*
	Candida albicans
CD4+ <200/μL	Cryptosporidiosis
	Kaposi's sarcoma
	Lymphoma
	Pneumocystis jaroveci
CD4+ <100/μL	Herpes simplex virus
	Toxoplasma gondii
	Cryptococcus neoformans
	Mucocutaneous candidiasis
CD4+ <50/μL	Cytomegalovirus retinitis
	Mycobacterium avium complex

The most common opportunistic pulmonary infections include *P. jaroveci*, *Mycobacterium avium* complex (a bacteria closely related to *M. tuberculosis*), and *Candida albicans*. The defect in cellular immunity also predisposes AIDS patients to nonopportunistic infections, such as bacterial infections, tuberculosis, coccidioidomycosis, and histoplasmosis (Table 17.3).[14] In addition to being prone to infections, patients with AIDS are at increased risk of some forms of

Table 17.3 Organisms that Frequently Cause Pneumonia in Patients with Defects of Cell-Mediated Immunity

Opportunistic Infections	Nonopportunistic Infections
Pneumocystis jaroveci	Pyogenic bacteria
Mycobacterium avium complex and other nontuberculous mycobacteria	Cryptococcus neoformans
Cytomegalovirus	Mycobacterium tuberculosis
Herpes simplex virus	Coccidioides immitis
Toxoplasma gondii	Histoplasma capsulatum

cancer, such as Kaposi's sarcoma[15] and lymphoma.[16] Interstitial pulmonary diseases, such as lymphoid interstitial pneumonitis or interstitial pneumonitis not associated with any identifiable infection, may also develop in AIDS patients.

AIDS patients may have constitutional symptoms such as fever, chills, malaise, and weight loss due to the HIV infection alone. Lymphadenopathy develops in the early stages of the disease. The lymph nodes enlarge throughout the body and are usually not tender when palpated. Most patients in the later stage of the disease experience severe weight loss. Many patients will also experience dyspnea on exertion if a pulmonary infection develops. These patients often have a cough, frequently productive, and occasionally have pleuritic chest pain. Fever may be absent in patients with pneumocystis pneumonia. Symptoms of pneumocystis pneumonia may be very subtle including simply a chronic cough and dyspnea on exertion. Uncommonly, a pneumothorax or large pleural effusion develops in patients with pulmonary infections associated with AIDS. Examination of the respiratory tract may reveal whitish plaques adherent to the tongue and mouth. These plaques are characteristic of mucocutaneous infection with *C. albicans* (oral thrush) and indicate that a form of immunocompromise is probably present. In patients with immunosuppression the Candida plaques may extend from the mouth to the throat and may involve the trachea and esophagus. Patients with HIV infection may have diffuse lymphadenopathy due to either the HIV infection itself or to an AIDS-related malignancy.

Patients with pneumocystis pneumonia often recover completely. The mortality for all cases of pneumocystis pneumonia in AIDS patients is approximately 10%.[17] However, patients who go into respiratory failure as a result of AIDS-associated pneumocystis pneumonia have a mortality of 80% to 90%.[17,18] Treatment of AIDS-associated pneumocystis infections is complicated by the inability of many AIDS patients to tolerate the commonly prescribed antibiotics. Adverse reactions to these medications may lead to a skin rash or more serious problems, such as neutropenia. When a severe reaction develops, the antibiotics must be changed. Unfortunately, the alternate drugs are often more toxic and no more effective than the initial medications.

Transplantation

Transplantation is an increasingly common treatment for patients with end-stage organ failure. Transplanting the organ of one person into a patient who is not genetically identical

Table 17.4 Pulmonary Infections Associated with Transplantation

Post-Transplantation Stage	Organism
Early (up to 30 days)	Pyogenic bacteria
	Fungi, particularly Aspergillus and Candida
	Viruses
Mid (30–100 days)	Cytomegalovirus
	Aspergillus
	P. jaroveci
	Pyogenic bacteria
Late (days)	Pyogenic bacteria
	Fungi
	Viruses
	P. jaroveci
	Mycobacteria

provides a stimulus for the recipient's immune system to attack the transplanted organ. The host's immune system recognizes the different pattern of MHC antigens on the surface of the transplanted organ and attacks it. This attack is called transplant rejection. A patient who has received a transplant takes immunosuppressive medications such as cyclosporin and corticosteroids to control transplant rejection. Although these immunosuppressive medications control transplant rejection, they also increase a patient's risk of pulmonary infection. The most common pulmonary infections seen in patients using immunosuppressive medications are listed in Table 17.4. The risk of pulmonary infection increases if the patient has received a bone marrow transplant or if high doses of immunosuppressive medications are required.

Symptoms of post-transplantation infection include a nonproductive cough, dyspnea, and fever. The fever may not be severe if the immunosuppression is significant. The chest examination findings may be localized (e.g., in pyogenic bacterial infections) or diffuse (e.g., in infections caused by cytomegalovirus or *P. carinii*).

Neutropenia

Cancer chemotherapy is designed to kill cells that are multiplying rapidly. Most cancers are made up of rapidly dividing cells. A large percentage of cancer cells are killed each time chemotherapy is used. Unfortunately, chemotherapy kills not only cancer cells but also some normal cells. Cells that generate hair and white blood cells are very sensitive to chemotherapy. For this reason, chemotherapy often causes hair loss and a low white blood cell (WBC) count (neutropenia). The number of circulating granulocytes may drop to very low levels when some forms of chemotherapy are given. Neutropenia occurs when the granulocyte count is less than 500/μL. Neutropenia may begin 7 days after chemotherapy is initiated and may continue for 2 to 3 weeks. During the period of neutropenia, a patient is prone to infection because of the small numbers of circulating phagocytic cells. These infections are generally caused by pyogenic bacteria or fungal organisms such as Aspergillus. An infection in a neutropenic patient advances quickly if the cause of the infection is not promptly treated. Fever is a very important sign of infection in a neutropenic patient and is often the initial clue of a serious infection. The patient will experience dyspnea and a cough if the lungs are the site of infection. Examination of the chest of a patient with neutropenia-associated pneumonia may disclose localized crackles or signs of consolidation.

Immunosuppressive Drugs

Many drugs used to treat inflammatory diseases such as rheumatoid arthritis, systemic lupus erythematosis, scleroderma, and asthma can suppress the immune system. Drugs such as corticosteroids, cyclophosphamide, and azathioprine increase the patient's risk of both opportunistic and nonopportunistic pneumonia.

TREATMENT

Empiric Therapy

In immunocompromised patients pneumonia can progress very rapidly, forcing clinicians to begin therapy without waiting for the results of diagnostic tests that determine the microorganism causing the infection (empiric therapy). A patient's particular type of immune defect helps predict which organisms are most likely to be responsible for the infection. Empiric therapy is selected on this basis. A patient with neutropenia is usually treated with antibiotics against pyogenic bacteria such as *Pseudomonas aeruginosa* and/or fungi such as Aspergillus organisms. Patients with AIDS are usually empirically treated with a combination of trimethoprim and sulfamethoxazole because they are likely to have pneumonia due to *P. jaroveci*.

> Treatment of opportunistic infections involves empirical selection of medication based upon the most likely pathogens or specific therapy based upon microbiologic tests.

Specific Therapy

Empiric therapy is replaced by treatment directed at the specific organism if diagnostic testing discloses which organism has caused the pneumonia. Patients with pyogenic bacterial infections are treated with at least one and frequently two antibacterial agents. The microbiology laboratory uses sensitivity testing to determine the best antibiotics to use for a given infection.

Pneumonia caused by *P. jaroveci* is diagnosed by identifying these small organisms with a high-powered microscope in specially stained lung secretions. These infections are usually treated with a combination of sulfa antibiotics. Patients who cannot tolerate sulfa antibiotics may be given pentamidine intravenously or by aerosol. Other treatment regimens have been developed, including dapsone, primaquine, atovaquone, and trimetrexate.[19] These drugs are usually reserved for patients who cannot tolerate either of the more common therapies. Patients who have moderate to severe pneumonia due to *P. jaroveci* benefit from high-dose corticosteroid treatments with methylprednisolone.[20,21]

Fungal pneumonia caused by Aspergillus organisms or other fungal infections is treated with antifungal antibiotics. Treatment is begun with amphotericin B for most immunocompromised patients with a fungal pneumonia. Oral antifungal agents classified as imidazoles are available. These drugs (e.g., itraconazole,[22] ketoconazole, fluconazole) are reserved for patients with mild infections or those who have responded well to amphotericin B but for whom further oral therapy is desired.

AIDS patients in whom tuberculosis develops require intensive therapy with multiple drugs. The first 2 months should include isoniazid, rifampin, pyrazinamide, and ethambutol. Isoniazid and rifampin are continued for 7 months.[23]

Prophylactic Therapy

Patients with immunodeficiencies such as AIDS are at risk for several forms of opportunistic pneumonia. As a preventive measure, it is often wise to institute prophylactic antibiotic therapy.[24] In AIDS cases prophylactic therapy is started either to follow an acute infection in order to prevent a recurrence or when the number of circulating CD4+ lymphocytes becomes so low that infection is likely. Antibiotics should be started to prevent pneumocystis pneumonia when the number of CD4+ lymphocytes is less than 200/μL. The first choice for prophylactic treatment is a daily tablet of trimethoprim-sulfamethoxazole. Aerosolized pentamidine or dapsone tablets may be used if a patient cannot tolerate sulfa antibiotics (e.g., trimethoprim-sulfamethoxazole). Rifampin and clarithromycin are recommended for prevention of *M. avium* complex if the CD4+ count is less than 50/μL.

MR. W

HISTORY

Mr. W is a 35-year-old man. Three years ago he was found to be infected with the HIV virus. Since the discovery of his infection, he has been well. He was started on anti retroviral medication shortly after diagnosis. He has lost 20 pounds over the past 2 months and experienced a progressive decrease in the number of circulating CD4+ lymphocytes. The most recent count revealed a CD4+ level of 97/μL. Two weeks prior to the office visit, he noticed mild dyspnea on exertion and a nagging, nonproductive cough. He did not experience fever or myalgias. A chest radiograph was normal, and his initial evaluation was unremarkable. Following that clinic visit, a diffusion capacity of the lung test (D$_{LCO}$) was ordered, and Mr. W was instructed to return for a follow-up visit in 2 weeks. During the next 2 weeks, Mr. W found that his cough persisted and his exercise tolerance progressively deteriorated. The D$_{LCO}$ was 42% of predicted.

QUESTIONS	ANSWERS
1. In what manner does HIV affect the immune system?	The human immunodeficiency virus attacks several cell types in the body. It most severely affects helper T lymphocytes, which are critical for the proper function of cellular immunity. As the helper T lymphocytes are destroyed, cellular immunity is destroyed along with them.
2. List several organisms that cause opportunistic pneumonia in patients infected with HIV.	Infections that would not normally occur in a person with a healthy immune system are called opportunistic infections. Table 17.2 lists several organisms that cause opportunistic pneumonia in patients with deficient cellular immunity; the most common is *P. jaroveci*. Other organisms include

M. avium complex, *Cryptococcus neoformans*, *Toxoplasma gondii*, cytomegalovirus, herpes simplex virus, and nontuberculous mycobacterial organisms.

3. How do you interpret the number of circulating CD4+ lymphocytes in Mr. W, and what is the significance?

Mr. W's CD4+ cell count is very low (normal levels are 800 to 1200/μL). This reduction in the number of circulating helper T cells indicates that Mr. W is at risk for several forms of opportunistic infections (see Box 17.2).

4. Mr. W has a nonproductive cough and dyspnea on exertion. What opportunistic infections can cause these symptoms?

Any pneumonia could cause dyspnea on exertion. Most pneumonias increase the mucus production of the pulmonary mucosa and therefore cause a productive cough. The cough may be nonproductive if there is little immune reaction to the infection or if the patient has an insufficient cough to expectorate the secretions.

5. What is the significance of the reduced D$_{LCO}$?

The reduction of D$_{LCO}$ indicates a functional decrease in the alveolar capillary surface area. A reduction in D$_{LCO}$ suggests that pulmonary disease is present, but it cannot specify which disease has caused Mr. W's pulmonary symptoms.

 More on Mr. W

PHYSICAL EXAMINATION

- **General.** A chronically thin, ill-appearing man who is in no acute distress; no respiratory distress exhibited at rest

- **Vital Signs.** Temperature 37.2°C (99.0°F), pulse 77/min, respiratory rate 21/min, blood pressure 125/76 mm Hg

- **HEENT.** Whitish plaques seen on tongue and palate; plaques firmly adhere to the mucosa and bleed when scraped. Diffuse, nontender lymphadenopathy in the neck; no jugular venous distention

- **Chest.** Normal configuration and resonance to percussion; normal expansion with respiration

- **Heart.** Regular, without murmurs or gallops

- **Lungs.** Air movement good, with harsh breath sounds over the entire chest; fine inspiratory crackles heard over both lungs diffusely, primarily in the bases

- **Abdomen.** Normal appearance; bowel sounds active, and abdomen nontender; no masses or organomegaly noted

- **Extremities.** Warm, well perfused, and without edema; pulses strong and symmetric

QUESTIONS	ANSWERS
6. Why does Mr. W have diffuse lymphadenopathy?	HIV infections cause a diffuse lymphadenopathy in most patients. This adenopathy is usually nontender and can be found in most lymph node–bearing regions. Another, less likely, possibility is that Mr. W has developed an HIV-associated lymphoma. HIV-associated lymphomas usually occur in extranodal sites[25] and can be of either the Hodgkin's or the non-Hodgkin's variety.
7. What does the distribution of inspiratory crackles over Mr. W's lungs indicate?	The distribution of crackles scattered diffusely over both lungs, primarily the bases, suggests that a diffuse process is affecting the lungs. Many pulmonary diseases associated with AIDS are diffuse. Possible diseases include lymphoid interstitial pneumonitis, idiopathic interstitial pneumonitis, and pneumonia due to *P. jaroveci*, cytomegalovirus, and many other organisms.
8. What is the most likely source of the whitish plaques on the oral mucosal surface?	The appearance of the oral mucosa is indicative of mucocutaneous candidiasis, caused by *C. albicans*. This is a frequent infection in patients who use corticosteroids (particularly inhaled) or who have depressed cellular immunity. Patients with severely depressed cellular immunity may have the Candida infection in the esophagus, trachea, bronchi, or lungs in addition to the mouth. The presence of mucocutaneous candidiasis suggests that Mr. W has a significant deficiency in cell-mediated immunity.
9. What is the most likely diagnosis for Mr. W's symptoms?	Mr. W probably has pneumonia. By far the most common cause of diffuse lung disease in AIDS patients is an infection. The most common pulmonary infection in patients with AIDS is pneumocystis pneumonia.
10. How can the suspected diagnosis be confirmed?	To confirm the diagnosis of pneumonia, a current chest radiograph should be reviewed. A stained sputum sample is useful to help establish the organism responsible for the pneumonia. If the patient cannot produce sputum, bronchoscopy can provide specimens for a definitive diagnosis.

More on Mr. W

Laboratory Evaluation

CBC

Measure	Value
WBC	3800/μL
Granulocytes	3150/μL
Monocytes	370/μL
Lymphocytes	280/μL
Hemoglobin	8.2 g/dL

Electrolytes

Measure	Value
Na^+	139 mEq/liter
K^+	4.3 mEq/liter
Cl^-	104 mEq/liter
CO_2	23 mEq/liter
Blood urea nitrogen	27 mg/dL
Creatinine	1.4 mg/dL

Arterial Blood Gases (ABGs)

Measure	Value
pH	7.45
Pa_{CO_2}	32 mm Hg
Pa_{O_2}	71 mm Hg
HCO_3^-	22 mEq/liter on room air

Chest Radiograph: See Figure 17.2
Sputum Gram Stain: Numerous squamous epithelial cells with occasional gram-positive rods, gram-positive cocci, and rare gram-negative rods; numerous yeasts and pseudohyphae seen

QUESTIONS	ANSWERS
11. How would you interpret the CBC results?	The WBC count is low, primarily because of a reduction in the number of circulating lymphocytes (lymphopenia). It is not uncommon for patients with AIDS to have a lymphopenia. Anemia is also present.
12. How would you interpret the ABG results? Are these ABGs normal for a man of this age?	The ABGs indicate a chronic respiratory alkalosis. In addition, the $P(A-a)_{O_2}$ is 39 mm Hg, which is far wider than one would predict for a 35-year-old man.

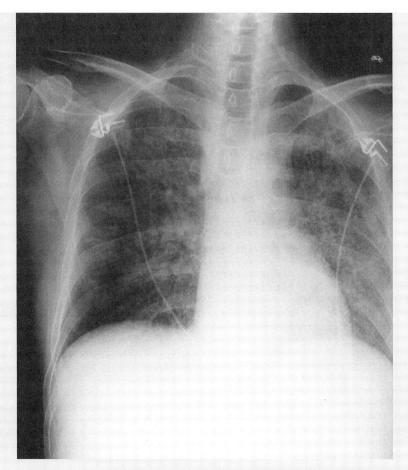

FIGURE 17.2 Chest radiograph from Mr. W.

13. How would you interpret the results of the chest radiograph?

The findings indicate a diffuse process. The possibilities for such a process include infections due to *P. jaroveci*, cytomegalovirus, or many other organisms or a form of interstitial lung disease. Tumors such as lymphoma and Kaposi's sarcoma rarely create lung disease as diffuse as Mr. W has developed.

14. What do the findings of the sputum Gram stain represent? Does the absence of *P. jaroveci* organisms on the Gram stain indicate that infection with *P. jaroveci* is unlikely?

The initial sputum Gram stain shows extensive contamination of the specimen with oral secretions. The large number of squamous epithelial cells come from the oral pharynx; thus, the sample is not representative of bronchial secretions. The bacterial organisms seen are probably from the mouth. The presence of yeast and pseudohyphae suggests that Mr. W has yeast organisms infecting or colonizing his mouth, and this correlates well with the physical examination findings. Pneumocystis organisms cannot be seen on a Gram stain, but require specialized stains.

15. Should Mr. W be admitted to the hospital, or could further evaluation and treatment be delivered to him as an outpatient?

Initial assessment and ABG data suggest that Mr. W is quite ill. Initial diagnostic studies and treatment could be done on an outpatient basis, but the rapid deterioration in his condition makes hospital admission reasonable. Once he is clearly stable, if the medication he needs can be administered at home, he can be discharged and cared for as an outpatient.

16. What are the best steps to take at this time to determine the source of Mr. W's pulmonary disease?

The diffuse lung disease that Mr. W has developed could be caused by an infection. The most common diffuse pneumonia in AIDS patients is due to *P. jaroveci*. An induced sputum specimen is likely to diagnose this and most other forms of pneumonia in AIDS patients. If, after a careful examination of an induced sputum specimen, no cause of the pulmonary disease is established, a bronchoscopy with bronchoalveolar lavage and possibly a transbronchial biopsy is often performed. If the diagnosis is still lacking after bronchoscopy, an open lung biopsy may be helpful.

17. If a repeat sputum sample is induced, what steps should be taken to ensure that the patient is properly prepared so that an optimal specimen can be obtained?

Specimens should be collected in the early morning, just after the patient has awakened. The patient should brush his teeth and oral cavity extensively and then gargle and rinse his mouth with water. Then a 3% saline solution is nebulized to induce the specimen. A high percentage of patients with AIDS-associated pneumonias can be diagnosed on the basis of such a specimen. By careful attention to proper patient preparation, the physician can avoid ordering invasive tests such as bronchoscopy.

 More on Mr. W

Mr. W is admitted to the hospital and placed in respiratory isolation. Sputum inductions are performed, and Mr. W begins treatment with trimethoprim-sulfamethoxazole. The day after admission, Mr. W experiences increasing respiratory distress. He appears diaphoretic, dusky in color, and is in moderate respiratory distress. He has inspiratory crackles scattered over his entire chest. His ABGs are pH 7.49, $Paco_2$ 27 mm Hg, Pao_2 46 mm Hg, and HCO_3^- 20 mEq/liter on room air. He is transferred to the intensive care unit (ICU), started on oxygen by a 50% entrainment mask and IV methylprednisolone. His respiratory distress improves and his ABGs on an Fio_2 of 0.50 are pH 7.39, $Paco_2$ 36 mm Hg, Pao_2 97 mm Hg, and HCO_3^- 21 mEq/liter.

QUESTIONS	ANSWERS
18. In the absence of blood or body fluid contamination of a health-care worker, Mr. W's HIV infection cannot be spread by casual contact, such as caring for a patient in the hospital. What is the value of placing this patient in respiratory isolation?	Respiratory isolation is of no benefit in protecting a health-care worker or family member from contracting an HIV infection. Many of the infections that patients with HIV disease get are opportunistic infections and cannot be spread to an immunocompetent health-care worker. The one pulmonary infection that can be spread to persons with a normal immunity is tuberculosis. If there is a question that a patient could be infected with *M. tuberculosis*, respiratory isolation should be instituted until the infection has either been partially treated or ruled out.
19. What is the purpose of administering trimethoprim-sulfamethoxazole?	The most likely pulmonary infection in an HIV-infected patient with a CD4+ lymphocyte count less than 100/μL is *P. jaroveci*. Trimethoprim and sulfamethoxazole are the drugs most often used for treatment of *P. jaroveci*. When Mr. W was first admitted, there were a number of signs that suggested that he was very ill with pneumonia. These signs included weight loss, the widened P(A-a)o_2 gradient, and the diffuse nature of the densities observed on the chest radiograph.
20. Interpret the results of both ABGs. What do the changes in Mr. W's ABG while in the ICU indicate in relation to the ABG findings on admission?	The initial ABG was measured on room air. There is an acute respiratory alkalosis with hypoxemia. The second ABG discloses a normal acid-base balance with no hypoxemia and a very wide P(A-a)o_2 gradient. These ABGs indicate that Mr. W's lung disease has progressed significantly.
21. Does the Pao_2 of 97 mm Hg on 0.50 Fio_2 indicate correction of the patient's hypoxemia? Is it an indication that the patient has stabilized or even improved?	Mr. W has a much better Pao_2 and is no longer hypoxemic on an Fio_2 of 0.50. Despite the improvement in his Pao_2, his gas exchange is much worse than it was on admission and indicates that his acute lung disease has not stabilized, but has progressed.

More on Mr. W

The sputum specimen that was induced on the first hospital day revealed organisms consistent with *P. jaroveci*. No acid-fast bacilli or fungal organisms were identified. Sputum culture had *C. albicans* and a mixture of organisms that normally colonize the upper respiratory tract. The chest radiograph taken the day Mr. W moved into the ICU showed a marked increase in the diffuse pulmonary opacification not unlike the pattern of acute respiratory distress syndrome (ARDS). Respiratory isolation was discontinued after three induced sputum specimens stained for acid-fast bacilli disclosed no tuberculosis-like organisms. After receiving a 1-week course of sulfa antibiotics, oxygen therapy, oral antifungal therapy, and antiretroviral therapy, Mr. W improved. He never required mechanical ventilation.

QUESTIONS	ANSWERS
22. What organisms are usually identified by an acid-fast stain?	Acid-fast stains are most useful in identifying Mycobacterial species such as *M. tuberculosis*. In addition, the acid-fast process will stain a few other organisms, such as Actinomyces and Nocardia.
23. The chest radiograph from the day Mr. W was admitted to the ICU indicated a diffuse pulmonary process. This process could be due to a diffuse pneumonia, ARDS, or cardiogenic pulmonary edema. How would a pulmonary artery catheter help you decide which of these problems is the most likely cause of Mr. W's pulmonary disease?	A pulmonary artery catheter provides many important hemodynamic measurements. One of these measurements is the pulmonary capillary wedge pressure (PCWP), which if elevated usually indicates left ventricular failure. Left ventricular failure is the most common cause of pulmonary edema. If a chest radiograph shows diffuse infiltrates but the PCWP is normal or low, pulmonary edema due to heart failure is unlikely; rather, ARDS or diffuse pneumonia is a more likely diagnosis (see Chapter 8).

Mr. W Conclusion

After 23 days of hospitalization, Mr. W improves enough to go home. He no longer has dyspnea on exertion. His lung examination improves, with only occasional inspiratory crackles. His chest radiograph clears. His room air ABGs are pH 7.42, $Paco_2$ 38 mm Hg, Pao_2 52 mm Hg, and HCO_3^- 24 mEq/liter. During the last days of treatment with trimethoprim-sulfamethoxazole, leukopenia develops. He is discharged home with instructions to receive a monthly treatment of aerosolized pentamidine.

QUESTIONS	ANSWERS
24. Should Mr. W receive supplemental oxygen at home?	Yes. Although he has improved markedly, he is still hypoxemic on room air.
25. What is the purpose of the aerosolized pentamidine?	Patients with AIDS frequently experience another pneumocystis pneumonia episode after their first infection. Mr. W could either receive trimethoprim-sulfamethoxazole or monthly aerosolized pentamidine. Pentamidine is the drug of choice for Mr. W because of the leukopenia he developed while receiving trimethoprim-sulfamethoxazole. ■

KEY POINTS

- Infections caused by organisms that do not usually affect people with a healthy immune system are called **opportunistic infections**.
- Defects in the immune system can be mild, causing only a slight increase in the frequency of infections, or severe, causing life-threatening infections. The source of the defect can be congenital (primary) or acquired (secondary).
- The immune system is a complex group of defense mechanisms designed to eliminate foreign organisms. Immunity has three principal characteristics that govern its behavior: ability to differentiate self from nonself, specificity, and memory.
- The immune system is made up of many different types of cells. Lymphocytes and monocytes comprise the majority of the immune cells.
- B lymphocytes can develop into antibody-secreting cells called plasma cells. Antibodies, also called immunoglobulins (Ig), are molecules that identify and bind to specific foreign antigens to assist the immune system in recognizing and destroying foreign invaders.
- Monocytes circulate in the blood and may migrate into tissue to become macrophages. Macrophages engulf foreign material and degrade it (phagocytosis).
- Neutrophils are the most common granulocytes. They are responsible for detecting invading microorganisms, phagocytosing them, killing them, and degrading their remains.
- When a portion of a patient's immune system is not functioning properly, the patient is prone to infection. Infections are frequently caused by organisms that are normally best controlled by the portion of the immune system that is damaged.
- A complete or partial absence of antibodies leads to repeated infections with bacteria such as *S. pneumoniae* or *Haemophilus influenzae* and other encapsulated bacteria. The respiratory tract is the usual target for these infections, but meningitis or septicemia can also develop.
- Cell-mediated immunity is the portion of the immune system provided by T lymphocytes. A good example of this immunity is the body's defense against intracellular pathogens, such as *M. tuberculosis*.
- AIDS is by far the most common acquired defect of cell-mediated immunity.
- Opportunistic pneumonia should be considered in any patient with recurrent bouts of pneumonia or a case of pneumonia that does not resolve with treatment.
- The physical examination of an immunocompromised patient with pneumonia will often reveal features of both the acute pulmonary infection and the immunosuppression. Localized crackles usually indicate localized pneumonia, whereas diffuse crackles indicate widespread infection. In an immunocompetent patient, an opportunistic pneumonia is more likely to be widespread.
- An abnormally low number of lymphocytes, particularly CD4+ cells, indicates a defect in cell-mediated immunity (e.g., AIDS).
- The chest radiograph of an immunocompromised patient with pneumocystis pneumonia usually reveals a diffusely increased density that often includes multiple portions of the lung.
- Culture and microscopic examination of the sputum are the least invasive and most readily available techniques for identifying infectious agents. Initially, a Gram stain and acid-fast stain are used to stain the sputum.

KEY POINTS (CONTINUED)

- HIV preferentially infects cells that have the CD4+ antigen. As the infection progresses, the helper T lymphocytes that express the CD4+ antigen are destroyed. The immune system becomes compromised when the number of helper T cells decreases from a normal concentration of 800 to 1200/μL to less than 600/μL.
- A patient's particular type of immune defect helps predict which organisms are most likely to be responsible for the infection. Empiric therapy is selected on this basis.
- A patient with neutropenia is usually treated with antibiotics against pyogenic bacteria such as *Pseudomonas aeruginosa* and/or fungi such as Aspergillus organisms.
- Patients with AIDS are usually empirically treated with a combination of trimethoprim and sulfamethoxazole because they are likely to have pneumonia due to *P. jaroveci.*
- Empiric therapy is replaced by treatment directed at the specific organism if diagnostic testing discloses which organism has caused the pneumonia.
- Pneumonia due to *P. jaroveci* is treated with a combination of sulfa antibiotics. Patients who cannot tolerate sulfa antibiotics may be given pentamidine intravenously or by aerosol.
- Patients with immunodeficiencies such as AIDS are at risk for several forms of opportunistic pneumonia. As a preventive measure, it is often wise to institute prophylactic antibiotic therapy.

REFERENCES

1. Notarangelo, L, Casanova, J, Fischer, A, et al: Primary immunodeficiency diseases: an update. *J Allergy Clin Immunol* 114:677, 2004.
2. Chapel, H, Geha, R, Rosen, F: Primary immunodeficiency diseases: an update. Clin Exp Immunol 132:9, 2003.
3. Suster, B, et al: Pulmonary manifestations in AIDS: review of 106 episodes. Radiology 161:87–93, 1986.
4. Mitchell, DM, et al: Pulmonary function in human immunodeficiency virus infection: a prospective 18 month study of serial lung function in 474 patients. Am Rev Respir Dis 146:745–751, 1992.
5. Vanarthos, WJ, et al: Diagnostic uses of nuclear medicine in AIDS. Radiographics 12:731–749, 1992.
6. Chaisson, R, et al: Tuberculosis in patients with AIDS: a population based study. Am Rev Respir Dis 136:570–574, 1987.
7. Small, PM, et al: Treatment of tuberculosis in patients with advanced human immunodeficiency virus infection. N Engl J Med 324:289–294, 1991.
8. Ng, VL, et al: The use of mucolysed induced sputum for the identification of pulmonary pathogens associated with human immunodeficiency virus infection. Arch Pathol Lab Med 113:488–493, 1989.
9. Wazir, JF, et al: EB9, a new antibody for the detection of trophozoites of Pneumocystis carinii in bronchoalveolar lavage specimens in AIDS. J Clin Pathol 47:1108–1111, 1994.
10. Murry, T, et al: Is transbronchial biopsy necessary for diagnosis of pulmonary infections with AIDS? Am Rev Respir Dis 133:A182, 1986.
11. Golden, JA, et al: Bronchoalveolar lavage as the exclusive diagnostic modality for Pneumocystis carinii pneumonia. Chest 90:18–22, 1986.
12. Milligan, SA, et al: Transbronchial biopsy without fluoroscopy in patients with diffuse roentgenographic infiltrates and the acquired immunodeficiency syndrome. Am Rev Respir Dis 137:486–488, 1988.
13. Fitzgerald, W, et al: The role of open-lung biopsy in patients with the acquired immunodeficiency syndrome. Chest 91:659–661, 1987.
14. Wallace, JM, et al: Respiratory illness in persons with human immunodeficiency virus infection. Am Rev Respir Dis 148:1523–1529, 1993.
15. Northfelt, DW: In Cohen, PT, et al (eds): *The AIDS Knowledge Base.* Little, Brown & Co, Boston, 1994.
16. Kaplan, LD, et al: AIDS associated non-Hodgkin's lymphoma in San Francisco. JAMA 261:719–724, 1981.
17. Hawley, PH, et al: Decreasing frequency but worsening mortality of acute respiratory failure secondary to AIDS-related Pneumocystis carinii pneumonia. Chest 106:1456–1459, 1994.

18. De Palo, VA, et al: Outcome of intensive care in patients with HIV infection. Chest 107:506–510, 1995.

19. Lane, HC, et al: NIH conference: Recent advances in the management of AIDS-related opportunistic infections. Ann Intern Med 120:945–955, 1994.

20. Bozzette, SA, et al: A controlled trial of early adjunctive treatment with corticosteroids for Pneumocystis carinii pneumonia in the acquired immunodeficiency syndrome: California Cooperative Treatment Group. N Engl J Med 323:1451–1457, 1990.

21. McLaughlin, GE, et al: Effect of corticosteroids on survival of children with acquired immunodeficiency syndrome and Pneumocystis carinii–related respiratory failure. J Pediatr 126:821–824, 1995.

22. Denning, D, et al: Treatment of invasive aspergillosis with itraconazole. Am J Med 86:791–800, 1989.

23. Centers for Disease Control, Advisory Committee for the Elimination of Tuberculosis: Recommendation for the elimination of tuberculosis. MMWR 38: 236–250, 1989.

24. Simonds, RJ, et al: Prophylaxis against Pneumocystis carinii pneumonia among children with perinatally acquired human immunodeficiency virus infection in the United States. Pneumocystis carinii Pneumonia Prophylaxis Evaluation Working Group. N Engl J Med 332:786–790, 1995.

25. Knowles, DM, et al: Lymphoid neoplasia associated with the acquired immunodeficiency syndrome (AIDS): The New York University Center experience with 105 patients (1981–1986). Ann Intern Med 108:744–753, 1988.

26. Treating opportunistic infections among HIV-infected adults and adolescents. MMWR 53:1–112, 2004.

27. Guidelines for preventing opportunistic infections among HIV-infected persons. MMWR 16:1371, 2002.

18

Sleep Disordered Breathing

Enrique Gil, MD, FCCP

CHAPTER OBJECTIVES:

After reading this chapter, you will be able to identify the:

- Incidence of sleep apnea/hypopnea syndrome in adults.
- Personal and medical problems associated with sleep disordered breathing (SDB).
- Key definitions associated with SDB.
- Normal stages of sleep and the changes in breathing seen with each stage.
- Physiologic effects of sleep apnea on daytime function and the cardiovascular system.
- Common clinical features seen in patients with SDB.
- Role of the polysomnogram in diagnosing the patient with SDB.
- Use of CPAP, surgery, and dental appliances in the treatment of obstructive sleep apnea.

INTRODUCTION

Sleep disordered breathing (SDB) is a condition characterized by partial or complete cessation of breathing during sleep. Breathing during sleep may decrease or stop either because of partial or complete airway obstruction (sleep apnea/hypopnea) or because of inadequate respiratory effort (central sleep apnea).

The vast majority of people with SDB have sleep apnea/hypopnea rather than central sleep apnea. Obstructive sleep apnea (OSA)/hypopnea syndrome causes sleepiness in approximately 4% of men and 2% of women between the ages of 30 and 60.[1] It is even more common in people over age 60. The problems caused by OSA/hypopnea syndrome fall into three main categories:

- Loud snoring, which can be a source of social embarrassment and marital distress.
- Excessive daytime sleepiness, which may interfere with job or school performance and even activities of daily living (such as eating). Motor vehicle crashes resulting from drowsiness are much more likely in individuals with sleep apnea.[2,3]
- Cardiovascular diseases, stroke, hypertension, and diabetes, which are all exacerbated by OSA/hypopnea syndrome.

Cardiovascular disease accounted for 38% of deaths in the United Sates in 2002.[4] There is increasing epidemiological evidence of a link between sleep apnea and cardiovascular diseases, including coronary artery disease,[5,6] congestive heart failure,[6,7] cor pulmonale, cardiac arrhythmias (including lone atrial fibrillation[8]), and pulmonary hypertension. Patients with

Box 18.1 Definitions Associated with Sleep Disordered Breathing

Apnea: Absence of air flow or breathing lasting at least 10 seconds during sleep
Apnea Index (AI): Number of apneas per hour
Apnea/Hypopnea Index (AHI): Number of apneas plus hypopneas per hour; 5 to 20 = mild, 21 to 40 = moderate, >41 = severe
Central Apnea: Cessation of airflow without breathing effort
Home Sleep Study: A sleep test performed at home variations include:

* Full portable polysomnogram with (attended) or without (unattended) a technician
* Cardiorespiratory sleep study: less comprehensive than a polysomnogram (no sleep stage monitoring)
* Dual- or single-channel monitoring device (i.e., sleep oximetry)

Hypopnea: Transient reduction in airflow during sleep
Maintenance of Wakefulness Test (MWT): Series of five tests lasting 5 minutes each, performed 2 hours apart to assess the ability to remain awake in a darkened room in a semi-reclined position
Mixed Apnea: Combination of both obstructive and central apnea
Multiple Sleep Latency Test (MSLT): Series of five naps lasting 20 minutes each, performed 2 hours apart the day after a polysomnogram to assess for sleepiness. Test is considered normal if sleep onset is more than 10 minutes; 5 to 10 minutes is consistent with pathological sleepiness; less than 5 minutes consistent with severe daytime sleepiness. Helpful for diagnosis of narcolepsy if REM sleep is observed in at least two of the naps
Obstructive Apnea: Cessation of airflow with continuing respiratory effort against a closed airway during sleep
Obstructive Hypoventilation: Reduction in airflow associated with hypoxemia without arousals
Polysomnogram (PSG): Continuous and simultaneous recording of physiological variables during sleep, i.e., electroencephalogram (EEG), electro-oculogram (EOG), electromyogram (EMG) (the three basic stage scoring parameters), EKG, respiratory air flow, respiratory excursion or effort, lower limb movement, chin tone, and other electrophysiological variables. Polysomnogram is the gold standard for diagnosis of sleep disordered breathing.
Respiratory Arousal Index (RAI) or Respiratory Disturbance Index (RDI): The sum of the apnea, hypopnea, and respiratory effort–related arousals per hour
Respiratory Effort–Related Arousal (RERA): Subtle reduction in airflow with subtle increase in respiratory effort leading to an arousal, usually without significant oxygen desaturations
Sleep Apnea Hypopnea Syndrome (SAHS) or Obstructive Sleep Apnea Syndrome (OSAS): Repetitive episodes of airway obstruction causing arousals and oxygen desaturations, usually leading to excessive daytime sleepiness
Sleep Disordered Breathing (SDB): Spectrum of breathing disorders related to sleep, including OSAS, **upper airway resistance syndrome,** and central apnea
Split All Night Study: A polysomnogram split in two parts; the first half used to establish a diagnosis, the second half to titrate CPAP
Upper Airway Resistance Syndrome (UARS): A mild variant of OSAS. Subtle reduction in airflow leading to arousals causing daytime sleepiness. These events can be detected by using an esophageal probe or by using a pressure transducer.

congestive heart failure and Cheyne-Stokes breathing have a worse prognosis than patients with congestive heart failure without Cheyne-Stokes breathing. Treatment of Cheyne-Stokes improves prognosis for patients with congestive heart failure.[9]

Stroke accounted for 1 of every 15 deaths in this country in 2002.[10] Up to 50% of stroke patients have SDB, and sleep apnea increases the likelihood of cerebrovascular accidents.[11–13]

Hypertension: affects nearly 1 in 3 adults. Approximately 33% of hypertensive patients also have sleep apnea.[14-16]

Diabetes mellitus was the sixth leading cause of death and had an estimated prevalence of 6.2% in 2002.[17,18] Sleep apnea may worsen diabetes by exacerbating insulin resistance whether or not the patient is obese.[19,20]

People with OSA/hypopnea syndrome have a higher mortality than age-matched peers, and their death rate decreases with treatment of the syndrome.[21,22]

Central sleep apnea is most often the result of other medical conditions rather than a primary medical problem. Common medical conditions resulting in central sleep apnea include congestive heart failure, extreme obesity, and neurologic injuries.

> The impact of SDB on general health is now believed to be potentially very harmful and may shorten the life-span significantly if not diagnosed promptly.

Many mechanisms appear to play a role in the development of cardiovascular disease in patients with sleep apnea. These include:

- Causing a hypercoagulable state[23]
- Causing hypoxia and hypoxia/reperfusion damage[24]
- Releasing inflammatory substances[25,26]
- Increasing sympathetic activity[27]

Box 18.1 provides definitions of terms related to SDB.

SLEEP AND BREATHING[28]

Sleep is divided into two states: rapid eye movement (REM) sleep and non–rapid eye movement (NREM) sleep. NREM sleep is further divided into four stages. Normal sleep begins with stage 1, which is characterized by relatively low-voltage, mixed-frequency activity, with slow eye movements usually preceding sleep onset (Figure 18.1). K complexes and sleep spindles with a similar background to that of stage 1 are characteristic of stage 2 (Figure 18.2). Stages 3 and 4 (slow-wave sleep) are characterized by the presence of high-voltage slow waves in 20% to 50% of the epoch in stage 3 and in more then 50% in stage 4 (Figures 18.3 and 18.4). REM sleep is characterized by rapid eye movements and absence of electromyographic activity (Figure 18.5). The normal adult sleeper alternates between NREM sleep and REM sleep approximately every 90 minutes throughout the night.

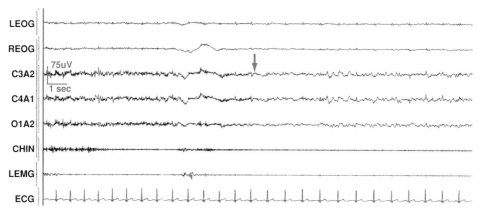

FIGURE 18.1 Polysomnogram demonstrating progression from wake to stage 1 sleep. Note the low-voltage activity seen in the EEG leads (C3A2 & C4A1) characteristic of stage 1 sleep (arrow).

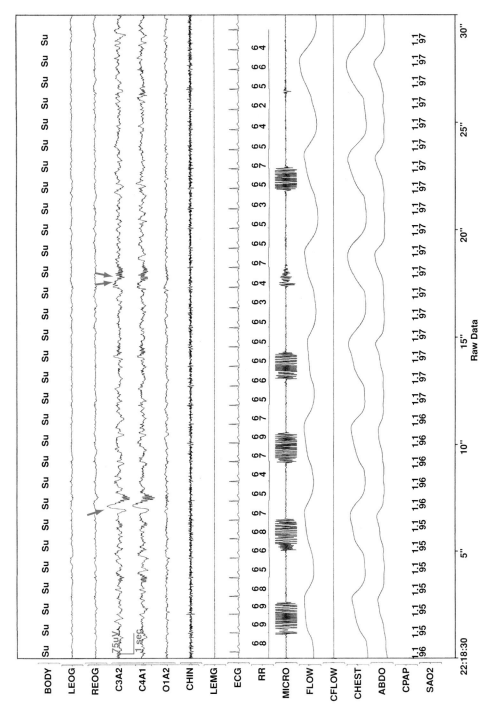

FIGURE 18.2 Polysomnogram demonstrating stage 2 sleep. Note the K complexes (single arrow) and sleep spindles (double arrow) in the EEG leads consistent with stage 2 sleep.

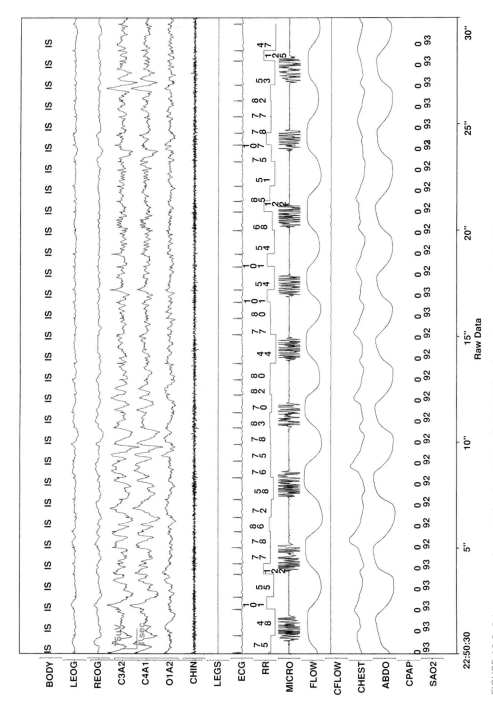

FIGURE 18.3 Polysomnogram demonstrating stage 3 sleep. Note the high-voltage slow waves seen in the EEG leads (C3A2, C4A1, O1A2).

409

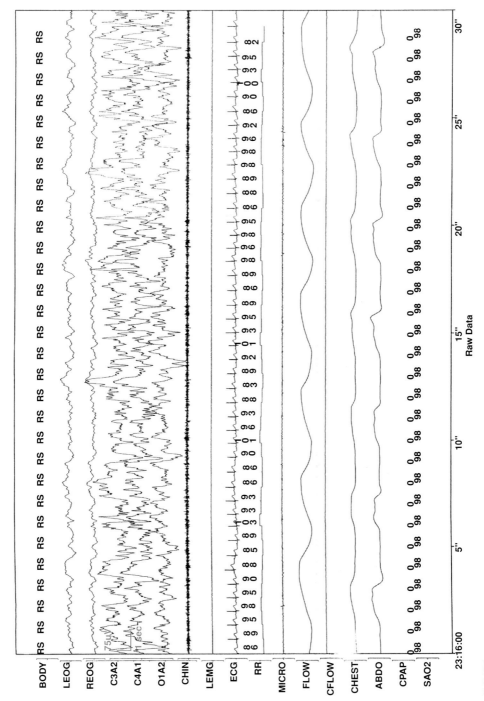

FIGURE 18.4 Polysomnogram demonstrating stage 4 sleep. Note the high-voltage slow waves seen in the EEG leads (C3A2, C4A1, O1A2).

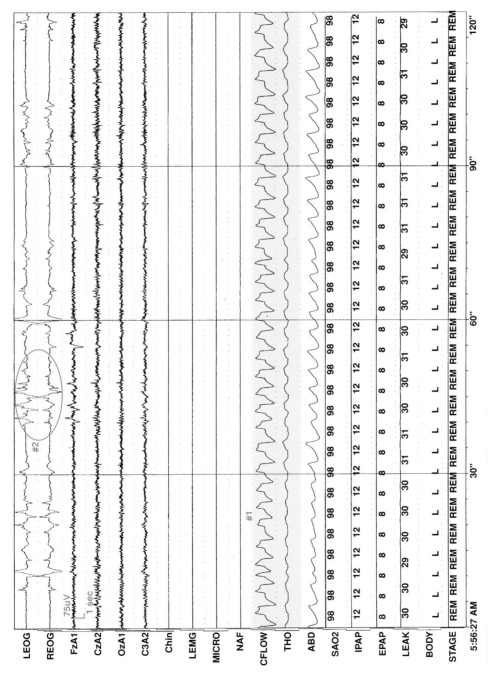

FIGURE 18.5 Polysomnogram demonstrating REM sleep. Note the large eye movements detected in the left and right eye oculogram tracings (LEOG and REOG) and the absence of EMG activity in the chin lead.

411

> Because breathing and gas exchange is normally less during sleep, patients with hypoxemia and hypercarbia while awake are at greater risk for severe hypoxemia and respiratory acidosis during sleep.

REM and NREM sleep states both cause changes in breathing, even in healthy individuals. Typically, during the lighter stages of NREM sleep (stages 1 and 2) the breathing pattern is irregular because of the decrease in respiratory drive associated with the stimulatory effect of wakefulness and the decreased metabolic rate associated with sleep. In the deeper stages of NREM sleep breathing is typically very regular; however, overall ventilation is reduced compared to that during wakefulness. During REM sleep the respiratory drive is irregular because of the transient decrease in ventilatory response to chemical and mechanical stimuli. The influence of sleep on the upper airway is similar to its effects on other skeletal muscles, resulting in a general loss of muscle tone and a reduction in tidal volume and minute ventilation.

PATHOPHYSIOLOGY

Obesity, by narrowing the airway, is the most common cause of OSA. Structural abnormalities such as micrognathia (small mandible), macroglossia (enlarged tongue), or enlarged tonsils or adenoids can be contributing factors. OSA may be present in nonobese patients as a result of inherited or acquired anatomic narrowing of the upper airway. In the patient with OSA whose airway is already compromised, the normal relaxation of the oropharyngeal muscles that occurs during sleep allows the airway to collapse even if the respiratory effort is normal or increased. The resultant hypoxemia and hypercapnia leads to a partial arousal that increases muscle tone and terminates the obstruction. Repeated arousals lead to sleep fragmentation that results in excessive daytime sleepiness.

Repeated episodes of hypoxemia during sleep result in adverse changes in people's hemodynamic system. Vagally mediated bradycardia may occur with the onset of hypoxemia. Tachycardia follows once breathing resumes. Systemic and pulmonary arterial blood pressures tend to rise during apneic episodes. The magnitude of the hypertension appears to be related to the degree of oxyhemoglobin desaturation. Vascular pressures usually return to baseline once ventilation resumes; however, sustained pulmonary hypertension and cor pulmonale may develop in patients with prolonged or severe OSA. The incidence of systemic hypertension is higher in OSA patients than in the general population, especially in young, morbidly obese OSA patients.

Most patients with central sleep apnea have an increased respiratory drive and hypocapnea. During sleep with hyperventilation, the low CO_2 periodically inhibits the respiratory drive, resulting in apneic events. This presentation is seen in patients with congestive heart failure who have Cheyne-Stokes breathing and in normal people at high altitude when hypoxemia leads to hyperventilation.

Some patients with central sleep apnea have a decreased respiratory drive and therefore may have CO_2 retention and hypoventilation. An example of this is very obese people whose chest walls are so heavy that they eventually accept hypoventilation and hypercapnea in exchange for expending less energy to breathe (obesity hypoventilation syndrome).

CLINICAL FEATURES

History

The main clinical features of SDB are loud snoring and excessive daytime sleepiness.[29] Loud snoring is caused by a relaxed and floppy airway. Excessive daytime sleepiness is caused by sleep fragmentation stemming from the frequent arousals necessary to relieve the obstructive events caused by an extremely relaxed and floppy airway. Reports of apneic or choking episodes and flailing arms or legs while the apneic patient attempts to regain consciousness are also common.

The assessment of abnormal breathing during sleep is usually made by the bed partner, family members, or friends who become concerned about the apneic events or cannot tolerate the patient's thunderous snoring. Occasionally the patient's problem is first recognized after a motor vehicle crash caused by drowsiness or after poor job or school performance is found to be associated with drowsiness.

Other problems associated with OSA include poor memory, depression, impotence, fatigue, morning headaches, dry mouth, sore throat upon waking, waking up in the mornings without feeling refreshed, and self-medicating with caffeine to wake up in the morning and stay awake during the day.

Physical Assessment

The typical patient with OSA is a middle-aged obese man, although age, obesity, and the male gender are not prerequisites for developing the disease. A neck circumference of 40 cm or more in the presence of snoring and hypertension suggests the diagnosis.[30,31] Nonobese patients may have anatomical defects of the upper airway that cause the disease, including micrognathia, nasal obstruction, tonsilar hypertrophy, elongated soft palate, a large uvula, or a large tongue. Unless obesity hypoventilation syndrome is present (in which case the arterial blood gas will reveal hypoxemia and hypercapnia), the daytime arterial blood gas (ABG) will usually be normal.

Patients with the following problems should be evaluated for OSA even if they deny excessive sleepiness or other symptoms associated with it:

- Poorly controlled hypertension in spite of multiple medications
- Polycythemia (from nocturnal hypoxemia)
- Pulmonary hypertension
- Congestive heart failure

EVALUATION FOR SLEEP APNEA

Sleepiness Scale

Sleepiness is very subjective and patients may adapt to sleep deprivation and even deny being drowsy. The Epworth sleepiness scale, although not very specific, is widely used to objectively evaluate for daytime sleepiness. A score above 10 suggests excessive daytime sleepiness (Table 18.1).

Sleep Studies

The definitive test for sleep apnea is the polysomnogram.[32] Performed in a sleep laboratory, this all-night recording of the patient's sleep is the gold standard for identifying the presence, type, and severity of sleep apnea. Using a multichannel recorder (polysomnograph), eye movements, airflow, respiratory movements, leg movements, electroencephalographic (EEG) readings, pulse oxymetry, electrocardiography (ECG) readings, and snoring are recorded. Home multichannel devices that record a limited number of parameters (e.g., respiratory movements, airflow, snoring, pulse oxymetry, ECG) are

Table 18.1 The Epworth Sleepiness Scale

Use this scale to choose the most appropriate number for each situation:
0 = would never doze
1 = slight chance of dozing
2 = moderate chance of dozing
3 = high chance of dozing
It is important that you circle a number (0 to 3) on each of the questions.

Situation	Chance of Dozing			
Sitting and reading	0	1	2	3
Watching television	0	1	2	3
Sitting inactive in a public place, for example, a theater or meeting	0	1	2	3
As a passenger in a car for an hour without a break	0	1	2	3
Lying down to rest in the afternoon	0	1	2	3
Sitting and talking to someone	0	1	2	3
Sitting quietly after lunch (when you've had no alcohol)	0	1	2	3
In a car while stopped in traffic	0	1	2	3
Total Score:				

available and may prove valuable in certain conditions, but the polysomnogram remains the gold standard.

The following findings are observed in the polysomnogram when OSA/hypopnea syndrome is present: frequent and repetitive apnea and hypopneas (Figures 18.6 and 18.7). The effort channels (usually chest and abdomen sensors) demonstrate increasing effort against an obstructed airway causing reduction or cessation or airflow (measured by a thermistor or a pressure transducer). The pulse oximeter shows oxygen desaturation leading to EEG evidence of arousals, documented by a transition from sleep to brief wake episodes, documented in the EEG channels. If the events are subtle, no desaturations or evidence of increased breathing effort are seen. The presence of crescendo snoring leading to an arousal suggests respiratory effort–related arousals. A pressure transducer or an esophageal balloon may help detect those subtle events not seen if a thermistor is used to detect air flow. **Upper airway resistance syndrome** can then be diagnosed.[33,34]

When central apneas are present, the airflow sensor shows absence of flow, and the effort channels show no effort to breathe (Figure 18.8). Cheyne-Stokes breathing (or periodic breathing) is characterized by a crescendo-decrescendo pattern in breathing effort and airflow without obstruction, but with clear apneas present between them.

> The best way to diagnose OSA is by use of the polysomnogram. The polysomnogram not only makes the diagnosis but also defines the severity and allows assessment of the proposed treatment.

If the polysomnogram is negative for sleep-related diseases, a multiple sleep latency test (MSLT) should be performed to objectively assess daytime sleepiness and to evaluate for narcolepsy or idiopathic hypersomnia.[35] Healthy subjects have a sleep latency of 10 to 20 minutes in the MSLT. The test is consistent with severe daytime sleepiness if sleep onset occurs within 5 minutes. The presence of REM sleep in two out of five naps is diagnostic of narcolepsy in the appropriate clinical setting.

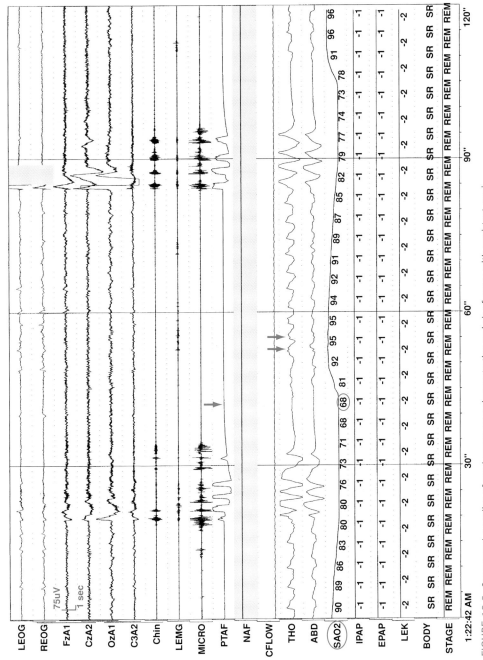

FIGURE 18.6 Compressed recording of a polysomnogram demonstrating periods of apnea with persistent respiratory effort of breathing typical for OSA. Note the periodic lack of air flow (arrow) lasting close to 60 seconds in spite of breathing efforts, as seen by movement in the chest and abdomen leads (double arrows). EEG shows arousals terminating the obstruction. Note the severe desaturations (seen in the Sao_2 lead) associated with the obstructive events.

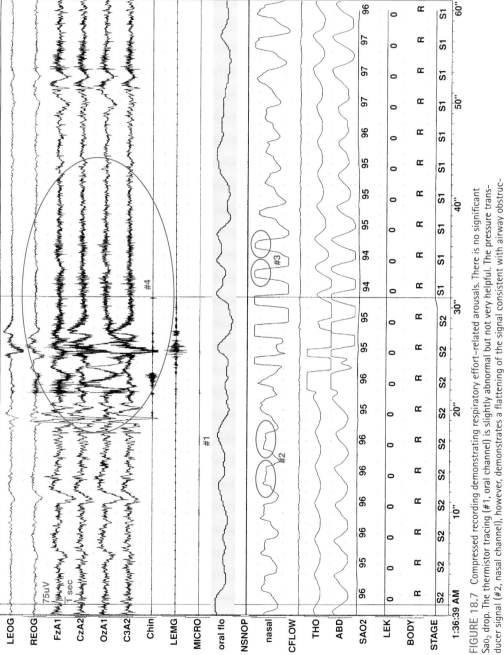

FIGURE 18.7 Compressed recording demonstrating respiratory effort–related arousals. There is no significant Sao$_2$ drop. The thermistor tracing (#1, oral channel) is slightly abnormal but not very helpful. The pressure transducer signal (#2, nasal channel), however, demonstrates a flattening of the signal consistent with airway obstruction, which disappears (#3, nasal channel) when flow is restored after an arousal (#4), seen clearly in the EEG channels. If a thermistor alone had been used, this event would have been scored as nonspecific, and a respiratory effort–related arousals would have been missed.

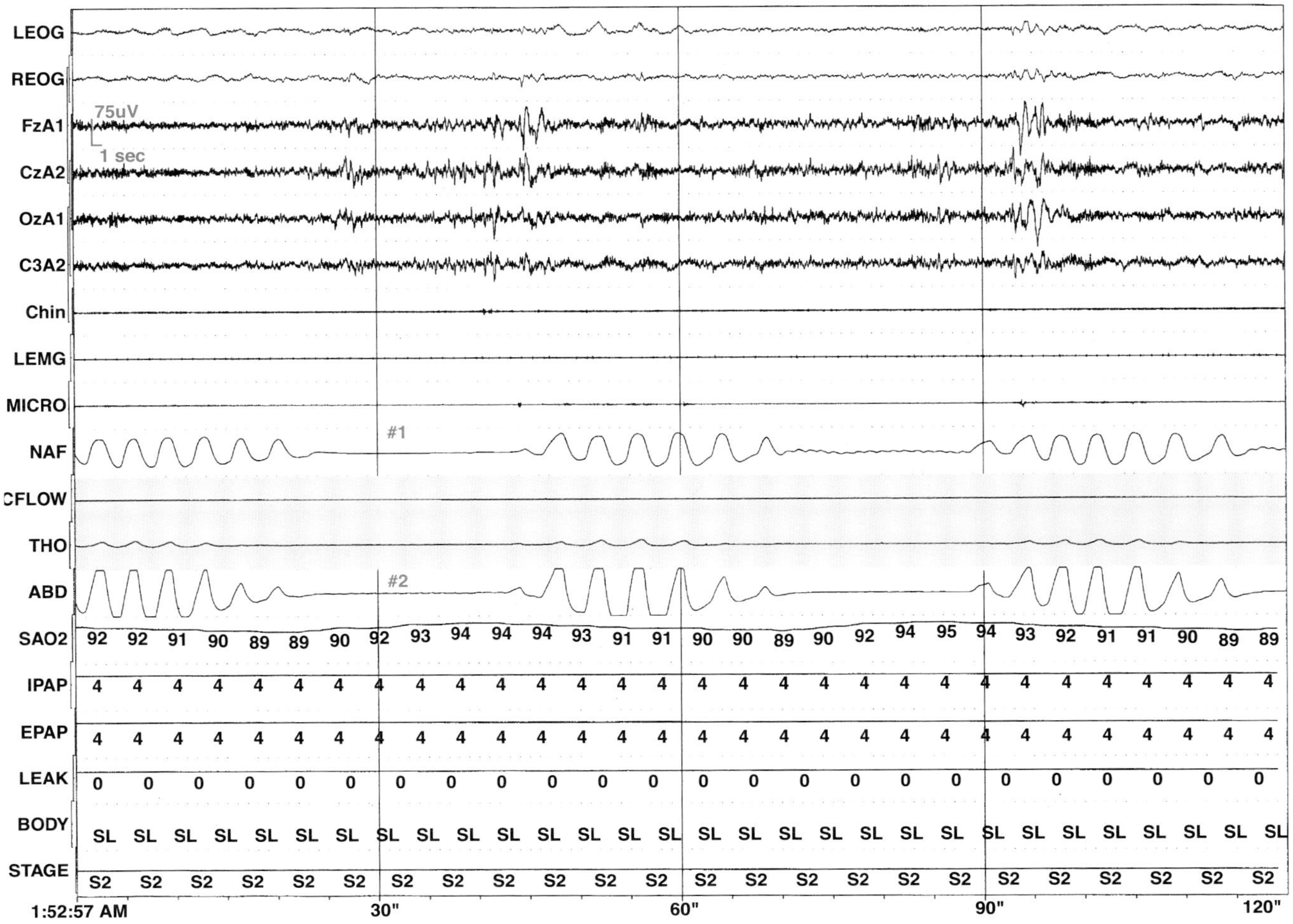

FIGURE 18.8 Compressed recording demonstrating central apneas. There is cessation of airflow (#1 NAF channel) in the absence of any respiratory effort (#2 THO and ABD channels). Note the crescendo–decrescendo pattern of the event.

417

TREATMENT

Obstructive Sleep Apnea

For many patients with mild OSA, a combination of weight loss, relief of nasal congestion, and avoidance of alcohol and sedatives is sufficient. Some patients have a strong positional component, with respiratory events present mainly while sleeping in the supine position. Sleeping on the other side could be very effective. Other patients have episodes of OSA only during REM sleep. These patients may improve with medication that decreases REM sleep.

More aggressive treatment is indicated if the respiratory disturbance index is higher than 20 or if the patient has excessive daytime sleepiness. It is important to remember, however, that patients with upper airway resistance syndrome may have a nondiagnostic polysomnogram, especially if a thermistor was used to measure air flow. Many sleep laboratories do not routinely use a pressure transducer, and an esophageal balloon is used only at a few laboratories. Therefore, a normal polysomnogram does not completely rule out OSA.

Patients with OSA have a higher risk of automobile crashes, and an important part of their treatment is to educate them regarding the risk of driving when drowsy. Weight loss is the most important treatment for obese patients with OSA. Unfortunately, available appetite suppressants are not very helpful. The phentermine and fenfluramine combination used to promote weight loss during the 1990s is no longer used because of the concern about pulmonary hypertension.

Three major treatments available for the treatment of OSA/hypopnea syndrome include continuous positive airway pressure (CPAP), dental appliances, and surgery (Table 18.2).

Table 18.2 Treatment Choices for Obstructive Sleep Apnea

Treatment	Pros	Cons
CPAP	• Highly effective regardless of severity • Noninvasive	Cumbersome; compliance problems Not everyone can tolerate it
Dental appliances	• Effective for mild to moderate apnea • May be a good choice for UARS • May be used in combination therapy, such as surgery. • When it works, patients prefer it to CPAP	• Not effective for severe cases • Expensive; not always covered by insurances • Long term compliance 50% at 5 years • Cannot be used in the presence of poor dentition, bruxism, or TemporoMandibular Joint (TMJ) pain
Surgery	• Effective in selected cases, especially when anatomical narrowing is significant	• Invasive • Potential postoperative complications
Bariatric Surgery	• Effective in morbid obesity	• Invasive • Potential postoperative complications

CPAP

The treatment of choice for moderate to severe OSA is nasal CPAP. Positive pressure works as a "pneumatic splint," preventing upper airway collapse and obstruction. The level of pressure needed to prevent obstruction (apnea and snoring) varies from patient to patient and must be determined by a sleep laboratory polysomnogram CPAP titration study. In certain cases an in-home automatic CPAP titrating device may be useful, particularly if the patient cannot sleep in the sleep laboratory, if pressure needs minor adjustment, or if compliance needs to be objectively measured. Using a variety of methods to detect airway obstruction and snoring, auto-CPAP units adjust pressure according to the degree of airway obstruction, which may change during the night and may be dependent of body position and sleep stage. These devices may also allow home CPAP titration in patients diagnosed by unattended multiple channel home studies. Anyone who could experience potential difficulties with CPAP use (poor coordination, mouth breathing, and severe nasal obstruction) would not be a good candidate for CPAP using one of these devices.

Several mask interfaces are available, including nasal masks, nasal pillows, full face masks, and at least one oral mask. All are effective, and their use depends on the patient's comfort and preference.

Standard CPAP units have a "ramp time" allowing for a slow increase in pressure until the prescribed level is reached in order to allow the patient to fall asleep before the maximum pressure is reached and thus minimize patient discomfort.

More sophisticated units record the actual time of CPAP use. This feature allows for a better measure of compliance, since it may not be possible to accurately assess compliance based exclusively on patients' self-reports.[36,37] In addition, patients' perceived benefit on their symptoms and discomfort from CPAP use impacted their long term compliance.[38-40] If compliance is poor, every effort should be made to address the problems and side effects of CPAP use. Poor mask fitting, excessively high pressures prescribed erroneously based on polysomnogram reports, dry air causing mucosal irritation, and social embarrassment are some of the issues that need to be addressed. If these issues cannot be corrected, alternative treatments should be considered.

Suboptimal patient compliance with CPAP remains a problem and an indication of our lack of a better treatment modality. Reported rates vary between 68% and 80%. Reported side effects include nocturnal awakenings and nasal dryness, congestion and discharge, and sneezing.[41] Nasal congestion may be corrected with the addition of a humidifier used in line with CPAP, although not all patients find it helpful. A heated humidifier is more effective than a nonheated or pass-through unit. Other simple measures that may be useful include the use of normal saline nasal spray and nasal corticosteroids.

Additional CPAP side effects include air leakage, causing ocular dryness and irritation; bruising of the bridge of the nose or gums; and facial irritation. Reported contraindications to the use of CPAP include pneumothorax,[42] hypotension with hypovolemia, uncontrolled emesis, unstable facial fractures, massive epistaxis, acute severe sinusitis, and nasal cerebrospinal fluid leak. Surprisingly, not much information regarding CPAP complications has been published, probably because CPAP is safe in the vast majority of patients.

Automatic CPAP titration devices adjust pressure throughout the night according to the degree of airway obstruction and pressure needed to relieve it. They may be helpful in patients who have difficulty tolerating CPAP.[43]

Of paramount importance in the treatment of OSA is patient education regarding the disorder and the associated health risks if it is left untreated. Regular follow-up by a

> CPAP can be very effective in treating OSA but often is not tolerated by the patient on the initial trial. Clinicians who apply the CPAP must coach the patient to be patient and stick with it.

knowledgeable practitioner is invaluable. We routinely ask our patients to bring their own equipment and visually evaluate mask/CPAP fit to ensure proper use at office visits. CPAP pressure is measured with a manometer. The need for new filters, hoses, or masks is evaluated. Careful patient follow-up also allows assessment of compliance and side effects or difficulties with its use.

Dental Appliances[44–47]

These devices relieve obstruction by repositioning of the tongue or advancement of the mandible. The devices are most effective in patients with mild to moderate sleep apnea. A dentist knowledgeable in sleep disorders is an invaluable addition to the sleep disorders team.

Surgery[48–51]

Surgical approaches for the treatment of OSA bypass the site of obstruction or increase the size of the airway. Tracheotomy is very effective but not frequently used, and it is reserved for patients with severe, life-threatening disease when other treatments have failed. In pediatric patients, removal of enlarged tonsils and adenoids removes the obstruction and is frequently effective.

Procedures targeted to the anatomical narrowing include nasal procedures if nasal obstruction is present, tonsillectomy if significant hypertrophy, glossectomy if a large tongue causes obstruction, and genioglossal advancement for hypo pharyngeal obstruction.

Uvulopalatopharyngoplasty (UPPP) has a reported success rate of approximately 50%.[52] UPPP may be useful in selected patients who fail to respond to nasal CPAP but may also interfere with CPAP use by increasing mouth leak due to velopharyngeal incompetence. Laser UPPP may be useful for snoring but not for clinically significant or severe sleep apnea.[53]

The Powell Riley protocol is a systematic approach to increasing the size of the airway and treating obstructions. It is usually performed in two phases.

Phase I

• For nasal obstruction: nasal surgery (septoplasty, turbinectomy)
• For pharyngeal obstruction: UPPP and tonsillectomy if needed.
• For hypopharyngeal obstruction: genioglossus advancement-hyoid myotomy and suspension (GAHMS)
• A follow-up polysomnogram is usually performed 6 months after surgery.

Phase II (only for persistent significant OSA)

• Maxillary and mandibular advancement (MMA)
• Alternative: Tongue reduction

Manufacturers promote newer procedures including the pillar palatal procedure for mild to moderate sleep apnea. This procedure involves the placement of three polyester inserts in the soft palate. The manufacturer's website mentions a 46-patient European trial in which 90 days after surgery, 64% of patients had an apnea/hypopnea index (AHI) below 10, but there is no mention of respiratory effort–related arousals and there is no information regarding long term follow-up.[54]

Somnoplasty (radiofrequency thermal ablation)[55] and snoreplasty (injection of sclerosing agents into the soft palate)[56] are used for primary snoring but are probably not effective in OSA.

Maxillofacial surgery should be considered in patients with craniofacial abnormalities.

Bariatric surgery leading to massive weight loss can lead to a dramatic improvement in SDB.[57]

Central Sleep Apnea

Medical management of congestive heart failure, if present, will often correct the Cheyne-Stokes breathing pattern associated with central sleep apnea. If treatment of congestive heart failure does not adequately correct central sleep apneas, then CPAP can be very effective and can potentially increase left ventricular function.[58,59] Some patients with congestive heart failure may benefit from bilevel noninvasive positive pressure (BiPAP) with a back up rate. BiPAP differs from CPAP in that it provides different inspiratory and expiratory pressures, while CPAP provides only a single sustained pressure.

Cardiac pacing may improve periodic breathing by increasing heart rate and cardiac output and by decreasing vagal tone.[60,61] A recent small study, however, failed to demonstrate significant benefit in sleep apnea,[62] although it may benefit some patients with Cheyne-Stokes breathing.[63]

Nocturnal supplemental oxygen improves central sleep apnea,[64,65] probably by reducing the hyperventilation response to nocturnal hypoxemia.

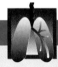

MR. A

HISTORY

Mr. A is a 50-year-old white man who was admitted to the hospital with chest pain. He is obese and has history of hypertension, which in the past few months, has been difficult to control in spite of multiple medications. While he was in the intensive care unit, the respiratory therapist noted a drop in oxygen saturation during sleep associated with snoring and gasping episodes. She reported it to the intensivist. Upon further questioning, Mr. A reported that he had been excessively sleepy for the past 6 months and has had difficulty concentrating at work. Two weeks ago he dozed off while driving and nearly had an accident on his way home after a long day at the office. He frequently has to stop to buy a cup of coffee in order to stay awake while driving.

Mr. A frequently drinks two to three beers in the evenings, and his wife has told him his snoring increases after he drinks in the evening.

QUESTIONS	ANSWERS
1. What is the likely explanation for Mr. A's daytime sleepiness?	The most common medical problem associated with excessive daytime sleepiness is OSA. Further evidence of OSA is that Mr. A has history of snoring, he is obese, and his blood pressure has been difficult to control.

2. What signs should the physician identify during the physical examination?	The upper airway should be evaluated carefully for any significant narrowing or obstruction. Neck size should be measured. Evidence of right heart failure should be looked for.
3. Is there a connection between Mr. A's use of alcohol and his symptoms?	Alcohol is known to worsen OSA symptoms. It also disrupts sleep.
4. Is there a connection between the lack of blood pressure control and the patient's excessive daytime sleepiness?	Yes, hypertension is common in patients with OSA. OSA causes excessive daytime sleepiness.
5. Which test should be ordered? What are the expected findings?	A polysomnogram should be ordered. Mr. A very likely has severe OSA with significant desaturations during the night.

More on Mr. A

PHYSICAL EXAMINATION

- **General.** Patient alert and oriented, in no distress; height 5 feet, 11 inches; weight 250 lb

- **HEENT.** No evidence of nasal obstruction; narrow posterior pharynx with large uvula

- **Neck.** 19 inches in diameter. No jugular venous distention (JVD) seen

- **Lungs.** Clear to auscultation

- **Heart.** Regular rhythm, with no evidence of murmurs or gallop. Normal heart sounds

- **Abdomen.** Markedly obese

- **Extremities.** 1+ ankle edema

POLYSOMNOGRAM RESULTS:

Sleep latency. 5 minutes

AHI. 70 (supine = 80, right side = 35)

Baseline SaO_2 levels. 90%; lowest SaO_2 = 69%; SaO_2 dropped below 90% during 40% of the recording.

Very loud snoring

CPAP titration. Recommended pressure: 14 cm H_2O

QUESTIONS	ANSWERS
6. What is the significance of the lack of JVD and normal heart sounds?	The lack of JVD could indicate that right heart failure has not occurred yet. Right heart failure will be likely if the nocturnal desaturations are not corrected. The lack of a loud P_2 during cardiac auscultation provides further evidence that right heart failure is not present.

7. How would you interpret the sleep latency and polysomnogram results?

A sleep latency of 5 minutes is very short and is consistent with excessive sleepiness (normal = 10 to 30 min.) An AHI of 70 is consistent with severe OSA. It is also worse with the supine position (normal: <5; mild 6 to 20; moderate 21 to 40; severe >40). Awake SaO_2 of 90% is slightly reduced, due either to obesity or to underlying cardiovascular disease. The lowest SaO_2 value of 69% indicates severe hypoxemia.

Mr. A Conclusion

A coronary angiogram shows single-vessel disease, and a coronary stent was placed. Mr. A has been able to lose only a few pounds. Nasal CPAP is started with good response and resolution of snoring at a CPAP level of 12 cm H_2O.

Mr. A is asked to return in 6 weeks for follow-up. In 6 weeks he appears much happier and states that his daytime sleepiness is nearly gone. His wife states that the snoring is completely resolved. His CPAP nasal mask is a bit uncomfortable and causes nasal dryness. He tolerates nasal pillows well, and a heated humidifier clears his nasal dryness. Blood pressure control improves. ∎

KEY POINTS

- Sleep disordered breathing (SDB) is a condition characterized by partial or complete cessation of breathing during sleep.
- Obstructive sleep apnea (OSA)/hypopnea syndrome causes sleepiness in approximately 4% of men and 2% of women between the ages of 30 and 60. It is even more common in people over age 60.
- Sleep is divided into two states: rapid eye movement (REM) sleep and non–rapid eye movement (NREM) sleep. NREM sleep is further divided into four stages.
- In the deeper stages of NREM sleep, breathing is typically very regular; however, overall ventilation is reduced compared to that during wakefulness.
- During REM sleep, the respiratory drive is irregular because of the transient decrease in ventilatory response to chemical and mechanical stimuli.
- The influence of sleep on the upper airway is similar to its effects on other skeletal muscles, resulting in a general loss of muscle tone.
- Obesity, by narrowing the airway, is the most common cause of OSA. Structural abnormalities such as micrognathia (small mandible), macroglossia (enlarged tongue), or enlarged tonsils or adenoids can be contributing factors.
- The incidence of systemic hypertension is higher in OSA patients than in the general population, especially in young, morbidly obese OSA patients.
- The main clinical features of SDB are loud snoring and excessive daytime sleepiness.

(key points continued on page 424)

KEY POINTS (CONTINUED)

- The typical patient with OSA is a middle-aged obese man, although age, obesity, and the male gender are not prerequisites for developing the disease. A neck circumference of 40 cm or more in the presence of snoring and hypertension suggests the diagnosis.
- The definitive test for sleep apnea is the **polysomnogram**. This test monitors many parameters during sleep including breathing, Sao_2, and ECG. The polysomnogram can determine the type and severity of any SDB problems.
- For many patients with mild OSA, a combination of weight loss, relief of nasal congestion, and avoidance of alcohol and sedatives is sufficient. Some patients have a strong positional component, with respiratory events present mainly while sleeping in the supine position.
- For patients with moderate to severe cases of OSA, CPAP, dental appliances, or surgery may be the best answer.

REFERENCES

1. Young, T, et al: The occurrence of sleep disordered breathing among middle aged adults. N Engl J Med 328:1230–1235, 1993.
2. Horstmann, S, Hess, CW, Bassetti, C, Gugger, M, Mathis, J: Sleepiness-related accidents in sleep apnea patients. Sleep 23(3):383–389, 2000.
3. Sassani, A, Findley, LJ, Kryger, M, Goldlust, E, George, C, Davidson, TM: Reducing motor-vehicle collisions, costs, and fatalities by treating obstructive sleep apnea syndrome. Sleep27(3): 453–458, 2004.
4. Javaheri, S, Parker, TJ, Wexler, L, Michaels, SE, Stanberry, E, Nishyama, H, Roselle, GA: Occult sleep-disordered breathing in stable congestive heart failure. Ann Intern Med 122(7):487–492, 1995. Erratum in Ann Intern Med 123(1):77, 1995.
5. Shamsuzzaman, AS, Gersh, BJ, Somers, VK: Obstructive sleep apnea: implications for cardiac and vascular disease. JAMA. 290(14):1906–1914, 2003.
6. Milleron, O, Pilliere, R, Foucher, A, de Roquefeuil, F, Aegerter, P, Jondeau, G, Raffestin, BG, Dubourg, O: Benefits of obstructive sleep apnea treatment in coronary artery disease: a long-term follow-up study. Eur Heart J 25(9):728–734, 2004.
7. Hanly, PJ, Millar, TW, Steljes, DG, Baert, R, Frais, MA, Kryger, MH: Respiration and abnormal sleep in patients with congestive heart failure. Chest 96(3):480–488, 1989.
8. Porthan, KM, Melin, JH, Kupila, JT, Venho, KK, Partinen, MM: Prevalence of sleep apnea syndrome in lone atrial fibrillation: a case-control study. Chest 125(3):879–885, 2004.
9. Takasaki, Y, Orr, D, Popkin, J, Rutherford, R, Liu, P, Bradley, TD: Effect of nasal continuous positive airway pressure on sleep apnea in congestive heart failure. Am Rev Respir Dis 140(6):1578–1584, 1989.
10. Heart disease and stroke statistics. 2005 Update, American Heart Association. Available at: http://www.americanheart.org/downloadable/heart/1105390918119HDSStats2005Update.pdf.
11. Palomaki, H: Snoring and the risk of ischemic brain infarction. Stroke 22(8):1021–1025, 1991.
12. Mohsenin, V: Is sleep apnea a risk factor for stroke? A critical analysis. Minerva Med 95(4):291–305, 2004.
13. Pressman, MR, Schetman, WR, Figueroa, WG, Van Uitert, B, Caplan, HJ, Peterson, DD: Transient ischemic attacks and minor stroke during sleep. Relationship to obstructive sleep apnea syndrome. Stroke 26(12):2361–2365, 1995.
14. Kales, A, Bixler, EO, Cadieux, RJ, Schneck, DW, Shaw, LC 3rd, Locke, TW, Vela-Bueno, A, Soldatos, CR: Sleep apnoea in a hypertensive population. Lancet 2(8410):1005–1008, 1984.
15. Jeong, DU, Dimsdale, JE: Sleep apnea and essential hypertension: a critical review of the epidemiological evidence for co-morbidity. Clin Exp Hypertens A 11(7):1301–1323, 1989.
16. Nieto, FJ, Young, TB, Lind, BK, Shahar, E, Samet, JM, Redline, S, D'Agostino, RB, Newman, AB, Lebowitz, MD, Pickering, TG: Association of sleep-disordered breathing, sleep apnea, and hypertension in a large community-based study. Sleep Heart Health Study. JAMA 283(14):1829–1836, 2000.
17. National center for Health Statistics. CDC (dm statistics) Available at http://www.cdc.gov/nchs/fastats/diabetes.htm.

18. National Center for Chronic Disease Prevention and Health Promotion. Diabetes Public Health Resource. (dm statistics) Available at http://www.cdc.gov/ diabetes/pubs/estimates.htm.

19. Babu, AR, Herdegen, J, Fogelfeld, L, Shott, S, Mazzone, T: Type 2 diabetes, glycemic control, and continuous positive airway pressure in obstructive sleep apnea. Arch Intern Med 165(4):447–4752, 2005.

20. Harsch, IA, Hahn, EG, Konturek, PC: Insulin resistance and other metabolic aspects of the obstructive sleep apnea syndrome. Med Sci Monit 11(3):RA70–RA75, 2005.

21. He, J, et al: Mortality and apnea index in obstructive sleep apnea: experience in 385 male patients. Chest 94:9–14, 1988.

22. Doherty, LS, Kiely, JL, Swan, V, McNicholas, WT: Long-term effects of nasal continuous positive airway pressure therapy on cardiovascular outcomes in sleep apnea syndrome. Chest 127(6):2076–2084, 2005.

23. Bokinsky, G, Miller, M, Ault, K, Husband, P, Mitchell, J: Spontaneous platelet activation and aggregation during obstructive sleep apnea and its response to therapy with nasal continuous positive airway pressure. Chest 108:625–630, 1995.

24. Lavie, L: Obstructive sleep apnoea syndrome: an oxidative stress disorder. Sleep Med Rev 7(1):35–51, 2003.

25. Minoguchi, K, Yokoe, T, Tazaki, T, Minoguchi, H, Tanaka, A, Oda, N, Okada, S, Ohta, S, Naito, H, Adachi, M: Increased carotid intima-media thickness and serum inflammatory markers in obstructive sleep apnea. Am J Respir Crit Care Med 172(5):625–630, 2005.

26. Vgontzas, AN, Zoumakis, E, Lin, HM, Bixler, EO, Trakada, G, Chrousos, GP: Marked decrease in sleepiness in patients with sleep apnea by etanercept, a tumor necrosis factor-alpha antagonist. J Clin Endocrinol Metab 89(9):4409–4413, 2004.

27. Somers, VK, Dyken, ME, Clary, MP, Abboud, FM: Sympathetic neural mechanisms in obstructive sleep apnea. J Clin Invest 96(4):1897–1904, 1995.

28. Rechtschaffen, A, Kales, A: A Manual of Standardized Terminology, Techniques and Scoring System for Sleep Stages of Human Subjects. NIH Publication #204, 1968.

29. Sleep-related breathing disorders in adults: recommendations for syndrome definition and measurement techniques in clinical research. Report of an American Academy of Sleep Medicine Task Force. Sleep. 23(2):151, 153, 2000.

30. Katz, I, Stradling, J, Slutsky, AS, Zamel, N, Hoffstein, V: Do patients with obstructive sleep apnea have thick necks? Am Rev Respir Dis 141:1228–1231, 1990.

31. Khoo, SM, Tan, WC, Ng, TP, Ho, CH: Risk factors associated with habitual snoring and sleep-disordered breathing in a multi-ethnic Asian population: a population-based study. Respir Med 98(6):557–566, 2004.

32. Practice Parameters for the indications for polysomnography and related procedures: an update for 2005. Sleep 28(4):449–521, 2005.

33. Guilleminault, C, et al: A cause of excessive daytime sleepiness: the upper airway resistance syndrome. Chest 104:781, 1993.

34. Norman, RG, Ahmed, MM, Walsleben, JA, Rapoport, DM: Detection of respiratory events during NPSG: nasal cannula/pressure sensor versus thermistor. Sleep 20(12):1175–1184, 1997.

35. Practice parameters for clinical use of the multiple sleep latency test and the maintenance of wakefulness test. Sleep 28 (1):113–121, 2005.

36. Rauscher, H, et al: Self reported vs measured compliance with nasal CPAP. Chest 103(6):1675–1680, 1993.

37. Reeves-Hoche, MK: Nasal CPAP: an objective evaluation of patient compliance. Am J Respir Crit Care Med 149:149–154, 1994.

38. Meurice, JC: Predictive factors of long term compliance with nasal CPAP treatment in sleep apnea syndrome. Chest 105:429–433, 1994.

39. McArdle, N, Devereux, G, Heidarnejad, H, Engleman, HM, Mackay, TW, Douglas, NJ: Long-term use of CPAP therapy for sleep apnea/hypopnea syndrome. Am J Respir Crit Care Med 159 (4 Pt 1):1108–1114, 1999.

40. Hoffstein, V, et al: Treatment of OSA with nasal CPAP: patient compliance, perception of benefits and side effects. Am Rev Respir Dis 145 (4 pt 1): 841–845, 1992.

41. Pepin, JL: Side effects of nasal CPAP in sleep apnea syndrome. Chest 107(2):375–381, 1995.

42. Branson, R: Mask CPAP, clinical indications and management. Caradyne.com, Vol. 10, 1999.

43. Hukins, C: Comparative study of autotitrating and fixed-pressure CPAP in the home: a randomized, single-blind crossover trial. Sleep 27(8):1512–1517, 2004.

44. Therapeutic efficacy of an oral appliance in the treatment of obstructive sleep apnea: a 2-year follow-up. Am J Orthod Dentofacial Orthop 121(3): 273–279, 2002.

45. Walker-Engstrom, ML, Tegelberg, A, Wilhelmsson, B, Ringqvist, I: 4-year follow-up of treatment with dental appliance or uvulopalatopharyngoplasty in patients with obstructive sleep apnea: a randomized study. Chest 121(3):739–746, 2002.

46. Ferguson, KA, Ono, T, Lowe, AA, Keenan, SP, Fleetham, JA: A randomized crossover study of an oral appliance vs nasal-continuous positive airway pressure in the treatment of mild-moderate obstructive sleep apnea. Chest 109(5):1269–1275, 1996.

47. Schmidt-Nowara, W: OA for OSA. Chest 109(5): 1269–1275, 1996.

48. Practice parameters for the treatment of OSA in adults. The efficacy of surgical modifications of the airway. Sleep 19:152–155, 1996.

49. Troell, RJ, Riley, RW, Powell, NB, Li, K: Surgical management of the hypopharyngeal airway in sleep disordered breathing. Otolaryngol Clin North Am 31(6):979–1012, 1998.

50. Li, KK, Powell, NB, Riley, RW, Troell, RJ, Guilleminault, C: Long-term results of maxillomandibular advancement surgery. Sleep Breath 4(3):137–140, 2000.

51. Li, KK, Riley, RW, Powell, NB, Troell, R: Overview of phase II surgery for obstructive sleep apnea syndrome. Ear Nose Throat J 78(11):851, 854–857, 1999.

52. Bettega, G, Pepin, JL, Veale, D, Deschaux, C, Raphael, B, Levy, P: Obstructive sleep apnea syndrome. fifty-one consecutive patients treated by maxillofacial surgery. Am J Respir Crit Care Med 162(2 Pt 1):641–649, 2000.

53. Littner, M, Kushida, CA, Hartse, K, Anderson, WM, Davila, D, Johnson, SF, Wise, MS, Hirshkowitz, M, Woodson, BT: Practice parameters for the use of laser-assisted uvulopalatoplasty: an update for 2000. Sleep 24(5):603–619, 2001.

54. The pillar procedure. A new first line treatment option for mild to moderate OSA. Available at http://www.restoremedical.com/docs/Clinical_Summary_WP_approved091404.pdf.

55. Boudewyns, A, Van De Heyning, P: Temperature-controlled radiofrequency tissue volume reduction of the soft palate (somnoplasty) in the treatment of habitual snoring: results of a European multicenter trial. Acta Otolaryngol 120(8):981–985, 2000.

56. Brietzke, SE, Mair, EA: Injection snoreplasty: extended follow-up and new objective data. Otolaryngol Head Neck Surg 128(5):605–615, 2003.

57. Bariatric surgery for obstructive sleep apnea. Verse, T Chest 128:485–487, 2005.

58. Javaheri, S: Effects of continuous positive airway pressure on sleep apnea and ventricular irritability in patients with heart failure. Circulation 101(4):392–397, 2000.

59. Cormican, LJ, Williams, A: Sleep disordered breathing and its treatment in congestive heart failure. Heart 91(10):1265–1270, 2005.

60. Garrigue, S, Bordier, P, Jais, P, Shah, DC, Hocini, M, Raherison, C, Tunon, De Lara, M, Haissaguerre, M, Clementy, J: Benefit of atrial pacing in sleep apnea syndrome. N Engl J Med 346(6):404–412, 2002.

61. Luthje, L, Unterberg-Buchwald, C, Dajani, D, Vollmann, D, Hasenfuss, G, Andreas, S: Atrial overdrive pacing in patients with sleep apnea with implanted pacemaker. Am J Respir Crit Care Med 172(1):118–122, 2005.

62. Pepin, JL, Defaye, P, Garrigue, S, Poezevara, Y, Levy, P: Overdrive atrial pacing does not improve obstructive sleep apnoea syndrome. Eur Respir J 25(2):343–347, 2005.

63. Gabor, JY, Newman, DA, Barnard-Roberts, V, Korley, V, Mangat, I, Dorian, P, Hanly, PJ: Improvement in Cheyne-Stokes respiration following cardiac resynchronisation therapy. Eur Respir J 26(1):95–100, 2005.

64. Sakakibara, M, Sakata, Y, Usui, K, Hayama, Y, Kanda, S, Wada, N, Matsui, Y, Suto, Y, Shimura, S, Tanabe, T: Effectiveness of short-term treatment with nocturnal oxygen therapy for central sleep apnea in patients with congestive heart failure. J Cardiol 46(2):53–61, 2005.

65. Javaheri, S: Central sleep apnea in congestive heart failure: prevalence, mechanisms, impact, and therapeutic options. Semin Respir Crit Care Med 26(1):44–55, 2005.

19

Tuberculosis

James R. Dexter, MD, FACP, FCCP
Robert L. Wilkins, PhD, RRT, FAARC

CHAPTER OBJECTIVES:

After reading this chapter, you will be able to identify:

- The incidence of tuberculosis infections around the world and in the United States.
- The way in which tuberculosis is spread from one person to another.
- The pathology and pathogenesis associated with primary and reactivation tuberculosis.
- The clinical features and radiographic findings associated with reactivation tuberculosis and the clinical significance of a positive TB skin test.
- The treatment of active and latent tuberculosis.

INTRODUCTION

According to the World Health Organization, tuberculosis (TB) is the number one cause of infectious disease–related deaths in the world. Globally, about 9 million new cases of TB were diagnosed in 2003 and in that same year TB killed 1.75 million people.[1] The majority of new cases were found in Southeast Asia (35%) and Africa (27%). About 4% of all new TB cases in the world in 2003 were diagnosed in the United States.

The incidence and mortality rates from tuberculosis have changed dramatically in the United States over the past 50 years. In 1953, when TB statistics were first reported, 84,304 new cases of TB were diagnosed in the United States and 19,707 deaths occurred. In 2003, 14,874 new cases of TB and about 800 deaths were reported in the United States.[2] The decline in incidence and mortality rates are the result of new medications, a better understanding of the disease, and important public health education. The decline in incidence of TB has not been steady since 1953. In fact, the incidence increased significantly between 1985 and 1992. This increase is believed to be due primarily to the increase in the incidence of HIV infection. HIV-infected patients have poor immunity and are highly prone to TB. TB is the leading killer of HIV-positive individuals, causing more than 30% of AIDS-related deaths.

The incidence of TB in the United States is affected by changes in population demographics (e.g., number of immigrants entering the United States from countries where TB is prevalent). Foreign-born individuals accounted for 53% of all new cases of TB in the United States in 2003.[2,3] The incidence is also influenced by the number of individuals who are highly susceptible to TB as a result of a poor immune system (e.g., organ transplant patients, cancer patients), malnutrition, and institutional housing (e.g., nursing homes, prisons, homeless shelters). For these reasons, in the United States TB has become a disease of the elderly, of foreign-born persons from high-prevalence countries, of nonwhite minorities, and of persons with immunodeficiency.

> About one-third of the world's population is infected with tuberculosis.

For a variety of reasons TB continues to be a health care problem in the United States and around the world. Active TB is sometimes difficult to diagnose, and many individuals have active disease without a diagnosis. Other individuals with TB do not seek medical care because of the gradual onset of the disease or because they belong to a segment of society that does not have ready access to medical care. Many who are diagnosed and started on treatment do not follow through with the medication regimen because it requires patient compliance for months. Failure to adequately treat TB has produced multi-drug-resistant tuberculosis (MDR-TB) that is difficult to treat.

ETIOLOGY AND TRANSMISSION

The organism that causes TB, *Mycobacterium tuberculosis*, is a nonmotile, nonsporulating, rod-shaped, acid-fast bacillus (AFB) with a dimension of approximately 0.2 $\times$ 5.0 mm. It is a slow-growing aerobe that multiplies faster in the presence of an abundant supply of oxygen. Therefore, it grows best in areas of the body where P_{O_2} is highest (lung apices) and immunity lowest (spinal discs).

M. tuberculosis is almost exclusively transmitted by very small, aerosolized droplets usually less than 8 to 10 microns in diameter. These minuscule particles are aerosolized into the environment by infected individuals through coughing, sneezing, and talking. The particles remain suspended in the air by brownian motion. Once inhaled by a susceptible person, they cause infection if they get deep into the lung, past the mucociliary transport system.

Other reported means of contracting the disease include ingestion of unpasteurized milk from cattle infected with the pathogen (usually *Mycobacterium bovis*); direct inoculation through the skin, as occurs in laboratory accidents and during postmortem examinations; and inhalation of aerosolized fluid from contaminated materials (e.g., urine, sinus drainage, feces, sputum) that are improperly handled. TB is not, however, contracted through contact with fomites, objects or material on which the bacteria are present, such as clothing, eating utensils, writing objects, and paper.

PATHOLOGY AND PATHOGENESIS

Primary Infection

Inhaled *Mycobacterium* particles initially settle in the distal parenchyma of the lung with the greatest amount of ventilation (i.e., the lung bases). The bacilli multiply despite the body's defense mechanisms and slowly migrate throughout the body by way of the lymph and circulatory systems. Approximately 6 to 8 weeks after this initial infection, the host's immune system causes localized inflammation and containment of the infection by forming granulomas.

A granuloma develops in the infected lung tissue and results in a fibrin mass; necrosis of this mass produces a cheesy material at the center, known as caseation. The regional lymph nodes also become infected and enlarged. The infection is often walled off by fibrosis. The initial lung lesion is called a **Ghon nodule**, and the combination of the initial lung lesion and the affected regional (hilar) lymph node is known as the **Ghon complex**. Although difficult to detect on a chest radiograph at this stage, the lesions may be seen as small, sharply defined opacities. This initial stage of TB usually heals completely in the majority of infected individuals, leaving only small scars that may later become calcified nodules.

The body's cell-mediated immune response is usually effective in controlling the infection at this point, but it does not often kill all the bacteria. Pockets of bacteria may lie dormant in either the primary (Ghon nodule) or the metastatic sites (which could be anywhere in the body), sometimes for many years, until some event precipitates reactivation of the infection. Between the primary and reinfection phases is a dormant, or "healthy," period known as tuberculosis infection without disease. Clinically there is no evidence of disease, except for a positive skin test and possibly residual scarring on the chest radiograph. This positive skin test reaction indicates the presence of live tuberculin bacilli in the body.

Postprimary or Reactivation Infection

Some time after the initial infection has occurred, reactivation of the infection may take place in up to 10% of infected individuals. Reactivation is most common within the first 2 years after initial infection but may occur up to several decades later. The exact cause of reactivation is poorly understood, but the following are among the known predisposing factors: aging, malnutrition, alcoholism, diabetes, immunocompromising diseases, silicosis, postpartum period, gastrectomy, chronic hemodialysis, and other chronic debilitating disorders. Because the bacilli grow best in an aerobic environment, they usually present as an infiltrate in the apical and posterior segments of the upper lobes, where the relative oxygen concentration is highest in the lung. Reactivation may also occur at extrapulmonary sites with a good oxygen supply or poor immune potential, to which the original infection had metastasized.

About 90% of TB patients in the non-HIV-infected population seen at medical clinics present with reactivated TB.[4] Extrapulmonary disease accounts for about 15% of active disease. Granulomas (or tubercules) with central caseation are typical pathological changes associated with reactivated TB. Fibrosis and cavity formation take place as the body continues its

> TB is usually considered a pulmonary infection, but 15% of TB infections develop in areas outside of the chest.

fight against the organism. Eventually fibrosis encases the granulomatous lesions, resulting in loss of lung volume. The affected lobe retracts and eventually collapses, and calcification may become evident. These retractions and morphological changes may cause the bronchi to become distorted and dilated.

In some cases a disseminated form of the disease may develop, known as miliary tuberculosis. This is usually an acute, generalized TB spread throughout the region or organ system characterized by the radiographic appearance of many small nodules. Miliary TB usually occurs in immunocompromised patients and predominantly involves newborns and older men. About half of the adult cases are associated with an underlying disease state such as chronic alcoholism, immunosuppression therapy (e.g., for organ transplantation), immunodeficiency diseases (e.g., AIDS), or neoplasia.

PATHOPHYSIOLOGY

The continuous destruction of infected lung parenchyma leads to scarring and loss of lung volume along with the destruction of blood vessels, which is why ventilation-perfusion ($\dot{V}/\dot{Q}$) mismatching is usually not seen. Hypoxemia and hypercapnia are unusual findings unless the patient has concurrent lung disease, such as chronic obstructive pulmonary disease (COPD). Pulmonary function is initially not greatly affected, but as the disease progresses, the lung volumes and flows decrease. Destruction of blood vessels may result in hemoptysis. Injury of the bronchi may result in bronchiectasis and chronic secondary infections of the airways.

CLINICAL FEATURES

History

The medical history is important in the patient suspected of having TB. The interview is done to determine whether (1) the patient has been exposed to TB, (2) the patient has risk factors for TB reactivation, and (3) symptoms are consistent with TB.

A careful history of the patient suspected of having TB must include recent travel outside the United States and travel of close family or friends who might be infected with TB. Other factors to identify are country of origin, immunosuppression, institutionalized care, and previous or current treatment for TB. Exposure of the patient to a person with active TB is extremely helpful to document, especially if this contact has been significantly close.

> Consider tuberculosis in every chronically ill patient, as the symptoms are very subtle.

TB is a chronic disease with an insidious onset. It may not be recognized as a serious illness by either the patient or the physician. The attending physician must document clues in the patient's medical history that are suggestive of TB, such as pleurisy with pleural effusion or a past diagnosis of prolonged pneumonia, such as chronic fevers, night sweats, weight loss, fatigue, cough, sputum, hemoptysis, or dyspnea. History of associated illnesses should also be documented, such as uncontrolled diabetes, alcoholism, malnutrition due to a variety of causes, immunosuppression, or occupational exposure to quartz dust or silica. It is important to note recent nursing home admission, incarceration, or institutional care.

TB patients commonly have the following complaints:

- Fatigue, low-grade fever, and night sweats
- Chronic cough, sputum production, and hemoptysis
- Pleuritic chest pain
- Weight loss

TB symptoms may progress so slowly over a period of weeks that they are recognized only in retrospect. Some patients may never have obvious symptoms, despite having extensive cavitation. Nonspecific systemic symptoms include progressive onset of fatigue, mild digestive disturbances, malaise, slow onset of weight loss, anorexia, irregular menses, night sweats, and low-grade fevers lasting for weeks to months. Fevers occur more often in the afternoon or evening and dissipate at night. Less common is an acute onset of spiking temperatures, chills, myalgia, sweating, and weakness in association with parenchymal infiltrates on the chest radiograph; this is usually attributed to a secondary pneumonia or viral illness.

Physical Examination

Physical examination findings in the patient with TB are not specific enough to make the diagnosis. Physical examination can, however, help determine the extent of the progression of the disease, and whether other areas of the body outside the chest are involved.

Vital signs are not initially suggestive of TB unless the infection is severe enough to produce changes in heart rate, respiratory rate, blood pressure, or body temperature. The pulmonary lesions associated with TB usually give rise to varying degrees of impaired resonance to percussion, bronchial breath sounds, and coarse crackles. Endobronchial disease or bronchial compression by lymph nodes (more common in children) may produce localized wheezing, which can be accentuated by forced expiration while the patient assumes different positions. The trachea may be deviated if the upper lobes have undergone loss in volume.

Evidence of extrapulmonary TB in other areas of the body (e.g., spine tenderness, swollen lymph nodes, joint tenderness, enlarged abdominal organs including the liver and spleen) should also be documented. Changes in skin color or blood pressure due to adrenocortical involvement may be present. Digital clubbing and hypertrophic osteoarthropathy are rare findings of TB.

A pleural effusion, whether or not it is associated with TB, is characterized by decreased resonance to percussion and absence of breath sounds over the affected region as well as diminished transmission of spoken or whispered sounds. The size of the effusion determines the degree of underlying lung compression and subsequent lung dysfunction.

Laboratory Findings

The microbiology laboratory provides the basis for TB diagnosis, but routine laboratory data are minimally helpful in the absence of any other underlying infections. The white blood cell (WBC) count is usually normal in primary pulmonary TB. A WBC count greater than 15 to 20×10^3/mL is generally suggestive of another type of infection except in cases of miliary TB (TB dissemination into the blood), which can result in significant leukocytosis. A mild anemia may be seen in chronic TB. The following laboratory data may be increased with TB, yet are considered nonspecific because other problems can also make them abnormal:

- Increase of immature WBCs (left shift) as the TB spreads
- Elevated erythrocyte sedimentation rate
- Elevated transaminases and alkaline phosphatase

Arterial Blood Gases

Arterial blood gas assessment is rarely helpful in evaluating the initial presentation of TB. In a mild infection the patient will compensate for mild $\dot{V}/\dot{Q}$ mismatching and hypoxemia by hyperventilation, which results in respiratory alkalosis. Respiratory acidosis and hypoxemia are seen only in end-stage TB patients in respiratory failure.

Chest Radiograph

Posteroanterior and lateral chest films show the extent of pulmonary involvement and location of the disease. Together with bacteriologic examinations of sputum and a positive skin test, the chest radiograph provides a valuable tool in the diagnosis of TB (Figure 19.1). Reactivation TB usually causes infiltrates in the apical-posterior segments of the upper lobes. In contrast, the most common abnormality on the chest radiograph of the patient with primary TB is hilar lymph node enlargement.[5]

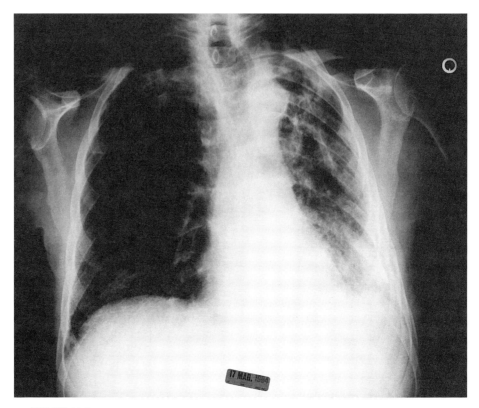

FIGURE 19.1 Typical chest radiograph for tuberculosis. Note the cavity lesion in the right upper lobe.

Fibronodular cavitations, atelectasis, pleural effusions, and empyema may be seen on the chest film.

Microbiology

Numerous nontuberculous strains of Mycobacteria can show up on AFB smears. Therefore, a culture of *M. tuberculosis* is a necessary test to confirm TB; unfortunately, these cultures take up to 6 weeks to complete. New innovations to circumvent this problem include DNA probe, polymerase chain reaction assay (from sputum), or mycolic acid pattern on high-pressure chromatography.

> It is relatively common for the purified protein derivative (PPD) skin test and the AFB smear and culture to be negative in patients with active TB.

An early morning collection of expectorated sputum is best for laboratory evaluation by stain and culture. The least invasive method of collecting sputum is to have the patient produce the sample by coughing. If the patient is unable to produce a sputum sample, a sputum induction can be done to collect the specimen. The health-care worker must be protected from exposure to TB during sputum collection and subsequent treatment of the patient. Whenever TB is suspected, universal precautions should be augmented by techniques to prevent micron size droplet inhalation to protect against potentially contaminated, aerosolized fluid. In sputum induction, aerosolized hypertonic saline is administered for 15 to 20 minutes to stimulate the patient to cough and produce sputum. Saline helps the patient produce sputum by providing moisture and stimulation of expectoration.

TB patients often swallow their sputum during sleep; thus, in some cases where the patient is unable to expectorate sputum, a gastric aspirate culture is helpful. A sample of stomach contents is aspirated in the early morning before the patient arises. The use of a gastric aspirate smear has limited value, however, because of the presence of nontuberculous AFB in the gastric contents.

Bronchoscopy may also be used to collect a sputum sample if other, less invasive techniques are not effective. Use of local anesthetics during bronchoscopy, such as xylocaine, can decrease the viability of the *M. tuberculosis* organism. Respiratory therapists (RTs) who assist physicians in the bronchoscopy procedure need to be aware of this and minimize the use of xylocaine in this setting.

Skin Testing

An estimated 10 to 15 million persons in the United States have dormant *M. tuberculosis* infection. The Mantoux skin test for TB is an intracutaneous injection of a standardized dose of purified protein derivative (PPD). A positive reaction is indicated by a visible or palpable induration (i.e., raised, hardened area) caused by prior sensitization to the TB organism. The Centers for Disease Control (CDC) classifies the positive skin test reactions for specific groups as follows:

5 mm or more

- Persons who have recently had close contact with an individual with infectious TB
- Persons whose chest radiographs showing fibrotic lesions are likely to represent old, healed TB
- Persons with known or suspected HIV infection

10 mm or more in those who do not meet the above criteria but have other risk factors

- Persons with other medical risk factors known to pose a substantially increased risk of TB once infection has occurred
- Foreign-born persons from high-prevalence countries
- Medically underserved, low-income populations, including high-risk minorities
- IV drug users
- Residents of long-term care facilities
- Populations that have been identified locally as having an increased prevalence of TB

15 mm or more

- All other persons

Older patients should have a repeat skin test in 2 to 4 weeks if the first skin test is negative. A positive second skin test indicates that the first test was a false-negative and that the patient has been infected with TB. Approximately 5% to 8% of the overall population is considered anergic (i.e., nonreactive to the PPD). In addition to the above populations, skin-test screening for TB infection is also recommended in high-risk populations, including the following:

- Persons with signs or symptoms, or both, that are suggestive of TB
- Individuals in close contact with persons known to have pulmonary TB

- Persons with medical conditions that increase the risk of TB (see later discussion)
- Alcoholics
- Health-care workers

It is important to remember that the absence of a reaction to the tuberculin test does not exclude the diagnosis of TB.

TREATMENT

After the diagnosis of active TB has been established by culture and the extent of the lung disease defined by chest radiograph, treatment can start. The decision about which treatment regiment should be used is based on the extent of the TB infection, the skin test reaction, and the sensitivity of the *M. tuberculosis* organism to the drug. The following are the basic principles of TB therapy:

- An effective multidrug regimen must be included in each program.
- Organisms must be susceptible to at least two of the drugs used.
- Bacteriologic response should occur within the expected time.
- A single drug should never be added to a program that is failing.
- Drug treatment must continue for a sufficient period of time.
- Patient compliance must be monitored.

Pharmacological Agents

The first-line drugs are relatively effective and pose a relatively low risk of toxic side effects. In addition to the above basic principles, the CDC has recommended the following treatment criteria:

> The current standard treatment regimen for TB is four drugs for 2 months followed by two drugs for 4 months.

- **6-month regimen:** 2-month period of daily isoniazid, rifampin, pyrazinamide, and either ethambutol or streptomycin, followed by isoniazid and rifampin given daily or twice weekly for 4 months
- **9-month regime:** 1 to 2 months of daily isoniazid and rifampin followed by twice-weekly isoniazid and rifampin for 9 months
- **Regimens of less than 6 months:** Not recommended

Side Effects

The most common side effect of rifampin, isoniazid, and pyrazinamide is chemical hepatitis. It can usually be avoided by stopping treatment when liver enzymes reach three to five times the upper limits of normal. Rifampin also has the further potential side effects of gastrointestinal upset, skin eruptions, flulike symptoms, and red-orange discoloration of urine and other body fluids (permanent discoloration of soft contact lenses may occur). Side effects of ethambutol are ocular toxicity (optic nerve); however, at the doses currently recommended, this condition is rare. During pregnancy, treatment should continue for a minimum of 9 months, and breastfeeding should not be discouraged.

Directly Observed Treatment

One of the most cost-effective methods of treating TB is called directly observed treatment (DOT). DOT calls for health-care workers to ensure appropriate treatment by watching their TB patients take each dose of their medications. New treatment regimens that require only 2 or 3 days of medication each week have made DOT a more practical approach.

Prophylactic Therapy

Patients without active disease but with a positive skin test can decrease their risk for the developing active disease by taking a 6- to 9-month course of isoniazid. Unfortunately, isoniazid-associated hepatitis increases in frequency in older patients; hepatitis will develop in nearly 2.5% of isoniazid-treated patients over the age of 65. The risk-benefit ratio thus mandates prophylactic therapy for 9 months for any patient with a positive TB skin test who is less than 35 years of age and for any patient older than 35 who has had a recent TB skin test conversion or has other risk factors for developing active disease such as diabetes, silicosis, achlorhydria, immunosupression, and so on.

> Six months of regular pill taking is so difficult to achieve that many public health departments are recommending DOT for all patients.

Mr. T

HISTORY

Mr. T is a 52-year-old mechanical engineer from Thailand who was referred to the pulmonary department by the public health service after his skin test was found to be positive. His brother, who lives with him, recently started a four-drug therapeutic course for a confirmed case of active TB. Mr. T denies having cough, sputum, fever, chills, night sweats, weight loss, change in exercise tolerance, or dyspnea. He reports, however, that in the early morning he has been producing one to two small globs of yellow sputum.

QUESTIONS	ANSWERS
1. What kind of immune reaction is responsible for the positive TB skin test?	Cellular immunity is responsible for the positive skin test.
2. Does the positive TB skin test prove that the patient has active TB?	No, the positive skin test does not prove that active TB is present. It indicates only that TB infection is present, which could be either dormant or active.
3. How would you determine whether Mr. T is merely infected with TB or has active disease?	Results of a sputum AFB smear and culture would determine whether active disease were present.
4. What further tests should be done to clarify the situation?	A positive skin test alone could occur with dormant disease; a positive skin test and a positive sputum TB culture indicates active TB.

5. Is Mr. T likely to be contagious, and should he be isolated from his family, friends, and coworkers?

The patient's contagiousness depends on the number of TB organisms in the lung, the amount of sputum production, and the severity of his cough. Mr. T does not need to be isolated, but until the chest radiograph and the sputum smear results are obtained, he should limit his exposure only to those family members with whom he has already had recent contact. A negative sputum smear but positive culture usually means that relatively few organisms are present in the sputum and that the risk of transmission is low. Those who are most susceptible to catching TB are the very young (especially infants) and the immunocompromised. If the smear and culture are negative, the patient may resume social activities.

 ## More on Mr. T

PHYSICAL EXAMINATION

- **General.** A thin, vigorous Asian man in no respiratory distress at rest

- **Vital Signs.** Temperature 37.0°C (98.6°F), heart rate 80/min, respiratory rate 14/min, blood pressure 120/72 mm Hg

- **HEENT.** Noncontributory to the current problem; neck supple with full, active range of motion; trachea midline and mobile with palpation; no stridor or wheezes; thyroid normal; carotid pulsations +2 and symmetrical with no bruits; no jugular venous distention; no cervicular or supraclavicular lymphadenopathy

- **Chest.** Anteroposterior diameter of chest normal; normal expansion of chest with respiration; chest nontender to palpation; normal resonance of chest with percussion; axillae without lymphadenopathy

- **Heart.** Regular rhythm; rate approximately 80/min without murmurs, gallops, or rubs

- **Lungs.** Clear on auscultation

- **Abdomen.** Soft, nondistended, and nontender to palpation; no masses noted; no organomegaly; bowel sounds present

- **Genitourinary.** Rectal examination is deferred at the patient's request

- **Extremities.** No cyanosis, clubbing, or edema; pulses and reflexes +2 and symmetrical; Homans' sign bilaterally negative

QUESTIONS	ANSWERS
6. Did the physical examination add any significant information to the history?	Yes, the physical examination suggests that if active disease is present, it is probably mild. There is no evidence of pleural effusion, lung collapse, or extensive tubercular pneumonia.

7. Has your impression changed about Mr. T's risk of simple dormant infection versus active disease?	The physical examination does not reveal any evidence of active disease, since the breath sounds are clear and the vital signs are normal. So far, the only evidence of any disease is the history of recent TB exposure, positive skin test, and morning sputum production. The recent exposure could result in either dormant or active disease. The sputum production suggests active TB or an unrelated problem, such as chronic bronchitis.
8. Should treatment be instituted at this time? If so, what sort of treatment?	No, treatment should not be started yet. Further evaluation is warranted. We must know whether the patient has had exposure without infection, exposure with dormant infection, or active infection before deciding on treatment.
9. Should Mr. T be isolated at this time? If so, for how long?	No, Mr. T should not be isolated yet. There is not enough evidence suggesting active disease. He should, however, be warned against visiting young, sick, or elderly persons. He should also be instructed to cover his mouth and nose with a tissue when he coughs.
10. What tests should be done now, and how soon can results be expected?	A chest radiograph is needed, and results should be available the same day. It is necessary to obtain a sputum AFB smear (results within about 3 days) and sputum AFB culture with rapid analysis techniques such as gene probe if it is positive (final results in 6 weeks).

More on Mr. T

LABORATORY EVALUATION

- CBC: WBC 8000/mm^3; hemoglobin 14.2 gm/dL; electrolytes normal; creatinine normal; normal liver profile (enzymes AST, ALT, and LDH normal)

- Chest Radiograph: See Figure 19.2

- AFB Stain (early morning sample): Few AFB organisms

- Gram Stain: 21 WBCs, 11 gram-positive cocci

- Sputum Culture: Normal flora

QUESTIONS	ANSWERS
11. Would you expect the WBC to become abnormal during a TB infection? Why or why not?	No, the WBC count is not expected to increase with TB infection. Generally, WBCs do not play a role in the body's fight against AFB.

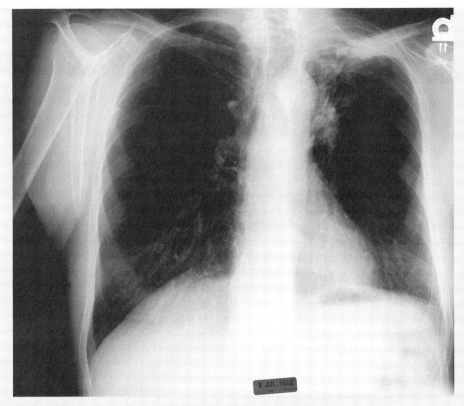

FIGURE 19.2 Pulmonary artery chest film for patient Mr. T.

12. The electrolytes, liver profile, and creatinine are normal. Is this more important for evaluating the tuberculous disease or for determining the dose of therapy?

The normal chemistry, liver profile, and creatinine are useful in determining the dose and risk of therapy. The liver and kidneys both play a role in breaking down the TB medications. If these organs are damaged, the dose must be reduced to prevent toxicity.

13. The liver enzymes are normal. Would this finding affect your choice of therapy? Why or why not?

Normal liver enzymes suggest that Mr. T should tolerate multiple drugs.

14. What are the typical chest radiograph abnormalities associated with TB infection?

The typical chest radiograph in the patient with primary TB shows pneumonia or a small peripheral nodule. In post-primary TB infection with active disease, upper lobe cavity is common.

15. Does Mr. T's chest radiograph show typical evidence of active TB infection?

Yes, Mr. T's chest film shows typical evidence of active disease: A small upper lobe cavity is present.

16. Does the presence of AFB organisms in the sputum smear prove that Mr. T has TB infection?

The presence of AFB organisms does not prove that TB is present. Other nontuberculous mycobacteria can be present in the sputum (especially in HIV patients, elderly patients, and those with chronic lung disease). These bacteria are called atypical organisms, and culture is required to distinguish them from *M. tuberculosis*.

17. Is the sputum Gram stain and culture helpful at this time?

Yes, the sputum Gram stain and culture are helpful at this time because they help rule out concurrent pneumonia.

18. What medications should be started at this time?

The physician should prescribe a combination of the four first-line drugs: isoniazid, rifampin, ethambutol, and pyrazinamide. Since Mr. T is Asian and foreign-born, he is at higher risk of having disease resistant to one or more of the first-line medications. The initial use of four drugs to start is consistant with ATS/CDC recommendations. The patient has no risk factors for drug complications.

19. Should Mr. T be isolated at this time?

Yes. The combination of exposure to TB, positive PPD, and positive CXR with positive sputum AFB smear is enough evidence to require isolation.

 ## More on Mr. T

Two months later Mr. T continues to feel well. Initial sputum AFB cultures were positive for TB, and the organism is sensitive to all drugs. No further sputum is produced. His liver profile reveals elevation of liver enzymes to approximately two times normal, and his chest radiograph is minimally changed from the initial film.

QUESTIONS	ANSWERS
20. Should the treatment be discontinued? If so, what new form of treatment should be instituted? If not, how should Mr. T be monitored?	No, treatment should not be discontinued. Normally, treatment is not discontinued until liver enzymes increase to 3 times normal. Monthly liver enzyme levels, sputum AFB, and chest x-ray are monitored.
21. Can any of the medications be stopped at this time?	Yes, the isoniazid and rifampin would be adequate for the treatment protocol.
22. How long should therapy be continued?	A classic treatment regimen calls for continuation of isoniazid and rifampin for 4 more months.

 ## Mr. T Conclusion

One month later, follow-up liver profiles slowly return toward normal levels, and Mr. T continues to feel well. His chest radiograph is not significantly changed, but he is not coughing and no longer produces sputum. ■

KEY POINTS

- According to the World Health Organization, tuberculosis (TB) is the number one cause of infectious disease-related deaths in the world. Globally, about 9 million new cases of TB were diagnosed in 2003 and in that same year TB killed 1.75 million people.
- The organism that causes TB, *Mycobacterium tuberculosis*, is a nonmotile, non-sporulating, rod-shaped, acid-fast bacillus (AFB) with a dimension of approximately 0.2×5.0 mm.
- *M. tuberculosis* is almost exclusively transmitted by very small, aerosolized droplets usually less than 8 to 10 microns in diameter.
- The initial lung lesion in TB is called a Ghon nodule, and the combination of the initial lung lesion and the affected regional (hilar) lymph node is known as the Ghon complex.
- The body's cell-mediated immune response is usually effective in controlling the initial lung infection, but it does not usually kill all the bacteria. Pockets of bacteria may lie dormant in either the primary (Ghon nodule) or metastatic sites.
- Some time after the initial infection has occurred, reactivation of the infection may take place in up to 10% of infected individuals. Reactivation is most common within the first 2 years after initial infection, but may occur up to several decades later.
- About 90% of TB patients in the non-HIV-infected population seen at medical clinics present with reactivated TB.
- TB patients may complain of fatigue, low-grade fever, night sweats, chronic cough, sputum production, hemoptysis, pleuritic chest pain, and/or weight loss.
- Reactivation TB usually causes infiltrates in the apical-posterior segments of the upper lobes. In contrast, the most common abnormality on the chest radiograph of the patient with primary TB is hilar lymph node enlargement.
- The Mantoux skin test for TB is an intracutaneous injection of a standardized dose of purified protein derivative (PPD). A positive reaction is indicated by a visible or palpable induration (i.e., raised, hardened area) caused by prior sensitization to the TB organism.
- The current standard treatment regimen for TB is four drugs for 2 months followed by two drugs for 4 months.
- The most common side effect of rifampin, isoniazid, and pyrazinamide is chemical hepatitis.
- One of the most cost-effective methods of combating TB is called directly observed treatment (DOT). DOT calls for health-care workers to ensure appropriate treatment by watching their TB patients take each dose of the medications over the full course of treatment.

REFERENCES

1. World Health Organization. WHO Report 2004: Global tuberculosis control. Geneva, Switzerland: World Health Organization, WHO/CDS/TB/2004. 331. Available at http://www.who.int/tb/publications/global_report/en/.
2. Trends in TB–U.S., 98–03, MMWR 53:209, 2004.
3. Bass, JB: Epidemiology of tuberculosis. Available at uptodate.com.
4. Basgoz, N: Clinical manifestations of pulmonary tuberculosis. Available at uptodate.com.
5. Krysl, J, Korzeniewska-Kosela, M, Muller, NL, FitzGerald, JM: Radiologic features of pulmonary tuberculosis: an assessment of 188 cases. Can Assoc Radiol J 45:101, 1994.

20

Lung Cancer

Gregory A. B. Cheek, MD, FCCP, MSPH

CHAPTER OBJECTIVES:

After reading this chapter you will be able to identify:

- The incidence, causes, and cell types of lung cancer.
- The most common clinical presentation for lung cancer.
- How the history and physical examination, laboratory studies, imaging techniques, and invasive diagnostic procedures are used in the evaluation of patients with lung cancer.
- The updated staging classification system for lung cancer and its implications on therapy and prognosis.
- The current treatment modalities recommended for lung cancer patients.

INTRODUCTION

Lung cancer, also called bronchogenic carcinoma, is now the most common fatal cancer in both men and women in the United States. According to the American Cancer Society, 172,500 new cases of lung cancer were diagnosed in 2005 and 163,510 deaths occurred due to the disease.[1] Currently, about 30% of all cancer deaths in men (90,000) and 25% of all cancer deaths in women (73,000) each year are due to lung cancer.[1] Despite advances in methods of diagnosis, staging, and therapy of lung cancer over the past 30 years, the overall 5-year survival rate still does not exceed 15% but is double compared to 8% survival in 1960.[2] Primary prevention, earlier diagnosis, and more effective therapy become ever more important as the worldwide incidence of lung cancer rises.

The term malignant denotes the lethal behavior of abnormal tissue that serves no purpose and spreads unchecked at the expense of healthy tissue. This chapter discusses those malignancies (four major types) that arise within the lung itself, called bronchogenic carcinoma (primary lung cancer), but not those that arrive in the lung from other tissues (metastatic malignancies).

ETIOLOGY

Most scientists agree that cigarette smoking causes lung cancer. There is a strong association between smoking exposure and the incidence of bronchogenic carcinoma.[3]

Between 10% and 20% of all smokers eventually get lung cancer, and over 80% of all lung cancer patients smoke, have smoked, or were chronically exposed to passive smoke.[4] The risk of lung cancer is related to the number of cigarettes smoked, the duration (in years) of smoking, the age at initiation of smoking, the depth of inhalation, and the tar

Table 20.1 Relative Risk of Lung Cancer

Patient History	Risk Ratio*
Never smoked; no significant industrial contact	1
Cigarette smoker:	
• <1/2 pack/day	15
• 1/2–1 pack/day	17
• 1–2 packs/day	42
• >2 packs/day	64
Cigar smoker	3
Pipe smoker	8
Ex-smoker	2–10
Nonsmoking spouse exposed to spouse's smoke	1.4–1.9
Asbestos worker	
• Nonsmoker	5
• Cigarette smoker	92
Uranium miner	
• Nonsmoker	7
• Cigarette smoker	38
Relatives of lung cancer patients	
• Nonsmokers	4
• Smokers	14

SOURCE: Adapted from Murray, JF, Nadel, JA: *Textbook of Respiratory Medicine.* WB Saunders, Philadelphia, 1988, p. 1177, with permission.
  *The risk ratio is the relative risk of developing lung cancer compared to the risk of comparable individuals without the listed exposure.

and nicotine content in cigarettes smoked. There is about a 10- to 25-fold greater risk of lung cancer among smokers than among life-long nonsmokers.[5] A person's lung cancer risk gradually declines for about 13 years after smoking cessation, but it never quite reaches a nonsmoker's risk level.[6]

A nonsmoker in the vicinity of a smoker inhales side-stream smoke that contains higher concentrations of carcinogens than the smoke inhaled by the smoker. There is about a 30% increased risk of lung cancer in individuals exposed to passive smoke.[6-8] Exposure to certain irritant fibers, ionizing radiation, and fumes from various chemicals has also been linked to an increased incidence of lung cancer. These agents include asbestos, chromium, nickel, uranium, vinyl chloride, bischloromethyl ether, and decay products of radon gas.[6,9] Many of these materials potentiate the effect of cigarette smoke in the induction of bronchogenic carcinoma. Asbestos exposure in nonsmokers has been associated with a seven-fold increase in the incidence of lung cancer, with a peak incidence 30 to 35 years after the exposure. Asbestos exposure in cigarette smokers is associated with a 92-fold increase in the incidence of lung cancer (Table 20.1).[6,10] Smoking cessation, reduction, and prevention are essential to reduce the rapidly growing worldwide epidemic of tobacco-related carcinogenesis and lung cancer.[11]

Other risk factors may include air pollution, cigar or pipe use, and lung scars.[4] The reducing type of pollutants (e.g., sulfur dioxide, carbonaceous particulate matter) are thought to be carcinogens, whereas oxidants (e.g., hydrocarbons, nitrous oxides) are not.

Exposure to combustion fumes from solid fuel (coal) used for indoor heating or cooking is associated with a 22% overall increased risk of lung cancer.[12]

A family history of lung cancer increases an individual's risk for developing the disease. Compared to the general population, lung cancer is three times more likely to develop in persons who have close relatives with the disease.[13,14] A personal or family history of malignancy suggests a genetic predisposition, that is, the presence (over-expression) of a tumor-growth promoting gene (oncogene) or a defective or absent tumor suppressor gene or both.[15] Sarcoidosis is associated with a threefold increase incidence of lung cancer.[16]

While several preventive agents, known as chemoprevention, including herbal and vitamin supplements (anti-oxidants) and drugs (e.g., celecoxib-Celebrex®), have been proposed to reduce the development of lung cancer in susceptible individuals, none can be advised at this time due to the lack of convincing evidence for benefit and data showing potential for harm with some agents (e.g., beta-carotene). Those agents that hold theoretical benefit are still being studied in clinical trials.[17,18] Interestingly, a diet high in fruits and vegetables appears to reduce the incidence of lung cancer compared to the general population.[6,19]

PATHOPHYSIOLOGY

The four major histological types of lung cancer are squamous cell carcinoma (29%), adenocarcinoma (32%), large-cell carcinoma (9%), and small-cell carcinoma (18%).[20,21] The clinical behavior of small-cell carcinoma is much different from that of the other three forms of lung cancer, which all act very much the same. Because of this difference, lung cancers are usually classified in terms of small-cell (SCLC) and non-small-cell lung carcinoma (NSCLC).[15,22]

Squamous cell carcinoma is named for the appearance of cells that resemble those of the skin (epidermis). These cells usually contain the skin protein keratin. Squamous cell carcinomas arise most often from the bronchial lining and may grow to obstruct air passages.[22]

Adenocarcinoma resembles poorly formed glandular tissue. It may be difficult to determine whether an adenocarcinoma is a primary lung cancer or a metastatic malignancy from elsewhere in the body. Many organs in the body can develop adenocarcinoma that may metastasize to the lungs.[22] The bronchoalveolar cell carcinoma is a unique subtype of adenocarcinoma that grows primarily along the walls of alveoli (air sacs) and airways and is associated with an improved surgical resectability and prognosis if diagnosed early.[23]

Large-cell carcinomas are characterized by a collection of poorly formed large cells that have abundant cytoplasm. These tumors may exhibit a gland-like structure and produce some mucin.[22]

Small-cell carcinomas generally arise from neuroendocrine cells of the lung and are characterized by very small cells with scant cytoplasm that resemble oats—hence the alternative name "oat cell cancer." Small-cell carcinoma is a very rapidly growing tumor that usually metastasizes to distant tissue (e.g., brain, liver, bone) while the tumor is quite small.[24]

Lung cancer can affect lung function in a variety of ways, depending on the size and location of the tumor. Small, peripheral lung tumors may not impair lung function in a noticeable way. Larger tumors may invade the lung parenchyma and reduce lung volume in an amount proportional to the size of the growth. Cancerous growths may obstruct a major airway and result in pooling of secretions and little or no gas exchange distal to the obstruction. The affected lung region will typically become atelectatic and susceptible to pneumonia.

CLINICAL PRESENTATION

A complete medical history and physical examination is essential when evaluating a patient for lung cancer. Emphasis is placed on identifying symptoms commonly associated with lung cancer (Table 20.2) and identifying (staging) the extent of organ systems involved by the disease. It is also important to identify functional limitations caused by concurrent cardiac or respiratory disease or other conditions that may adversely influence the patient's ability to undergo resective (curative) surgery or receive other therapies.

History

The clinical presentation of lung cancer depends on several variables, including cell type, growth rate, where in the lung it originates, and the integrity of the host immune system.

Table 20.2 Clinical Manifestations of Bronchogenic Carcinoma

Cough	74%
Weight loss	68%
Dyspnea	58%
Chest pain	49%
Sputum production	45%
Hemoptysis	29%
Malaise	26%
Bone pain	25%
Lymphadenopathy	23%
Hepatomegaly	21%
Fever	21%
Clubbing	20%
Neuromyopathy	10%
Superior vena cava syndrome	4%
Dizziness	4%
Hoarseness	3%
Asymptomatic	12%

SOURCE: Adapted from Doyle, LA, Aisner, J: Clinical presentation of lung cancer. In Roth, JA, Ruckdeschel, JC, Weisenburger, TH (eds): *Thoracic Oncology.* WB Saunders, Philadelphia, 1989, p. 53.

Approximately 10% to 15% of patients are asymptomatic at the time of diagnosis (e.g., an incidental lung nodule seen on chest radiograph or computerized tomography).[25,26] Over 70% of all lung cancer patients present with symptoms that are due either to local intrathoracic or to distant metastatic effects of tumor.[25,27]

Pulmonary symptoms associated with lung cancer may include a change in cough or sputum production, hemoptysis, wheezing, dyspnea, stridor, chest pain, or fever. These findings may provide the first clue that lung cancer is present and would indicate that the cancer is obstructing airways and lymphatics.

Cough and sputum production are not specific symptoms, as the majority of lung cancer patients have chronic bronchitis and emphysema from cigarette smoking. However, a change in the character of the cough, a change in the quality and quantity of sputum, or unresponsiveness to previously effective therapy (e.g., bronchodilators, antibiotics, steroids) should raise the suspicion that a tumor may be present.

Shortness of breath may be associated with lung cancer when the tumor obstructs a large airway. Large pleural effusions or paralysis of a hemidiaphragm resulting from phrenic nerve involvement may contribute to the patient's complaint of dyspnea.

Hemoptysis associated with lung cancer is caused by ulceration of the bronchial mucosa. The quantity of blood is usually small, but it can become massive and life-threatening. Hemoptysis usually prompts the patient to seek medical attention and should raise suspicion of endobronchial tumor.

Chest pain in lung cancer may indicate local invasion of the pleura, ribs, and nerves. It may be dull, constant, and debilitating or intermittent and sharp, varying with the respiratory cycle. It may localize to the chest wall, or radiate to the mid-back, scapula, shoulder, or arm on the side of the tumor. Chest pain may decrease as a pleural effusion develops and grows.

Physical Examination

Physical examination of the patient with lung cancer may be relatively normal when the tumor is small and located peripherally. Auscultation may reveal wheezing if an airway is partially obstructed. The wheezing is usually monophonic, is localized, and does not disappear after a cough. Wheezing may be heard on inhalation and exhalation. Percussion will reveal diminished resonance over lung tissue affected by a large tumor, pleural effusion, or pneumonia (consolidation). Careful examination may reveal distant metastasis to skin or regional lymph nodes. Clubbing of the fingers or toes or both may indicate hypertrophic pulmonary osteoarthropathy (paraneoplastic syndrome) caused by subperiosteal new bone formation of the extremities associated with lung cancer (mostly adenocarcinoma).[28]

Physical examination may also reveal evidence of tumor spread, which precludes surgical resection. Hoarseness suggests left vocal cord paralysis caused by recurrent laryngeal nerve compression by tumor. Facial edema with distended veins of the upper chest suggests compression of the superior vena cava by tumor.[29] Tumor compression of the cervical sympathetic nerve plexus causes Horner's syndrome, which is ptosis (drooping eyelid), myosis (pinpoint pupil), and anhydrosis (lack of sweating of the cheek). Arm and shoulder pain suggests a superior sulcus tumor invading the brachial nerve plexus (called Pancoast's syndrome when combined with Horner's syndrome).[30] Bone pain suggests metastasis to the bone. Change in mental status, emotional status, or coordination suggests brain metastasis.

> The clinical symptoms of patients presenting with lung cancer are related to (1) local effects of the primary lesion on the lung and airways; (2) intrathoracic spread of the tumor to pleura, chest wall, nerves, vascular structures or vital organs; (3) distant metastases, for example, to adrenals, brain, or bones; or (4) a paraneoplastic syndrome.

Metastatic Disease

Clues to metastatic disease may include chest wall or distant bone pain, seizures from brain metastasis, stroke from tumor emboli, paraplegia from spread to the spinal cord, or weight loss associated with liver metastasis.

Patients with advanced lung cancer may present with the following:

- Nonspecific systemic symptoms
- Signs and symptoms of intrathoracic spread
- Signs and symptoms of extrathoracic extension
- Classic systemic paraneoplastic syndromes

Nonspecific Systemic Symptoms

Nonspecific systemic symptoms include weight loss, anorexia, nausea, vomiting, and weakness. Systemic symptoms do not necessarily indicate that the tumor is unresectable but this is generally a poor prognostic sign.

Intrathoracic Spread

Signs of tumor spread or metastases within the chest may include (1) pleural effusion, (2) superior vena cava syndrome, (3) brachial neuritis, (4) hoarseness, (5) pericardial effusion, (6) diaphragm elevation, and (7) malignant central airway obstruction.

1. Pleural effusion is a collection of fluid in the pleural space around the lung. It may be caused by direct extension of the lung tumor to the pleural surface, by blockage of lymphatic ducts, or by pneumonia associated with malignancy. Tumor cells invading lymphatics obstruct normal lymph flow in the lung and result in the accumulation of fluid in the pleural space.
2. Superior vena cava syndrome is caused by tumor compression or direct invasion of the great veins in the thoracic outlet. It is associated with dyspnea, headache, and periorbital, facial, neck, and upper trunk edema. Collateral circulation across the upper thorax and neck is usually prominent and very distended.

3. Brachial neuritis is typically caused by a superior sulcus tumor (most often squamous cell carcinoma located in the lung apex, which may be pleural based) called Pancoast's tumor that grows through the parietal pleura and invades the brachial plexus. Involvement of the last cervical and first thoracic (C7 to T2) segment of the sympathetic nerve trunk results in a triad of clinical findings called Horner's syndrome (see physical examination for definition).

4. Pressure on the recurrent laryngeal nerve from tumor or enlarged lymph nodes causes nerve disruption resulting in left vocal cord paralysis and hoarseness.

5. Pericardial effusion (fluid in the sac around the heart) is a serious complication of thoracic cancer caused by metastasis or direct tumor extension into the pericardium and epicardium. It causes neck vein distension, cardiac arrhythmias, and cardiac tamponade (fluid compressing on the heart muscle preventing it from pumping blood, which may be fatal).

6. Unilateral hemidiaphragmatic paralysis with paradoxic motion (upward motion on rapid inspiration) on fluoroscopy may occur as a result of phrenic nerve involvement.

Extrathoracic Spread

Symptoms of extrathoracic spread or distant metastases depend on the sites involved. Common sites of spread include lymph nodes, brain and spinal cord, liver, adrenal glands, bone, bone marrow, and skin. Bone and central nervous system (CNS) spread usually results in symptomatic disease, whereas liver and adrenal gland metastases may be asymptomatic.

Paraneoplastic Syndromes

A constellation of symptoms and signs at a site distant from the primary tumor, unrelated to local effects or metastases, is termed a *paraneoplastic syndrome*. These may serve as the first sign of disease because they often occur before evidence of the primary tumor. The cancer produces its effects on one or multiple organ systems, including endocrine, hematologic, renal, cutaneous, and neurologic, often through poorly understood mechanisms. The more common (well-studied) syndromes include ectopic production of peptide proteins (hormones) or immunologic mechanisms. Examples include the ectopic production of antidiuretic hormone (SIADH) or parathyroid hormone-related protein (humoral hypercalcemia of malignancy) and antibodies formed against channels in the neuromuscular junction causing myasthenia gravis-like symptoms (Lambert-Eaton syndrome). Their prognostic implications are varied, and paraneoplastic effects may occur without evidence of gross extrathoracic disease or spread. Scientists believe that unraveling the mechanisms that produce these syndromes will lead to insight into tumor biology that will be translated into novel approaches for early detection and therapy.[31]

DIAGNOSIS

Early Detection and Screening for Lung Cancer

The overall 5-year survival rate for patients presenting with carcinoma of the lung is only about 10% to 15%.[2] This dismal statistic reflects the fact that the disease is usually advanced when first detected. Based on all the evidence collected to this point, routine or frequent screening with sputum cytology and chest radiographs has not yet proved to alter the mortality rate and is not cost-effective, but trials sponsored by the National Cancer Institute (NCI) are ongoing. The evidence for screening high-risk populations with low-dose computerized tomography (LDCT) of the chest appears more promising (but final results of the studies are not yet available), since the technology is able to identify lung cancer at an earlier stage, theoretically improving treatment options and odds of survival.[32–35] Evidence is not yet convincing enough to warrant a general recommendation regarding the cost-effectiveness and survival benefit, and clinical trials are ongoing to better define the role of LDCT in the evaluation of asymptomatic high-risk individuals.[36–37] No professional or governmental organization currently recommends the routine screening of asymptomatic patients at risk for lung cancer with LDCT or other methods.[38]

Other proposed screening tools to assist in early detection of lung cancer in the high-risk population include autofluorescence bronchoscopy, analysis of exhaled volatile organic compounds in the breath, and immunostaining of sputum or serum for specific proteins or genetic markers of tumors.[15,39–41]

Diagnostic Studies

Further investigative testing is appropriate in patients with symptoms or clinical manifestations suggesting the presence of lung cancer, particularly if known risk factors are present, adding to clinical suspicion.[42]

In patients with lung cancer, the abnormal components of the history and physical examination are used to direct further diagnostic studies to eventually establish a tissue diagnosis and clinical stage. Essential diagnostic tools include imaging techniques, noninvasive laboratory studies, and invasive procedures. The initial aims of diagnostic testing are twofold: (1) to confirm the clinical diagnosis by cytology (cells) or histology (tissue) and (2) to establish the extent of dissemination (stage) of the disease. This information will be used to direct suitable treatment (e.g., surgery, chemotherapy, irradiation, or best-supportive/palliative or hospice care and determine prognosis.

IMAGING TECHNIQUES
Several imaging techniques play an important role in the diagnosis and staging of patients with lung cancer, including standard chest radiography, computerized tomography (CT) scanning, and magnetic resonance imaging (MRI). In recent years, the 5-flurodeoxy glucose-positron emission tomography (FDG-PET) scan, which measures the uptake of radiolabled glucose substrate by tissue with a high metabolic (growth) rate has made a significant contribution to the diagnosis and staging process, especially when combined with CT scan findings.[43]

Radiographic Imaging
The chest radiograph plays a pivotal role in the recognition of lung cancer. The chest radiograph may demonstrate asymptomatic lung cancer but is almost always abnormal when the patient is symptomatic. A tumor nodule must be at least 3 to 5 mm before it is visible on a chest radiograph. The *solitary pulmonary nodule* (SPN) is a focal lesion seen on chest radiograph, located in the lung tissue or parenchyma (surrounded by aerated lung) described in terms of margins (well or poorly marginated), shape (roughly circumscribed, round, or oval shaped) and size (measuring less than 3 cm in diameter). Lesions 3 cm in diameter or greater are called lung masses.

A common dilemma with the SPN, also called "coin lesion," found incidentally on imaging studies done for other reasons, is whether it represents a small bronchogenic cancer or a more benign process (infectious, inflammatory, vascular, traumatic, or congenital lesion). Clues as to the probability of malignancy include growth rate, margin configuration, and presence of calcification. Malignant tumors grow at a rate such that the number of

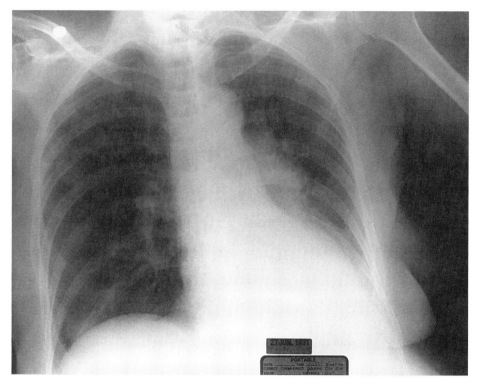

FIGURE 20.1 Chest radiograph demonstrating tumor obstruction of left lower lobe bronchus ("cutoff sign") leading to atelectasis distal to obstruction and mediastinal shift toward the lung volume loss.

cells in the tumor doubles at least every 120 days, but not more often than every 30 days.[26] Careful measurement is important because a tumor or granuloma is a three-dimensional sphere, so doubling of its volume changes its diameter only by a factor of 1.27. Tumor margins are most often irregular and indistinct because tumors invade neighboring tissue, whereas granulomas often develop around a central area of inflammation and therefore have very smooth, distinct borders. Tumors rarely develop asymmetric calcification, whereas granulomas develop central, well-defined calcification. A rare benign tumor called a hamartoma is noted for developing a pattern of calcification with a "popcorn ball" configuration.

Given the inconsistencies of plain chest radiographic technique with inherent inaccuracies in the identification and measurement, referral for chest CT is standard for nearly all newly suspected SPNs and lung masses. Chest CT offers more accurate size comparisons (especially with smaller nodules) and discrimination of margins and may reveal hidden calcifications, satellite nodules, and lymphadenopathy.[44,45]

The heart and other thoracic structures obscure large portions of the lung tissue, and it is important to evaluate both a frontal and side view before calling a chest radiograph "normal." The four most common types of bronchogenic carcinoma (squamous cell, adenocarcinoma, small cell, and large cell) present with slightly different chest radiographic patterns, but there is so much overlap that only biopsy and histological examination provide reliable evidence about the cell type.

Obstruction of a main or segmental bronchus may be associated with atelectasis. Atelectasis causes a shift of the mediastinum toward the lesion and is best seen on a maximal inspiratory chest radiograph (Figures 20.1, 20.2, and 20.3).

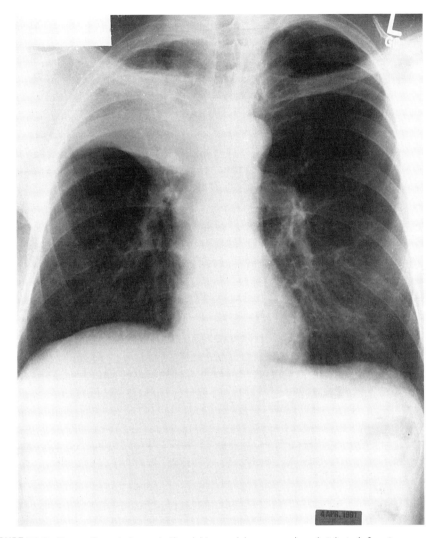

FIGURE 20.2   Chest radiograph demonstrating right upper lobe pneumonia and atelectasis from tumor obstruction of a major airway.

Chest Computed Tomography

Chest CT has become the major imaging modality of choice for evaluation of patients with lung cancer. CT is much more sensitive than radiographs to detect calcifications, satellite nodules, direct extension of the primary tumor, or regional lymph node enlargement, suggesting spread (Figure 20.4). However, given the limited specificity of chest CT, abnormal mediastinal lymph node findings alone in an otherwise operable patient should never preclude thoracotomy for surgical resection, without biopsy confirming tumor spread.[46]

Axial CT views using "soft tissue" windows can show the location of lymph nodes or masses adjacent to the airways to direct future bronchoscopic or percutaneous needle biopsies. A high-resolution (thin-section) CT may be reformatted with specialized software into a three-dimensional image to more precisely demonstrate the airway anatomy, called an "airway study." The airway study also demonstrates the location (which airways are involved), the type (extrinsic compression and/or endobronchial growth), extent (length), and severity of narrowing due to a lung cancer growth causing airway stenosis (Figure 20.5).

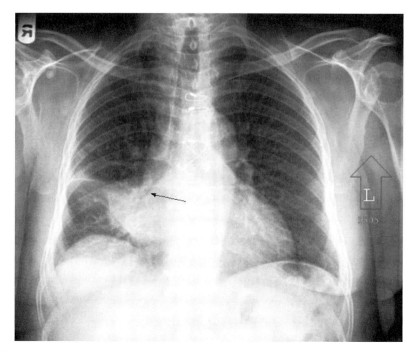

FIGURE 20.3 Chest radiograph demonstrating atelectasis of the right middle lobe due to a tumor obstructing the segmental bronchus, causing an obscured border of the right cardiac shadow. Note tapering of the right bronchus intermedius airway (arrow).

Magnetic Resonance Imaging

MRI is not better than CT for evaluating pulmonary nodules or mediastinal metastases and is more expensive. However, MRI is better able to show chest wall invasion and has greater specificity than CT regarding invasion of vascular structures in the mediastinum. MRI is more sensitive than CT in imaging the brain, especially when looking for small metastases.[46]

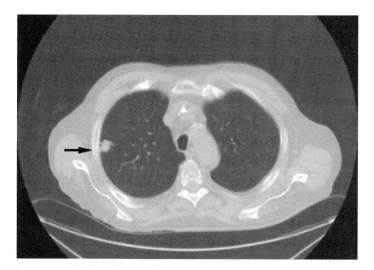

FIGURE 20.4 Chest CT showing SPN with irregular or spiculated margins, suggesting malignancy.

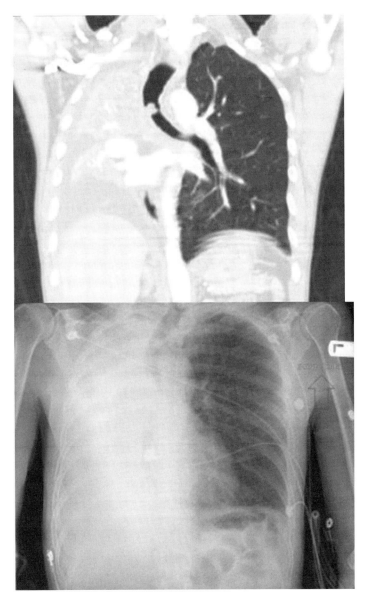

FIGURE 20.5 Chest radiograph paired with a chest CT, coronal reconstruction view in the same patient seen in Figure 20.3 as the tumor progressed, demonstrating complete right lung obstruction with airway tumor protruding from the right main bronchus into the trachea.

Positron Emission Tomography

The role for the PET (positron emission tomography) scan, which uses FDG (5-fluoro-deoxy glucose) tagged with a radionucliide to assess metabolic activity of soft tissues is evolving, in particular regarding the SPN and lymphadenopathy. The PET scan is a metabolic imaging technique based on the function of a tissue rather than its anatomy and has proven more sensitive and specific than CT for staging the mediastinum (presence of nodal disease) and showing distant metastases. When it is coupled (fused) with a CT scan, more accurate and useful staging information is obtained. Tissue biopsy is needed to confirm a positive scan in a patient who would be otherwise operable/resectable. The greatest benefit of PET appears to be a reduction in "futile" (unnecessary) surgery (41% down to 21%) by detecting occult metastases (more sensitive and specific than bone scan for bony metastases). The PET scan is also being tested as a screening tool combined with LDCT for evaluating and following lung nodules of $\geq$7 mm in size over time.

Limitations include false positives (inflammation or infection) and false negatives (bronchoalveolar cell carcinoma, carcinoid and lesions <1 cm). In the past most patients with evidence of mediastinal lymphadenopathy (nodes >1 cm) and central or large (>6 cm) peripheral lesions have had a diagnostic mediastinoscopy pre- or intra-operatively before curative resection is attempted.[47–49]

Laboratory Studies

Other diagnostic tests that may reflect local, metastatic, or paraneoplastic effects of lung cancer include serum chemistry, complete blood count (CBC), liver function, arterial blood gas (ABG), the 12-lead electrocardiogram (ECG), and pulmonary function tests. Hyponatremia occurs in the presence of ectopic (hormone produced by tumor cells) antidiuretic hormone (ADH), most often from small-cell carcinoma. Hypercalcemia in lung cancer occurs either from metastatic tumor spread to bone or from a parathyroid hormone-like substance most often associated with squamous cell carcinoma. Alkaline phosphatase may be elevated in the presence of bone or liver metastases. Liver dysfunction may occur because of intrahepatic spread and/or extrahepatic obstruction from metastatic disease. Anemia (low hemoglobin), thrombocytopenia (low platelet count), leukoerythroblastic (immature blood cell forms resembling leukemia) peripheral blood pattern, and even pancytopenia (low count of all blood cell types) may occur from metastatic spread of tumor to bone marrow.

The ECG may show low voltage or pulsus alternans (amplitude of QRS waveform varies with respiration) from pericardial effusion or a conduction block from metastatic disease. A murmur may indicate marantic endocarditis (noninfectious vegetations on heart valves) or spread of tumor via pulmonary vein to form an intracardiac mass. Pulmonary function tests may indicate restrictive disease owing to lymphatic spread or effect of the tumor compressing the lung tissue or airways. ABGs may show hypoxemia resulting from ventilation-perfusion abnormalities or shunting.

Diagnostic Procedures

Methods currently utilized for providing a definitive diagnosis and clinical staging of bronchogenic carcinoma include sputum cytology, fiberoptic bronchoscopy (including washings, brushings, forceps biopsy of mucosa and lung tissue, or transbronchial needle aspiration biopsies), trans-esophageal endoscopic ultrasound-guided needle aspiration, image-guided percutaneous transthoracic needle aspiration (TTNA) (also called fine-needle aspiration [FNA]), thoracentesis, pleural biopsy, thoracoscopy, mediastinoscopy, and video-assisted thoracoscopic surgery (VATS). Each method has its unique usefulness and diagnostic yield, as well as potential risks and technical limitations.

> The primary goals of the diagnostic evaluation in lung cancer include (1) confirming the presence and tissue type of the malignancy and (2) defining the clinical stage or spread of the tumor to determine surgical resectability.

Diagnosis and Clinical Staging

Noninvasive Diagnostic Testing

Sputum cytology is most useful for diagnosing central airway (e.g., squamous cell) carcinomas. Potential problems in accurately interpreting sputum cytology specimens include:

- Inadequate specimen without alveolar macrophages (less than 3 to 4/high-power field [hpf]) or greater than 5 to 10 epithelial cells/hpf.
- Degeneration of malignant cells before examination
- Purulent samples
- Inexperience of cytologist-technician (bronchial squamous cell metaplasia frequent in chronic bronchitis makes distinction of malignancy difficult)
- Cell clumps that resemble adenocarcinoma possibly present in asthma patients
- Lipoid pneumonia and pulmonary infarction that may produce cellular changes and are easily confused with malignancy.[50]

The sensitivity of sputum cytology for central airway lesions is about 70% and decreases to about 50% for peripheral lesions. Cytologic evaluation of sputum offers little help to patients with peripheral lesions or solitary pulmonary nodules, due to the very low reported yield.[51]

Invasive Diagnostic Procedures
Flexible Fiberoptic Bronchoscopy
The flexible fiberoptic bronchoscope is a small-bore, *flexible* tube with a light source going to the tip (*fiberoptic*) and a port for suctioning secretions, flushing with saline, and passing small instruments for sampling cytology or tissue (e.g., brush, forceps, needle) or as a part of providing other interventions (e.g., electrocautery, laser, balloon dilators) in the trachea or bronchial airways. The angle, direction, and location of the tip of the bronchoscope is controlled by the operator's thumb movement, wrist rotation, and relative depth of passage into the airway (via nose or mouth) (Figure 20.6). It may be performed using local anesthesia with or without IV (moderate) sedation in the outpatient setting. A specially trained respiratory therapist assists the physician during the procedure, while the patient's vital signs are monitored closely. The location and extent of tumor spread within the airways is assessed by direct observation, allowing more accurate diagnosis and staging of visible endobronchial tumors. Findings that suggest malignancy may include widening of the carina, narrowing or obstruction of the airway from endobronchial (exophytic) growth or (submucosal) infiltration, extrinsic compression, or a combination of both. The involved airway often shows erythema, loss of bronchial markings, and thickening or nodular appearance of the bronchial mucosal lining.

A tissue diagnosis (or cytology) is essential to determine tumor histology. Endoscopic diagnostic (sampling) techniques include bronchial washings, brushings,

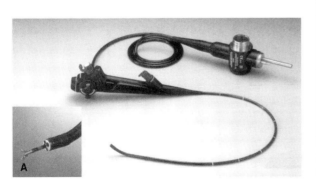
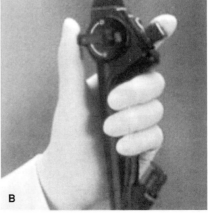

FIGURE 20.6 (A) Flexible fiberoptic bronchoscope; (B) view of hand control mechanism.

endobronchial needle aspiration and forceps biopsy, transbronchial needle aspiration and transbronchial forceps (lung tissue) biopsy, and bronchoalveolar lavage. When lesions are visible (central) in the bronchial airway, *bronchial washings* have a diagnostic yield of approximately 68%; *bronchial brushings* and *bronchial mucosal forceps biopsy* samples provide a "tissue-type" diagnosis in roughly 70% to 80% percent of visualized tumors and up to 90% when combining techniques for exophytic airway lesions.[52]

False-negative results may occur in deeper submucosal lesions owing to the inability to grasp and sample directly. Transbronchial forceps (lung tissue) biopsies using fluoroscopic guidance plus brushings and washings can diagnose more peripheral, parenchymal lesions up to 60% to 70% of the time, for lesions >2 cm. The sensitivity of bronchoscopy is usually poor for peripheral lesions that are <2 cm in diameter. Transbronchial lung tissue (forceps) biopsies carry a higher risk of bleeding (occasionally massive) and pneumothorax.[53] Bronchoalveolar lavage provides between a 33% and 69% yield for peripheral lesions.[52]

Transbronchial Needle Aspiration (TBNA)

Transbronchial needle aspiration (TBNA) may obtain a sample of tumor cells or tissue "core" capable of providing a diagnosis and mediastinal staging of lung cancer.[54] TBNA uses a 19-, 21-, or 22-gauge needle-tipped catheter passed through a flexible bronchoscope and entered directly into a submucosal lesion in the airway or across the tracheal/bronchial wall into enlarged lymph nodes or masses adjacent to the airways (e.g., below the main carina), using prior chest CT/PET scan results for guidance. One of a variety of entry methods may be used for passing the needle across the airway wall, including the jabbing, piggyback, cough, or "hub against the wall" methods.[55] The yield ranges between 30% and 70% and is subject to variable operator experience and on-site sampling and processing techniques. A higher yield of up to 75% is obtained when TBNA is consistently performed using (1) ultrasound guidance (*endobronchial ultrasound-EBUS*) to direct the needle across the wall of the trachea/bronchus toward a lesion, (2) rapid on-site evaluation (ROSE) to confirm adequate cellularity of the samples, and (3) immediate quick-prep fixation of the specimen once acquired.[52,56,57]

Radiographic guidance using fluoroscopy and chest CT during bronchoscopy for transbronchial biopsy or sampling of peripheral lung lesions, while shown to improve diagnostic yield, exposes the patient and medical personnel to considerable radiation. Endobronchial ultrasound technology, while shown to improve the yield of extrabronchial lesions (especially <3 cm), is demanding, and the probes cannot easily be steered beyond the visible parts of the airways. A new innovative technique called *superDimension*® bronchoscopy, recently tested in humans under general anesthesia, offers real-time, electromagnetic guidance using a retractable sensor probe (locatable guide) for navigation, coupled with preprocedure, digitalized and downloaded, three-dimensional CT images to create a "virtual" roadmap. While not widely available, it has been shown to be a feasible and safe method for obtaining transbronchial lung biopsies of peripheral lesions.[58]

Transthoracic Needle Aspiration (TTNA)

Transthoracic needle aspiration (TTNA) biopsy offers the highest overall diagnostic yield (up to 95%) for peripheral solitary pulmonary nodules as small as 2 cm that prove to be malignant.[52] Tumors located away from mediastinal vascular structures and emphysematous bullae are most suitable for this technique, with "core tissue" samples obtained using a 20-gauge needle. A fine-bore needle (e.g., 25 gauge) is often used if lesions are near high-pressure vascular structures. Tumors up to 12 cm deep can be reached by this method. The incidence of pneumothorax is 15% to 35% but varies widely and is more common in emphysematous patients. Only about 5% to 10% of patients with TTNA require any kind of thoracostomy tube placement for lung reexpansion after biopsy. Fluoroscopic guidance is adequate for nodules that are 2 cm or greater in diameter and visible on both frontal and lateral chest radiographs.[59] Nodules smaller than 2 cm in diameter are usually aspirated under CT guidance.[52] Bronchoscopy carries less risk of pneumothorax (less than 5% with transbronchial biopsy) and may be performed before TTNA.[60] Cytology samples can accurately distinguish between SCLC and NSCLC.[53]

A TTNA may be indicated before a thoracotomy to establish that a lesion is not small-cell carcinoma. Also, in a patient who is a poor surgical candidate (or refuses surgery) it may provide adequate cytologic diagnosis and obviate the need for exploratory thoracotomy.

Thoracentesis

A positive pleural fluid cytology may provide a diagnosis and show the spread of malignancy to the pleural space. Definitive diagnosis may be obtained from a cell block of centrifuged pleural fluid or positive histology from pleural biopsy. Thoracentesis and pleural biopsy combined provide up to a 90% diagnostic yield in patients with malignancy.[61] Most malignant pleural effusions are exudative. An exudative effusion has a pleural protein level of greater than 3.5 g/dL and a lactate dehydrogenase (LDH) level of greater than 200; pleural/serum protein ratios are greater than 0.5, and pleural/serum LDH ratios are greater than 0.6.

Mediastinoscopy

Historically, patients with evidence of mediastinal lymphadenopathy (lymph nodes greater than 1 cm) and with central or large (greater than 6 cm) peripheral lesions have usually had a diagnostic mediastinoscopy before undergoing a thoracotomy.[62] A mediastinal lymph node of any size or location showing increased metabolic activity on a PET scan in the presence of a known lung cancer should be biopsied before or during surgery to reassess the clinical stage before the patient undergoes a full thoracotomy to resect the tumor.[63] Mediastinal lymph nodes are involved on initial presentation in about 30% to 44% of all lung cancer patients.[56]

Mediastinoscopy has long been the gold standard among staging tests of mediastinal lymph nodes and offers direct visualization and biopsy with overall less risk than an exploratory thoracotomy. It is performed in the operating room, usually under general anesthesia on a stand-alone, outpatient basis or performed as a part of invasive diagnostic staging immediately prior to a scheduled thoracic surgical resection of a lung cancer. The procedure involves an incision just above the suprasternal notch, insertion of a mediastinoscope alongside the trachea, and biopsy of mediastinal lymph nodes. The average sensitivity to detect mediastinal lymph node involvement from lung cancer is about 80% to 85%, with an average false negative rate about 10%.[63]

Cancers in the left upper lobe (LUL) have a predilection for involving the lymph nodes in the aortopulmonary window (APW) station. These mediastinal lymph nodes are not accessible by standard cervical mediastinoscopy. The Chamberlain procedure (anterior mediastinotomy) is the usual method of assessing lymph nodes in this area, which involves an incision in the second or third intercostal space just to the left of the sternum with about an 87% sensitivity (10% false negative) rate.[63]

Mediastinoscopy and other invasive staging methods have decreased the percentage of unnecessary thoracotomies by accurately upstaging lung cancers with clinical evidence of mediastinal lymph node spread, particularly as PET scanning becomes more available.[64]

Trans-Esophageal Ultrasound-Guided Endoscopic Needle Aspiration

Trans-esophageal ultrasound-guided fine needle aspiration (EUS-FNA) is a valuable and minimally invasive method of evaluating mediastinal lymph nodes that are not accessible by TTNA, flexible bronchoscopy (TBNA), or cervical mediastinoscopy with an overall sensitivity of about 76%, but a false-negative rate of up to 26%.[56] While EUS-FNA provides a highly reliable alternative method of sampling APW lymph nodes, the false negative rate may be an issue.

Recent findings suggest that EUS-FNA, when added to mediastinoscopy, improves the preoperative staging of lung cancer and reduces unnecessary thoracotomies due to the complementary reach in detecting mediastinal lymph node metastases and the ability to assess mediastinal tumor invasion.[65]

Thoracoscopy

Thoracoscopy, or video-assisted thoracoscopic surgery (VATS), improves the diagnostic yield of a pleural effusion, usually exudative, caused by lung cancer. Biopsy specimens are taken under direct vision with a diagnostic yield of 93% to 96% for malignant pleural effusions.[66] VATS offers the most reliable and accurate alternative approach to invasively staged mediastinal lymph nodes not accessible on mediastinoscopy, especially among patients with potentially resectable lung cancer before a full thoracotomy is performed.[56]

> Invasive techniques used for mediastinal lymph node staging prior to a thoracotomy include (1) transbronchial needle aspiration, (2) transthoracic needle aspiration, (3) endoscopic ultrasound with needle aspiration, (4) mediastinoscopy, (5) Chamberlain procedure, and (6) video–assisted thoracoscopic surgery.

Pathologic Staging

Surgical thoracotomy with wedge resection, lobectomy, or pneumonectomy, provides a definitive diagnosis with pathologic staging and may offer the definitive treatment for patients with lung cancer. Diagnostic thoracotomy is performed in some patients with good lung function and early clinical stage, potentially resectable lung cancer (nodule) for both diagnosis and treatment. Systematic mediastinal lymph node dissection is routinely performed during surgical resection of lung cancer. The pathologist evaluates all the specimens resected to offer more precise pathologic staging information and allow physicians to formulate a more accurate prognosis to guide future therapy.

Staging Classification System

Staging the extent of lung cancer is essential for selecting appropriate therapy and avoiding unnecessary surgery. The staging classification system developed by the American Joint Committee and the Union Contre le Cancer in 1986 and modified in 1997 to more accurately reflect prognosis and outcomes of treatment provides a nomenclature that is accepted by specialists around the world.[67,68]

This system is based on the TNM system (T = primary *tumor*; N = regional lymph *nodes*; M = distant *metastasis* [spread of cancer to distant site identified on biopsy]). T describes the size of the tumor (Table 20.3). N describes the lymph node buds involved (Table 20.4). M is either present (M1) or absent (M0) (Table 20.5).

Table 20.3 Definition of Primary Tumor (T) Characteristics in Lung Cancer According to TNM System

Descriptor	Definition
TX	Primary tumor cannot be assessed or tumor proven by the presence of malignant cells in sputum or bronchial washings but not visualized on imaging studies or bronchoscopy
T0	No evidence of primary tumor
TIS	Carcinoma in situ
T1	A tumor that is 3.0 cm or less in greatest dimension, surrounded by lung or visceral pleura, and without bronchoscopic evidence of invasion more proximal than the lobar bronchus* (i.e., not in the main bronchus)
T2	A tumor with *any* of the following features of size or extent: More than 3.0 cm in greatest dimension Involves main bronchus, 2 cm or more distal to the carina Invades the visceral pleural Associated with atelectasis or obstructive pneumonitis that extends to the hilar region but does not involve entire lung
T3	A tumor of any size with direct invasion into the chest wall (including superior sulcus tumors), diaphragm, mediastinal pleura, or parietal pericardium without involving the heart, great vessels, trachea, esophagus, or vertebral body; or a tumor in the main bronchus within 2 cm of the carina without involving the carina; or associated atelectasis or obstructive pneumonitis of the entire lung
T4	A tumor of any size that directly invades any of the following: mediastinum, heart, great vessels, trachea, esophagus, vertebral body, or carina; separate (satellite) tumor nodule (s) within the same lobe as the primary tumor, ipsilateral lung; or tumor with a malignant pleural effusion** or pericardial effusion

*The uncommon superficial tumor of any size with its invasive component limited to the bronchial wall, which may extend proximal to the main bronchus, is also classified as T1.

**Most pleural effusions associated with lung cancer are due to tumor. However, there are a few patients in whom multiple cytopathologic examinations of pleural fluid are negative for tumor. In these cases fluid is nonbloody and is not an exudate. Such patients may be further evaluated by videothoracoscopy (VATS) and direct pleural biopsies. When these elements and clinical judgment dictate that the effusion is not related to the tumor, the effusion should be excluded as a staging element and the patient should be staged T1, T2, or T3.

Table 20.4 Definition of Nodal Involvement (N) in Lung Cancer by TNM Classification

Descriptor	Definition
NX	Regional lymph nodes cannot be assessed
N0	No demonstrable metastasis to regional lymph nodes
N1	Metastasis to lymph nodes in the peribronchial or ipsilateral hilar region, or both, including direct extension
N2	Metastasis to ipsilateral mediastinal lymph nodes and subcarinal lymph nodes
N3	Metastasis to contralateral mediastinal lymph nodes, contralateral hilar lymph nodes, ipsilateral or contralateral scalene or supraclavicular lymph nodes

All regional nodes are above the diaphragm. They include the intrathoracic, scalene, and supraclavicular nodes.

Table 20.5	Definition of Distant Metastasis (M) in Lung Cancer by TNM Classification
Descriptor	Definition
MX	Distant metastasis cannot be assessed
M0	No (known) distant metastasis
M1	Distant metastasis present; specify site(s). This includes separate tumor nodule(s) in the nonprimary tumor lobe(s) of the lung (ipsilateral or contralateral)

The TNM classification is used as a basis upon which to formulate seven stages of severity of lung cancer (Table 20.6). This system is primarily used in the management of NSCLC and provides a standard nomenclature for ongoing clinical trials.

SCLC is either *limited* disease (contained within the hemithorax, including ipsilateral hilar/mediastinal, or supraclavicular lymph nodes) or *extensive* disease (all others). Bone marrow evaluation is often performed if extensive disease is suspected.

TREATMENT AND PROGNOSIS

Most patients with lung cancer present with extensive disease and have a poor prognosis. The choice of therapy and the survival rate are related to the histological *cell type* of the tumor (i.e., NSCLC vs. SCLC), *clinical stage* of the lung cancer (i.e., I–IV), concurrent medical disease, and performance status at the time of diagnosis. SCLC acts as a systemic disease but may respond significantly to chemotherapy in limited stages, so the cornerstone of therapy is chemotherapy (see below). On the other hand, NSCLC may be cured surgically or require chemotherapy with or without radiation therapy to prolong life and reduce symptoms from the disease, depending on the clinical stage.

In "occult stage" (TX, N0, M0) NSCLC a diagnostic evaluation, including imaging studies and selective bronchoscopy, is required with close follow-up to identify the site and nature of the primary tumor. When discovered, these tumors are generally early stage and curable by surgery. Stage 0 NSCLC is the same as *carcinoma in situ* of the lung, noninvasive by definition, and should be curable with surgical resection. Surgical resection using the least extensive technique possible (segmentectomy or wedge resection) to preserve maximum normal pulmonary tissue is advised because these patients are at high risk for a second primary lung cancer (many unresectable).[69]

Endoscopic photodynamic therapy (PDT) uses a hematophorphyrin derivative injected into the blood, which is activated by direct exposure to a special light source being placed

Table 20.6 TNM Stage Grouping for Lung Cancer

Stage	TNM Subsets		
	T	N	M
Occult carcinoma	TX	N0	M0
0	TIS	Carcinoma in situ	
IA	T1	N0	M0
IB	T2	N0	M0
IIA	T1	N1	M0
IIB	T2	N1	M0
	T3	N0	M0
IIIA	T3	N1	M0
	T1-3	N2	M0
IIIB	Any T	N3	M0
	T4	Any N	M0
IV	Any T	Any N	M1

Above staging tables from flash card provided by: The Staging of Cancer: Staging for Lung Carcinoma", 6th edition, American Cancer Society, American Joint Committee on Cancer (AJCC), American College of Surgeons (ACS), American Society of Clinical Oncology (ASCO) (Form No. 3485.25-Rev. 1/03).

in the airway to create oxygen radicals that locally destroy tumor tissue. PDT is under clinical evaluation as an alternative to surgical resection in carefully selected patients with stage 0 NSCLC.[70] It appears most effective for very early central tumors that extend <1 cm within a bronchus, but its efficacy remains to be proven.[71]

In stages I and II the cancer is considered surgically resectable. Stage IIIA cancer may be surgically curable, but the perioperative risk is high and the survival benefit marginal. Cancers in stage IIIB are not surgically resectable and usually receive a combination of chemotherapy with radiotherapy. Stage IV lung cancer is treated primarily with chemotherapy.

In summary, treatments recommended for stages I to IV NSCLC are as follows:

- For stage IA and IB, the treatment is surgery.
- For stage IIA and IIB, the treatment is surgery.
- For stage IIIA, the treatment is surgery for some, neoadjuvant therapy followed by surgery for some, and chemotherapy and radiation therapy for some.
- For stage IIIB, except for some (T4N0M0-Pancoast), the treatment is chemotherapy and radiation therapy, preferably concurrently if possible.
- For stage IV, the treatment is best supportive care or chemotherapy.

Only 20% to 30% of all lung cancers (NSCLC type) are considered surgically resectable at the time of presentation. Postoperative survival primarily depends on the lung cancer stage at the time of surgical resection. The 5-year survival following surgery for stage I is 60% to 70%, which drops to 30% to 50% for stage II. For untreated stage IV disease the median survival is 4 months, and 1-year survival rate is 10%. With state of the art treatment the median survival rate improves.[72,73]

One of the most important indices of long-term survival in patients receiving therapy for lung cancer is their performance status at the time the lung cancer is diagnosed. The performance status is a fairly objective assessment of cardiopulmonary reserve and the effect the cancer and other concurrent medical illness have on the patient's ability to carry on with daily activities and work. Two scales are widely used in the United States: the Karnofsky Performance Scale and the Eastern Cooperative Oncology Group (ECOG), or Zubrod, Performance Scale.[74] A poor performance status with a low-stage lung cancer indicates that the cancer may be more widespread than believed or that the patient's physiological status is such that he or she will not tolerate therapy well. There is a very strong relationship between performance index and length of survival. Chronologic age is not an independent risk factor for patients being considered for lung cancer resection.[75]

Preoperative Pulmonary Evaluation

For patients undergoing thoracotomy for diagnosis or cure, several parameters must be measured to estimate

> Treatment decisions are based on three factors: (1) the tissue or cell type of the tumor (small–cell vs. non–small cell carcinoma), (2) surgical resectability or clinical stage of the tumor, and (3) medical operability based on performance status (cardiopulmonary reserve) and concurrent medical diseases. Age is not an independent risk factor for patients being considered for surgery.

> All patients with early stage disease (stages I and II) should have surgical resection if medically feasible; otherwise definitive radiotherapy may be considered. Patients with potentially resectable stage IIIA disease (N2 ipsilateral/subcarinal lymphadenopathy) should receive careful assessment to look for N3 disease to avoid unnecessary surgical intervention.

Preoperative cardiopulmonary evaluation is necessary when considering lung cancer resection surgery to assess medical operability (surgical risk). The most important variables of lung function are the FEV_1 and DLCO. Differential lung perfusion scan allows estimation of predicted postoperative lung function. Exercise study assessing VO_2 max helps discriminate the overall risk of surgical resection of lung cancer in patients with borderline lung function.

the patient's risk of perioperative pulmonary complications. One of the most important prognostic indicators is pulmonary function. Postoperative survival depends on adequate preoperative pulmonary reserve. The desired postoperative forced expiratory volume in 1 second (FEV_1) is greater than 0.8 liter. In patients with borderline or poor lung function, a differential lung perfusion study helps predict postoperative effective FEV_1. The percent of flow to the "good" lung that is to remain is multiplied by the preoperative FEV_1 to estimate postoperative FEV_1. This estimate is most helpful when large portions of lung are to be removed. Exercise testing is performed in some patients considered at high risk for surgery (i.e., preoperative FEV_1 and/or diffusion capacity of the lung [DLCO] <40 % predicted or $PaCO_2$ >45 mm Hg and PaO_2 <50 mm Hg on room air) to measure oxygen consumption at peak exercise. A peak oxygen consumption value (VO_2 max) of ≥20 mL/kg per min carries an "acceptable" risk of perioperative cardiopulmonary complications and death, while the risk is "indeterminant" for a value between 10 and 20 mL/Kg per min and "prohibitve" for a value <10 mL/kg per min (only nonsurgical treatement is advised).[76-79]

Radiation Therapy

Radiation therapy is an effective form of primary treatment in early stage NSCLC in patients who are medically inoperable. However, it is not a comparable alternative to surgical therapy for cure. These patients should have a good performance status and be able to tolerate postirradiation pulmonary fibrosis based on pre-treatment lung function. Radiotherapy does not improve survival after complete surgical resection of stages IA or IB.

Chemotherapy

Chemotherapy is generally not used as a primary form of treatment for NSCLC, except in more advanced cases (stages IIIB-IV). Chemotherapy is the primary treatment for SCLC (see below).

Adverse side effects of chemotherapy depend on the drug regimen chosen. The most common side effects include bone marrow suppression, nausea, vomiting, renal and liver toxicity, and neuropathy. Bone marrow suppression will cause the patient to be neutropenic (low white blood cells) and susceptible to numerous bacterial, viral, and opportunistic infections. Nausea and emesis will lead to weight loss and a miserable quality of life unless treated. Some agents cause severe tissue necrosis if leaked into the skin around the IV catheter site. Dysrhythmias, red urine, and permanent cardiac dysfunction may result from the use of some older agents, now rarely used.

Newer chemotherapeutic agents have been developed that are less toxic for most individuals and better tolerated (e.g., Paclitaxel and Carboplatin). Hormonal growth factors have been synthesized and may be used to stimulate the bone marrow production of white and red blood cells. Neutropenia is now better controlled and reversed more quickly with granulocyte-colony stimulating factor (G-CSF/Neupogen®) injections, avoiding the severity and length of immunosuppression due to chemotherapy. Anemia can be controlled with fewer blood transfusion requirements using synthetic Erythropoetin (Epogen®) injections.

Stronger anti-emetics are now available to treat nausea and improve overall tolerance of chemotherapy.

Treatment of Small Cell Disease

Limited Disease

Chemotherapy (platinum-based regimen) is much more effective for small-cell carcinoma than for NSCLC. The overall initial response rate measured by remission of tumor growth or shrinkage of primary tumor mass, or both, with limited small-cell disease ranges from 60% to 90%. A complete response occurs in 45% to 75%, with a long-term complete remission (cure) rate of about 20% percent.[80]

Concurrent radiation therapy of the thorax may decrease incidence of local recurrence. Prophylactic cranial radiation is used in patients with complete response because metastasis to the brain is common and chemotherapy does not cross the blood-brain barrier.

Extensive Disease

Systemic chemotherapy results in an overall initial response rate of 60% to 70%, with complete response in 20% to 30%. Unfortunately, complete response rates are temporary (median 4 months), and chemotherapy becomes palliative due to the eventual recurrence of tumor. The median survival rate ranges from 9 to 12 months.[80]

> SCLC is treated primarily with chemotherapy for both limited and extensive stage disease. Concurrent thoracic irradiation is given for limited stage disease to improve local clinical response if the patient's health status allows.

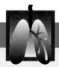

Mr. D

HISTORY

Mr. D is a 72-year-old man who presents with fever, chills, progressive dyspnea, and cough. The cough had produced one-quarter cup of yellow-green sputum each day for 2 weeks and had been blood-tinged for 2 days. He has had decreasing exercise tolerance for the past 6 months but never sought medical attention. He had noticed a 30-lb weight loss over 6 months. He had smoked two packs of cigarettes per day for 40 years, but quit 4 months ago because "they didn't taste good anymore." He admits to difficulty swallowing solids for 4 months and hoarseness for 3 months. He had been seen in the emergency department two days earlier for a diagnosis of "pneumonia" and given a course of oral antibiotics.

- Surgical: Transurethral resection of the prostate (TURP) 2 years earlier; basal cell carcinoma of the lip removed 1 year earlier

- Medications: Augmentin 875 mg twice a day; Albuterol/Ipratropium (Combivent) inhaler two puffs every 4 hours as needed, Fluticasone/Salmeterol (Advair) one inhalation twice a day

- Exposure: Worked in the boiler room on a ship in the navy for 3 years during the Korean War, then as a sandblaster in a shipyard for 2 years; denies symptoms of tuberculosis (TB) and fungal disease, as well as exposure to these diseases

- Occupation: Car mechanic and garage manager

QUESTIONS

1. What risk factors for bronchogenic carcinoma in Mr. D's history can you identify? How many pack-years has he smoked?

2. What symptoms in the history suggest lung cancer?

3. Would old granulomatous disease increase the risk of lung cancer?

4. What would the following symptoms suggest in a patient suspected of having lung cancer?

   a. Chest pain
   b. Bone pain
   c. Hoarseness
   d. Dysphagia (difficulty swallowing)
   e. Weakness of extremities or change in mental status

ANSWERS

Age is a significant risk factor for lung cancer.

Tobacco smoking is the most significant risk factor for developing bronchogenic carcinoma. The number of pack-years is calculated by multiplying the packs smoked per day times the number of years smoked. This patient has an 80-pack-year smoking history. Over 10% of long-term smokers get lung cancer and over 80% of all patients with lung cancer smoke or have smoked.

Asbestos exposure (working in a boiler room without protective respiratory apparatus) is a risk factor for lung cancer; concurrent smoking and asbestos exposure vastly increases the risk (up to approximately 90-fold). Exposure to silicates (sandblasting) also increases the risk of lung cancer in smokers.

Change in cough and sputum production may be a sign of lung cancer. Hemoptysis has many causes, including acute bronchitis, tuberculosis, pulmonary embolus, trauma, or tumor, but tumor is a likely cause of the bleeding in this case.

Progressive dyspnea may be due to large airway obstruction from a tumor or worsening of underlying emphysema. Other possible causes for the dyspnea include pleural effusion, diaphragmatic paralysis, pulmonary embolus, or pericardial effusion.

Unexplained weight loss should prompt a search for hidden malignancy.

Old granulomatous lung disease is associated with a slightly higher risk of lung cancer, especially if extensive scarring is present.

In the patient suspected of having lung cancer, specific symptoms may be suggestive of intrathoracic or extrathoracic spread, including:

Lung tissue does not have pain receptors; therefore, chest pain indicates spread of the lung cancer to parietal pleura, ribs, or other chest wall structures.

Bone pain may indicate bone metastasis or osteoarthropathy.

The recurrent laryngeal nerve travels from the neck around the aorta and back to the vocal cord. Compression of the recurrent laryngeal nerve by tumor or enlarged para-aortic lymph nodes may cause hoarseness. Hoarseness often indicates that the tumor has involved vital structures and is unresectable.

Dysphagia (difficulty swallowing) may indicate esophageal compression from mediastinal adenopathy or invasion by lung tumor.

Arm or leg weakness or change in mental status suggests metastasis to the brain. Tumor in the brain may be manifest initially by relatively subtle signs, but these signs gradually progress to clear evidence of mental, emotional, or physical dysfunction.

 ## More on Mr. D

PHYSICAL EXAMINATION

- **General.** Lethargic, thin, chronically ill-appearing white man who appears older than stated age, with mild respiratory distress; patient alert but mildly confused (disoriented to place and time) and unable to provide a coherent history

- **Vital Signs.** Temperature 37.68°C (99.78°F), pulse 102/min, respiratory rate 22/min, blood pressure 110/50 mm Hg; height, 5 feet 8 inches; weight, 120 lb

- **HEENT.** Pupils equally round and responsive to light and accommodation; no ptosis, fundoscopically normal; tympanic membranes clear bilaterally; edentulous; no jugular venous distention, facial edema, or adenopathy

- **Chest.** Chest wall nontender; regular rhythm, no murmur, gallop, or rub; point of maximum impulse (PMI) below xiphoid process; markedly decreased breath sounds over lower right lung with inspiratory coarse crackles; localized, monophonic expiratory wheeze in right midlung; no pleural rub; right lower lobe dull to percussion.

- **Abdomen.** Soft, nondistended, with bowel sounds active; slightly enlarged liver at 4 cm below right costal margin

- **Extremities:** Abnormally small muscle mass; no edema or cyanosis; mild enlargement (clubbing) of distal fingertips

QUESTIONS	ANSWERS
5. What do the vital signs and general appearance indicate?	Low-grade fever is consistent with pneumonia. Respiratory rate is elevated slightly, indicating compromised respiratory mechanics, compromised gas exchange, psychogenic stress (anxiety) or a combination of these. There is no evidence of accessory respiratory muscle use or paradoxic breathing to indicate diaphragmatic fatigue (i.e., impending respiratory failure). Weight loss in conjunction with tumor is a poor prognostic sign. Confusion and lethargy suggest one or more of the following: cerebral metastasis, hypoxia, hypercapnia, or chemical imbalance.

6. What does the decreased resonance to percussion over the right lower lobe indicate?

Dullness to percussion indicates lung consolidation, atelectasis or pleural effusion.

7. What does the monophonic wheeze indicate?

The localized right monophonic wheeze indicates partial airway obstruction of a single, large conducting airway in the right lung.

8. What would be the significance of facial edema?

Tumor-related facial edema is most often caused by compression of the superior vena cava by an enlarging tumor.

9. What would be the significance of ptosis (drooping of the eyelid)?

Eye ptosis is a sign of Horner's syndrome, which is caused by tumor compression of the sympathetic nerves (from lower cervical and upper thoracic spinal nerves).

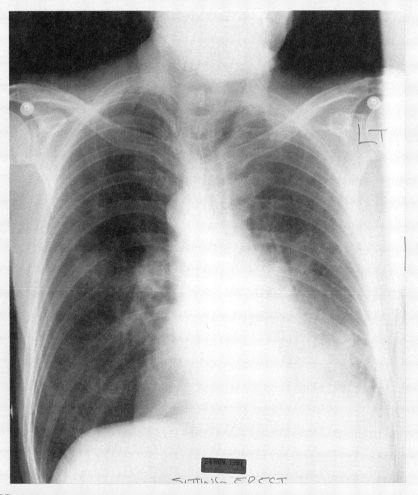

FIGURE 20.7 Chest radiograph taken two days earlier in an emergency room visit shows right lower lobe pneumonia with patchy infiltrate in the left lower lobe.

More on Mr. D

Diagnostic Data

Chest Radiographs: See Figures 20.7 and 20.8.
Esophagograms: See Figures 20.9 and 20.10.
Chest CT: See Figure 20.11.

Laboratory Data

ABGs on room air

pH	7.38,
$PaCO_2$	48 mm Hg
PaO_2	60 mm Hg
HCO_3^-	28 mEq/liter
SaO_2	94%

Electrolytes (see Appendix for normal values)

Na^+	144 mEq/liter
K^+	3.7mEq/liter
Cl^-	108 mEq/liter
Total CO^2	29 mEq/liter
Blood urea nitrogen (BUN)	20 mg/dL
Creatinine	0.9 mg/dL

CBC (see Appendix for normal values)

White blood cells (WBCs)	16,500/mm³
Granulocytes	64%
Bands	14%
Lymphocytes	12%
Monocytes	4%
Eosinophils	2%
Basophils	1%
Hemoglobin (Hb)	12.1 g/dL
Platelets	415,000/mm³
Ca++	12.5 mg/dL (8.5 to 10.5 mg/dL)
Liver function tests normal	
Lactate dehydrogenase (LDH)	240 IU/liter (100 to 190 IU/liter)
Total protein	5.2 g/dL (6 to 8 g/dL)
Albumin	3.0 (3.5 to 5.5 g/dL)

Sputum Gram Stain for Culture and Sensitivities

4+ polymorphonuclear neutrophils (pus)
3+ gram-negative rods
1+ budding yeast with hyphae
Epithelial cells less than 3 to 5 per hpf

Spirometric Studies (2 months before this visit):

Prebronchodilator
• Forced vital capacity (FVC) 3.4 liters (68% predicted)
• FEV_1 1.7 liters (55% predicted)
• FEV_1/FVC 50%
Postbronchodilator
• FVC 3.6 liters (72%)
• FEV_1 1.9 liters (60%)
• FEV_1/FVC 53%

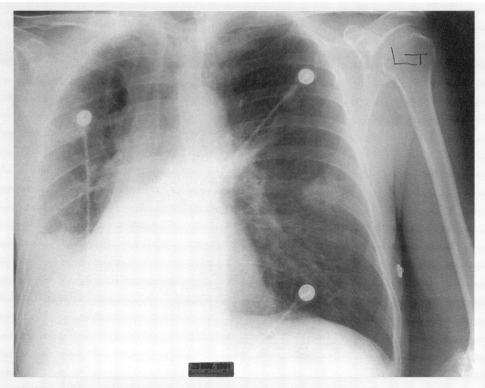

FIGURE 20.8 Chest radiograph (frontal view) of Mr. D taken on day of admission demonstrates considerable atelectasis of the right middle and lower lobes with right pleural effusion due to obstruction of right bronchus intermedius. Evidence of bilateral metastatic disease most likely represents bronchogenic carcinoma.

QUESTIONS	ANSWERS
10. How would you interpret the ABG values?	The ABG is consistent with mild hypoxemia on room air. The acid-base status indicates compensated respiratory acidosis.
11. What do the chest radiographs tell you about Mr. D's pulmonary condition?	Comparison of the admission chest radiograph to that of the day before suggests a right bronchus inter-medius obstruction, likely from a tumor. There is also evidence of a cavitating metastasis to the left lung.
12. What did the CT scan and esophagogram add to the information provided by the chest radiograph?	The CT scan of the chest demonstrates a mass in the right middle lobe and probable mediastinal and left lung metastases. The tumor appears to have involved the esophagus on esophogram, causing high-grade obstruction to food passage. Overall, the stage of cancer appears to be locally advanced within the thorax.
13. What pulmonary abnormality do the pulmonary function data suggest in Mr. D?	The pulmonary function data indicate moderate obstructive pulmonary disease. The mild decrease in lung volumes may be due to air trapping or tumor. Mr. D demonstrates minimal spirometric improve-ment with bronchodilator therapy.

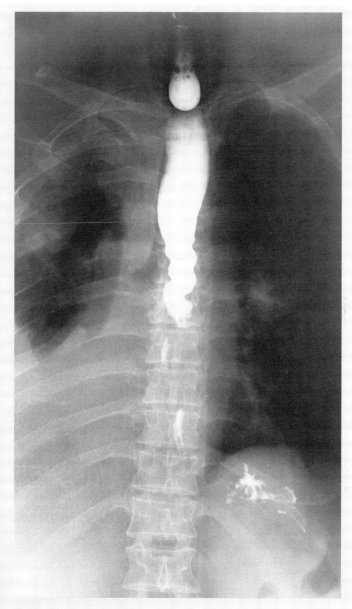

FIGURE 20.9 Frontal view of an esophagogram reveals high-grade obstruction of midesophagus, likely due to extensive mediastinal adenopathy or tumor invasion.

14. What is the significance of the elevated serum calcium?

The elevated serum calcium may be responsible for Mr. D's confusion and lethargy. Squamous cell carcinomas are the tumors most commonly associated with hypercalcemia due to production of parathyroid-related hormone, a paraneoplastic syndrome. Bone metastases can also cause elevated serum calcium levels.

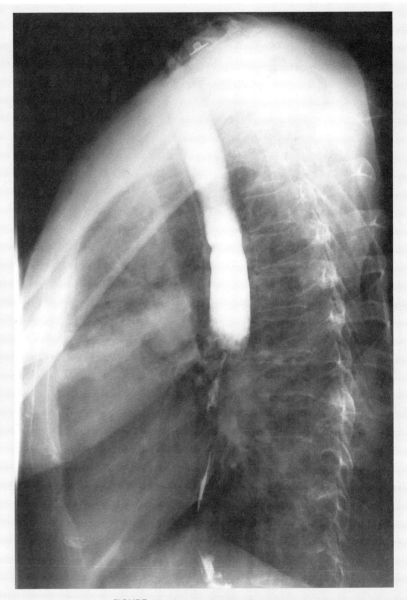

FIGURE 20.10 Lateral view of Figure 20.9.

15. What evidence indicates pneumonia in this case?

Indicators of pneumonia in Mr. D are the elevated white blood cell count with increased band cells (left shift to earlier white cell forms produced in response to significant infection), fever, right lower lung opacification on chest radiograph, and sputum Gram stain positive for pus cells with predominance of gram-negative rod organisms.

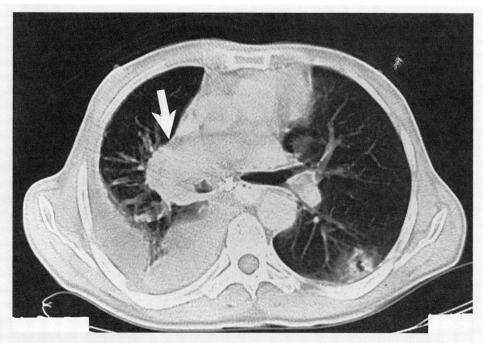

FIGURE 20.11 Computerized tomography of the chest shows a right hilar mass greater than 5 cm (arrow). A cavitary metastatic lesion is seen in the posterior left lung. There is evidence of pretracheal lymphadenopathy with 2.5- to 3-cm lymph nodes. A moderate right pleural effusion is also visualized.

16. What diagnostic procedure(s) would be most appropriate at this time?

Bronchoscopy would quickly distinguish between common pneumonia and a cancer partially obstructing a bronchus, causing a postobstructive pneumonia. Not every patient with pneumonia needs bronchoscopy. In Mr. D, with evidence of weight loss, pneumonia, and a monophonic right lower lobe wheeze suggesting partial obstruction of a large airway, bronchoscopy would have a high diagnostic yield for malignancy (overall around 88%).

Sputum cytology is much less sensitive than bronchoscopy for diagnosing lung cancer and when positive does not define the extent of airway involvement. However, it may provide a (cytology) diagnosis in the presence of central airway lesions up to 50% to 70% of the time.

Clinical staging is necessary to accurately assess prognosis and direct future lung cancer therapies. This may include the use of imaging studies (e.g., fused PET/CT, body CT, brain MRI) and an invasive procedure, such as TBNA, EUS-FNA, thoracentesis, mediastinoscopy, or thoracoscopy.

17. Should Mr. D be hospitalized? Why?

Mr. D should be hospitalized because of the presence of pneumonia, hypercalcemia, and symptoms suggesting lung cancer. The lung cancer alone would not require hospital admission, but the combination of pneumonia and hypercalcemia requires IV drug therapy and close observation; antibiotics for the pneumonia and IV saline, furosemide (a diuretic to assist in urinary dumping of calcium), and pamidronate (inhibits release of calcium from bones) for the treatment of severe hypercalcemia.

More on Mr. D

Mr. D is given IV antibiotics for the pneumonia and IV saline, furosemide (lasix), and pamidronate for the hypercalcemia. Flexible fiberoptic bronchoscopy is performed after 2 days of therapy. Bronchoscopy shows an endobronchial tumor totally obstructing the right bronchus intermedius (unable to pass scope) with a mucosal lesion within 2 cm of the carina. Analysis of tumor specimens reveals squamous cell carcinoma.

QUESTIONS	ANSWERS
18. What is the TNM classification of this lung cancer, and what is its stage? (See Tables 20.3, 20.4, 20.5, and 20.6 for the classification systems.)	The TNM classification is T4 (tumor greater than 3 cm in diameter indicated by chest CT, within 2 cm of carina and involving the esophagus); N2 (2 cm mediastinal lymphadenopathy); M1 (evidence of metastasis to contralateral lung). A T4N2M1 classification is equivalent to cancer stage IV.
19. Is Mr. D a surgical candidate? What therapy is recommended?	Surgical resection is not an option for stage IV lung cancer. Chemotherapy is recommended to help shrink the primary tumor, reduce symptoms from local and distant tumor spread, and provide an overall better quality of life with a small survival benefit compared with best supportive care. Radiotherapy is given as palliative treatment in advanced lung cancer to reduce tumor compression effects on major airways and neural and vascular structures. Also, it is given focally to bone and brain metastases to reduce pain and mass effects, respectively.
20. What intervention(s) may be considered to restore or maintain airway patency?	Assessing the patency of the right bronchial airways is essential to evaluate for a post-obstructive pneumonia. If a central airway shows narrowing or obstruction by endobronchial tumor growth, tumor ablation using the argon plasma coagulator (APC), electrocautery, or Nd–YAG laser photocoagulation therapy may be performed to open it. Balloon bronchoplasty is used to dilate the airway before placing a covered wire mesh (nitinol) stent or a silicon stent to maintain airway patency (prevent re-occlusion).

This procedure is usually performed through a rigid bronchoscope in the operating room with general anesthesia, before palliative chemo or radiotherapy is started. Nonemergent endobronchial interventions to reduce tumor size and growth in the airway include cryotherapy, brachytherapy, and photodynamic therapy.

More on Mr. D

Mr. D is evaluated for tumor ablation therapy and a stent procedure. He receives APC therapy to reduce endobronchial tumor growth in the right bronchus intermedius followed by balloon bronchoplasty to dilate the airway. Unfortunately, the airways beyond the bronchus intermedius appear significantly involved with tumor growth and are collapsed. The right mainstem has no significant stenosis from tumor and the right upper lobe is patent and uninvolved, so no stent is placed at that time.

   Mr. D receives local radiation therapy to the chest to reduce compression effects on the airways and vital mediastinal structures from the tumor mass (palliative therapy), followed by a course of chemotherapy. Two months after finishing external-beam irradiation therapy to the thorax and mediastinum, Mr. D returns to the emergency department for a sudden onset of massive hemoptysis. Mr. D coughs up about 800 mL of bright red blood over a 30-minute period. After he is placed on his right side, he is taken to the operating room for emergent rigid bronchoscopy. The airway is cleared of blood, a large clot is removed from the right mainstem bronchus, and tamponade with packing is successful. The packing is removed after about 15 minutes, and there is no further bleeding. After recovery from bronchoscopy, he is sedated with lorazepam and morphine to prevent coughing and transferred to the intensive care unit for observation.

QUESTIONS	ANSWERS
21. Why was Mr. D laid on his right side during the massive hemoptysis event?	The massive hemoptysis is most likely from a ruptured blood vessel supplying the bronchial mucosa (bronchial arterial source). Radiation induces necrosis of the tumor, which leads to sloughing and ulceration of bronchial mucosa and walls in regions affected by tumor growth. This can lead to hemoptysis, significant at times, especially if the tumor invades through a bronchial wall or into a large blood vessel. Laying him on the side of the "bad lung" (probable source) protects the "good" lung from filling up with blood, thus avoiding complete asphyxiation, respiratory failure, and death.
22. What additional palliative therapy may be offered if the bleeding recurs?	Bronchial arterial embolization therapy is a highly effective, nonsurgical means of controlling and reducing the recurrence of massive hemoptysis in patients with advanced lung cancer. Interventional radiology performs pulmonary and bronchial arteriography to locate the "feeder" vessels and injects

material to embolize and obstruct or block off the offending vessel(s). If his condition deteriorated rapidly, he may be selectively intubated into the left mainstem bronchus to provide adequate ventilation and oxygenation until the source of bleeding is controlled.

Mr. D Conclusion

Mr. D undergoes bronchial arterial embolization therapy with resolution of his hemoptysis. He experiences two months of relatively stable health outside of the hospital, except for weight loss and monthly chest infections. After a fair initial clinical response to palliative radiation and chemotherapy with partial re-opening of his airways, his tumor begins to grow again, causing compression of his right middle and lower lobes, distally. He decides against further bronchoscopic interventions. Two weeks later, Mr. D acquires a postobstructive pneumonia (Figure 20.12), which persists despite treatment with oral antibiotics. He enrolls in an outpatient hospice program and is kept comfortable with supplemental oxygen, inhaled bronchodilators and oral and transdermal narcotics. A few days later he dies peacefully at home from respiratory failure with family members at his bedside. ■

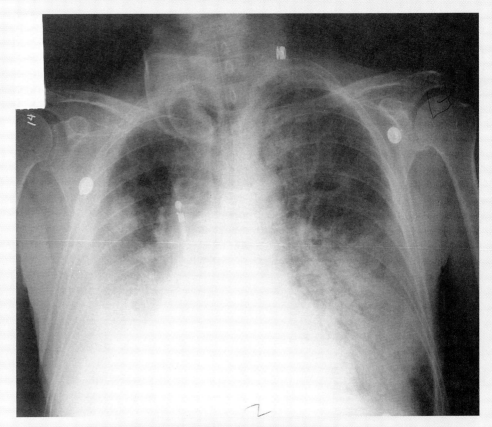

FIGURE 20.12 Chest radiograph (frontal view) shows pneumonia advanced to the lower left lobe with progressive postobstructive pneumonitis in the right lower and middle lobes.

Ms. F

HISTORY

Ms. F, a 42-year-old Korean female is transferred from a local hospital for a higher level of care in acute respiratory failure with inability to wean from mechanical ventilator support due to malignant central airway obstruction from a large mediastinal mass. Four years prior she was diagnosed with limited stage SCLC in the central chest and treated with local irradiation and chemotherapy (Etoposide and cis-platinum) with a good initial clinical response. She has received chemotherapy (Taxotere) over the past year for recurrent tumor growth with poor response of late, having already received maximum allowable doses of chest irradiation. She has recently required a pericardial window to drain a malignant pericardial effusion and had bilateral pulmonary emboli followed by inferior vena cava filter placement.

Before this event Ms. F experienced several weeks of progressive dyspnea and cough with bark-like quality and difficulty clearing secretions. She had an audible inspiratory and expiratory "hissing" noise from the throat with breathing and central chest discomfort with deep breathing. She had chronic hoarseness from right vocal cord paralysis. She had weight loss of 15 pounds in the past 3 months with poor appetite, generalized weakness and fatigue, and chronic "low" blood pressure and anemia.

- Surgical: Pericardial drainage with "window" formation.

- Medications: Albuterol/Atrovent pre-mix solution via med neb every 4 hours as needed, Piperacillin/Tazobactam 3.375 GM intravenously every 6 hours, Epogen 40,000 units via subcutaneous injection every week, Famotidine 20 mg IV twice a day, Midazolam IV drip for titrated for sedation, and morphine sulfate 2 to 4 mg IV every 4 hours as needed for pain control

- Tobacco Exposure: 20 pack-year history; quit 4 years ago; denies asbestos, toxic chemical fume, dust or significant smoke inhalation exposure

QUESTIONS	ANSWERS
1. What symptoms suggest progressive central airway obstruction due to malignancy in Ms. F?	Her worsening dyspnea suggests progressive resistance to airflow due to narrowing that reduces the airway caliber to 50% or less. The length of airway involved with stenosis exponentially worsens airway resistance and work of breathing. Her cough may suggest irritation from tumor growth in the airway, retention of mucus or secretions or inflammation in the lungs. An audible hissing sound with deep respiration is caused by turbulent airflow through a stenosis in the thoracic airway, occurring with both inspiration and expiration. Chronic hoarseness suggests damage to the recurrent laryngeal nerve that supplies the right vocal cord, probably from tumor and/or radiation.

2. Why is Ms. F unable to receive any more radiation to her large chest mass?

Ms. F has already received the maximum allowable cumulative radiation dose to her mediastinum from her initial treatment of limited disease plus a boost given at the time of recurrence one year ago. The tissue integrity and function of vital vascular, airway, esophageal, and spinal organs may be compromised if more radiation is given.

3. What is a pericardial window? Why did Ms. F receive it?

A fluid collection containing malignant cells may develop within the pericardial sac around the heart due to the spread of lung cancer. If the fluid builds up enough pressure, cardiac tamponade occurs from reduced venous blood return to the heart. This leads to circulatory compromise and may lead to a sudden drop in cardiac output, refractory cardiogenic shock, and death if not recognized and treated immediately. A pericardial window is a method of treatment and preventing recurrence of tamponade from malignant pericardial effusion.

More on Ms. F

PHYSICAL EXAMINATION

- **General.** Intubated with #7.5 endotrachal tube, taped at 26 cm at the upper lip, sedated but arouses easily to voice, follows commands and answers questions appropriately with head gestures

- **Vital Signs.** Temperature 36.8°C, pulse 86/min, respirations 16/min, blood pressure 92/58 mm Hg; height 5 feet 2 inches; weight 98 pounds

- **Ventilator Settings.** Assist control mode, rate 12, tidal volume 500 cc, FIO_2 30%, PEEP 5 cm H_2O

- **Chest.** Chest wall: nontender to palpation; heart: regular rhythm, no murmur, gallop, or rub; PMI nondisplaced; lungs: transmitted bronchial sounds in right chest with an inspiratory squeak and end-expiratory low-pitched wheeze over right mid-chest, slight inpiratory crackles lower right lung; left lung clear with ventilator-produced breath sounds

- **Abdomen.** Bowel sounds present, but reduced activity to auscultation; nontender and soft, nondistended with no organomegaly or masses to palpation

- **Extremities.** Muscular atrophy, pulses 1+ bilaterally symmetric upper and lower; no clubbing, cyanosis or edema

DIAGNOSTIC DATA:

CBC. (WBC 13.6, Hgb 12.4, Plt 285, normal differential) and electrolytes within normal limits, (BUN 10/ CR 0.4). Prothrombin time/partial thromboplastin time (PT/PTT) within normal limits. albumin 2.8 (low), liver function tests show mild elevation of transaminases, otherwise WNL; LDH 220

ABG. 7.43/34/88/23, showing normal oxygenation and ventilation indices, on above ventilator settings; 12-lead ECG shows normal sinus rhythm, no ST or T wave abnormalities, normal R-wave progression and voltage

Chest Radiograph. ETT in place; lungs show overall good expansion, except for a small right pleural effusion with volume loss (atelectasis) in the right lung base

Chest CT axial view and three-dimensional reconstruction airway study. Shows evidence of ETT and stenosis/obstruction distal trachea/right main take off at level of carina

QUESTIONS	ANSWERS
4. What are the important findings of the physical examination? Why?	**Mentation:** Although sedated, Ms. F is easily aroused and able to participate and guide in the decision-making process, to discuss intended quality of life benefits and the potential risks and complications of any future palliative interventions. **Size of ETT:** #7.5 internal diameter limits the ability to ventilate around a larger bronchoscope during a procedure, especially a "therapeutic" sized bronchoscope that offers a larger instrument port. The ETT is about 4 cm "deeper" than normal, which offered the best flow into her lungs according to the bedside respiratory therapist, suggesting the ETT may be helping keep the trachea from collapse or obstructing. **Chest:** The entire right lung has reduced air exchange, inspiratory squeak, and an end-expiratory low-pitched wheeze suggesting an obstruction affecting the right mainstem bronchus.
5. What do the laboratory studies tell us?	The labs do not suggest active infection or coagulation defects. Despite recent bilateral pulmonary emboli, Ms. F's oxygenation and respiratory acid-base status are close to normal. The 12-lead ECG indicates no dysrhythmia or signs of ischemic heart disease. Chest x-ray does not suggest pneumonia, pulmonary edema, or significant effusion as the cause of Ms. F's respiratory failure. There is atelectasis in the right lung base with a small effusion, suggesting poor airflow from airway obstruction.
6. What does the chest CT and airway imaging study tell us about Ms. F's obstruction?	The airway study is useful in evaluating the viability and structure of airways beyond points of obstruction, especially when unable to pass the bronchoscope for direct visual inspection.
7. What diagnostic study would be most appropriate now and why?	A diagnostic flexible bronchoscopy to further evaluate the size, severity (diameter and length), and type (extrinsic vs. intrinsic vs. both) of airway stenosis would be appropriate.

More on Ms. F

Bronchoscopy is performed and reveals a crescent-shaped narrowing of the distal trachea down to about 2 to 3 mm width and around 4 cm in length, beginning at the main carina with right mainstem bronchial orifice collapse, mostly from external compression (mass effect) and some submucosal thickening and irregularity. The distal endotracheal tube serves to maintain partial airway patency.

QUESTIONS	ANSWERS
8. What type of intervention is needed, and what are the potential benefits?	The dilemma faced by Ms. F is ventilator dependence due to central airway obstruction from a recurrent, locally advanced, "terminal," SCLC that is not responding well to chemotherapy. Options include comfort care with narcotic (and benzodiazepine) drips for relief of dyspnea, pain, and anxiety, followed by extubation with subsequent death or attempt at palliative interventional bronchoscopy with the goal of liberation from mechanical ventilator support, relief of dyspnea and cough, and prevention of postobstructive processes such as pneumonitis or pneumonia.
9. What factors are considered in the patient assessment before palliative intervention?	Pre-procedure patient assessment includes a full understanding of the indications and expected benefits (short- and long-term) balanced with the overall risk of intervention and potential for complications. The potential for overall benefit should outweigh the risks of palliative intervention. Potential benefits (indications) may include liberation from mechanical ventilation, prevention of postobstructive pneumonia, relief of dyspnea and cough, discharge from the hospital, and possibly a longer survival time (days, weeks, or months). Quality of life benefit will depend on tumor behavior, the status of nonairway tumor-related symptoms or those from concurrent disease, patient tolerance of future palliative therapies, and the effect on overall performance status. The patient should not be septic or have uncontrolled infection. Hemodynamics should be stable with no significant dysrhythmias or active myocardial ischemia present. Oxygen requirements should be no greater than FiO_2 of 40% to avoid risk of fire when using APC, electrocautery, or laser photocoagulation. Ventilator pressures should not be high, with PEEP $\leq$5 cm H_2O and not on pressure

control with reverse I:E ratio or high-frequency oscillator, since the patient would not tolerate periods of apnea. Overall life expectancy based on non-airway disease processes should be factored into the decision determining overall benefit of the palliative procedure.

10. What are some of the potential risks and complications in performing interventional bronchoscopy?

The potential for destabilization of current status is high with most patients presenting with acute respiratory failure due to advanced lung cancer. The risks of intervention should be discussed, understood, and accepted by the patient or surrogate decision-maker before any procedure is performed. Potential risks and complications of interventional bronchoscopy include bleeding from the airways or lungs, sometimes massive or difficult to control but rarely lethal; loss of the airway, either due to stent dislodgment, dysfunction, massive bleeding, or rupture or laceration or inability to re-establish an airway. Prolonged mechanical ventilator dependence is possible after an intervention, especially if underlying lung disease such as COPD, extensive intrathoracic tumor spread, or pneumonia is present. Pneumonia with sepsis with or without septic shock may occur following an intervention. Cardiac dysrhythmias are common and sometime can be serious. Hypoxemia is usually transient but may be severe and prolonged, leading to end-organ ischemia and anoxic damage. Pneumothorax may occur, requiring a chest tube. Injury to the cervical spine (vertebral fracture or spinal cord injury) may occur, especially if the patient has cervical arthritis and stiffness. Injury to the lips, gums, teeth, back of throat, or vocal cords may occur. Laryngeal edema may cause stridor and require reintubation.

 More on Ms. F

Ms. F undergoes rigid bronchoscopy with sequential balloon tracheal-bronchoplasty. A significant extrinsic compressive process is noted with strong dynamic recoil and collapse of the tracheal wall/lumen back to a 3-mm crescent-shaped stenosis, despite balloon multiple balloon dilations up to 15-mm diameter. The anterior wall appears to have fractured cartilaginous rings. No endobronchial tumor ablation therapy is needed. No significant bleeding occurs. The interventional pulmonologist initially uses a covered wire (nitinol) self-expanding stent in the distal trachea and right mainstem bronchus and is soon able to extubate the patient. However, over the course of a couple days the tracheal-covered wire stent migrates proximally away from the distal stenosis above the main carina, and the right mainstem stent migrates distally with every cough, allowing airway obstruction to recur.

QUESTION	ANSWER
11. In light of the current problem of stent migration, what is the next best intervention?	The best stent for maintaining Ms. F's central airway patency will need to support the regions of the distal trachea, main carina, and right mainstem bronchial orofice. This trifurcation of the central airway is most critical and calls for a unique airway stent called the Tracheal-Y stent. A variety of stent types are available, including the Dumon and Hood (silicone) stents or the Rusch-Freitag dynamic stent. The dynamic Rusch-Freitag Tracheal-Y stent is a hybrid of steel struts providing anterior support mimicking the cartilaginous rings and a thin, pliable, silastic posterior membrane mimicking the dynamic tracheal physiology to promote secretion clearance. The stent is deployed using a specialized forceps delivery device with which the apneic and anesthetized patient is intubated after the airway is assessed and prepared. Fluroscopy is used for guiding correct stent orientation and placement followed by bronchoscopy to confirm.

Ms. F Conclusion

The intubated patient undergoes general anesthesia in the OR, where a Rusch-Freitag dynamic Tracheal-Y stent of appropriate size is successfully deployed with the assistance of fluoroscopy. In addition, because of the strong compressive forces in the distal trachea, a dilating balloon catheter is utilized to direct the right bronchial arm into position over a guidewire.

Over the next 24 hours Ms. F is successfully weaned and extubated. She requires several therapeutic bronchoscopies to remove hemorrhagic and mucopurulent secretions from a viral (herpetic) tracheobronchitis, having just been treated for *E. coli* pneumonia. She has some dysphagia, odonyphagia, and pleuritic quality chest discomfort "deep" in the center of her chest. One week later she is discharged to a skilled nursing facility for rehabilitation and two weeks later goes home. Two weeks after that, she is treated successfully for a left upper lobe cavitary pneumonia with IV antibiotics at home. Four weeks later she is hospitalized for a brisk upper GI bleed and is found to have tumor metastasis to her stomach. Bleeding is difficult to control. She experiences worsening anemia and septic shock. After deciding to be DNR/DNI status, she is placed on continuous morphine drip for control of dyspnea and pain. She dies peacefully during that hospitalization.

In summary, interventional bronchoscopy was used to successfully re-establish Ms. F's airway, liberate her from mechanical ventilation, provide relief for symptoms of dyspnea and cough, and prevent postobstructive processes in her airways. She was discharged from hospital and allowed to spend some quality time at home with her family and eventually died of a nonairway effect of the lung cancer. ■

KEY POINTS

- Lung cancer, also called bronchogenic carcinoma, is now the most common fatal cancer in both men and women in the United States.
- Most scientists agree that cigarette smoking causes lung cancer. There is a strong association between smoking exposure and the incidence of bronchogenic carcinoma.
- There is about a 30% increased risk of lung cancer in individuals exposed to passive smoke.
- The four major histological types of lung cancer are squamous cell carcinoma (29%), adenocarcinoma (32%), large-cell carcinoma (9%), and small-cell carcinoma (18%).
- Pulmonary symptoms associated with lung cancer may include a change in cough or sputum production, hemoptysis, wheezing, dyspnea, stridor, chest pain, or fever.
- Physical examination of the patient with lung cancer may be relatively normal when the tumor is small and located peripherally. Auscultation may reveal wheezing if an airway is partially obstructed.
- Physical examination may also reveal evidence of tumor spread, which precludes surgical resection.
- Symptoms of extrathoracic spread or distant metastases depend on the sites involved. Common sites of spread include lymph nodes, brain and spinal cord, liver, adrenal glands, bone, bone marrow, and skin.
- The overall 5-year survival rate for patients presenting with carcinoma of the lung is only about 10% to 15%.
- The chest radiograph plays a pivotal role in the recognition of lung cancer. The chest radiograph may demonstrate asymptomatic lung cancer but is almost always abnormal when the patient is symptomatic.
- Chest CT offers more accurate size comparisons (especially with smaller nodules) and discrimination of margins and may reveal hidden calcifications, satellite nodules, and lymphadenopathy.
- Sputum cytology is most useful for diagnosing central airway (e.g., squamous cell) carcinomas. The sensitivity of sputum cytology for central airway lesions is about 70% and decreases to about 50% for peripheral lesions.
- The flexible fiberoptic bronchoscope is a small-bore, *flexible* tube with a light source going to the tip (*fiberoptic*) and a port for suctioning secretions, flushing with saline, and passing small instruments for sampling cytology or tissue (e.g., brush, forceps, needle). This device is very useful for evaluating the patient suspected of having lung cancer.
- Most patients with lung cancer present with extensive disease and have a poor prognosis.
- For stage IA and IB, the treatment is surgery.
- For stage IIA and IIB, the treatment is surgery.
- For stage IIIA, the treatment is surgery for some, neoadjuvant therapy followed by surgery for some, and chemotherapy and radiation therapy for some.
- For stage IIIB, except for some (T4N0M0-Pancoast), the treatment is chemotherapy and radiation therapy, preferably concurrently if possible.
- For stage IV, the treatment is "best supportive care" or chemotherapy.
- One of the most important prognostic indicators for patients needing surgery is pulmonary function. Postoperative survival depends on adequate preoperative pulmonary reserve. The desired postoperative forced expiratory volume in 1 second (FEV_1) is greater than 0.8 liter.
- Chemotherapy (platinum-based regimen) is much more effective for small-cell carcinoma than for NSCLC.

REFERENCES

1. American Cancer Society: Cancer Facts and Figures 2005. Atlanta, GA: American Cancer Society, 2005.

2. Jemal, A, Thomas, A, Murray, T, et al: Cancer statistics, 2002. CA Cancer J Clin 52:23, 2002.

3. Doll, R, Hill, AB: Smoking and carcinoma of the lung. BMJ 2:739–748, 1950.

4. Bilello, KS, Murin, S, Matthay, RA. Epidemiology, etiology, and prevention of lung cancer. Lung Cancer Clin Chest Med 23(1):1–25, 2002.

5. Filderman, AE, et al: Bronchogenic carcinoma. In Brandstetter, RD (ed): *Pulmonary Medicine*. Medical Economics, Oradell, NJ, 1989, pp. 525–549.

6. Alberg, AJ, Samet, JM. Epidemiology of lung cancer. Chest 123(suppl):S21–S49, 2003.

7. Hirayama, T: Passive smoking and lung cancer: Consistency of association. Lancet 2:1425,1983.

8. Weiss, ST: Passive smoking and lung cancer: what is the risk? (editorial) Am Rev Respir Dis 133:1–3, 1986.

9. Warnock, M, Churg, A: Association of asbestos and bronchogenic carcinoma in a population with low asbestos exposure. Cancer 35:1236, 1975.

10. Hammond, EC, et al: Asbestos exposure, cigarette smoking, and death rates. Ann NY Acad Sci 330:473–490, 1979.

11. Godtfredsen, NS, Prescott, E, Osler, M: Effect of smoking reduction on lung cancer risk. JAMA 294:1505–1510, 2005.

12. Lissowska, J, Bardin-Mikolajczak, A, Fletcher, T, et al: Lung cancer and indoor air pollution from heating and cooking with solid fuels. The IARC International Multicentre Case-Control Study in Easter/Central Europe and the United Kingdom. Am J Epidemiol 162:326–333, 2005.

13. Samet, JM, et al: Personal and family history of respiratory disease and lung cancer risk. Am Rev Respir Dis 134:466–470, 1986.

14. Ooi, WL, Elston, RC, Chen, VW, et al: Increased familial risk for lung cancer. J Natl Cancer Inst 76:217–222, 1986.

15. Fong, KM, Minna, JD: Molecular biology of lung cancer: clinical implications. Clin Chest Med 23(1):83–101, 2002.

16. Brincker, H, Wilbek, E. The incidence of malignant tumors in patients with sarcoidosis. Br J Cancer 29:247, 1974.

17. Dragnew, KH, Stover, D, Dmitrovsky, E: Lung cancer prevention: the guidelines. Chest 123(suppl):60S–71S, 2003.

18. Keith, RL, Miller, YE: Lung cancer: genetics of risk and advances in chemoprevention. Curr Opin Pulm Med 11(4):265–271, 2005.

19. Schabath, MB, Hernandez, LM, Wu, X, et al: Dietary phytoestrogens and lung cancer risk. JAMA 294:1493–1504, 2005.

20. The World Health Organization histological typing of lung tumors, 2nd ed. Am J Clin Pathol 77:123, 1982.

21. Travis, WD, Travis, LB, Devesa, SS: Lung cancer. Cancer 75:191–202, 1995. Erratum. Cancer 75(12):2979, 1995.

22. Travis, WD. Pathology of lung cancer. Clin Chest Med 23(1):65–81, 2002.

23. Yokose, T, Suzuki, K, et al: Favorable and unfavorable morphologic prognostic factors in peripheral adenocarcinoma of the lung 3 cm or less in diameter. Lung Cancer 29:179–188, 2000.

24. Johnson, BE. Management of small cell lung cancer. Clin Chest Med 23(1):225–239, 2002.

25. Doyle, LA, Aisner, J: Clinical presentation of lung cancer. In Roth, JA, Ruckdeschel, JC, Weisenburger, TH (eds): *Thoracic Oncology*. WB Saunders, Philadelphia, *1989, p 53.*

26. Leef, JL 3rd, Klein, IS: The solitary pulmonary nodule. Radiol Clin North Am 40:123–143, 2002.

27. Midthun, DE, Jett, JR: Clinical presentation of lung cancer. In: Pass, HI, et al (eds): *Lung Cancer: Principles and Practice*, Lippincott-Raven, Philadelphia 1996, p. 421.

28. Sridhar, KS, Lobo, CF, Altman, RD: Digital clubbing and lung cancer. Chest 114:1535, 1998.

29. Hyde, L, Hyde, CI. Clinical manifestations of lung cancer. Chest 65:299, 1974.

30. Pancoast, HK: Superior sulcus pulmonary tumor: Tumor characterized by pain, Horner's syndrome, destruction of bone, and atrophy of hand muscles. JAMA 99:1391, 1932.

31. Gerber, RB, Mazzone, P, Arroliga, A: Paraneoplastic syndromes associated with bronchogenic carcinoma. Clin Chest Med 23(1): 257–264, 2002.

32. Henschke, CI, McCauley, DI, Yankelevitz, DF, et al: Early Lung Cancer Action Project: overall design and findings from baseline screening. Lancet 354:99–105, 1999.

33. Henschke, CI, Naidich, DP, Yankelevitz, DF, et al: Early Lung Cancer Action Project: initial findings on repeat screening. Cancer 92:153–159, 2001.

34. Henschke, CI, Yankelevitz, DF, Libby, D, et al. Computed tomography screening for lung cancer. Chest Clin 23(1):49–57, 2002.

35. Mulshine, JL. New developments in lung cancer screening. J Clin Oncol 23:3198–3202, 2005.

36. Swenson, SJK, Jett, JR, Sloan, JA, et al: Screening for lung cancer with low-dose spiral computed tomography. Am J Respir Crit Care Med 165:508–513, 2002.

37. Bach, PB, Kelley, MJ, Tate, RC, McCrory, DC: Screening for lung cancer: a review of the current literature. Chest 123(suppl):72S–82S, 2003.

38. Bach, PB, Niewoehner, DE, Black, WC: Screening for lung cancer. Chest 123(suppl):83S–88S, 2003.

39. Mulshine, JL, Sullivan, DC: Lung cancer screening. NEJM 352:2714–2720, 2005.

40. Jett, JR, Midthun, DE: Screening for lung cancer: current status and future directions. Chest 125(suppl):158S–162S, 2004.

41. Phillips, M, Cataneo, RN, Cummin, ARC, et al: Detection of lung cancer with volatile markers in the breath. Chest 123(6):2115–2123, 2003.

42. Beckles, MA, Spiro, SG, Colice, GL, Rudd, RM: Initial evaluation of the patient with lung cancer: symptoms, signs, laboratory tests, and paraneoplastic syndromes. Chest 123(suppl):97S–104S, 2003.

43. McLoud, T: Imaging techniques for diagnosis and staging of lung cancer. Clin Chest Med 23(1):123–136, 2002.

44. Tan, BB, Flaherty, KR, Kazerooni, EA, Iannettoni, MD: The solitary pulmonary nodule. Chest 123 (suppl):89S–96S, 2003.

45. Ost, D, Fein, A: Evaluation and management of the solitary pulmonary nodule. Am J Respir Crit Care Med 162:782–787, 2000.

46. Silvestri, GA, Tanoue, LT, Margolis, ML, Barker, J, Detterbeck, F: The noninvasive staging of non-small cell lung cancer. Chest 123(suppl): 147S–156S, 2003.

47. Kelly, RF, Tran, T, Holmstrom, A, et al: Accuracy and cost-effectiveness of (18F)-2-fluoro-deoxy-D-glucose-positron emission tomography scan in potentially resectable non-small cell lung cancer. Chest 125:1413–1423, 2004.

48. Vansteenkiste, JF: PET scan in the staging of non-small cell lung cancer. Lung Cancer 42(suppl 1):S27–S37, 2003.

49. Gould, MK, Kuschner, WG, Rydzak, CE, et al: Test performance of positron emission tomography and computed tomography for mediastinal staging in patients with non-small cell lung cancer. Ann Intern Med 139:879–892, 2003.

50. Koss, LG: *Diagnostic Cytology*, 3rd ed. JB Lippincott, Philadelphia, 1979, pp. 534–606.

51. Schreiher, G, McCrory, DC: Performance characteristics of different modalities for diagnosis of suspected lung cancer: summary of published evidence. Chest 123(suppl):115S–128S, 2003.

52. Mazzone, P, Jain, P, Arroliga, AC, Matthay, RA: Bronchoscopy and needle biopsy techniques for diagnosis and staging of lung cancer. Clin Chest Med 23(1):137–158, 2002.

53. Schreiber, G, McCrory, DC: Performance characteristics of different modalities for diagnosis of suspected lung cancer. Chest 123(suppl):115S–128S, 2003.

54. Wang, KP, Terry, PB: Transbronchial needle aspiration in the diagnosis and staging of bronchogenic carcinoma. Am Rev Respir Dis 127:344, 1983.

55. Minai, OA, Dasgupta, A, Mehta, AC: Transbronchial needle aspiration of central and peripheral lesions. In Bolliger CT, Mathur PN (eds): *Progress in Respiratory Research-Interventional Bronchoscopy*. Karger, Basel, Switzerland, 1999.

56. Toloz, EM, Harpole, L, Detterbeck, F, McCrory, DC: Invasive staging of non-small cell lung cancer: a review of the current evidence. Chest 123(suppl): 157S–166S, 2003.

57. Diacon, AH, Schuurmans, MM, Theron, J, et al: Transbronchial needle aspirates: comparison of two preparation methods. Chest 127:2015–2018, 2005.

58. Becker, HD, Herth, F, Ernst, A, Schwarz, Y: Bronchoscopic biopsy of peripheral lung lesions under electromagnetic guidance. J Bronchol 12(1):9–13, 2005.

59. Chaffey, MH: The role of percutaneous lung biopsy in the work up of a solitary pulmonary nodule. West J Med 148:176, 1988.

60. Fletcher, EC, Levin, DC. Flexible fiberoptic bronchoscopy and fluoroscopically guided transbronchial biopsy in the management of solitary pulmonary nodules. West J Med 136:477, 1982.

61. Filderman, AE, et al: Bronchogenic carcinoma. In Brandstetter, RD (ed): *Pulmonary Medicine*. Medical Economics, Oradell, NJ, 1989, pp. 525–549.

62. Carr, DT, Holoye, PY: Bronchogenic carcinoma. In Murray, JF, Nadel, JA (eds): *Textbook of Respiratory Medicine*. WB Saunders, Philadelphia, 1988, pp. 1174–1250.

63. Detterbeck, FC, DeCamp, MM, Kohman, L, Silvestri, GA: Invasive staging: the guidelines. Chest 123(suppl):167S–175S, 2003.

64. van Tinteren, H, Hoekstra, O, Smit, E, van de bergh, J, et al: Effectiveness of positron emission tomography in the preoperative assessment of patients with suspected non-small cell lung cancer: the PLUS Multicentre Randomised Trial. Lancet 359:1388–1393, 2002.

65. Annema, JT, Versteegh, MI, Veselic, M, et al: Endoscopic ultrasound added to mediastinoscopy for preoperative staging of patients with lung cancer. JAMA 294:931–936, 2005.

66. Menzies, R, Charbonneau, M: Thoracoscopy for the diagnosis of pleural disease. Ann Int Med 114:271, 1991.

67. Mountain, CF: Revisions in the international system for staging lung cancer. Chest 111: 1710–1717, 1997.

68. Mountain, CF, Dresler, CM: Regional lymph hode classification for lung cancer staging. Chest 111: 1718–1723, 1997.

69. Woolner, LB, Fontana, RS, Cortese, DA, et al: Roentgenographically occult lung cancer: pathologic findings and frequency of multicentricity during a 10-year period. Mayo Clin Proc 59(7):453–466, 1984.

70. Edell, ES, Cortese, DA. Photodynamic therapy in the management of early superficial squamous cell carcinoma as an alternative to surgical resection. Chest 102(5):1319–1322, 1992.

71. Furuse, K, Fukuoka, M, Kato, H, et al: A prospective phase II study on photodynamic therapy with phofrin for centrally located early-stage lung cancer. The Japan Lung Cancer Photodynamic Therapy Study Group. J Clin Oncol 11(11):1852–1857, 1993.

72. Alberts, WM: Lung Cancer. In ACCP Pulmonary Board Review, Course Syllabus, pp. 29–48, 2004.

73. Alberts, WM, Colice, GL, et al: Diagnosis and management of lung cancer: ACCP evidence-based guidelines. Chest 123(suppl):1S–335S, 2003.

74. Carr, DT, Holoye, PY: Bronchogenic carcinoma. In Murray, JF, Nadel, JA (eds): *Textbook of Respiratory Medicine*. WB Saunders, Philadelphia, 1988, pp. 1174–1250.

75. Sawada, S, Komori, E, Nogami, N, et al: Advanced age is not correlated with either short-term or long-term postoperative results in lung cancer patients in good clinical condition. Chest 128:1557–1563, 2005.

76. Beckles, MA, Spiro, SG, Colice, GL, Rudd, RM: The physiologic evaluation of patients with lung cancer being considered for resectional surgery. Chest 123(suppl):105S–114S, 2003.

77. Schuurmans, MM, Diacon, AH, Bolliger, CT. Functional evaluation before lung resection. Clin Chest Med 23(1):159–172, 2002.

78. Jett, J, Feins, R, Kvale, PA, et al: Pretreatment evaluation of non-small cell lung cancer. Am J Respir Crit Care Med 156:320–332, 1997.

79. British Thoracic Society: Guidelines on the selection of patients with lung cancer for surgery. Thorax 56:89–108, 2001.

80. Simon, GR, Wagner, H: Small cell lung cancer. Chest 123(suppl):259S–271S, 2003.

Glossary

α_1-protease inhibitor: A protein substance produced by the liver that blocks the action of the enzyme elastase; lack of this substance leads to a breakdown of the lung parenchyma and results in emphysema

A_2: Aortic component of the second heart sound

Abdominal paradox: Abnormal inward movement of the abdomen with inspiratory effort; occurs with diaphragm fatigue or paralysis

Acidosis: An abnormal increase in the hydrogen ion concentration, which leads to a decrease in the measured pH

Acquired immune deficiency syndrome (AIDS): An immune disorder caused by infection with the human immunodeficiency virus (HIV), which reduces the body's ability to fight infections

Acrocyanosis: Cyanosis of the extremities

Acute lung injury: a syndrome characterized by persistent lung inflammation seen at the level of the alveolar-capillary membrane with increase vascular permeability

Acute postinfectious polyneuropathy: Progressive ascending paralysis caused by inflammation of the myelin sheath around peripheral nerves; also known as Guillain-Barré syndrome

Acute respiratory distress syndrome (ARDS): Acute onset of respiratory failure due to increased permeability of the alveolar-capillary membrane and diffuse pulmonary edema

Adventitious lung sounds: Abnormal sounds, such as crackles and wheezes, superimposed on the breath sounds

Aerobic: Able to live or metabolize only in the presence of oxygen

Afterload: The resistance to blood flow out of the ventricle during ventricular contraction

Air bronchogram: An abnormal finding on the chest film seen when air-filled bronchi are visible as a result of surrounding consolidation

Alkalosis: An abnormal decrease in the hydrogen ion concentration leading to elevation of the serum pH

Amniotic fluid: A liquid produced by the fetal membranes that surround the fetus throughout pregnancy

Amyotrophic lateral sclerosis (ALS): A progressive, fatal neurologic disease due to loss of motor neurons in the anterior horn cell; also known as Lou Gehrig's disease

Anabolic metabolism: The constructive process by which the body converts simple substances into more complex compounds

Anaerobic: Able to live or metabolize in the absence of oxygen

Anatomical shunt: Blood bypassing the lung through anatomical channels; such blood is poorly oxygenated

Anemia: An abnormal reduction in the number of circulating red blood cells

Angina: Severe chest pain associated with coronary artery disease

Angiography: The visualization of coronary arteries by x-ray after injection of radiopaque contrast medium

Anion gap: The mathematical difference between the positive and negative ions of the blood

Anorexia: Loss of appetite

Anticholinergics: Medications designed to inhibit activity of the parasympathetic nervous system

Anticoagulation: The process of inhibiting blood from clotting

Antigens: Uniquely shaped molecules that are recognized by the immune system and stimulate a specific immune response

Aortic rupture: The sudden fracture of the aorta caused by trauma

Apnea: Cessation of spontaneous breathing for more than 10 seconds

Arrhythmia: An abnormal rhythm of the heartbeat

Arterial blood gases (ABGs): Measurements of oxygen, carbon dioxide, and pH in the arterial blood sample

Asbestosis: A condition of pulmonary fibrosis related to the chronic inhalation of asbestos fibers

Ascites: The accumulation of serous fluid in the peritoneal cavity

Aspergillus: A fungal organism that may infect the immunosuppressed patient

Asphyxia: Cessation of life due to lack of effective gas exchange in the lungs

Aspiration: Drawing in or out by the application of suction. In respiratory care patients, the term aspiration is often used to indicate the inhalation of vomitus into the trachea

Asthma: A pulmonary disease characterized by reversible obstruction of the airways

Atelectasis: Collapsed or airless condition of the lung

Atopy: A term used clinically to apply to a group of diseases of an allergic nature; they differ from most allergies in that (1) they are inherited; (2) the antibody produced, called atopic reagin or skin-sensitizing antibody, is deposited in cutaneous tissues and may enter the blood stream; and (3) the primary reaction is edema, as occurs in hay fever or rhinitis; principal atopic manifestations are bronchial asthma, vasomotor rhinitis, and chronic urticaria

Atrophy: A reduction in the size of a body part due to disease

Auto-PEEP: The inadvertent build-up of positive end-expiratory pressure (PEEP) in the lung during mechanical ventilation as a result of inadequate expiratory time

Autoimmune disease: Disease of the immune system that attacks the host

Autonomy: Ability to function independently

Autosomal recessive: A genetic feature that is not dominant

Bands: Immature neutrophils that are recognized by the lack of neutrophil segmentation

Barrel chest: An abnormal condition in which the anteroposterior diameter of the chest is increased because of loss of lung recoil; often seen with emphysema

Beck's Triad: a set of clinical signs that help recognize the onset of cardiac tamponade; the clinical signs include distended neck veins, hypotension, diminished heart sounds

Blunt chest trauma: a blow to the chest area that does not penetrate the skin. The underlying lung or other structures often are bruised as a result of the trauma

Bradycardia: Abnormally slow heart rate; less than 60/min in the adult

Bradypnea: Abnormally slow breathing rate

Bronchial breath sounds: Abnormal breath sounds heard over consolidated lung; sounds have equal inspiratory and expiratory components and are louder than vesicular breath sounds

Bronchial provocation: Testing of the patient's airway responsiveness; asthmatics are known to have increased bronchospasm when exposed to the stimulating agent

Bronchiectasis: Permanent dilatation of a portion of a bronchus due to structural weakness in the wall of the airway after infection

Bronchiolitis: Inflammation of the bronchioles; most often occurs in infants and children

Bronchitis: Inflammation of the bronchi, usually due to infection

Bronchodilators: Medication designed to cause the smooth muscles of the airways to relax

Bronchogenic carcinoma: primary lung cancer; malignancies that arise within the lung itself

Bronchopleural fistula: An abnormal opening between the lung and the pleura that leads to a continuous leak of air into the pleural space

Bronchopneumonia: A type of bacterial pneumonia that has segmental distribution

Bronchoscopy: The process of placing a scope into the tracheobronchial tree for the purpose of diagnosis or therapy

Bronchospasm: An abnormal contraction of the smooth muscles lining the intrathoracic airways

Bruit: An adventitious sound of venous or arterial origin heard on auscultation and produced by turbulent blood flow

Cachexia: A state of ill health, malnutrition, and wasting; may occur in many chronic diseases (e.g., certain malignancies, advanced chronic pulmonary disease)

Carbon monoxide poisoning: Significant contamination of the blood with carbon monoxide, leading to reduced oxygen content of the arterial blood and tissue hypoxia when severe

Carboxyhemoglobin (Hbco): Hemoglobin bound with carbon monoxide

Carcinogens: Agents known to produce cancer

Cardiac contusion: Trauma to the myocardium leading to tissue damage

Cardiac index: The cardiac output divided by the patient's body surface area in meters squared. Normal cardiac index is 2.5 to 4.0 liters/min per m^2

Cardiac output: The quantity of blood pumped out of the left ventricle per minute. Normal values in the adult are 4 to 8 liters/min

Cardiac tamponade: Compression of the heart due to a build-up of blood in the pericardium

Cardiomegaly: Hypertrophy (enlargement) of the heart

Cardiomyopathy: Disease of the heart muscle

Catabolic metabolism: The destructive process by which the body breaks down more complex compounds into more simple substances

Central cyanosis: Bluish discoloration of the oral cavity due to hypoxemia

Central sleep apnea: Pauses in breathing during sleep due to an inadequate drive to breathe

Central venous pressure (CVP): Blood pressure in the central veins

Chemotherapy: The use of chemical agents to treat cancer

Chest pain: Abnormal pain in the region of the chest; may be of pleuritic or cardiac origin

Chest physical therapy: Therapeutic procedures designed to improve expectoration of mucus from the tracheobronchial tree

Chest trauma: injury to the chest as a result of a penetrating wound or blunt force deceleration

Cheyne-Stokes breathing: An abnormal pattern of breathing characterized by periods of apnea lasting 10 to 60 seconds, followed by gradually increasing depth and frequency of breathing

Chronic obstructive pulmonary disease (COPD): A chronic lung disease characterized by the presence of airflow obstruction; most often associated with emphysema and chronic bronchitis

Circulatory failure: Inability of the circulatory system to meet the metabolic needs of the body; *see* shock

Clubbing: Abnormal enlargement of the distal phalanges

Community-acquired pneumonia: bacterial infection in the lung acquired outside the hospital. Usually due to a gram positive organism and responsive to antibiotics

Complete blood count (CBC): A laboratory test in which the red blood cell and white blood cell counts in the circulatory blood are reported

Congestive heart failure (CHF): A clinical syndrome associated with left ventricular failure and diffuse pulmonary edema due to increased hydrostatic pressure in the pulmonary capillaries

Consolidation: The process of becoming denser; often used in reference to the lung tissue when pneumonia is present

Continuous positive airway pressure (CPAP): The provision of supra-atmospheric end-expiratory pressure to the spontaneously breathing patient

Contractility: The ability to contract or shorten

Contusion: An injury to the body in which the skin is not broken; a bruise

Copious: Large amounts

Cor pulmonale: A condition of right ventricular failure due to chronic lung disease

Corticosteroid: Medication designed to reduce inflammation; often given to the patient with reversible obstruction of the airways, such as the asthmatic during an acute attack

Cough: A sudden, forceful expiratory effort designed to expel mucus or foreign material from the lung and airways

Crackles: Discontinuous adventitious lung sounds produced by the sudden opening of collapsed airways or by the movement of excessive airway secretions or fluid

Crepitus: A dry, crackling sound or sensation

Cromolyn sodium: A medication that inhibits mast cells from releasing mediators that cause bronchospasm; primarily useful in the prevention of asthma attacks

Cyanosis: Slightly bluish, grayish, slatelike, or dark-purple discoloration of the skin due to the presence of abnormal amounts of reduced hemoglobin in the blood; may not appear in patients with severe anemia, even though their blood is poorly oxygenated, because there is not enough reduced hemoglobin present to cause the blue color to be visible

Cystic fibrosis: A chronic inherited disease that affects the exocrine glands of the body, including the pancreas, lungs, and sweat glands

Cytology: The study of cells through the use of a microscope

Defibrillation: The application of direct electric shock to the chest in an effort to return the heart rhythm to normal

Delayed hypersensitivity: The reaction of the cell-mediated immune system to an antigen

Diaphoresis: Profuse sweating

Diplopia: Double vision

Disseminated intravascular coagulation (DIC): The abnormal diffuse form of coagulation that consumes several clotting factors, leading to generalized bleeding

Diuresis: The excretion of large amount of urine

Diuretic: An agent that increases the excretion of urine

Drowning: Suffocation resulting from submersion

    a. **near drowning:** Drowning involving successful resuscitation after submersion
    b. **dry drowning:** Drowning without aspiration
    c. **wet drowning:** Drowning with aspiration

Drug-induced lung disease: Disease of the lung that occurs as a side effect of certain medications

Ductus arteriosus: An opening between the pulmonary artery and the aorta in the fetus; normally closes after birth

Dysphagia: Difficulty swallowing

Dysphonia: Difficulty speaking; hoarseness

Dyspnea: Air hunger resulting in labored or difficult breathing; sometimes accompanied by pain; normal when due to vigorous work or athletic activity

Edema: Abnormal collection of fluid in the tissues

Ejection fraction: The portion of the ventricular volume ejected during contraction of the ventricle (systole); normally approximately 70%

Electrocardiogram (ECG): A recording of the electrical activity of the heart

Emphysema: A chronic obstructive pulmonary disease associated with abnormal dilatation of the distal airspaces

    a.   **panlobular:** All the airways distal to the terminal bronchioles are involved

    b.   **centrilobular:** Distal lung units are spared and only the more central airways are involved

Empyema: The collection of pus in the pleural cavity

End-diastolic volume: The amount of blood in the ventricle at the end of the diastolic period; represents the amount of blood available for ejection during the subsequent contraction of the ventricles

Endogenous: Produced within or caused by factors within the organism

Enuresis: Involuntary urination

Epiglottitis: A bacterial infection of the epiglottis

Epoch: A portion of the polysomnogram representing a 30-second period of time

Erythema: Redness of the skin due to congestion of the capillaries

Escharotomy: The surgical removal of burned skin that has formed scabs or dry, crusted tissue

Excessive daytime sleepiness: Abnormal sleepiness during the day that leads to decreased ability to function

Exercise-induced asthma: Asthma attacks caused by exertion

Exocrinopathy: Disease of the exocrine glands

External respiration: Gas exchange between the lung and an inhaled gas

Extrinsic asthma: Asthma due to allergic reactions

Exudates: Accumulations of fluid in a cavity; matter that penetrates through vessel walls into adjoining tissue; or pus or serum

Fasciculations: Involuntary contraction or twitching of muscle fibers

Fetid: Foul smelling

Fever: An abnormal elevation of body temperature due to disease

Fibrosis: The formation of fibrous tissue

Fistula: An abnormal tubelike passage from a normal cavity or tube to another cavity or tube

Flail chest: A condition of the chest wall due to two or more fractures on each affected rib that result in a "free-floating" portion of the rib cage; affected region moves in a paradoxical fashion with breathing; *see* paradoxical respiration

Flash over: A wall of fire extending down from the ceiling and billowing out of open doors or windows

Foramen ovale: An opening between the two atria of the heart in the fetus; normally closes after birth

Forced vital capacity (FVC): The volume of air that is exhaled after full inspiration during a forceful expiratory maneuver

Frank-Starling response: Increases in the force of myocardial contraction following increases in the stretching of the myocardium

Functional residual capacity (FRC): The amount of gas in the lungs at the end of a normal tidal volume exhalation; represents a combination of the residual volume and the expiratory reserve volume

Gallop: An abnormal rhythm of the heart characterized by an extra sound heard during diastole; this extra sound, added to the normal first and second heart sounds, results in a rhythm that resembles the pattern produced by the hooves of a horse during a gallop

Ghon complex: The combination of the initial lung lesion and the affected lymph node in the patient with tuberculosis

Ghon nodule: the initial lung lesion

Glasgow coma scale: A scoring system used to document the neurological condition of the patient

Granuloma: A granular growth or tumor

Guillain-Barré syndrome: *See* acute postinfectious polyneuropathy

Hb: Hemoglobin

HbCN: Hemoglobin bound with cyanide

Heave: An abnormal pulsation on the chest as the result of ventricular hypertrophy

HEENT: Head, ears, eyes, nose, and throat

Helper T lymphocytes: White blood cells that promote the development of antibodies; play a key role in cell-mediated immunity

Hemolysis: The breakdown of red blood cells resulting in the release of hemoglobin into the plasma

Hemopneumothorax: blood and air trapped in the pleural space

Hemoptysis: Expectoration of blood arising from hemorrhage of the larynx, trachea, bronchi, or lungs

Hemothorax: An abnormal build-up of blood in the pleural space

Heparin: A medication designed to reduce blood clotting

Hepatojugular reflex: A physical examination finding of jugular venous distention occurring shortly after pressure is applied over the liver; this finding suggests that the liver is engorged

Hepatomegaly: Enlargement of the liver

Hilum: A depression in an organ in which nerves and blood vessels enter or exit the lung

History of present illness: The section of the medical history that describes the details about the patient's current medical problem; details such as when the symptom first started, its level of intensity, and its location are included

Honeycomb lung: A radiographic finding seen in end-stage interstitial lung disease caused by the formation of cysts

Hoover's sign: An abnormal breathing pattern, seen in patients with severe emphysema, in which the lateral portions of the chest wall move inward with each inspiratory effort

Horner's syndrome: A clinical syndrome caused by tumor compression of the cervical nerves

Hypercapnia: An abnormal increase in carbon dioxide in the arterial blood ($Paco_2$ >45 mm Hg)

Hyperkalemia: An abnormal increase in the serum potassium level

Hypernatremia: An abnormal increase in the serum sodium level

Hyperpnea: Deep breathing

Hypersensitivity pneumonitis: A form of interstitial lung disease due to inhalation of organic dusts

Hypersomnolence: An abnormal degree of sleepiness; *see* excessive daytime sleepiness

Hypertension: An abnormal increase in systemic blood pressure

Hypertrophy: Enlargement of an organ or a part of the organ

Hypocapnia: Reduction of the Pa_{CO_2} level below 35 mm Hg

Hypoglycemia: An abnormal decrease in blood glucose levels

Hypokalemia: An abnormal decrease in the potassium level in plasma of the circulating blood

Hyponatremia: An abnormal decrease in the level of sodium in the plasma of the circulating blood

Hypoplasia: Underdevelopment of a tissue or organ

Hypopnea: Shallow breathing

Hypotension: An abnormal decrease in systemic blood pressure

Hypothermia: An abnormally low body temperature

Hypoxemia: Insufficient oxygenation of the arterial blood

Hypoxia: Insufficient oxygenation at the tissue level

ICU: Intensive care unit

Idiopathic: Disease occurring without a known cause

Ileus: An obstruction of the intestines

Infarction: Formation of an infarct; an area of tissue in an organ or body part that undergoes necrosis after cessation of blood supply

Inotropes: Medications or compounds that affect the contractility of the heart muscle

Insomnia: The inability to sleep

Intermittent mandatory ventilation (IMV): A mode of mechanical ventilation in which the patient can take spontaneous tidal volumes in between the machine-delivered breaths

Intermittent positive-pressure ventilation (IPPV): The application of positive pressure to the airway during inspiration

Internal respiration: Gas exchange between the blood and tissues

Intrinsic asthma: Asthma that is unrelated to allergic disorders

Intubation: The process of placing an endotracheal tube into the trachea

Ischemia: Local and temporary anemia due to obstruction of the circulation to a body part

Jugular venous distention (JVD): Abnormal filling of the veins of the neck due to heart failure

Kyphoscoliosis: Abnormal deviation of the spine laterally and from anterior to posterior

Kyphosis: Excessive posterior curvature of the spine; gives rise to a condition commonly known as humpback or hunchback

Lactic acidosis: A disturbance in the lactic acid balance of the body

Laryngotracheobronchitis: *See* croup

Leukocyte: A white blood cell

Leukocytopenia: An abnormal decrease in the number of white blood cells in the circulation

Leukocytosis: A transient increase in the number of white blood cells in the blood

Leukopenia: Abnormal decrease in the number of white blood corpuscles, usually below $5000/mm^3$

Loud P_2: Refers to an abnormally loud second heart sound that occurs as the result of an abnormally forceful closure of the pulmonic valve; often the result of pulmonary hypertension

Lou Gehrig's disease: *See* amyotrophic lateral sclerosis

Lung contusion: An injury to the lung that is the result of a blunt trauma, causing pathological changes; similar to a bruise

Lymphadenopathy: Disease of the lymph nodes

Lymphocytosis: An excess of lymphocytes in the blood or an effusion

Macroglossia: An enlarged tongue

Macrognathia: Abnormal size of jaw

Maximum inspiratory pressure (MIP): A test typically used to determine the strength of the patient's inspiratory muscles and their potential ability to wean from mechanical ventilation

Mechanical ventilation: The application of positive-pressure breathing to a patient's lungs to maintain adequate gas exchange

Metaplasia: The change in body cells from normal to abnormal for that type of tissue

Metastatic malignancy: A tumor that is the result of a malignancy that has spread beyond the primary site

Metered-dose inhaler (MDI): A device designed to deliver a specific dose of an aerosolized medication for inhalation

Microemboli: Very small blood clots

Micrognathia: Abnormal smallness of the jaws, especially the lower jaw

Miliary tuberculosis: A uniquely disseminated form of tuberculosis that involves both lungs; *see* tuberculosis

Mixed apnea: When both central and obstructive apnea are present in the same patient

Mixed venous Po_2 ($P\bar{v}O_2$): The partial pressure of oxygen in the plasma of the venous blood in the right atrium, right ventricle, or pulmonary artery

Morbidity: The condition of being diseased or unhealthy

Mortality: The condition of being subject to death; often used to refer the death rate of a specific illness

Mucoid: Clear, thick mucus from the tracheobronchial tree

Mucus: Secretions from the tracheobronchial tree

Murmur: A soft blowing or rasping sound heard on auscultation of the heart

Myasthenia gravis: A neuromuscular disease associated with abnormal conduction of the nerve impulse through the neuromuscular junction

Mycobacterium: A genus of acid-fast organisms responsible for the lung infection known as tuberculosis

Myocardium: The muscle making up the walls of the heart

Myopathy: Disease of the muscles

Narcolepsy: A chronic ailment consisting of recurrent attacks of drowsiness and sleep

Nasal flaring: Flaring outward of the external nares with each inspiratory effort; usually indicates an increase in the work of breathing

Nasal polyps: An abnormal growth protruding from the mucous membranes of the nasal passages

Necrosis: The death of areas of tissue surrounded by healthy tissue

Necrotizing: Causing death of areas of tissue or bone surrounded by healthy parts; *see* infarction

Neoplasm: An abnormal growth of new tissue; can be benign or malignant

Night sweats: Excessive sweating during sleep that often soaks the patient's pillow and pajamas and is the result of rapid decreases in body temperature following a fever

Nitric oxide (NO): A pharmacological gas that causes pulmonary vasodilatation in low doses

Nocturnal dyspnea: Shortness of breath that occurs during sleep; most often associated with congestive heart failure

Non–rapid eye movement (NREM) sleep: Sleep not involving rapid eye movements, having four stages and making up the majority of sleep time in healthy people

Normocephalic: Normal configuration of the head

Nosocomial: Pertaining to or originating in a hospital; usually used in reference to an infection acquired by a patient while in a hospital

Obstructive sleep apnea: The cessation of breathing for more than 10 seconds due to obstruction of the upper airway

Obtunded: A condition of reduced response to stimuli

Occupational asthma: Asthma attacks associated with a stimulant in the work place

Oliguria: Diminished amount of urine formation

Opportunistic infection: Infection caused by an organism that does not infect persons with a healthy immune system

Optimal PEEP: The level of positive end-expiratory pressure (PEEP) that causes adequate oxygenation of the arterial blood without impeding cardiac output

Oral thrush: Fungus infection of mouth or throat, characterized by formation of white patches and ulcers, frequently with fever and gastrointestinal inflammation

Organomegaly: Abnormal enlargement of an organ in the body

Orthopnea: Shortness of breath that occurs in the reclining position

Oxygenation failure: Inability of the lungs to maintain adequate oxygenation of the arterial blood despite the use of supplemental oxygen

Oxyhemoglobin: Hemoglobin bound with oxygen

P_2: Pulmonic component of the second heart sound. A loud P_2 is suggestive of pulmonary hypertension

Paradoxical pulse: Pulse that is abnormally suppressed during each inspiration

Paradoxical respiration: Most often used to describe a condition seen with diaphragm fatigue or paralysis in which the diaphragm ascends with inspiration; seen as an inward sinking motion of the abdominal wall with each inspiratory effort by the patient; can also be used to describe a traumatized portion of the chest wall that sinks inward with inspiration in the patient with a flail chest; *see* flail chest

Parenchyma: The essential parts of an organ that are concerned with its function; lung parenchyma refers to the distal portions of the lung involved with gas exchange

Paresthesia: Sensation of numbness, prickling, or tingling, often in the extremities

Paroxysmal nocturnal respiration (PNR): A sudden onset of difficulty breathing that typically occurs during sleep; associated with congestive heart failure

Partial pressure of mixed venous oxygen: the partial pressure of oxygen in the pulmonary artery; normally the $P\bar{v}O_2$ is 38–42 mm Hg

Pectus carinatum: Abnormal protrusion of the sternum

Pectus excavatum: Abnormal concavity of the sternum

Pedal edema: Abnormal collection of fluid in the soft tissues around the ankles; often due to heart failure

Penetrating chest trauma: trauma to the chest that results in an open wound and internal injuries

Perfusion: Passing of a fluid through spaces

Pericardial tamponade: Compression of the heart due to a build-up of blood in the pericardial sac around the heart

Pericarditis: Inflammation of pericardium (the double membrane sac enclosing the heart and the origins of the great blood vessels)

Perihilar: Pertaining to the tissues around the hilum of the lung; the hilum is the opening that gives entrance to the pulmonary artery and veins for each lung

Peristalsis: The rhythmic, coordinated contraction of smooth muscle that moves a substance through a canal; for example, peristalsis of the bowel moves food through the intestinal tract

Peritoneal: Concerning the peritoneum, which is a serous membrane lining the abdominal cavity

Permissive hypercapnia: The process of allowing the $PaCO_2$ to increase above normal by reducing the volume of the delivered tidal volume from the ventilator or by reducing the number of breaths per minute; done to reduce the negative impact of elevated mean intrathoracic pressure associated with mechanical ventilation

PERRLA: A mnemonic for pupils equal, round, and reactive to light and accommodation; part of the neurological component of the physical examination of the patient

Phagocytosis: The engulfing and destruction of foreign organisms by macrophages

Pharyngitis: Inflammation of the pharynx

Physiological shunt: Blood flow through the lung that passes by unventilated alveoli

Plasmapheresis: The removal of plasma from withdrawn blood and replacement of the formed elements back into the patient

Platypnea: Difficulty breathing in the upright position

Pneumoconiosis: Disease of the lung caused by the chronic inhalation of dust, often of occupational origin

Pneumonia: Inflammation of the pulmonary parenchyma

   a. **lobar pneumonia:** A form of bacterial pneumonia that affects a specific lobe as seen on the chest radiograph
   b. ***Pneumocystis carinii* pneumonia:** A pneumonia often seen in AIDS patients

Pneumoplasty: A surgical procedure done to remove abnormal, hyperinflated lung tissue; also known as lung volume reduction surgery

Pneumothorax: The presence of air in the pleural space

Point of maximum impulse (PMI): Impulse generated by the contraction of the left ventricle

Polycythemia: An excess of red blood cells; often due to chronic hypoxemia

Polyphonic: A sound made up of multiple notes

Polysomnogram: An all-night sleep study designed to help diagnose a patient's sleep problems

Positive end-expiratory pressure (PEEP): The application and maintenance of positive pressure in the airways throughout the expiratory phase of mechanical ventilation

Precordium: The surface of the chest wall overlying the heart

Preload: The volume of blood filling the ventricle just before ventricular contraction

Pressure-support ventilation: A method of ventilary support in which the patient's spontaneous breathing is assisted by the ventilator at a preset level of inspiratory pressure

Primary blast injury: a form of blunt chest trauma caused by an explosive blast and the resulting wave of energy

Primary hypoventilation: A disease caused by insufficient respiratory drive that leads to chronic elevation of the Pa_{CO_2}

Primary lung cancer: A lung tumor that originates in the lung

Ptosis: Drooping of an organ such as the upper eyelid as a result of paralysis

Pulmonary capillary wedge pressure (PCWP): The pressure used to evaluate left ventricular filling (preload)

Pulmonary contusion: Trauma to the pulmonary tissue due to sudden impact

Pulmonary fibrosis: A chronic lung disease associated with permanent fibrotic changes in the connective tissues of the lung following inflammation

Pulmonary hypertension: Abnormal elevation of the pressure in the pulmonary artery

Pulse pressure: The difference between the systolic and diastolic blood pressures

Pulsus alternans: A pulse characterized by a regular alternation of weak and strong beats

Pulsus paradoxus: An abnormal decrease in the systolic pressure during inspiration; associated with a significant increase in the patient's work of breathing

Purified protein derivative (PPD): Used in the Mantoux skin test to diagnose tuberculosis

Purulent: Containing pus; indicates the presence of bacterial infection

Pyrogenic: Producing fever

Radiolucency: Property of being partly or wholly permeable to radiant energy. Structures that are radiolucent (e.g., lungs) allow the x-ray beam to easily penetrate and result in a dark shadow on the film.

Radiopaque: Impenetrable to x-ray beams; for example, bones are usually impenetrable to x-ray beams and leave a white shadow on the radiograph

Rales: A discontinuous type of adventitious lung sound heard on auscultation of the chest; *see* crackles

Rapid eye movement (REM) sleep: sleep stage in which a person dreams and has rapid eye movements

Refractory hypoxemia: Hypoxemia that does not respond adequately to significant increases in fraction of inspired oxygen

Replication: To reproduce genetic material

Respiratory alternans: An abnormal pattern of breathing where the patient alternates for short periods of time between breathing with accessory muscles and breathing with the diaphragm

Respiratory disturbance index: Obtained by dividing the total number of abnormal events during a night of sleep by the total sleep time in hours; indicates the severity of a patient's sleep disturbance

Respiratory failure: Failure of the lungs to maintain adequate oxygenation with or without an elevated P_{CO_2}

Retinopathy: Any noninflammatory disease of the retina

Retractions: A visible sinking inward of the skin and soft tissues surrounding the bones of the thorax with each inspiratory effort; indicates that the work of breathing is significantly increased

Rhinorrhea: Thin, watery discharge from the nose

Rhonchus: A low-pitched, continuous type of adventitious lung sound heard during auscultation of the chest

S_1: First heart sound; produced by the closure of the mitral and tricuspid valves

S_2: Second heart sound; produced by the closure of the aortic and pulmonic valves

S_3: Third heart sound; may be normal in young persons, but usually indicates heart disease in adults

S_3 gallop: An abnormal third heart sound

S_4: Fourth heart sound; often heart in adult patients with heart disease

Sarcoidosis: A disease of unknown etiology characterized by widespread granulomatous lesions that may affect any organ in the body, but more often the lungs

Scoliosis: Abnormal lateral curvature of the spine

Segmented neutrophils: Mature neutrophils

Sensorium: Portion of the brain that functions as a center of sensations

Sepsis: Pathologic state, usually febrile, resulting from the presence of microorganisms or their poisonous products in the blood stream

Shock: A clinical condition resulting from inadequate blood flow to the vital organs; often characterized by a reduced urine output, diminished level of consciousness, hypotension, peripheral cyanosis, and tachycardia

    a.   **anaphylactic:** shock due to injection of a protein substance to which the patient is sensitized
    b.   **hypovolemic:** shock due to inadequate blood volume
    c.   **septic:** shock that occurs in septicemia, when endotoxins are released from certain bacteria in the blood stream; characterized by hypotension from a significant drop in systemic vascular resistance
    d.   **toxic:** severe, acute shock brought on by infection with strains of *Staphylococcus aureus*

Shunt: Blood that passes from the right side of the heart to the left side without coming into contact with gas exchange units of the lung

Silicosis: Pulmonary fibrosis due to inhalation of silica dust

Simple pneumothorax: a small pneumothorax that does not result in significant physiologic impairment

Sleep apnea: Temporary pauses in breathing during sleep lasting at least 10 seconds

Sleep hypopnea: A period of decreased airflow during sleep defined as a 50% or greater reduction in thoracoabdominal movement lasting at least 10 seconds

Sputum: An aggregation of secretions from the tracheobronchial tree and mouth

Stable asthma: Asthma that has not caused an increase in symptoms over the past 4 weeks

Static compliance: The lung compliance calculated by using the static pressure in the airways during an expiratory hold maneuver; results reflect the compliance of the lung and chest wall

Status asthmaticus: Persistent and intractable asthma unresponsive to conventional treatment

Stenotic: Abnormal narrowing of a body passage or opening

Stridor: Harsh or high-pitched sound heard most often during inhalation; due to obstruction of upper airway

Stroke volume: The amount of blood ejected by the left ventricle with each beat

Subcutaneous emphysema: An abnormal accumulation of air in the subcutaneous tissues due to a leak from the lung

Surfactant: a liquid substance in the peripheral lung units that acts to maintain alveolar patency

Sweat chloride: The level of the chloride ion in the sweat of the patient; a sweat chloride test is done to assist the physician in the diagnosis of cystic fibrosis

Sympathomimetic: Medications that stimulate the sympathetic nervous system; often given in an attempt to dilate the smooth muscle of the airways in patients with obstructive pulmonary disease

Tachycardia: Abnormal increase in heart rate

Tachyphylaxis: Rapid immunization against the effect of toxic doses of an extract by previous injection of small doses of it

Tachypnea: Abnormal increase in the respiratory rate

Tamponade: Pathological compression of a body part

Tension pneumothorax: air trapped in the pleural space under pressure. Often causes a diminished cardiac and pulmonary function until the pressure is release

Tetany: A nervous system problem characterized by spasms of the muscles, typically in the extremities

Theophylline: A xanthine type of bronchodilator

Thromboembolism: A blood clot that has broken loose from its site of origin and is traveling in the vascular system; often lodges in the lung

Thrombosis: The formation of a blood clot

Thyromegaly: Enlargement of the thyroid gland

Tracheal tugging: The physical examination finding in which the trachea is seen or felt to tug downward with each inspiratory effort; indicates an increase in the work of breathing

Tram tracks: Abnormal findings on the chest film associated with hypertrophy of the bronchial walls; often seen in patients with cystic fibrosis

Tuberculosis: Infection due to *Mycobacterium*; often involves the lungs but can occur in most body tissues

Universal precautions: The practice of treating all patients as though they were infected with a blood-borne infection; requires the use of precautionary measures such as wearing latex gloves, a gown, and a mask whenever contact with a patient's blood or secretions could occur

Unstable asthma: Asthma that has caused an increase in symptoms during the past 4 weeks

Upper airway resistance syndrome: A form of obstructive sleep hypopnea in which narrowing of the upper airway partially limits airflow, leading to an arousal

Uvulopalotopharyngoplasty (UPPP): A surgical procedure designed to remove redundant tissue from the upper airway and therefore reduce the likelihood of hypopneas or obstructive events during sleep

Vasopressor: A medication given to increase peripheral vascular resistance in an attempt to elevate blood pressure

Ventilatory failure: Inadequate ventilation that causes an increase in Pa_{CO_2}

Ventricular hypertrophy: Abnormal enlargement of one or both of the ventricles of the heart

Vesicular breath sounds: Normal breath sounds occurring over the lung; represent filtered bronchial breath sounds produced by turbulent airflow in the larger airways

Viral pneumonia: Viral infection in the lung most often associated with inflammation of the interstitial tissues

Virulent: Very poisonous

Vital capacity (VC): The volume of air a person is able to exhale after a maximum inspiratory effort

Weaning: The process of gradually discontinuing mechanical ventilation from a patient

Wheeze: A high-pitched, continuous type of adventitious lung sound resulting from narrowing of the intrathoracic airways.

    a.   **monophonic:** wheeze with a single tone
    b.   **polyphonic:** wheeze with multiple notes occurring at the same time

REFERENCE

Taber's Cyclopedic Medical Dictionary, 19th ed. F.A. Davis Company, Philadelphia, 2001.

Normal Laboratory Values

ADULT

Arterial Blood Gases (ABGs)	
pH	7.35–7.45
$Paco_2$	35–45 mm Hg
Pao_2	90–100 mm Hg
HCO_3^-	22–26 mEq/liter
Base excess (BE)	–2 to +2
Arterial saturation with oxygen (Sao_2)	>95 percent

Complete Blood Count (CBC)	
Red blood cell (RBC) count	
Men	4.6–6.2 million/mm^3
Women	4.2–5.4 million/mm^3
Hemoglobin (Hb)	
Men	13.5–16.5 g/dL
Women	12.0–15.0 g/dL
Hematocrit (Hct)	
Men	40–54%
Women	38–47%
Erythrocyte index	
Mean cell volume (MCV)	80–96 μ^3
Mean cell hemoglobin (MCH)	27–31 pg
Mean cell hemoglobin concentration (MCHC)	32–36%
White blood cell (WBC) count	4,500–10,000/mm^3
Differential of WBCs	
Neutrophils	40–75%
Bands	0–6%
Eosinophils	0–6%
Basophils	0–1%
Lymphocytes	20–45%
Monocytes	2–10%
Platelet count	150,000–400,000/mm^3

Chemistry

Na$^-$	137–147 mEq/liter
K+	3.5–4.8 mEq/liter
Cl$^-$	98–105 mEq/liter
CO_2	25–33 mEq/liter
Blood urea nitrogen (BUN)	7–20 mg/dL
Creatine	0.7–1.3 mg/dL
Total protein	6.3–7.9 g/dL
Albumin	3.5–5.0 g/dL
Cholesterol	150–220 mg/dL
Glucose	70–105 mg/dL

Hemodynamic Values

Variable	Abbreviation	Normal
Cardiac output	Q̇T	4–8 liters/minute
Cardiac index	CI	2.5–4.0 liters/minute/m^2
Stroke volume	SV	60–130 mL
Ejection fraction	EF	65–75%
Central venous pressure	CVP	0–6 mm Hg
Pulmonary artery pressure	PAP	25/10 mm Hg
Pulmonary capillary wedge pressure	PCWP	6–12 mm Hg
Systemic vascular resistance	SVR	900–1400 dynes/second/cm^5
Pulmonary vascular resistance	PVR	110–250 dynes/second/cm^5

Pulmonary Function Tests

Variable	Abbreviation	Normal
Forced vital capacity	FVC	>80% of predicted
Slow vital capacity	SVC	80–120% of predicted
Forced expiratory volume in 1 second	FEV$_1$	>80% of predicted
Forced expiratory volume in 1 second/Forced vital capacity	FEV$_1$/FVC	>75%
Forced expiratory flow	FEF$_{25-75\%}$	>80% of predicted
Carbon monoxide diffusing capacity	D$_{LCO}$	25 mL CO/minute/mm Hg
Total lung capacity	TLC	6000 mL
Functional residual capacity	FRC	2400 mL
Residual volume	RV	1200 mL
Vital capacity	VC	4800 mL

Vital Signs

	Normal Range
Temperature range	36.1–37.5°C
Heart rate	60–100/minute
Respiratory rate	12–20/minute
Blood pressure range	120/80 mm Hg
	Systolic 95–140 mm Hg
	Diastolic 60–90 mm Hg

B

GOLD Standards for Diagnosing and Treating Patients with COPD

The Global Initiative for Chronic Obstructive Lung Disease (GOLD) works with health care professionals and public health officials around the world to raise awareness of Chronic Obstructive Pulmonary Disease (COPD) and to improve prevention and treatment of this lung disease.

GOLD was launched in 1997 in collaboration with the *National Heart, Lung, and Blood Institute, National Institutes of Health*, USA, and the *World Health Organization*.

Following are three tables from the GOLD website that address when to admit the COPD patient with an exacerbation, a summary of the recommended treatment at each stage of COPD, and commonly used medications for treating the COPD patient. The entire GOLD standards can be found at www.goldcopd.org

Table B.1 Indications for Hospital Admission for Exacerbations

- Marked increase in intensity of symptoms, such as sudden development of resting dyspnea
- Severe background COPD
- Onset of new physical signs (e.g., cyanosis, peripheral edema)

- Failure of exacerbation to respond to initial medical management
- Significant comorbidities
- Newly occurring arrhythmias
- Diagnostic uncertainty
- Older age
- Insufficient home support

From Global Strategy for the Diagnosis, Management, and Prevention of COPD. NHLBI and WHO, 1998.

Table B.2 Summary of Characteristics and Recommended Treatment at Each Stage of COPD

Therapy at Each Stage of COPD					
			II: Moderate		
Old	0: At Risk	I: Mild	IIA	IIB	III: Severe
New	0: At Risk	I: Mild	II: Moderate	III: Severe	IV: Very Severe
Characteristics	• Chronic symptoms • Exposure to risk factors • Normal spirometry	• $FEV_1/FVC < 70\%$ • $FEV_1 \geq 80\%$ • With or without symptoms	• $FEV_1/FVC < 70\%$ • $50\% \leq FEV_1 < 80\%$ • With or without symptoms	• $FEV_1/FVC < 70\%$ • $30\% \leq FEV_1 < 50\%$ • With or without symptoms	• $FEV_1/FVC < 70\%$ • $FEV_1 < 30\%$ or $FEV_1 < 50\%$ predicted plus chronic respiratory failure
	Avoidance of risk factor(s); influenza vaccination				
		Add short-acting bronchodilator when needed			
			Add regular treatment with one or more long-acting bronchodilators *Add* rehabilitation		
				Add inhaled glucocorticosteroids if repeated exacerbations	
					Add long-term oxygen if chronic respiratory failure *Consider* surgical treatments

From Global Strategy for the Diagnosis, Management, and Prevention of COPD. NHLBI and WHO, 1998.

Table B.3 Commonly Used Formulations of Drugs for COPD

Drug	Inhaler (μg)	Solution for Nebulizer (mg/ml)	Oral	Vials for Injection (mg)	Duration of Action (hours)
β2-agonists					
Short-acting					
Fenoterol	100–200 (MDI)	1	0.05% (Syrup)		4–6
Salbutamol (albuterol)	100, 200 (MDI & DPI)	5	5 mg (Pill) Syrup 0.024%	0.1, 0.5	4–6
Terbutaline	400, 500 (DPI)	–	2.5, 5 (Pill)	0.2, 0.25	4–6
Long-acting					
Formoterol	4.5–12 (MDI & DPI)				12+
Salmeterol	25–50 (MDI & DPI)				12+
Anticholinergics					
Short-acting					
Ipratropium bromide	20, 40 (MDI)	0.25–0.5			6–8
Oxitropium bromide	100 (MDI)	1.5			7–9
Long-acting					
Tiotropium	18 (DPI)				24+
Combination Short-acting β₂-agonists Plus Anticholinergic in One Inhaler					
Fenoterol/ Ipratropium	200/80 (MDI)	1.25/0.5			6–8
Salbutamol/ Ipratropium	75/15 (MDI)	0.75/4.5			6–8
Methylxanthines					
Aminophylline			200-600 mg (Pill)	240 mg	Variable, up to 24
Theophylline (SR)			100-600 mg (Pill)		Variable, up to 24
Inhaled Glucocorticosteroids					
Beclomethasone	100, 250, 400 (MDI & DPI)	0.2–0.4			
Budesonide	100, 200, 400 (DPI)	0.20, 0.25, 0.5			
Fluticasone	50-500 (MDI & DPI)				
Triamcinolone	100 (MDI)	40		40	
Combination Long-acting β₂-agonists Plus Glucocorticosteroids in One Inhaler					
Formoterol/ Budesonide	4.5/80, 160 (DPI) (9/320) (DPI)				
Salmeterol/ Fluticasone	50/100, 250, 500 (DPI) 25/50, 125, 250 (MDI)				
Systemic Glucocorticosteroids					
Prednisone			5-60 mg (Pill)		
Methyl- prednisolone	10-2000 mg		4, 8, 16 mg (Pill)		

MDI = metered dose inhaler; DPI = dry powder inhaler

From Global Strategy for the Diagnosis, Management, and Prevention of COPD. NHLBI and WHO, 1998.

Websites Useful for Learning Information About the Diagnosis and Treatment of Lung Diseases

- CHAPTER 1 Introduction to Patient Assessment
  www.antiquemed.com

- CHAPTER 2 Introduction to Respiratory Failure

- CHAPTER 3 Asthma
  www.nlm.nih.gov.medlineplus/asthma.html
  www.cdc.gov/asthma
  http://www.pulmonologychannel.com/asthma/

- CHAPTER 4 Chronic Obstructive Pulmonary Disease
  www.goldcopd.org
  http://www.pulmonologychannel.com/copd/

- CHAPTER 5 Cystic Fibrosis
  www.cff.org (cystic fibrosis foundation)
  http://www.nlm.nih.gov/medlineplus/cysticfibrosis.html
  http://www.pulmonologychannel.com/cf/

- CHAPTER 6 Hemodynamic Monitoring and Shock

- CHAPTER 7 Pulmonary Thromboembolic Disease
  http://www.nlm.nih.gov/medlineplus/pulmonaryembolism.html
  http://www.ahrq.gov/clinic/tp/dvttp.htm

- CHAPTER 8 Heart Failure
  http://www.cardiologychannel.com/chf/
  http://www.heartsite.com/html/chf.html

- CHAPTER 9 Smoke Inhalation Injury and Burns
  http://www.coheadquarters.com/
  http://www.cdc.gov/co/

•CHAPTER 10 Near Drowning

•CHAPTER 11 Acute Respiratory Distress Syndrome
http://www.ardsnet.org/
http://www.pulmonologychannel.com/ards/

•CHAPTER 12 Chest Trauma

•CHAPTER 13 Postoperative Atelectasis

•CHAPTER 14 Interstitial Lung Disease
http://www.pulmonologychannel.com/sarcoidosis/

•CHAPTER 15 Neuromuscular Diseases
http://www.alsa.org/

•CHAPTER 16 Bacterial Pneumonia
http://www.nlm.nih.gov/medlineplus/pneumonia.html

•CHAPTER 17 Pneumonia in the Immunocompromised Patient
http://www.nlm.nih.gov/medlineplus/aids.html

•CHAPTER 18 Sleep Disordered Breathing
http://www.nlm.nih.gov/medlineplus/sleepapnea.html
http://www.pulmonologychannel.com/osa/

•CHAPTER 19 Tuberculosis
http://ntcc.ucsd.edu
tbetn@ced.gov
www.cdc.gov/tb
www.findtbresources.org

•CHAPTER 20 Lung Cancer
http://www.nlm.nih.gov/medlineplus/lungcancer.html
http://www.pulmonologychannel.com/lungcancer/

Index

Page numbers followed by *f* indicate figures; page numbers followed by *t* indicate tables.